Pain Imaging

Maria Assunta Cova · Fulvio Stacul
Editors

Pain Imaging

A Clinical-Radiological Approach to Pain Diagnosis

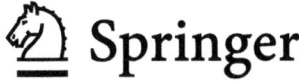

Editors
Maria Assunta Cova
Department of Radiology
Cattinara Hospital
University of Trieste
Trieste
Italy

Fulvio Stacul
Department of Radiology
Maggiore Hospital
Trieste
Italy

ISBN 978-3-319-99821-3   ISBN 978-3-319-99822-0   (eBook)
https://doi.org/10.1007/978-3-319-99822-0

Library of Congress Control Number: 2019932989

This Springer imprint is published by the registered company Springer Nature Switzerland AG
The registered company address is: Gewerbestrasse 11, 6330 Cham, Switzerland

To Gabrio

Foreword

Writing a radiological book dedicated to a symptom, rather than to an organ or a disease process, is quite unusual. It is, however, a much needed new way to present radiology. As a matter of fact, patients come to the Radiology Department complaining of symptoms and signs and with a request for imaging in order to identify their origin. I do really believe that the better the radiologist understands his/her patient's complaints, the better he/she is able to choose the correct imaging modalities to evaluate them and to provide a correct interpretation of their findings. The editors of this volume have prepared a radiological textbook that takes into consideration the patient's symptoms first: in this case, the book is dedicated to the symptom of pain.

Our discipline has a central role in healthcare: all diagnoses and decisions on patients' management are mostly based on the results of imaging, and image-guided procedures allow minimally invasive therapies in many cases. However, the radiologist is almost unknown to the patient, and many people do not even know that we are physicians.

It is quite important to learn how to work through this "clinical-radiological approach." On one side, it makes us able to provide a better service to our patients; on the other, it teaches how to get closer to patients, to understand better their symptoms, and to link them to our results. This underlines our role as physicians and, I am sure, makes it perceived by our patients too.

Clinical chapters are written by clinicians, and this reinforces the "clinical-radiological approach" of the book by providing information on what clinicians want from our examinations. I am sure this volume will prove useful not only to radiologists but also to emergency medicine physicians and to colleagues of other specialties who want to understand which are the best tests to use to identify the causes of pain in different areas of the body and what are the results they can expect from them.

M. A. Cova and F. Stacul have to be thanked for guiding the preparation of this book through a novel way and for helping the authors of the different chapters in following it. I am sure this is the starting point of a new teaching method in radiology.

January 2019

Lorenzo E. Derchi
Department of Health Sciences (DISSAL)
University of Genoa
Genoa, Italy

Preface

Pain can be a major clinical challenge. Its correct assessment is often related to a careful analysis of the patient history, to an accurate physical examination, to the evaluation of laboratory data, and to an appropriate referral to diagnostic imaging.

This book addresses pain imaging aspects in both neuro and body, thus updating the international literature scenario on the topic. Actually, books on pain imaging published so far provided a partial approach to this issue, considering specific fields only. The book aims to provide a comprehensive clinical-radiological approach, and it underlines the need of a close cooperation among clinicians and radiologists. It offers differential diagnoses for a number of painful syndromes, as many of them can mimic one other, and it aims to help in the diagnostic management of these patients, suggesting the most appropriate diagnostic algorithm.

The book is structured into sections for each anatomical macro-area (the brain, spine, thorax, abdomen, and pelvis), and dedicated chapters cover the topics from both a clinical and radiological point of view.

Following introductive chapters considering mechanisms of pain and the brain imaging of pain, the neurological section approaches headache, trigeminal neuralgia, and spine pain. As to the thorax, both vascular and nonvascular causes of pain are addressed. A number of disease possibly responsible of abdominal pain are considered, including biliary colic and cholecystitis, pancreatitis, renal colic, pyelonephritis, bowel obstruction, bowel perforation, inflammatory bowel disease, and vascular disease. Finally, some diseases causing pelvic pain are addressed, namely, uterine disease, ovarian disease, endometriosis, and testicular disease.

The chapters offer a state-of-the-art approach to clinical challenging situations and provide up-to-date knowledge on the present contribution of imaging techniques, thanks to the newest technological developments.

The book provides electronic supplementary material including radiological images that allow a comprehensive evaluation of some cases that were included in the chapters. This approach allows the reader to consider a full set of images, thus getting an overall view of the anatomical involvement by the disease overcoming the limit of evaluating just a single selected image.

We strongly hope the book could be a valuable tool for radiologists, neuroradiologists, neurologists, clinicians, and surgeons, working in general hospitals and teaching hospitals, from residents to consultants.

Trieste, Italy   Maria Assunta Cova
                                                                  Fulvio Stacul

Contents

Paolo Manganotti and Stefano Tamburin

Neuropathic pain (NP) afflicts 6–8% of the general population and has a severe burden on quality of life, sleep, and mood and a heavy impact in terms of disability [1]. Although its prevalence overlaps to that of very common pathologies, such as diabetes mellitus and bronchial asthma, NP still represents a difficult condition to diagnose and treat, both for the general practitioner and for the specialist in neurology, pain therapy, or physical and rehabilitation medicine.

NP is defined as "pain that arises as a direct consequence of a lesion or disease involving the somatosensory system" [2]. This definition allows a clear distinction with nociceptive pain, which is caused by an actually or potentially dangerous stimulus for a tissue or organ, in the presence of a normal functioning of the somatosensory system.

The site of the injury or disease also allows to classify the NP in either peripheral or central (Table 1.1).

Table 1.1 Some common neuropathic pain conditions according to the site of damage of the somatosensory system

Peripheral nervous system—mononeuropathy
Post-traumatic mononeuropathy
Entrapment mononeuropathy (e.g., carpal tunnel syndrome)
Postsurgical mononeuropathy
Trigeminal neuralgia
Cervical and lumbosacral radiculopathy
Diabetic painful monoradiculopathy and mononeuropathy
Postherpetic neuralgia
Peripheral nervous system—multineuropathy
Brachial and lumbosacral plexopathy
Vasculitic multineuropathy
Peripheral nervous system—polyneuropathy
Diabetic symmetrical and small fiber polyneuropathy
Metabolic neuropathy
Immune-mediated polyneuropathy
Chemotherapy-induced polyneuropathy
HIV-related polyneuropathy
Central nervous system—spinal cord lesions
Traumatic lesions of the spinal cord
Inflammatory myelopathy
Spondylotic myelopathy
Central nervous system—brain
Central post-stroke pain
Central nervous system—multiple sites of lesions
Multiple sclerosis-related neuropathic pain

Based on the evidence from animal models and the clinical conditions of NP, the pathophysiological mechanisms of NP are traditionally classified into peripheral and central ones (Table 1.2).

P. Manganotti (✉)
Clinical Neurology Unit, Department of Medical, Surgical and Health Sciences, University of Trieste, Trieste, Italy
e-mail: pmanganotti@units.it

S. Tamburin
Clinical Neurology Unit, Department of Neurosciences, Biomedicine and Movement Sciences, University of Verona, GB Rossi Hospital, Verona, Italy

© Springer Nature Switzerland AG 2019
M. A. Cova, F. Stacul (eds.), *Pain Imaging*, https://doi.org/10.1007/978-3-319-99822-0_1

Table 1.2 Some pathophysiological mechanisms of neuropathic pain according to the site of the nervous system

Site of the nervous system		Mechanism
Peripheral nervous system	Peripheral nerve Dorsal root ganglion	Release of pain-related inflammatory mediators Upregulation of transient potential receptors Increased activity or increased expression in voltage-gated sodium and potassium channels Hyperexcitability of neuronal soma Increased synthesis of proinflammatory cytokines Infiltration of activated macrophages
Central nervous system	Dorsal horn neuron (spinal cord) Descending systems (brainstem) Brain	Increased release of glutamate and substance P Increased expression of voltage-gated sodium and calcium channels Loss of γ-aminobutyric acidergic neurons Functional reorganization of nociceptive neurons Hyperactivation of N-methyl-D-aspartate or glutamate metabotropic receptors Microglial activation Loss of function in inhibitory opioidergic, serotoninergic, and noradrenergic pathways Functional reorganization in the somatosensory thalamic and cortical nociceptive neurons

1.1 Peripheral Mechanisms

The alterations affecting the peripheral nerve involve the unmyelinated C and small-caliber myelinated Aδ nociceptive fibers, but some studies also suggest the involvement of large-caliber myelinated fibers, which do not carry the nociceptive information.

Different type of nerves and receptors can carry pain sensation. For example, the epidermal mechanoreceptors for touch are composed of Meissner corpuscles, Merkel cells, and free nerve endings. In the dermis, there are Ruffini endings and Pacinian corpuscles in a glabrous (or hairless) skin, whereas there is a complex combination of mechanoreceptors and their associated nerves and hair follicle receptors in a hairy skin [3]. The low-threshold mechanoreceptors (LTMR) were found to be the major activators of Aβ and C fibers, and LTMR around hair follicles were posited to activate C fibers. These mechanoreceptors are selectively connected to the nerves. Meissner corpuscles connect to Aα and β fibers for stroking, Merkel cells connect to Aα and β fibers for pressure, and Ruffini corpuscles connect to Aα and β fibers during skin stretching. The primary sensory afferents innervating the human skin are connected to the nerves as follows: discriminative touch nociceptors for pain

are connected to Aβ fibers, nociceptors for pain connect to Aδ fibers, and polymodal nociceptors for pain, emotional touch, and itch connect to C fibers [4]. Pacinian corpuscles and a part of the lanceolate endings surrounding hair roots sometimes show rapidly adapting firing responses. From this, we posit that to achieve a long-lasting effect, vibration may be the most potent type of stimulation. These mechanoreceptors have various types of mechanosensitive (TRP) channels: TRPV1–TRPV4, TRPA1, TRPM8, and TRPCs in keratinocytes. Many signaling chemicals have been proposed including NGF, bradykinin, 5-HT, ATP, H+, glutamate, somatostatin, and GABA. Among them, only ATP and H+ are known to be associated with TRP channel activation. In the dorsal root ganglion (DRG) and dorsal horn (DH), essential modification of the pain signal may occur through interactions among astrocytes, microglia, and presynaptic and postsynaptic neurons. Peripheral nerve fibers show alterations of voltage-dependent sodium and potassium channels and an abnormal expression of receptors of the transient receptor potential family. Similar alterations have been documented in the dorsal root ganglia, the site cell bodies of the first-order sensory neurons, which give rise to peripheral nerve fibers. Following a painful stimulus, if sufficient numbers of a particular type, or types, of nociceptor are activated, an afferent volley will be produced. The afferent volley travels along the peripheral nociceptor and enters the spinal cord via the dorsal horn [5]. The whole of these alterations leads to a hyperexcitability of the peripheral nerve and the dorsal root ganglion, which can be responsible for both spontaneous and evoked pain to either Tinel maneuvers or root stretching (i.e., Lasegue and Wassermann maneuvers).

1.2 Spinal Mechanisms

Beyond the peripheral nociceptor and dorsal horn, depending on the type of nociceptor activated, pain-related information ascends in the contralateral spinothalamic tract (STT), but there are also direct connections to the medulla and brainstem via the spino-reticular (SRT) and spino-mesencephalic (SMT) tracts and to the hypothalamus via the spino-hypothalamic tract (SHT). Outside of the thalamus, there are spinal projections to the ventrolateral medulla, parabrachial nucleus, periaqueductal gray (PAG), and brainstem reticular formation. Of particular interest is the role of these structures in both inhibiting and facilitating nociceptive transmission and subsequent pain perception [6].

Numerous animal models have documented abnormalities in second-order nociceptive neurons, which are found in the dorsal horn of the spinal cord. These alterations include changes in the calcium channels and neurotransmitters and neuromediators. These changes, together, shift the spinal excitability balance toward excitation rather than inhibition and result in a set of phenomena that characterize the so-called spinal sensitization [7, 8].

Changes in neuroplastic receptive fields at spinal level may be responsible for phenomena such as the extraterritorial expansion of pain and sensory symptoms, for example, in patients with simple carpal tunnel syndrome [7].

A reduction in the strength of opioidergic, serotoninergic, and noradrenergic pain control descending systems, which are located in the brainstem and project to the dorsal horn of the spinal cord, has been documented in animal models of chronic NP [1].

The drugs that are currently available for the treatment of NP aim to correct the alterations listed above, which occur mainly at the neuronal level. For example, some antiepileptic drugs (e.g., phenytoin, carbamazepine) can reduce the hyperexcitability of the peripheral nerve by blocking the voltage-dependent sodium channels. The drugs that are active on the $\alpha 2\delta$ subunit of calcium channels (i.e., gabapentin, pregabalin) can reduce spinal sensitization. Opioids and serotonin-noradrenaline reuptake inhibitor antidepressants (i.e., duloxetine, venlafaxine) may potentiate pain control descending inhibitory systems. Tricyclics (e.g., amitriptyline) may control NP through multiple mechanisms. Meta-analyses and guidelines document that these classes of drugs are effective in reducing NP, although in a limited number of patients [2] and with an unfavorable side effect profile in a consistent number of cases.

1.3 Central Mechanisms and Pain Matrix

Neuroimaging studies have revolutioned the understanding of the involvement of the cortex in pain sensation. Not only is the pain primarily being represented in the primary somatosensory cortex (S1), but large distributed brain networks were found to be active during painful stimulation [9–12]. The cortical and subcortical brain regions found to be commonly activated from these early studies by nociceptive stimulation included anterior cingulate cortex, insula, frontal cortices, S1, second somatosensory cortex (S2), and amygdala and are often referred to as the "pain matrix" [13].

Because pain signals are important for survival, it is as important to regulate pain signaling in the central nervous system. The brainstem has a tonic regulatory influence from the spinal cord dorsal root level (Table 1.2). There are also strong suggestions that the analgesic system is heavily related to the endogenous opioid systems. The brainstem integrates information from autonomic, homeostatic, affective, and limbic brain centers and can participate to the descending control of pain [14]. The relationship between reported pain intensity and the peripheral stimulus that evokes it depends on many factors such as the level of arousal, anxiety, depression, attention, and expectation or anticipation. These factors are in the process of being characterized on the physiological and pharmacological levels by means of functional imaging. These "psychological" factors are in turn regulated by overt and covert information as well as more general contextual cues that establish the significance of the stimulus and help determine an appropriate response to it. Simple manipulations with attention alter the subjective pain experience as well as the corresponding pattern of activation during painful stimulation [15]. Functional and connectivity analyses in neuroimaging suggest that the increased activity within prefrontal and cingulate cortices during distraction decreases pain perception via the descending pain modulatory system, presumably via anti-nociceptive pathways [16].

The complex mechanism of pain at spinal and central system based on sensitization and modulation can explain in most occasions the limited efficacy of current NP treatments. The first, and probably the most important reason, is that many of the evidence in favor of the mechanisms described above come from animal models of NP, where the main outcome is usually the reduction of pain evoked by mechanical or thermal stimuli [17]. Indeed, this type of outcome cannot capture the complexity and multidimensional features of pain in humans, whereby the main complaint is spontaneous pain [17]. The second reason is that the treatment of pain should aim to reduce the negative effects of pain on mood, sleep and quality of life, features that are difficult to explore in animal models. The third reason is that current models do not allow to understand the complex mechanisms that take place in patients with NP in several brain areas, which include thalamic and cortical areas that cannot be explored in animal models [18, 19] and have been just studied by neuroimaging in humans.

References

1. Magrinelli F, Zanette G, Tamburin S. Neuropathic pain: diagnosis and treatment. Pract Neurol. 2013;13:292–307.
2. Finnerup NB, Haroutounian S, Kamerman P, Baron R, Bennett DL, Bouhassira D, Cruccu G, Freeman R, Hansson P, Nurmikko T, Raja SN, Rice AS, Serra J, Smith BH, Treede RD, Jensen TS. Neuropathic pain: an updated grading system for research and clinical practice. Pain. 2016;157:1599–606.
3. Lumpkin EA, Caterina MJ. Mechanisms of sensory transduction in the skin. Nature. 2007;445:858–65.
4. Zimmerman A, Bai L, Ginty DD. The gentle touch receptors of mammalian skin. Science. 2014;346:950–4.
5. Basbaum A, Jessell T. The perception of pain. In: Principles of neural science. Amsterdam: Elsevier; 2000. p. 472–91.
6. Tracey I, Dunckley P. Importance of anti- and pronociceptive mechanisms in human disease. Gut. 2004;53:1553–5.
7. Zanette G, Cacciatori C, Tamburin S. Central sensitization in carpal tunnel syndrome with extraterritorial spread of sensory symptoms. Pain. 2010;148:227–36.
8. Finnerup NB, Attal N, Haroutounian S, McNicol E, Baron R, Dworkin RH, Gilron I, Haanpää M, Hansson P, Jensen TS, Kamerman PR, Lund K, Moore A, Raja SN, Rice AS, Rowbotham M, Sena E, Siddall P, Smith BH, Wallace M. Pharmacotherapy for neuropathic pain in adults: a systematic review and meta-analysis. Lancet Neurol. 2015;14:162–73.
9. Porro C, Cettolo V, Francescato MP, Baraldi P. Temporal and intensity coding of pain in human cortex. J Neurophysiol. 1998;80:3312–20.
10. Craig A, Chen K, Bandy D, Reiman E. Thermosensory activation of insular cortex. Nat Neurosci. 2000;3:184–9.
11. Price DD. Psychological and neural mechanisms of the affective dimension of pain. Science. 2000;288:1769–72.
12. Tracey I, Becerra L, Chang I, et al. Noxious hot and cold stimulation produce common patterns of brain activation in humans: a functional magnetic resonance imaging study. Neurosci Lett. 2000;288:159–62.
13. Ingvar M. Pain and functional imaging. Philos Trans R Soc Lond Ser B Biol Sci. 1999;354:1347–58.
14. Suzuki R, Rygh LJ, Dickenson AH. Bad news from the brain: descending 5-HT pathways that control spinal pain processing. Trends Pharmacol Sci. 2004;25:613–7.
15. Petrovic P, Petersson KM, Ghatan PH, Stone-Elander S, Ingvar M. Pain-related cerebral activation is altered by a distracting cognitive task. Pain. 2000;85:19–30.
16. Valet M, Sprenger T, Boecker H, et al. Distraction modulates connectivity of the cingulo-frontal cortex and the midbrain during pain—an fMRI analysis. Pain. 2004;109:399–408.

17. Colloca L, Ludman T, Bouhassira D, Baron R, Dickenson AH, Yarnitsky D, Freeman R, Truini A, Attal N, Finnerup NB, Eccleston C, Kalso E, Bennett DL, Dworkin RH, Raja SN. Neuropathic pain. Nat Rev Dis Primers. 2017;3:17002.

18. Tamburin S, Maier A, Schiff S, Lauriola MF, Di Rosa E, Zanette G, Mapelli D. Cognition and emotional decision-making in chronic low back pain: an ERPs study during Iowa gambling task. Front Psychol. 2014;5:1350.

19. Tamburin S, Borg K, Caro XJ, Jann S, Clark AJ, Magrinelli F, Sobue G, Werhagen L, Zanette G, Koike H, Späth PJ, Vincent A, Goebel A. Immunoglobulin g for the treatment of chronic pain: report of an expert workshop. Pain Med. 2014;15:1072–82.

Brain Imaging of Pain

Massimo Caulo, Valerio Maruotti, and Antonio Ferretti

2.1 Introduction

Pain is not just a warning symptom informing our body of actual or potential damage to the tissue, but it is an unpleasant sensation with sensory, emotional, and cognitive dimensions occurring after nervous system lesions. Neuroimaging techniques provide a tool for understanding the mechanisms involved in perception and modulation of the pain experience. Brain functional magnetic resonance imaging shows that multiple pain conditions are associated with changes within large-scale distributed networks involved in sensory, motor, autonomic, cognitive, and emotional functions. The importance of the

brain for pain perception derives from patients with cerebral lesions. Traditionally pain has been conceptualized as the neural substrate that passively reflects peripheral changes following injury. Today it is clear that the conscious perception of a sensory stimulus cannot be completed in sensory areas, but rather there is an extensive, interconnected network of cortical and subcortical areas. The group of brain structures jointly activated by painful stimuli is commonly called "the pain matrix." Generally, the ascending pain processes divide signals into localization and emotional/motivation centers (Fig. 2.1). The brain regions involved in processing pain depend on the type of pain experienced (acute and chronic pain) and on the different pathologies.

Electronic Supplementary Material The online version of this chapter (https://doi.org/10.1007/978-3-319-99822-0_2) contains supplementary material, which is available to authorized users.

M. Caulo (✉) · A. Ferretti
Department of Neuroscience, Imaging and Clinical Sciences, University "G. d'Annunzio" of Chieti, Chieti, Italy

ITAB - Institute of Advanced Biomedical Technologies, University "G. d'Annunzio" of Chieti, Chieti, Italy
e-mail: caulo@unich.it

V. Maruotti
ITAB - Institute of Advanced Biomedical Technologies, University "G. d'Annunzio" of Chieti, Chieti, Italy

Neurology Department, IRCCS Neuromed, Pozzilli, Isernia, Italy

2.2 Structural and Functional Neuroimaging Techniques

2.2.1 Magnetic Resonance Imaging (MRI)

MRI uses a strong static magnetic field and radio-frequency (RF) waves to create multiplanar cross-sectional images. The main parameters on which the image contrast is based are T1 and T2. T1 (the longitudinal relaxation time) is a measure of how long atomic nuclei take to realign longitudinally with the main magnetic field, after they have been knocked over by an RF pulse. T2 (the transverse relaxation time) is a measure of how long a group

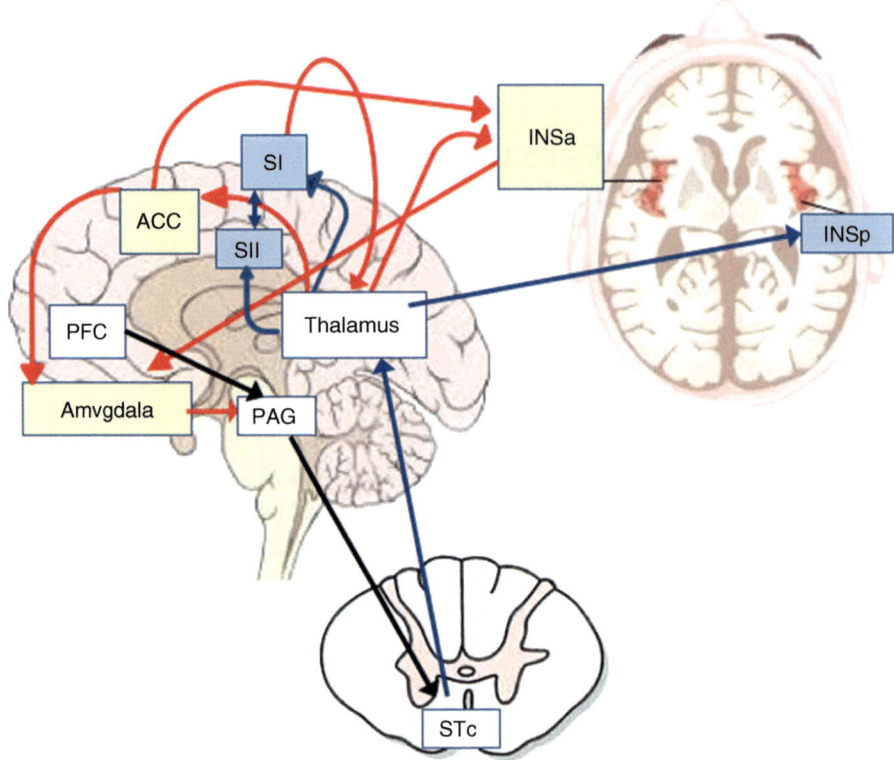

Fig. 2.1 Schematic representation of the pain matrix. Nociceptive inputs enter the spinal dorsal horn and ascend through the contralateral spinothalamic tract (STc) to the thalamus. The medial pathway (yellow square and red arrows) projects from the medial thalamus to the anterior cingulate cortex (ACC), anterior insular cortex (INSa), and amygdala; the medial pathway processes the affective-motivational component of pain. The lateral pathway (light blue square and blue arrows) projects from the lateral thalamus to the primary and secondary somatosensory cortices (SI and SII) and posterior insular cortex (INSp); the lateral pathway processes the corporal specificity of bodily pain. Inhibitory projections (black arrows) descend from the prefrontal cortex (PFC), via the periaqueductal gray matter (PAG), to the spinal cord

of atomic nuclei that have been knocked over by an RF pulse take to become maximally disordered in the transverse plane. Different tissues have different T1 and T2. Images with T2 weighting are most commonly used when looking for pathology, while T1-weighted images are more commonly used to highlight anatomy [1].

2.2.2 Functional Magnetic Resonance Imaging (fMRI)

Beyond the study of normal and pathological brain anatomy, MRI has been used during the last 20 years to investigate brain functions with a technique generally defined as functional MRI (fMRI). Since its introduction [2] fMRI has become an indispensable tool in neuroscience research and in clinical neurological and neurosurgical practice. fMRI is classically performed using the blood-oxygen-level-dependent contrast (BOLDc) technique. The functional contrast is based on deoxyhemoglobin which acts as an endogenous contrast medium. Deoxyhemoglobin is a paramagnetic molecule, thus creating magnetic field distortions within and around the blood vessels that affect T2*- and T2-weighted images. fMRI is based on the hemodynamic response triggered by an increase of neuronal activity related to a given stimulus or task. Briefly, an increased neuronal activity triggers a local vasodilation (the neurovascular coupling mechanism), altering cerebral blood flow (CBF) and cerebral blood volume (CBV). These physiological responses are needed to support the increased oxygen metabolism of activated neuronal pools. These hemodynamic and metabolic changes alter the local deoxyhemoglobin content, producing a slight alteration in the MR signal [3]. fMRI is usually performed using T2*-weighted echo-planar imaging sequences that are the most sensitive to the BOLD effect, allowing to map regional brain activation robustly and with good spatial resolution. The BOLD technique can also be used to study the brain at rest by mapping temporally synchronous, spatially distributed, spontaneous signal fluctuations and generating measures of functional connectivity [4].

BOLD fMRI has enough temporal resolution (around 1 s) to allow the study of acute pain with paradigms alternating short periods of pain followed by short periods that are pain-free, causing a hemodynamic response in the activated brain regions. However these paradigms are not well suited to study chronic or sustained pain since these conditions cannot be easily switched on and off [5]. Furthermore, due to its complex nature, the BOLD signal is not able to offer quantitative physiological measurements referred to a particular brain condition. In these and similar applications, fMRI based on arterial spin labeling (ASL) can be more appropriate.

ASL [6] provides a direct measure of cerebral blood flow using magnetically labeled water in the blood to act as an endogenous diffusible tracer. The blood water is magnetically labeled in the main cerebral feeding arteries with radiofrequency pulses that invert the direction of nuclei magnetic moment. When the bolus of magnetically inverted blood reaches the different brain regions, it will affect the MRI signal according to the local CBF. ASL is able to measure both absolute levels of CBF and perfusion changes triggered by neuronal activity [7–9]. Despite a lower sensitivity and temporal resolution with respect to BOLD, these features make ASL fMRI an ideal technique to study brain functioning when control and stimulus conditions cannot be rapidly alternated. In addition, compared with BOLD, ASL offers increased spatial specificity to neuronal activity due to the capillary/tissue origin of the signal [10]. fMRI ASL techniques have consequently been used to assess the central processing of pain in patients with migraine [11] and chronic pain [12].

2.2.3 PET

Positron emission tomography (PET) can measure changes in hemodynamic, metabolic, or chemical events at receptor and neurotransmitter reuptake sites or neurotransmitter precursor uptake in living tissues.

Although PET is an invasive technique requiring the injection of a radioactive tracer (e.g., $H_2^{15}O$ or ^{18}F-FDG) and suffers from low spatial and temporal resolution with respect to fMRI, it can quantify regional CBF, oxygen uptake, and glucose metabolism in physiological units. Thus, PET can be used to indirectly and directly measure different aspects of the neuronal response to painful stimuli. PET is also unique in its ability to evaluate the neurochemical components of central pain processing by using tracers which directly measure events within the central opioid and dopaminergic systems [13].

2.2.4 MEG

Magnetoencephalography (MEG) is an electrophysiological technique that has higher temporal resolution than fMRI and PET, but lacks good spatial resolution.

MEG detects the tiny magnetic field generated by postsynaptic ionic currents of synchronically active pyramidal cortical neurons, oriented in palisade. These postsynaptic potentials reflect the integrative information processing of signals coming from the thalamus, brainstem, and other cortical areas. The magnetic currents are detected by arrays of superconducting quantum interference devices (SQUIDs) in a magnetically shielded room. Heavy magnetical shielding is necessary to attenuate external magnetic fields, since neuromagnetic fields are very weak. These technical requirements make the MEG device relatively expensive [14]. MEG studies are often used to evaluate separate temporal components of the cerebral pain response, for instance, in relation to expectation [15, 16] or the processing of first and second pain due to the varying conduction times by A and C fibers [17].

2.2.5 NIRS

Near-infrared spectroscopy (NIRS) is a noninvasive, relatively inexpensive portable optical imaging technique based on the principle that diffusion and absorption of light in the near-infrared (NIR) range (700–1000 nm) is sensitive to blood oxygenation. This light is able to pass through the skin, soft tissue, and skull with relative ease and can penetrate brain tissue to a depth of up to 8 cm in infants and 5 cm in adults. It measures the hemodynamic response to neural activity based on the different absorption properties of biological chromophores. The hemodynamic signal obtained with the NIRS technique is based on the absorption of NIRS light depending on the oxygenation state of hemoglobin circulating through the tissues. NIRS quantifies levels of oxygenated and deoxygenated hemoglobin in brain tissue and allows for calculation of absolute changes in blood flow and cerebral blood volume [18]. Functional NIRS research is rapidly expanding across a wide range of areas. This technique can be usefully applied to assess cerebral hemodynamic changes associated with pain in infants and in non-collaborative patients [19].

2.3 Structural Neuroimaging of Pain

Neuropathic pain can arise as a direct consequence of a lesion or disease affecting the somatosensory system at central and peripheral level.

2.3.1 Central Post Stroke Pain

Central pain results from a primary lesion or dysfunction of the central nervous system in different pathologies: stroke, multiple sclerosis, spinal cord injury, syringomyelia, vascular malformations, infections, and traumatic brain injury.

Déjerine and Roussy described initially patients with severe, persistent, paroxysmal, and often intolerable pains on the hemiplegic side related to lesions of the thalamus and parts of the posterior limb of the internal capsule [20].

Central post stroke pain (CPSP) can develop after both hemorrhagic and ischemic lesions in sensory pathway of the central nervous system [21]. The onset is usually within the first few months, but it can occur some years later, and it is often gradual coinciding with improvements in sensory loss [22]. Abnormalities in either thermal (particularly cold) or pain (e.g., pinprick) sensation are found in more than 90% of patients, whereas sensory loss in other modalities (such as touch and vibration) is less frequent [23]. Pain can be localized within the entire area of sensory abnormalities or within a fraction of this area [24]. Non-sensory findings depend on the localization and severity of the cerebrovascular lesion. Pain is characterized by an intense spontaneous or evoked pain, typically constant and often made worse by touch, movement, emotions, and temperature changes. It is often described as constant burning or aching, with paresthesia and intolerable intermittent stabbing. Allodynia and hyperalgesia are usually present [25].

The stroke can be anywhere along the somatosensory system from the cortex to spinal cord, although lateral medullary (Wallenberg syndrome) and thalamic infarctions have the highest incidence. Wallenberg syndrome is the most frequent ischemic stroke in posterior circulation (Fig. 2.2). It is most often secondary to intracranial vertebral artery or posterior inferior cerebellar artery (PICA) occlusion due to atherothrombosis, embolism, and sometimes to spontaneous dissection of the vertebral arteries. A complete Wallenberg syndrome is not common. Facial pain is homolateral to lesion. Different combinations of the following homolateral (ataxia, vertigo, diplopia, nystagmus, Horner's syndrome, hiccups, hoarseness, dysphonia, dysphagia, dysarthria, decreased gag reflex) and contralateral deficits (loss of pain and temperature sensation over the side of body) may all be found. The thalamus plays an important role in the underlying mechanisms of central pain, and CPSP is common after lesions affecting the thalamus. The thalamus may be involved by ischemic and hemorrhagic stroke, in particular in hypertension (Fig. 2.3). Ischemic stroke is most often secondary to intracranial occlusion due to atherothrombosis of the posterior cerebral artery. In thalamic lesions pain is located in the contralateral hemibody. The side of lesion is not a consistent predictor of pain [26]. Lesions can be located in the posterolateral, ventral posterior lateral, and medial nuclei [27].

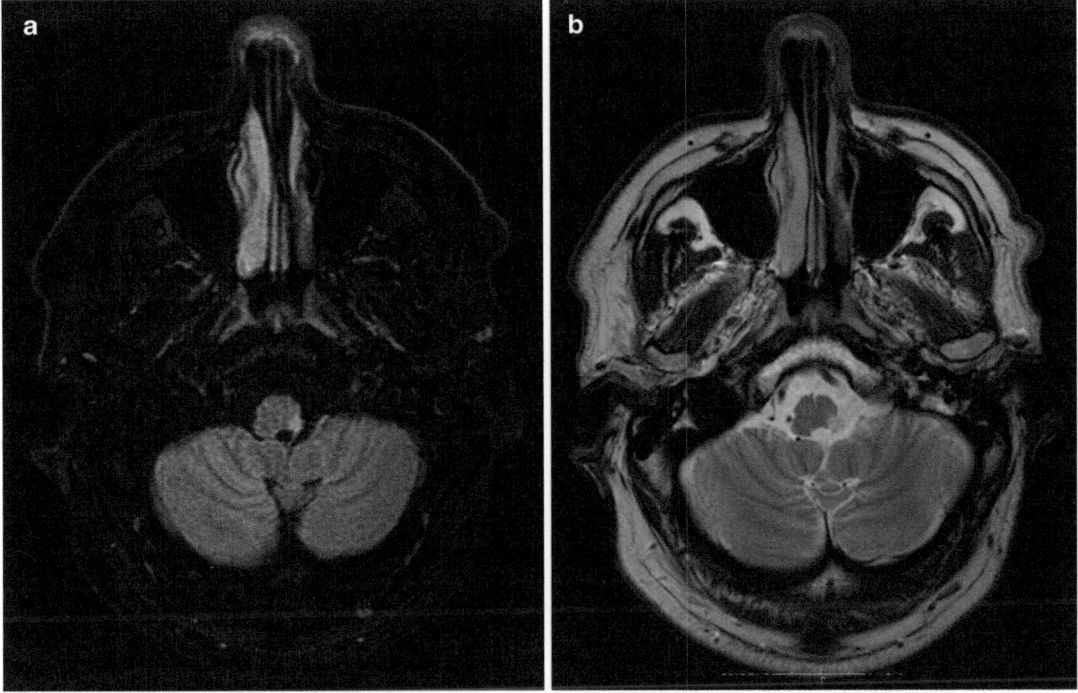

Fig. 2.2 Wallenberg syndrome: axial FLAIR (**a**) and T2 (**b**) MR images showing a hyperintense ischemic lesion in the left posterolateral medulla oblongata

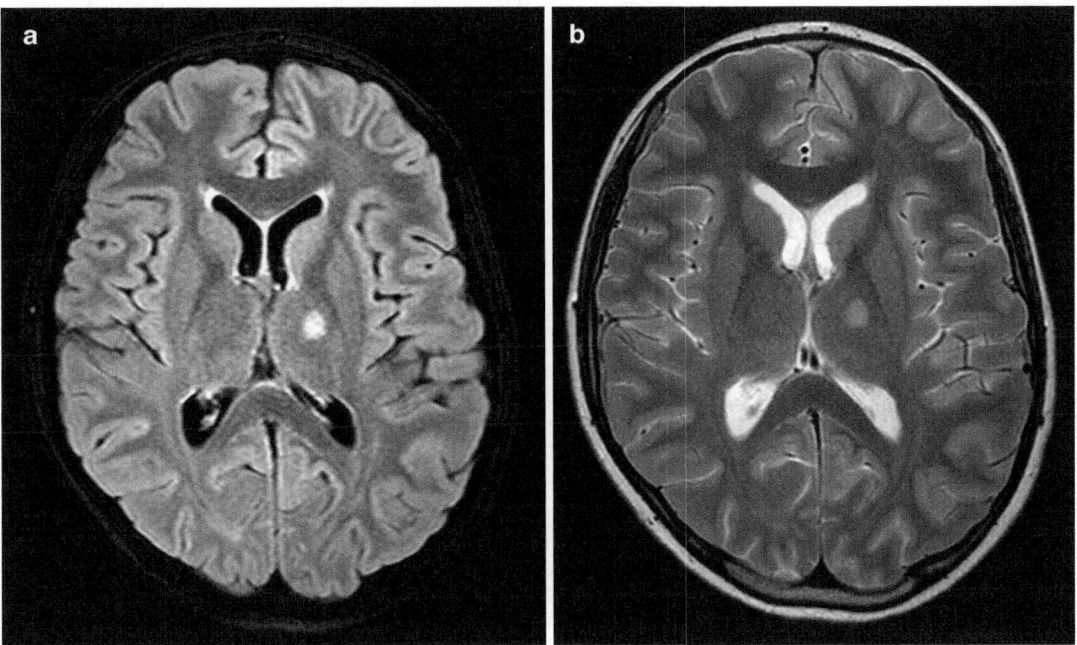

Fig. 2.3 Thalamic stroke: axial FLAIR (**a**) and T2 (**b**) MR images showing a hyperintense ischemic lesion in the left lateral thalamus

In addition to Wallenberg syndrome, trigeminal nuclei can be involved in hypertensive hemorrhage, cavernous angiomas, arteriovenous malformations (AVMs), or trauma (Duret's hemorrhage) [28]. The most common cause is hypertension in middle-aged elderly patients and cavernous angiomas in young.

2.3.2 Multiple Sclerosis

Multiple sclerosis (MS) is an unpredictable autoimmune and neurodegenerative disease of the central nervous system characterized by demyelination and axonal loss. It is a heterogeneous disease with a variety of sign and symptoms depending on the site of lesions that leads to motor, sensory, and cognitive impairment [29].

Chronic pain is one of the most frequent MS-associated symptoms that dramatically reduces the quality of life. Pain in multiple sclerosis (MS) has a variable prevalence of 20–90%. Patients usually have more disability at expanded disability severity score (EDSS), depression, and anxiety. Imaging studies showed that lesions are most commonly reported in the brainstem and less commonly in the spinal cord [30].

MS patients can suffer from nociceptive pain (such as pain resulting from musculoskeletal problems), neuropathic pain, or a mixed nociceptive/neuropathic pain (e.g., tonic painful spasms or spasticity). The most common MS-associated chronic neuropathic pain conditions are dysesthetic pain in the lower extremities, paroxysmal pain, (Lhermitte's phenomenon and trigeminal neuralgia), migraine, and tension-type headache.

Lhermitte's phenomenon, defined as a transient short-lasting sensation related to neck flexion in the back of the neck, the spine, and into the legs and arms, has a prevalence from 9 to 41%. It is frequently associated with posterior columns lesions of the cervical spinal cord (Fig. 2.4).

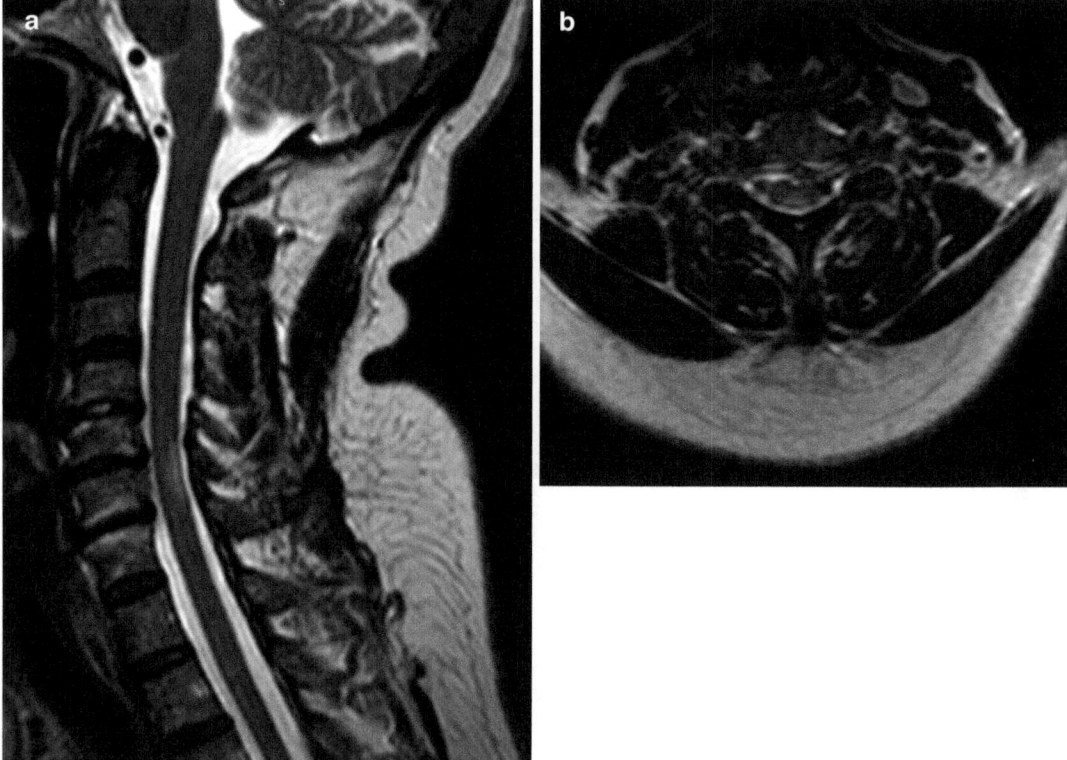

Fig. 2.4 Cervical spinal cord lesion in a patient with multiple sclerosis. Sagittal (**a**) and axial (**b**) T2 MR images showing a hyperintense demyelinating lesion in the posterior columns

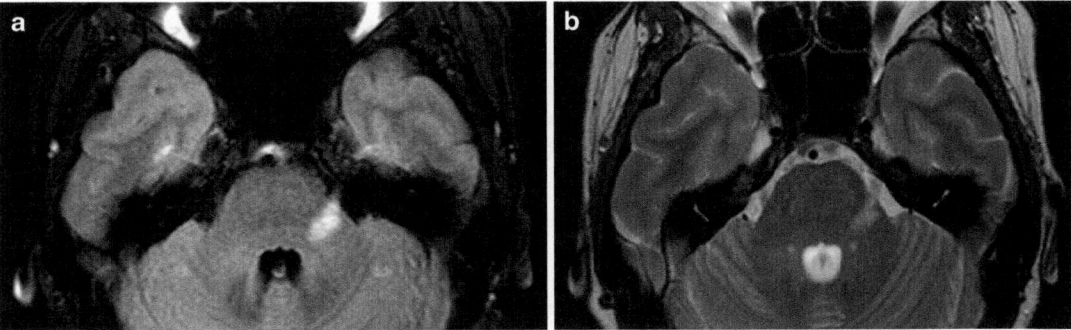

Fig. 2.5 Trigeminal neuralgia in a patient with multiple sclerosis. Axial FLAIR (**a**) and T2 (**b**) MR images showing a demyelinating lesion in the left lateral pons near the root entry zone

Hyperexcitability resulting by miscommunication between the lesioned nerves is considered as the main pathophysiological mechanism.

The pathophysiology of trigeminal neuralgia (TN) in MS patients involves CNS demyelination along the fifth cranial nerve at "entry zone" or at the main sensory nucleus. If a patient under the age of 50 presents face pain, MS is the most common etiology. In MS patients, the facial neuropathic pain syndrome is similar to classic TN. While classic TN is caused by neurovascular compression of the fifth cranial nerve (CN V), MS-related lesions correlate with MRI lesions in the trigeminal nucleus, nerve, and brainstem. Conventional MRI, better high-resolution MRI at 3 T, demonstrates demyelination in the trigeminal root entry zone and intrapontine tracts (Fig. 2.5) that could extend in either direction to the trans-cisternal part of the nerve and to both ascending and descending trigeminal nuclei [31].

2.4 Functional Neuroimaging of Pain

The first half of the twentieth century was dominated by the idea that pain integration in the central nervous system was limited to subcortical structures, not extending beyond the thalamus.

Further studies suggested that the pain experience reflected interacting sensory, affective, and cognitive dimensions that could influence each other and implied that it could only be conceived as a conscious sensation.

The first human brain imaging studies of pain using PET and SPECT indicated that multiple cortical and subcortical regions are activated by noxious stimuli in normal subjects [13]. Since then many other functional hemodynamic and neurophysiologic studies (PET, MEG fMRI, ASL) confirmed that pain activates several brain regions. The group of brain structures jointly activated by painful stimuli is commonly described as "the pain matrix." The pain matrix includes the thalamus, basal ganglia, anterior cingulate cortex (ACC), insula, amygdala, primary and secondary somatosensory cortices (S1 and S2), prefrontal cortex (PFC), and the periaqueductal gray (PAG) [32] (Fig. 2.6).

A division of function between the lateral and medial components of the human pain processing system of the brain was yet proposed several decades ago [33]. The lateral pain system is formed by the lateral thalamic nuclei, the primary and secondary somatosensory cortices (SI and SII, respectively), and posterior insula [34]. Activation of these areas is thought to support the corporal specificity of bodily pain and transmits information about the intensity, location, and duration of noxious stimuli. The medial pain system is formed by medial thalamic nuclei, anterior cingulate cortex (ACC), amygdala, and anterior insula and participates in affective and attentional concomitants of pain sensation or perceiving pain as an unpleasant experience [32].

Also the descending pain modulation system includes the PFC and ACC and exerts its

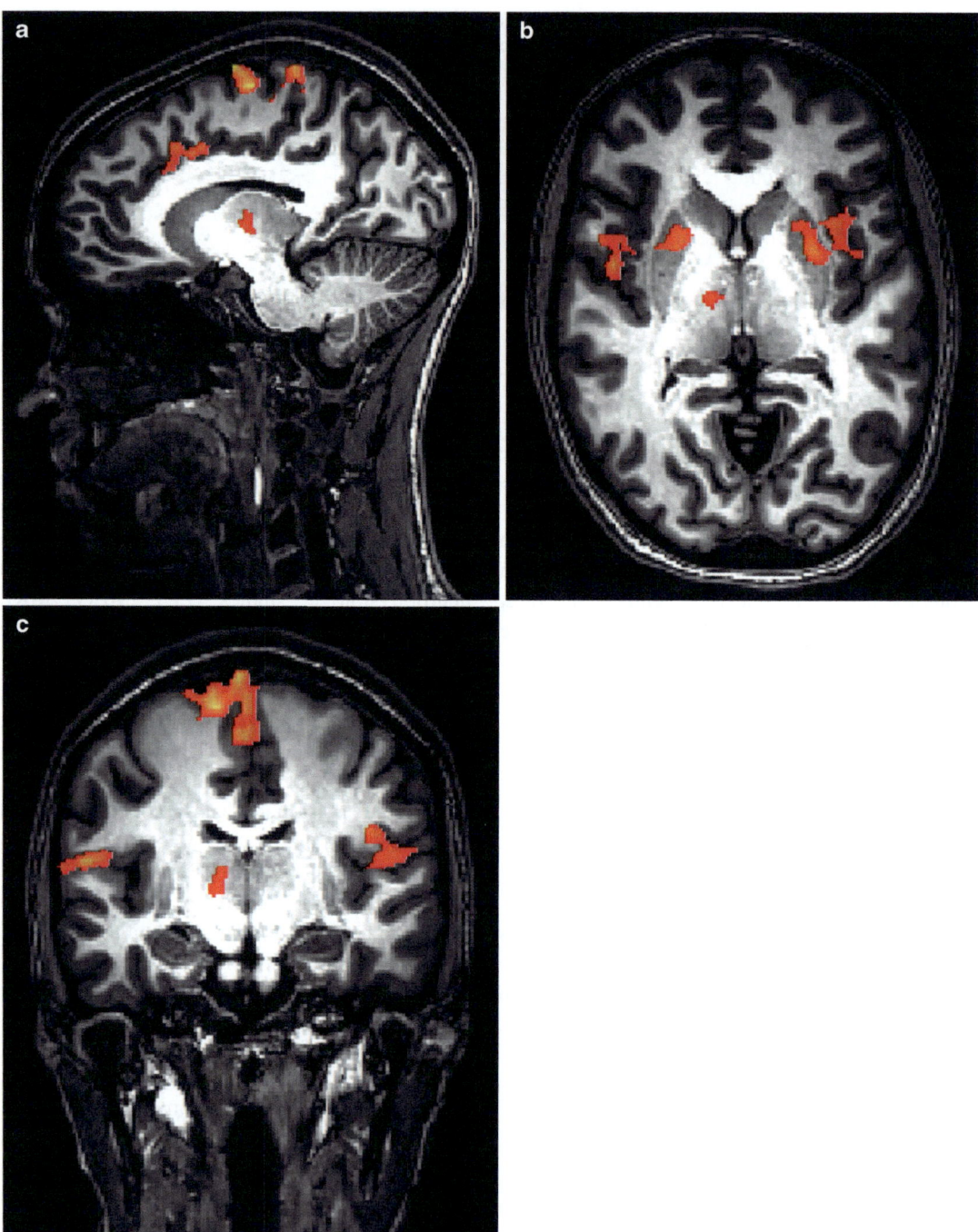

Fig. 2.6 BOLD fMRI activations during painful electrical stimulation of the left ankle. (**a**) Sagittal view: SI, anterior cingulate and thalamus activations. (**b**) Axial view: putamen, bilateral insula, and left thalamus activations. (**c**) Coronal view: left SI, bilateral SII, and left thalamus activations. Images are displayed using the neurological convention, i.e., right is right, left is left. (Courtesy of Piero Chiacchiaretta PhD, University of Chieti, Italy)

influence on the periaqueductal gray matter and thalamus [35].

SI is located posteriorly to the central sulcus, across the surface of the postcentral gyrus and seems to have the same somatotopy in the processing of nonpainful and painful somatosensory stimuli [36]. SII is hidden in the upper bank of the lateral sulcus in the parietal operculum. It has a functional segregation of the subregions involved in the processing of nonpainful and painful somatosensory stimuli [16]. Indeed, the posterior but not the anterior SII increases its activation as a function of the stimulus intensity from nonpainful to painful levels [37] (Fig. 2.7).

No clear somatotopic organization has been reported for painful input, but a topographic organization of SII is reported for nonpainful somatosensory input [38].

In the somatosensory system, SI is presumed to receive the peripheral afferents involved in the encoding of spatial and sensory-discriminative aspects and to dispatch the received input to higher order cortical areas, such as contralateral SII. Contralateral SII sends transcallosal fibers to ipsilateral SII [39].

The nociceptive system has a parallel structure in which SI and SII would receive in parallel painful stimuli [40]. Also pain sensory informations

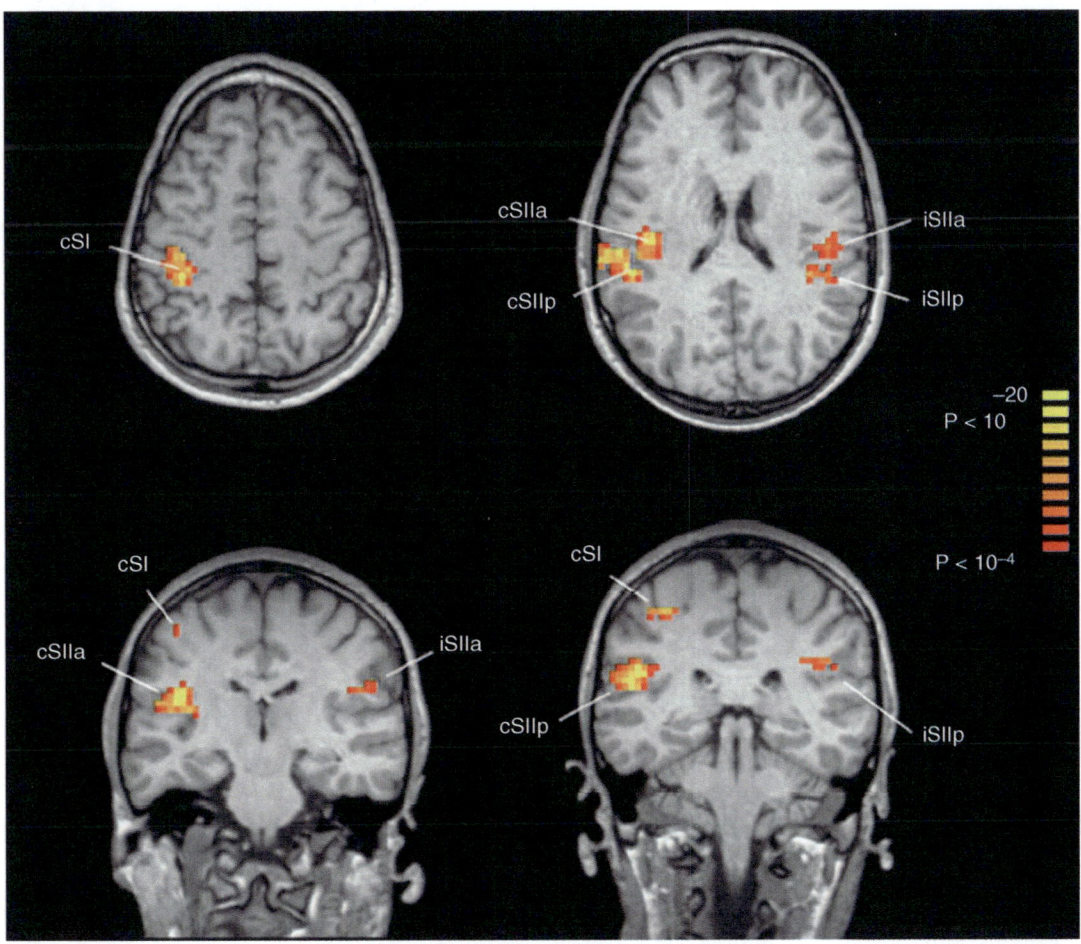

Fig. 2.7 Activated areas in the somatosensory cortex during painful electrical stimulation of the right median nerve, obtained from a group of healthy individuals. The activations are superimposed onto structural images of an individual brain using the neurological convention, i.e., right is right, left is left. Top left, contralateral SI; top right, bilateral SII anterior and posterior subregions; bottom left, anterior SII areas and contralateral SI; bottom right, posterior SII areas and contralateral SI. Reproduced from Ferretti et al. [37] with permission

are processed bilaterally by the two SII areas [41]. This parallel organization bypasses several cortico-cortical and transcallosal connections shortening the processing time of the painful stimulus. SII is consistent with the complexity of thalamic projections from several relays within a multifunctional network involved in noxious stimulus recognition, learning, and memory, autonomic reactions to noxious stimuli, affective aspects of pain-related learning, and memory [38].

ACC has a robust activation across different stimulus modalities and measurement techniques although the locus of this activation varies among studies. The perigenual or rostral ACC seems to be related to affective reactions to pain, while mid-cingulate is related to cognitive processes [42]. After cingulotomy subjects may feel pain but they are not disturbed by it. The insula shows the highest incidence of activity during painful stimulation. The activations of the posterior portion of the insula may be more related to sensory aspects of pain, while the more anterior portion is more related to emotional, cognitive, and memory characteristics of pain perception (Fig. 2.8). In addition, a somatotopic representation exists in the posterior insula for nociceptive stimuli [43]. Strong evidences suggest that the posterior operculo-insular cortex is the only known cortical region where direct stimulation can induce acute physical pain [44] and focal cortical injury to that region entails selective deficits of pain and temperature sensations while leaving other somatosensory modalities intact [45].

Emotional state is a large factor in how pain is perceived, with negative emotions enhancing pain-evoked activity in ACC and insula and pain perception [46].

In the absence of physical stimulus, expecting or anticipating pain activates SI, ACC, insula, PAG, PFC, and ventral striatum [47]. Also, attending to pain is related to stronger pain impact [48]. fMRI studies show that in attention-demanding task while experiencing pain, there is decreased activity in SII, PAG/midbrain, thalamus, and insula resulting in reduced pain perception [49]. The complexity of a task plays also a relevant role on the subjective pain rating [35].

Habituation also occurs in pain network. Repetitive applications of identical painful stimuli decrease pain ratings and decrease BOLD responses to painful stimuli in the thalamus, insula, and SII, mediated by the rACC [50].

Cortical activation has been studied related to different types of painful stimuli: cutaneous noxious cold, muscle stimulation using electric shock or hypertonic saline, capsaicin, colonic distension, rectal distension, gastric distension, esophageal distension, ischemia, cutaneous electric shock, ascorbic acid, and laser heat. These stimuli produce many similar activations in cortical and subcortical areas [51].

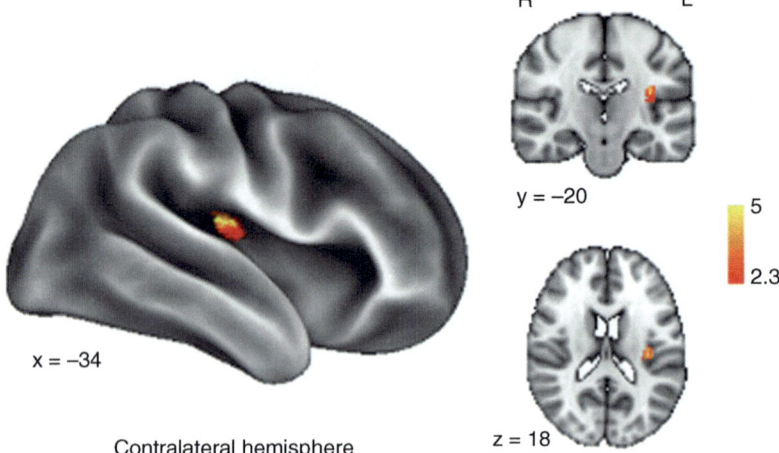

Fig. 2.8 Perfusion MRI study with ASL technique (pCASL sequence) after capsaicin application in the anteromedial aspect of the lower right leg. Note the increased CBF in the dorsal insula of the left hemisphere. Modified from Segerdahl et al. [43] with permission

2.4.1 Pain Network and Connectivity

Painful stimuli induce a robust activation directly proportional to the intensity of the stimulus into the pain matrix. Connectivity in the pain matrix revealed synchronous activity in the bilateral SI cortex, mid-cingulate cortex, posterior insula, and bilateral SII, but not in ACC, one of the brain regions most consistently associated with affective dimension of pain. Similar results were obtained placing a seed in SII. When ACC and anterior insula are used as the seed regions for connectivity analysis, significant synchronous activity is observed in several brain regions including bilateral ACC, mid-cingulate cortex, bilateral anterior and middle insula, thalamus, caudate, orbital PFC, LPFC, and cerebellum, but not in SI or SII. These data confirm a functional segregation of lateral and medial pain system, supporting different functions [52, 53].

In addition, painful stimulation induces a simultaneous decrease in activation in several brain regions, including some of the "core structures" of the default mode network (DMN) [54]. The DMN maintains its typical temporal properties during painful stimulation although an increase of connectivity was found between the left prefrontal cortex and posterior cingulate cortex-precuneus and a decrease in the lateral parietal cortex [55] (Fig. 2.9).

Functional connectivity analyses indicate that the activity of areas displaying pain-evoked changes in the same direction is highly correlated, though there are no significant correlations between brain activations and deactivations indicating that activations and deactivations might underlie different aspects of the pain experience [52].

2.4.2 Pain in Infants

Most of the tools that have been developed for assessing pain perception in infants encompass either behavioral (brow bulge, eye squeeze, nasolabial furrow, qualities of infant cry, flexion of fingers and toes) or physiological (heart rate, arterial oxygen saturation, and blood pressure) responses or combine both into a composite measure. Behavioral responses, particularly facial actions, are the most sensitive and specific pain indicators in infants. NIRS response to painful stimuli found a significant increase over the somatosensory cortex in oxyhemoglobin, total hemoglobin, and deoxyhemoglobin. Biobehavioral pain scores found a significant correlation with NIRS response. Also the areas of BOLD response to painful stimulation are similar in infants and adults, with amygdala and the orbitofrontal cortex not activated in infants. The cortical response depends on the age, the gestational age, and awake/sleep states of the infants. It is directly associated with postnatal age and inversely correlated with gestational age. Less robust cortical responses are also observed in neonates asleep versus awake [56].

2.4.3 Chronic Pain

Painful conditions that usually end without treatment or that respond to simple analgesic measures may also become intractable and develop into a long-lasting condition: chronic pain. Chronic pain (CP) is considered as a condition affecting normal brain function and causing cognitive impairment, depression, sleeping disturbances, and decision-making abnormalities. Altered cortical dynamics have been demonstrated using functional magnetic resonance imaging in patients with CP [57]. A prominent difference between acute and chronic pain consists in the major activation, in the latter, of brain regions involved in cognitive and/or emotional pain processing. Evidence of frontal-limbic dysfunction comes also from PET studies suggesting abnormal opioidergic transmission within frontal-limbic regions in patients with CP [41]. CP disrupts the dynamics of the default mode network. Various types of CP (chronic back pain complex, regional pain syndrome, knee osteoarthritis, diabetic neuropathy, fibromyalgia) are associated with MR functional connectivity changes within the DMN [52]. The most common reorganization consists in an

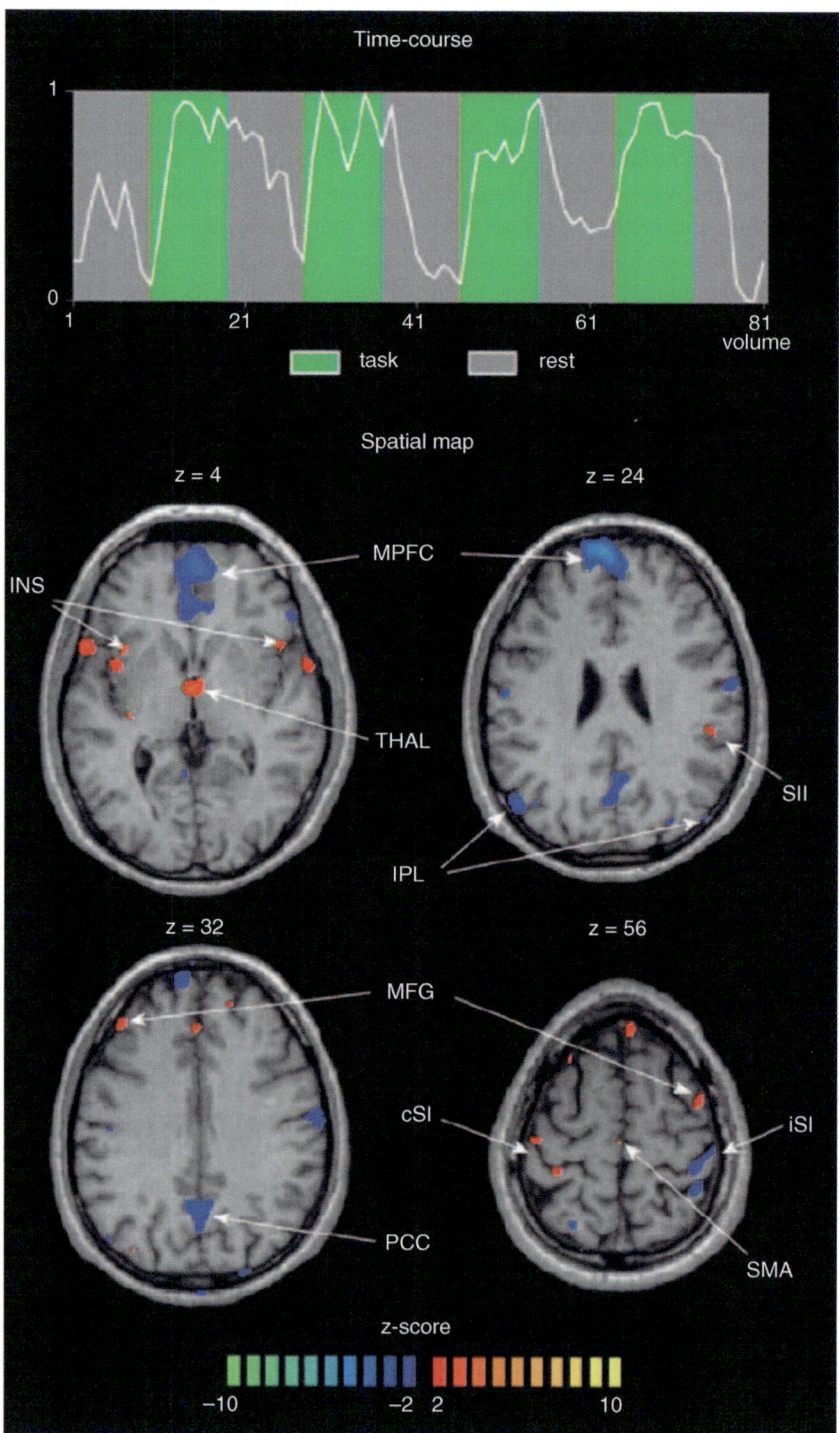

Fig. 2.9 Modulation of the DMN during painful electrical stimulation of the right median nerve. DMN was separated from a single-subject functional MR imaging data set at independent component analysis. Brain areas of the DMN are colored in yellow-orange or azure in case of a positive or negative correlation with the task. *cSI* contralateral primary somatosensory area, *INS* insula, *IPL* inferior parietal lobule, *iSI* ipsilateral primary somatosensory area, *MFG* middle frontal gyrus, *MPFC* medial prefrontal cortex, *PCC* posterior cingulate cortex-precuneus, *SII* secondary somatosensory area, *SMA* supplementary motor area, *THAL* thalamus. Images are displayed using the neurological convention, i.e., right is right, left is left. Reproduced from Mantini et al. [55] with permission

increased association of the medial prefrontal cortex (MPFC) with the insula and dissociation from the posterior components of the DMN (precuneus). The precuneus is involved in autobiographical and episodic memory retrieval and mentalizing. It is primarily involved in elaborating and integrating information rather than directly processing stimuli [52]. The functional correlation of insular regions with portions of the MPFC correlates with the intensity and the extent of pain and decreases after successful treatment of pain [58].

The decreased MPFC connectivity with the precuneus is directly related to the increased connectivity with the insular cortex, suggesting that chronic pain might modulate higher cognitive processes by altering normative functions of the DMN.

The extent of this reorganization is a function of the intensity of the chronic pain and the duration, with functional changes occurring after more than a decade living with chronic pain. In addition an increase of functional connectivity between the PFC and nucleus accumbens predicts pain persistence, suggesting that the frontal-striatal connection is involved in the transition from acute to chronic pain.

Prolonged pain can lead to neuroplastic changes at the cortical level, which induce central sensitization [46].

2.4.4 Phantom Limb Pain (PLP)

Arm amputation often can be followed by pain sensation in the missing limb (PLP). It occurs in up to 80% of amputees and may be exacerbated by many physical (e.g., temperature changes) and psychological (e.g., stress) factors. It is usually described as stabbing, throbbing, burning, or cramping and commonly starts in the first week after amputation. The duration of PLP is unpredictable, resolving in months or persisting for years.

The cause of phantom pain experience has commonly been attributed to maladaptive plasticity of the primary sensorimotor cortex contralateral to the amputation. The representations of body parts adjacent to the missing limb expand and invade the deprived

cortex leading to phantom limb pain. The degree of cortical reorganization appears to be directly related to the degree of phantom pain, and imaging studies have correlated greater extent of somatosensory cortex changes with more intense phantom limb experience. A greater phantom pain is associated with more local activity and more structural integrity within the phantom cortex and with disrupted interregional functional connectivity of the primary sensorimotor cortex of the other body parts [59].

References

1. Atlas SW. Magnetic resonance imaging of the brain and spine. Philadelphia: Wolters Kluwer Health; 2008. p. 1923. [cited 2018 Feb 26]. https://books.google.it/books?hl=it&lr=&id=Mu7MmTXkPeAC&oi=fnd&pg=PA2&dq=Atlas+SW+et+al+magnetic+Resonance+Imaging+of+the+brain+and+spine&ots=r0IH3g6Olm&sig=IXU6TlWiEAXchZFdJGb3IPEQZ3s#v=onepage&q=Atlas&f=false.

2. Ogawa S, Tank DW, Menon R, Ellermann JM, Kim SG, Merkle H, et al. Intrinsic signal changes accompanying sensory stimulation: functional brain mapping with magnetic resonance imaging. Proc Natl Acad Sci U S A. 1992;89(13):5951–5. [cited 2018 Feb 26]. http://www.ncbi.nlm.nih.gov/pubmed/1631079.

3. Buxton RB, Uludağ K, Dubowitz DJ, Liu TT. Modeling the hemodynamic response to brain activation. NeuroImage. 2004;23:S220–33. [cited 2018 Feb 26]. http://www.ncbi.nlm.nih.gov/pubmed/15501093.

4. Fox MD, Raichle ME. Spontaneous fluctuations in brain activity observed with functional magnetic resonance imaging. Nat Rev Neurosci. 2007;8(9):700–11. [cited 2018 Apr 9]. http://www.nature.com/articles/nrn2201.

5. Peyron R, Laurent B, García-Larrea L. Functional imaging of brain responses to pain. A review and meta-analysis. Neurophysiol Clin. 2000;30(5):263–88. [cited 2018 Feb 26]. http://www.ncbi.nlm.nih.gov/pubmed/11126640.

6. Detre JA, Leigh JS, Williams DS, Koretsky AP. Perfusion imaging. Magn Reson Med. 1992;23(1):37–45. [cited 2018 Apr 8]. http://www.ncbi.nlm.nih.gov/pubmed/1734182.

7. Alsop DC, Detre JA, Golay X, Günther M, Hendrikse J, Hernandez-Garcia L, et al. Recommended implementation of arterial spin-labeled perfusion MRI for clinical applications: a consensus of the ISMRM perfusion study group and the European consortium for ASL in dementia. Magn Reson Med. 2015;73(1):102–16. [cited 2018 Apr 8]. http://www.ncbi.nlm.nih.gov/pubmed/24715426.

8. Diekhoff S, Uludağ K, Sparing R, Tittgemeyer M, Cavuşoğlu M, von Cramon DY, et al. Functional localization in the human brain: gradient-echo, spin-echo, and arterial spin-labeling fMRI compared with neuronavigated TMS. Hum Brain Mapp. 2011;32(3):341–57. [cited 2018 Apr 8]. https://doi.org/10.1002/hbm.21024.

9. Tjandra T, Brooks JCW, Figueiredo P, Wise R, Matthews PM, Tracey I. Quantitative assessment of the reproducibility of functional activation measured with BOLD and MR perfusion imaging: implications for clinical trial design. NeuroImage. 2005;27(2):393–401. [cited 2018 Apr 8]. http://www.ncbi.nlm.nih.gov/pubmed/15921936.

10. Raoult H, Ferr J, Petr J, Bannier E, Stamm A, Barillot C, et al. Functional arterial spin labeling: optimal sequence duration for motor activation mapping in clinical practice. J Magn Reson Imaging. 2012;36(6):1435–44. [cited 2018 Apr 8]. https://doi.org/10.1002/jmri.23782.

11. Youssef AM, Ludwick A, Wilcox SL, Lebel A, Peng K, Colon E, et al. In child and adult migraineurs the somatosensory cortex stands out … again: an arterial spin labeling investigation. Hum Brain Mapp. 2017;38(8):4078–87. [cited 2018 Feb 26]. http://www.ncbi.nlm.nih.gov/pubmed/28560777.

12. Wasan AD, Loggia ML, Chen LQ, Napadow V, Kong J, Gollub RL. Neural correlates of chronic low back pain measured by arterial spin labeling. Anesthesiology. 2011;115(2):364–74. [cited 2018 Feb 26]. http://www.ncbi.nlm.nih.gov/pubmed/21720241.

13. Jones AKP, Brown WD, Friston KJ, Qi LY, Frackowiak RSJ. Cortical and subcortical localization of response to pain in man using positron emission tomography. Proc R Soc B Biol Sci. 1991;244(1309):39–44. [cited 2018 Feb 26]. http://www.ncbi.nlm.nih.gov/pubmed/1677194.

14. Babiloni C, Pizzella V, Del Gratta C, Ferretti A, Romani GL. Chapter 5 fundamentals of electroencefalography, magnetoencefalography, and functional magnetic resonance imaging. Int Rev Neurobiol. 2009;86:67–80. [cited 2018 Feb 26]. http://www.ncbi.nlm.nih.gov/pubmed/19607991.

15. Ploner M, Gross J, Timmermann L, Schnitzler A. Cortical representation of first and second pain sensation in humans. Proc Natl Acad Sci U S A. 2002;99(19):12444–8. [cited 2018 Feb 26]. http://www.ncbi.nlm.nih.gov/pubmed/12209003.

16. Torquati K, Pizzella V, Babiloni C, Del Gratta C, Della Penna S, Ferretti A, et al. Nociceptive and non-nociceptive sub-regions in the human secondary somatosensory cortex: an MEG study using fMRI constraints. NeuroImage. 2005;26(1):48–56. [cited 2018 Feb 28]. https://www.sciencedirect.com/science/article/pii/S1053811905000352.

17. Brown CA, Seymour B, Boyle Y, El-Deredy W, Jones AKP. Modulation of pain ratings by expectation and uncertainty: behavioral characteristics and anticipatory neural correlates. Pain. 2008;135(3):240–50. [cited 2018 Feb 26]. http://www.ncbi.nlm.nih.gov/pubmed/17614199.

18. Hillman EMC. Optical brain imaging in vivo: techniques and applications from animal to man. J Biomed Opt. 2007;12(5):51402. [cited 2018 Feb 26]. http://www.ncbi.nlm.nih.gov/pubmed/17994863.

19. Boas DA, Elwell CE, Ferrari M, Taga G. Twenty years of functional near-infrared spectroscopy: introduction for the special issue. NeuroImage. 2014;85:1–5. [cited 2018 Feb 26]. http://www.ncbi.nlm.nih.gov/pubmed/24321364.

20. Wilkins RH, Brody IA. The thalamic syndrome. Arch Neurol. 1969;20(5):559–62. [cited 2018 Feb 26]. http://www.ncbi.nlm.nih.gov/pubmed/5767614.

21. Weimar C, Kloke M, Schlott M, Katsarava Z, Diener H-C. Central poststroke pain in a consecutive cohort of stroke patients. Cerebrovasc Dis. 2002;14(3-4):261–3. [cited 2018 Feb 27]. http://www.ncbi.nlm.nih.gov/pubmed/12403962.

22. Andersen G, Vestergaard K, Ingeman-Nielsen M, Jensen TS. Incidence of central post-stroke pain. Pain. 1995;61(2):187–93. [cited 2018 Feb 27]. http://www.ncbi.nlm.nih.gov/pubmed/7659428.

23. Bowsher D. Central pain: clinical and physiological characteristics. J Neurol Neurosurg Psychiatry. 1996;61(1):62–9. [cited 2018 Feb 27]. http://www.ncbi.nlm.nih.gov/pubmed/8676164.

24. Vestergaard K, Nielsen J, Andersen G, Ingeman-Nielsen M, Arendt-Nielsen L, Jensen TS. Sensory abnormalities in consecutive, unselected patients with central post-stroke pain. Pain. 1995;61(2):177–86. [cited 2018 Feb 27]. http://www.ncbi.nlm.nih.gov/pubmed/7659427.

25. Leijon G, Boivie J, Johansson I. Central post-stroke pain—neurological symptoms and pain characteristics. Pain. 1989;36(1):13–25. [cited 2018 Feb 27]. http://www.ncbi.nlm.nih.gov/pubmed/2919091.

26. Bowsher D, Leijon G, Thuomas KA. Central poststroke pain: correlation of MRI with clinical pain characteristics and sensory abnormalities. Neurology. 1998;51(5):1352–8. [cited 2018 Feb 27]. http://www.ncbi.nlm.nih.gov/pubmed/9818859.

27. Kim JS. Pure sensory stroke. Clinical-radiological correlates of 21 cases. Stroke. 1992;23(7):983–7. [cited 2018 Feb 27]. http://www.ncbi.nlm.nih.gov/pubmed/1615549.

28. Parizel PM, Makkat S, Jorens PG, Özsarlak Ö, Cras P, Van Goethem JW, et al. Brainstem hemorrhage in descending transtentorial herniation (Duret hemorrhage). Intensive Care Med. 2002;28(1):85–8. [cited 2018 Feb 27]. http://www.ncbi.nlm.nih.gov/pubmed/11819006.

29. Murphy KL, Bethea JR, Fischer R. Neuropathic pain in multiple sclerosis—current therapeutic intervention and future treatment perspectives. In: Multiple sclerosis: perspectives in treatment and pathogenesis. Brisbane: Codon Publications; 2017. [cited 2018 Mar 9]. http://www.ncbi.nlm.nih.gov/pubmed/29261265.

30. Seixas D, Foley P, Palace J, Lima D, Ramos I, Tracey I. Pain in multiple sclerosis: a systematic review of neuroimaging studies. Neuroimage Clin. 2014;5:322–31. [cited 2018 Mar 8]. http://creativecommons.org/licenses/by-nc-nd/3.0/.

31. Mazhari A. Multiple sclerosis-related pain syndromes: an imaging update. Curr Pain Headache Rep. 2016;20(12):63. [cited 2018 Mar 9]. http://www.ncbi.nlm.nih.gov/pubmed/27864731.

32. Treede RD, Kenshalo DR, Gracely RH, Jones AK. The cortical representation of pain. Pain. 1999;79(2-3):105–11. [cited 2018 Feb 26]. http://www.ncbi.nlm.nih.gov/pubmed/10068155.

33. Melzack R. From the gate to the neuromatrix. Pain. 1999;82(Suppl 6):S121–6. [cited 2018 Feb 26]. http://www.ncbi.nlm.nih.gov/pubmed/10491980.

34. Kulkarni B, Bentley DE, Elliott R, Youell P, Watson A, Derbyshire SWG, et al. Attention to pain localization and unpleasantness discriminates the functions of the medial and lateral pain systems. Eur J Neurosci. 2005;21(11):3133–42. [cited 2018 Feb 28]. https://doi.org/10.1111/j.1460-9568.2005.04098.x.

35. Wiech K, Seymour B, Kalisch R, Enno Stephan K, Koltzenburg M, Driver J, et al. Modulation of pain processing in hyperalgesia by cognitive demand. NeuroImage. 2005;27(1):59–69. [cited 2018 Feb 28]. http://www.ncbi.nlm.nih.gov/pubmed/15978845.

36. Omori S, Isose S, Otsuru N, Nishihara M, Kuwabara S, Inui K, et al. Somatotopic representation of pain in the primary somatosensory cortex (S1) in humans. Clin Neurophysiol. 2013;124(7):1422–30. [cited 2018 Feb 28]. http://www.ncbi.nlm.nih.gov/pubmed/23415452.

37. Ferretti A, Babiloni C, Del Gratta C, Caulo M, Tartaro A, Bonomo L, et al. Functional topography of the secondary somatosensory cortex for nonpainful and painful stimuli: an fMRI study. NeuroImage. 2003;20(3):1625–38. [cited 2018 Mar 13]. https://www.sciencedirect.com/science/article/pii/S1053811903004385.

38. Ferretti A, Del Gratta C, Babiloni C, Caulo M, Arienzo D, Tartaro A, et al. Functional topography of the secondary somatosensory cortex for nonpainful and painful stimulation of median and tibial nerve: an fMRI study. NeuroImage. 2004;23(3):1217–25. [cited 2018 Feb 28]. http://www.ncbi.nlm.nih.gov/pubmed/15528121.

39. Chen TL, Babiloni C, Ferretti A, Perrucci MG, Romani GL, Rossini PM, et al. Human secondary somatosensory cortex is involved in the processing of somatosensory rare stimuli: an fMRI study. NeuroImage. 2008;40(4):1765–71. [cited 2018 Feb 27]. http://www.ncbi.nlm.nih.gov/pubmed/18329293.

40. Ploner M, Schmitz F, Freund H-J, Schnitzler A. Parallel activation of primary and secondary somatosensory cortices in human pain processing. J Neurophysiol. 1999;81(6):3100–4. [cited 2018 Feb 28]. https://doi.org/10.1152/jn.1999.81.6.3100.

41. Apkarian AV, Bushnell MC, Treede R-D, Zubieta J-K. Human brain mechanisms of pain perception and regulation in health and disease. Eur J Pain. 2005;9(4):463. [cited 2018 Feb 27]. http://www.ncbi.nlm.nih.gov/pubmed/15979027.

42. Vogt BA, Berger GR, Derbyshire SWG. Structural and functional dichotomy of human midcingulate cortex. Eur J Neurosci. 2003;18(11):3134–44. [cited 2018 Feb 28]. http://www.ncbi.nlm.nih.gov/pubmed/14656310.

43. Segerdahl AR, Mezue M, Okell TW, Farrar JT, Tracey I. The dorsal posterior insula subserves a fundamental role in human pain. Nat Neurosci. 2015;18(4):499–500. [cited 2018 Feb 28]. http://www.nature.com/articles/nn.3969.

44. Mazzola L, Isnard J, Peyron R, Mauguière F. Stimulation of the human cortex and the experience of pain: Wilder Penfield's observations revisited. Brain. 2012;135(2):631–40. [cited 2018 Mar 11]. http://www.ncbi.nlm.nih.gov/pubmed/22036962.

45. Garcia-Larrea L, Perchet C, Creac'h C, Convers P, Peyron R, Laurent B, et al. Operculo-insular pain (parasylvian pain): a distinct central pain syndrome. Brain. 2010;133(9):2528–39. [cited 2018 Mar 11]. https://doi.org/10.1093/brain/awq220.

46. Morton D, Jones A, Sandhu J. Brain imaging of pain: state of the art. J Pain Res. 2016;9:613–24. [cited 2018 Feb 26]. http://www.ncbi.nlm.nih.gov/pubmed/27660488.

47. Porro CA, Baraldi P, Pagnoni G, Serafini M, Facchin P, Maieron M, et al. Does anticipation of pain affect cortical nociceptive systems? J Neurosci. 2002;22(8):3206–14. [cited 2018 Feb 28]. http://www.ncbi.nlm.nih.gov/pubmed/11943821.

48. Arntz A, de Jong P. Anxiety, attention and pain. J Psychosom Res. 1993;37(4):423–31. [cited 2018 Feb 28]. http://www.ncbi.nlm.nih.gov/pubmed/8510069.

49. Bantick SJ, Wise RG, Ploghaus A, Clare S, Smith SM, Tracey I. Imaging how attention modulates pain in humans using functional MRI. Brain. 2002;125(Pt 2):310–9. [cited 2018 Feb 28]. http://www.ncbi.nlm.nih.gov/pubmed/11844731.

50. Bingel U, Schoell E, Herken W, Büchel C, May A. Habituation to painful stimulation involves the antinociceptive system. Pain. 2007;131(1):21–30. [cited 2018 Feb 28]. http://www.ncbi.nlm.nih.gov/pubmed/17258858.

51. Iannetti GD, Mouraux A. From the neuromatrix to the pain matrix (and back). Exp Brain Res. 2010;205(1):1–12. [cited 2018 Feb 26]. https://doi.org/10.1007/s00221-010-2340-1.

52. Kong J, Loggia ML, Zyloney C, Tu P, LaViolette P, Gollub RL. Exploring the brain in pain: activations, deactivations and their relation. Pain. 2010;148(2):257–67. [cited 2018 Feb 28]. http://www.ncbi.nlm.nih.gov/pubmed/20005043.

53. Wilcox CE, Mayer AR, Teshiba TM, Ling J, Smith BW, Wilcox GL, et al. The subjective experience of pain: an FMRI study of percept-related models and functional connectivity. Pain Med. 2015;16(11):2121–33. [cited 2018 Apr 10]. http://www.ncbi.nlm.nih.gov/pubmed/25989475.

54. Perrotta A, Chiacchiaretta P, Anastasio MG, Pavone L, Grillea G, Bartolo M, et al. Temporal summation of the nociceptive withdrawal reflex involves deactivation of posterior cingulate cortex. Eur J Pain. 2017;21(2):289–301. [cited 2018 Apr 8]. http://www.ncbi.nlm.nih.gov/pubmed/27452295.

55. Mantini D, Caulo M, Ferretti A, Romani GL, Tartaro A. Noxious somatosensory stimulation affects the default mode of brain function: evidence from func-

tional MR imaging. Radiology. 2009;253(3):797–804. [cited 2018 Feb 28]. http://www.ncbi.nlm.nih.gov/pubmed/19789220.

56. Benoit B, Martin-Misener R, Newman A, Latimer M, Campbell-Yeo M. Neurophysiological assessment of acute pain in infants: a scoping review of research methods. Acta Paediatr. 2017;106(7):1053–66. [cited 2018 Mar 11]. http://www.ncbi.nlm.nih.gov/pubmed/28326623.

57. Tagliazucchi E, Balenzuela P, Fraiman D, Chialvo DR. Brain resting state is disrupted in chronic back pain patients. Neurosci Lett. 2010;485(1):26–31.

[cited 2018 Feb 28]. http://www.ncbi.nlm.nih.gov/pubmed/20800649.

58. Baliki MN, Mansour AR, Baria AT, Apkarian AV. Functional reorganization of the default mode network across chronic pain conditions. PLoS One. 2014;9(9):e106133. [cited 2018 Feb 28]. https://doi.org/10.1371/journal.pone.0106133.

59. Jutzeler CR, Curt A, Kramer JLK. Relationship between chronic pain and brain reorganization after deafferentation: a systematic review of functional MRI findings. Neuroimage Clin. 2015;9:599–606. [cited 2018 Mar 10]. http://www.ncbi.nlm.nih.gov/pubmed/26740913.

Headache: Clinical Features

Antonio Granato and Paolo Manganotti

Headache is one of the most common medical complaints of civilized humans; nevertheless severe and chronic headaches are only infrequently caused by organic disease. Although the overall headache prevalence figures vary, in most studies headache prevalence lifetime is over 70%, and it is higher in women than men, partly due to the high female preponderance of migraine, tension-type headache and several other types of headache [1, 2]. The female preponderance of headache disorders has been attributed to a possible influence of female hormones. In cross-sectional studies the prevalence of headache decreases after middle age, probably because subjects may become headache-free with increasing age [1].

In 1988, for the first time, the International Headache Society (IHS) instituted a classification system for headache that became a standard for headache diagnosis and clinical research. The current IHS classification (the International Classification of Headache Disorder, third edition

[ICHD-3]) provides operational definitions for all headaches types [3]. It divides headaches into two broad categories: the primary (Table 3.1) and secondary headache disorders (Table 3.2). Most headaches seen in practice belong to the category of primary headaches, where there is no underlying structural cause identifiable. Less than 10% headaches in practice belong to the category of secondary headaches where there is an underlying condition that can sometimes be ominous and life-threatening.

The first task in evaluating a headache patient is to identify or exclude secondary headache based on the history, the general medical and the neurologic examination. If suspicious features are present, diagnostic testing may also be necessary. Once secondary headaches are excluded, the task is to then diagnose one, or more than one, specific primary disorder. Thus, the diagnosis of primary headache disorder is based on the patient's report of symptoms of previous attacks, and accurate diagnosis requires explicit rules about the required symptom features.

A. Granato (✉)
SC (UCO) Clinica Neurologica, Azienda Sanitaria Universitaria Integrata di Trieste (ASUITS), Trieste, Italy
e-mail: antonio.granato@asuits.sanita.fvg.it

P. Manganotti
SC (UCO) Clinica Neurologica, Dipartimento di Scienze Mediche, Chirurgiche e della Salute, Università degli Studi di Trieste, Azienda Sanitaria Universitaria Integrata di Trieste (ASUITS), Trieste, Italy
e-mail: pmanganotti@units.it

3.1 Primary Headaches

3.1.1 Migraine

Migraine is an important and fascinating disorder due to its high prevalence and disabling severity. The total sum of suffering caused by migraine is

Table 3.1 The primary headaches (first two classification levels) [3]

1. Migraine
1.1 Migraine without aura
1.2 Migraine with aura
1.3 Chronic migraine
1.4 Complications of migraine
1.5 Probable migraine
1.6 Episodic syndromes that may be associated with migraine
2. Tension-type headache (TTH)
2.1 Infrequent episodic tension-type headache
2.2 Frequent episodic tension-type headache
2.3 Chronic tension-type headache
2.4 Probable tension-type headache
3. Trigeminal autonomic cephalalgias (TACs)
3.1 Cluster headache
3.2 Paroxysmal hemicrania
3.3 Short-lasting unilateral neuralgiform headache attacks
3.4 Hemicrania continua
3.5 Probable trigeminal autonomic cephalalgia
4. Other primary headache disorders
4.1 Primary cough headache
4.2 Primary exercise headache
4.3 Primary headache associated with sexual activity
4.4 Primary thunderclap headache
4.5 Cold-stimulus headache
4.6 External-pressure headache
4.7 Primary stabbing headache
4.8 Nummular headache
4.9 Hypnic headache
4.10 New daily persistent headache (NDPH)

Table 3.2 The secondary headaches (first classification level) [3]

5. Headache attributed to trauma or injury to the head and/or neck
6. Headache attributed to cranial and/or cervical vascular disorder
7. Headache attributed to non-vascular intracranial disorder
8. Headache attributed to a substance or its withdrawal
9. Headache attributed to infection
10. Headache attributed to disorder of homoeostasis
11. Headache or facial pain attributed to disorder of the cranium, neck, eyes, ears, nose, sinuses, teeth, mouth, or other facial or cervical structures
12. Headache attributed to psychiatric disorder

Table 3.3 Diagnostic criteria of migraine without aura [3]

A. At least five attacks fulfilling criteria B–D
B. Headache attacks lasting 4–72 h (when untreated or unsuccessfully treated)
C. Headache has at least two of the following four characteristics
1. Unilateral location
2. Pulsating quality
3. Moderate or severe pain intensity
4. Aggravation by or causing avoidance of routine physical activity (e.g. walking or climbing stairs)
D. During headache at least one of the following
1. Nausea and/or vomiting
2. Photophobia and phonophobia
E. Not better accounted for by another ICHD-3 diagnosis

probably higher than that of any other kind of headache. Migraine is essentially a common episodic headache with a 1-year prevalence of approximately 15–18% in women, 6–12% in men, and 4% in children. The different types of migraine are shown in Table 3.1. Migraine without aura is the most common form (more than 85% of the migraine pathology). The frequency of migraine with aura in the general population is about 8%, while the frequency of migraineurs in which migraine without aura and migraine with aura are associated is 37%. Migraine prevalence is consistently higher in women than men, both in migraine without aura (15–18% female; 10–12% male) and in migraine with aura (3.8–9% female; 1.3–4% male) [4]. Diagnostic criteria for migraine without and with aura are shown in Tables 3.3 and 3.4.

The migraine attack can be divided into four phases: premonitory (prodrome), which occurs hours or days before the headache; the aura, which immediately precedes the headache; the headache; and the postdrome.

3.1.1.1 Premonitory Phase

Premonitory phenomena occur 2–48 h before headache onset in about 7–88% of migraineurs. They consist of psychologic, neurologic, or general (constitutional, autonomic) symptoms and can be divided into excitatory and inhibitory phenomena (Table 3.5) [5]. Each patient, before a migraine attack, can perceive more than one

Table 3.4 Diagnostic criteria of migraine with aura [3]

A. At least two attacks fulfilling criteria B and C
B. One or more of the following fully reversible aura symptoms
1. Visual
2. Sensory
3. Speech and/or language
4. Motor
5. Brainstem
6. Retinal
C. At least three of the following six characteristics
1. At least one aura symptom spreads gradually over 5 min
2. Two or more aura symptoms occur in succession
3. Each individual aura symptom lasts 5–60 min
4. At least one aura symptom is unilateral
5. At least one aura symptom is positive
6. The aura is accompanied, or followed within 60 min, by headache
D. Not better accounted for by another ICHD-3 diagnosis

Table 3.5 Premonitory symptoms in migraine

Excitatory symptoms	Inhibitory symptoms
Irritability	Apathy
Physical hyperactivity	Psychophysical slowing, weakness
Insomnia	Drowsiness
Craving for carbohydrates	Anorexia
Euphoria	Depressed mood
Diarrhoea	Constipation
Increased diuresis	Abdominal swelling
Yawning	Slowed speech
Thirst	Difficulty in concentration
	Cold sensation

Table 3.6 Factors precipitating migraine attack

Psychological factors	Hormonal changes
Emotions	Menstruation
Stress	Ovulation
Relaxation after stressful period	Contraception
Changes in mood	
Environmental factors	Other factors
Climatic factors	Deficiency or excess of sleep
Altitude	Hypoglycaemia
Exposure to the sun or bright light	Fatigue
Noise	Fever
Intense smell	Irregular feeding
Smoke	
Food and eating habits	Drugs
Alcohol	Nitroglycerine
Nitrates, glutamate, tyramine, phenylethylamine	Reserpine
Vinegar, citrus, tea, coffee	Fenfluramine
Aspartame	Oestrogens

sufferers are sensitive to any specific factor. Precipitants appear to be more common in patients with migraine without aura than in those with migraine with aura. Trigger factors are shown in Table 3.6, the most common being menstruation, dietary factors (alcoholic drinks, chocolate, cheese, citrus fruit, fried fatty foods), stress, and mental tension [6].

3.1.1.2 Aura

A pathophysiologic disturbance (probably cortical spreading depression or its human analogue) that gradually spreads through the cerebral cortex underlies the aura symptoms.

Migraine with aura is defined in ICHD-3 as recurrent attacks, lasting minutes, of unilateral fully reversible visual, sensory, or other central nervous system symptoms that usually develop gradually and are usually followed by headache and associated migraine symptoms [3] (Table 3.4). The criterion of the gradual development of symptoms over a period of more than 5 min is essential; particular attention must be paid to diagnosing an acute-onset migrainous aura, since it may mimic another potentially dangerous cerebral disease (e.g. cerebrovascular disorder or epileptic seizure). Epidemiological

premonitory symptom, on average 3–12. Changes in mood and behaviour are the most typical and frequent symptoms. In 82% of patients, the warning symptoms are followed by a migraine attack in more than 50% of cases. Headache appears after more than 24 h in 19% of cases and between 6 and 24 h in 68%.

Precipitating factors, alone or in combination with other exogenous exposures, can induce headache attacks in susceptible individuals. Multifactorial trigger mechanism for individual attacks are suggested, because the presence of a factor does not always precipitate an attack in the same individual and only subgroups of headache

and population studies have shown that, in most cases, the duration of visual, sensory, and aphasic symptoms is less than 60 min, and often the visual and sensory aura has a duration of 30 min. The headache following the aura may have migraine (54%) or non-migraine (40%) features, or in some cases the algic phase may also be absent (9%) [7, 8]. Visual aura is the most common (98%), followed by sensory (36%) and aphasic aura (10%) [8]. Two or more aura symptoms occur in 60% of patients with typical aura with migrainous headache, in 70% with typical aura with non-migrainous headache, in 33% with typical aura without headache, and in 81% with migraine with brainstem aura [7]. The aura always requires careful investigation to discriminate secondary pathologies.

It is often difficult for patients to describe retrospectively the temporal relationships between aura and headache. Viana et al. [8] reported that headache started when the aura stopped or after a free interval of time after the end of aura in 49% of patients, during aura in 38%, and rarely before aura (12%).

With increasing age, there is often a reduction in the duration and intensity of the algic phase until its disappearance (typical aura without headache). The disappearance of headache with persistence of the aura may be observed also during pregnancy.

Types of Aura Symptoms

Visual Aura

Visual typical aura begins as a "patch" or as unilateral zigzag lines (fortification spectra) (81%), often trembling (87%), white (47%) or coloured (33%), or rarely colourless (14%) or black (3%). The fortification slowly moves away from the centre of vision while expanding in size and finally disappeared at the extreme lateral margin of the visual field (Figs. 3.1 and 3.2) [9–11]. A scotoma is left in the wake of the expanding visual disturbance about 50% of the time. In 3–4%, visual symptoms develop in the reverse order, starting laterally in the visual field. The localization of the aura is more frequently unilateral (69%). In the majority of patients

(69%), the visual aura is characterized by the gradual development of symptoms (within 5–30 min in 82% of cases, within 31–60 min in 11%, and in more than 60 min in 4%).

Sensory Aura

Sensory aura is second in frequency to visual symptoms. The typical sensory aura is unilateral (84%) and it has a cheirooral distribution. In fact it begins at the level of the hand (97%) and then enlarges to the arm (78%) and then affects the face (67%) and the tongue (62%), more rarely legs and feet (24%) and the rest of the body (18%) [7]. Sensory symptoms tend to progress in less than 30 min (82%), and the total duration is usually less than 1 h (80%). When occurring with motor aura, the symptoms tend to last longer.

Language Aura

Not infrequently, patients report that speech occurs as the spreading paraesthesias reach the face or the tongue, and in many cases it is difficult to decide whether dysarthria or aphasia is present. The aphasic aura is characterized by the presence of paraphasias (>70%) or by difficulties in understanding the speech or reading (about 30%). Dysarthria is rarely described and often in association with motor aura [12, 13].

Motor Aura

Weakness or paralysis is an uncommon migrainous aura and, when it occurs, is transient, resolving without evidence of infarction. Paresis usually develops focally and gradually spread to involve more and more muscles. Quite often it is associated with unilateral impaired coordination; visual disturbances (bright flashes or scotomas); sensory, aphasic, or brainstem symptoms; and rarely consciousness disorders. Each non-motor aura symptom lasts 5–60 min, and motor symptoms last <72 h [3]. This form of migraine with aura is rare (prevalence of 0.01% in general population), and it is defined *familial hemiplegic migraine* (if at least one first- or second-degree relative has migraine aura including motor weakness) or *sporadic hemiplegic migraine* (if no first- or second-degree relative has migraine aura including motor weakness).

Fig. 3.1 Fortification spectra [9]

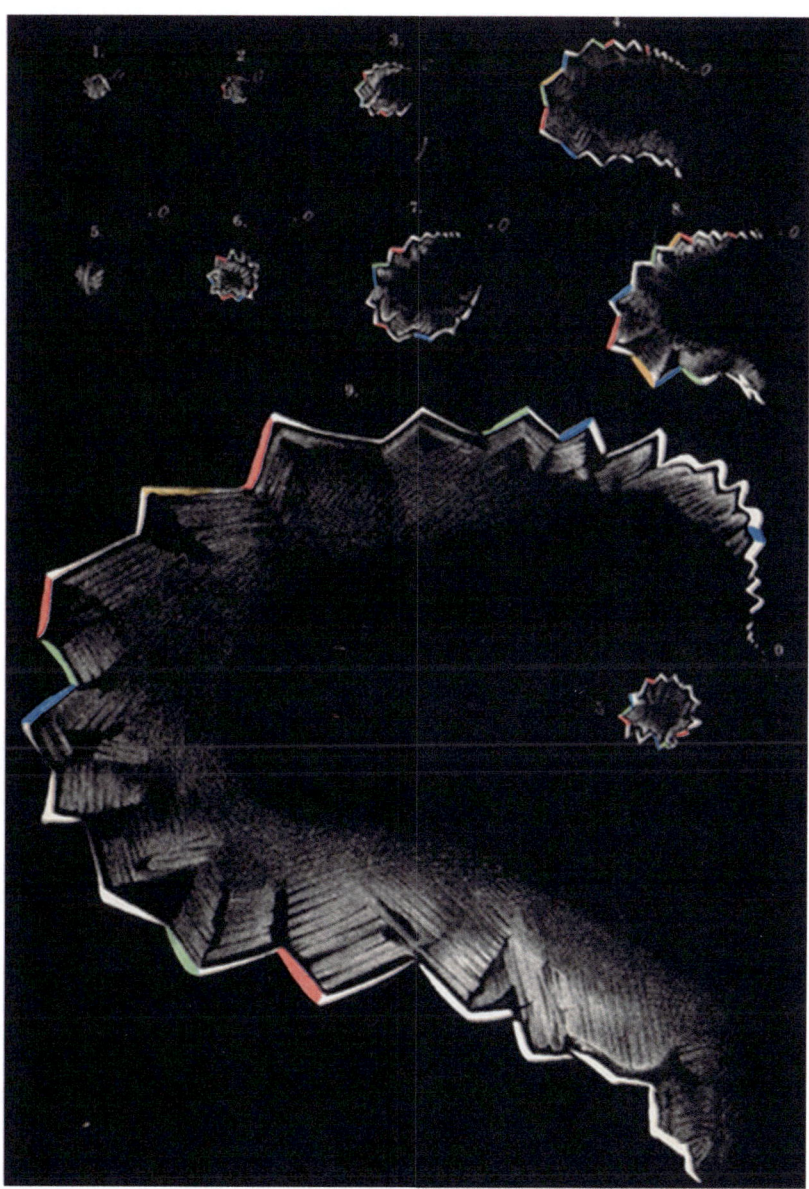

Less Typical Aura Symptoms

Symptoms less frequently occurring in the aura are reported in Table 3.7. Such symptoms suggest the involvement, by the spreading depression, of cortical and subcortical areas different from those interested in the classics symptoms of the aura.

3.1.1.3 Headache

Migraine is a recurrent headache disorder manifesting in attacks lasting 4–72 h, with pain characterized by unilateral localization, pulsating quality, moderate or severe intensity, aggravation by routine physical activity, and association with nausea and/or photo- and phonophobia [3].

The onset is usually gradual and often the patient is not able to identify the location of the pain and to define its characteristics. Within about an hour, the intensity becomes severe and limits the patient's activities. Headache may begin during sleep by waking up the patient when the intensity is already moderate or severe. More frequently it occurs in the morning or at the

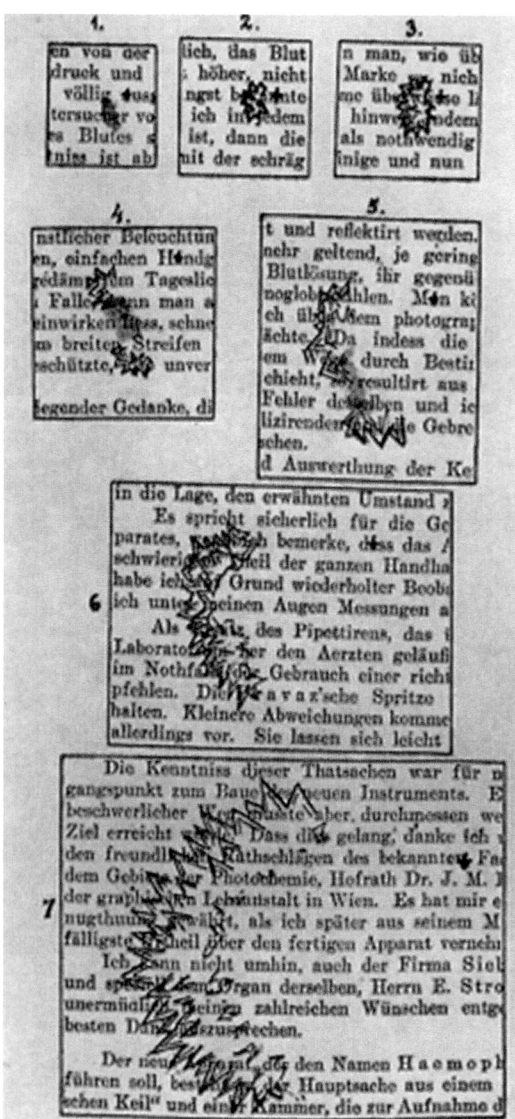

Fig. 3.2 Fortification spectra [10]

Table 3.7 Less typical aura symptoms

Visual symptoms	Other symptoms
Macropsia	Olfactory hallucinations
Micropsia	Gustatory hallucinations
Pelopsia	Oscillacusis
Teleopsia	Acalculia
Rotated vision	Neglect
Mosaic vision	Automatic behaviour
Allaesthesia	Disorientation
Polyopia	Depersonalization
Déjà vu	Transient global amnesia
Jamais vu	Anxiety
Palinopsia	
Reduction of visual attention	
Achromatopsia	

in order to exclude a secondary pathology. Headache has pulsating quality in 73.5%, burning in 73.8%, pressing in 75.4%, and stubbing in 42.6% of attacks [16]. Pain varies greatly in intensity, ranging from annoying to incapacitating, although most migraineurs report at least moderate pain; it reaches the acme in an hour or less in 48.1% of attacks [17]. Physical activity or simple head movement commonly aggravates the pain. Patients prefer to lie down in a quiet, dark room, pressing their head on the side of the pain or tightening a band around the head. About 90% of patients feel nauseated during their migraine headache and 75% of them vomit during some attacks. Most patients are aware of an exaggeration of brightness of light and some feel pain on exposure to light (photophobia). Moreover, about 80% of patients are subject to phonophobia; in particular they complain that their hearing becomes more acute during migraine so that the faintest sound seems to be louder and more disturbing. A heightened sense of smell is also common. Drummond found that the mean pupil diameter in migraine patients was smaller during headache than that of normal controls and was significantly smaller on the affected side in patients with unilateral headache [18].

3.1.1.4 Postdrome
Remaining symptoms are found in about 80% of migraineurs. A feeling of exhaustion and lethargy may remain for several days after the cessation of

beginning of the afternoon [14]. Pain is bilateral in 40% and unilateral in 60% of cases; it consistently occurs on the same side in 20% of patients [15]. Migraineurs whose headache alternates sides do not develop more consistently lateralized headache with the passage of time. Pain usually begins at the ocular and frontotemporal area and then spreads to the rest of the head. Less frequently, the initial localization is in the occipital region and in the neck. Occipital pain is rare in child and requires particular diagnostic attention,

headache. The patient may have impaired concentration or feel tired, washed out, irritable, and listless. Some people feel unusually refreshed or euphoric after an attack. Muscle weakness, aching, and anorexia or food cravings can occur [5].

3.1.2 Tension-Type Headache

Tension-type headache (TTH) is by far the most common form of headache. In Russel's review the 1-year prevalence of tension-type headache ranges from 11% to 93% [19]. Differences in definitions and methodology may be largely responsible for this variation. The highest percentage found in industrialized countries, especially in Denmark, ranges between 75% and 83% in women and around 68% in men [20]. Genetics is not very important in episodic TTH, while concordance appears high in case of high-frequency TTH [21]. In general, TTH is slightly more prevalent in women than men (male-to-female ratio about 1:1.3). The sex distribution of episodic TTH is controversial; on the contrary, frequent or chronic TTH consistently shows female predominance (sex ratio F/M is 1.16 in episodic TTH and 2.0 in chronic TTH) [22]. In both sexes, the prevalence seems to peak between the ages of 30 and 39 years and then to decline with age.

IHS define the criteria that must be present to diagnose TTH (Table 3.8) and distinguish it from migraine [3]. Neither premonitory symptoms nor neurologic aura symptoms occur with TTH. In contrast to migraine, the typical pain characteristics of TTH are not pulsating, not unilateral, not severe in intensity, and not aggravated by routine physical activity.

Typically, pain is bilateral in almost 90% of subjects [20], strictly unilateral pain accounts for 4–12.5%, and in order of frequency, the location of TTH is occipital, parietal, temporal, and frontal. A band-like topography, including frontal and occipital areas, is rather typical.

Headache is usually dull and persistent and undulates in intensity during the day. It is often described as a feeling of heaviness, pressure, weight on the head, or tightness rather than pain. Some patients experience sudden jabs of pain on one side or at the back of the head superimposed on a general background of discomfort. The intensity of headache varies with the mood, the symptoms being more severe when the patient is depressed. In the chronic form, the patient either awakens with headache or notices it shortly after getting up, and it remains throughout the day, without regard to the emotional content of the day's activities.

The intensity of headache is typically mild or moderate in 87–99% of subjects, but severity increases markedly with increasing frequency [1].

Lack of aggravation of pain by physical activity is almost always present in TTH and is one of the best criteria to distinguish it from migraine.

TTH is not accompanied by nausea and vomiting, and their presence actually rules out the diagnosis. Nevertheless, 18% of patients with TTH can report mild or moderate anorexia during the pain. Photophobia or phonophobia may be present, but the presence of both symptoms is not allowed in the ICHD-3 criteria.

Psychometric tests in patients with TTH and controls reveal significantly higher levels of anxiety, depression, and suppressed anger in TTH patients [23]. The frequency of TTH rises with increasing frequency of daily annoyances, and at least one psychosocial stress event or psychiatric disorder is noted in 85% of patients with TTH [24].

Table 3.8 Diagnostic criteria of tension-type headache (adapted from [3])

A. Headache lasting from 30 min to 7 days
B. At least two of the following four characteristics
1. Bilateral location
2. Pressing or tightening (non-pulsating) quality
3. Mild or moderate intensity
4. Not aggravated by routine physical activity such as walking or climbing stairs
C. Both of the following
1. No nausea or vomiting
2. No more than one of photophobia or phonophobia
D. Not better accounted for by another ICHD-3 diagnosis

3.1.3 Trigeminal Autonomic Cephalalgias (TACS)

The trigeminal autonomic cephalalgias (TACs) are a group of primary headache disorders that share similarities. The primary feature common to all is attacks of severe or extreme, strictly unilateral headache of different durations, accompanied by prominent cranial parasympathetic autonomic symptoms, which include conjunctival injection, lacrimation, periorbital oedema, aural fullness, rhinorrhoea, facial flushing, or pallor. Meiosis and ptosis, an incomplete Horner's syndrome, are mediated by third-order sympathetic fibres surrounding the ipsilateral carotid artery. This sympathetic activation may be a downstream effect of an increase in local parasympathetic tone [25].

TACs consist of cluster headache (CH), paroxysmal hemicrania (PH), short-lasting unilateral neuralgiform headache attacks with conjunctival injection and tearing (SUNCT)/short-lasting neuralgiform headache attacks with cranial autonomic features (SUNA), and hemicrania continua (HC) [3]. These conditions are distinguished by their attack duration and frequency, as well as response to treatment. The primary differentiating features of TACs are described in Table 3.9 [26].

3.1.3.1 Cluster Headache

Cluster headache may be defined as a severe unilateral head of facial pain, which lasts from 15 min to 3 h, associated commonly with ipsilateral conjunctival injection, lacrimation, nasal congestion, eyelid oedema, forehead and facial sweating or flushing, miosis or ptosis, and sense of agitation, usually recurring once or more daily for a period of weeks or months (Table 3.10).

The term "cluster headache" derives from the tendency of the pain to appear in bouts, separated by intervals of complete freedom.

The episodic form recurs in periods lasting 7 days to 1 year, separated by pain-free periods lasting at least 1 month. Commonly, bouts last between 2 and 12 weeks and most patients have one or two clusters per year [27]. About 10–15% of patients have chronic CH, with attacks occurring for more than 1 year without remission or with remission periods lasting less than 1 month.

Lifetime and 1 year prevalence are 124 and 53 cases per 100,000 population, respectively; the incidence is approximately 2–10 per 100,000 per year, and the illness usually starts in the second to fourth decades of life [28, 29]. CH is predominantly a male disease, with a male-to-female ratio of 4.3; it was higher in chronic (15.0) compared with episodic form (3.8) [29].

Table 3.10 Diagnostic criteria of cluster headache [3]

A. At least five attacks fulfilling criteria B–D
B. Severe or very severe unilateral orbital, supraorbital, and/or temporal pain lasting 15–180 min (when untreated)
C. Either or both of the following
1. At least one of the following symptoms or signs, ipsilateral to the headache
(a) Conjunctival injection and/or lacrimation
(b) Nasal congestion and/or rhinorrhoea
(c) Eyelid oedema
(d) Forehead and facial sweating
(e) Miosis and/or ptosis
2. A sense of restlessness or agitation
D. Occurring with a frequency between one every other day and eight per day
E. Not better accounted for by another ICHD-3 diagnosis

Table 3.9 Characteristics of the individual TACs (adapted from [26])

	Cluster headache	Paroxysmal hemicrania	SUNCT	Hemicrania continua
Attacks/day	1–8	1–40	3–300	Continuous
Attack duration	15–180 min	2–30 min	1–600 s	Hours to days
Pain intensity	Very severe	Very severe	Severe	Varying
Typical pain location	Orbital, frontotemporal	Orbital, frontotemporal	Trigeminal	Orbital, frontotemporal
Typical age of onset	20–40	20–70	35–65	35–50
Male/female	2.5/1	1/1	2/1	1/2,8
Restlessness	90%	80%	65%	During exacerbation

Cluster attacks usually have their onset once or twice a day, usually in the same hours, with peaks between 1–2 a.m., 1–3 p.m., and 9 p.m. The main "entraining" factors of cluster attacks can be considered some phases of sleep, REM in particular.

Pain attacks are typically unilateral, extremely severe, localized deeply in and around the eye, commonly radiating to the supraorbital region, temple, maxilla, and upper gum on the same side of the face. In some patients the ipsilateral nostril aches and burns, and a few complain of aching in the roof of the mouth. In other patients, the lower gums, jaw, or chin is also involved. Presentation with pain in the gums or jaw may be interpreted as toothache. In 15% of patients, pain may change side from one cluster to another, more rarely (5%) within the same cluster period [27]. The quality of pain is constant, boring, pressing, or burning when reaching its peak. During attacks and more rarely between attacks, patients may be supersensitive to touch in the affected areas; in some patient discomfort persists in the symptomatic area between attacks. A minority of patients describe the pain as throbbing or pulsating. The severity of attacks usually increases in the first few days or weeks. The intensity of pain increases rapidly, reaching the peak in less than 10 min. The maximum intensity lasts about 30 min and tends to decrease in 40 min. During the crisis the patient is restless and tends to isolate himself, walk, and continually change the position of the body.

In certain patients cluster periods occur at regular intervals or fixed seasons; in particular, the incidence is higher in February and June and lower in August and November.

Accompanying signs and symptoms are mostly described on the pain side and suggest a disturbance in the function of the autonomic nervous system. They are typical for CH attacks and must be considered for the diagnosis. The frequency, which can vary in percentage according to the studies (Table 3.11), and the intensity of the autonomic features seem to correlate mainly to the severity of pain during the attack. All the accompanying autonomic symptoms are transient, lasting only for the

Table 3.11 Frequency of autonomic signs and symptoms in cluster headache

Autonomic signs and symptoms	
Lacrimation	80–84%
Conjunctival injection	58–84%
Incomplete Horner's syndrome	57–69%
Rhinorrhoea	38–76%
Nasal congestion	38–54%
Eyelid oedema	10–21%
Facial sweating	6.5–21%
Nausea	40%
Phonophobia	12–39%
Photophobia	5–72%
Osmophobia	7%

duration of the attack, with the exception of a partial Horner's syndrome with ptosis or meiosis, both of which may persist after many acute attacks, although this is rare. Lacrimation and conjunctival injection are the most common local signs of autonomic involvement; less frequent are nasal stuffiness and rhinorrhoea. Forehead sweating, facial flushing, and oedema are rare. Cardiovascular accompanying findings are increase in heart rate at the onset of the attacks, rhythm disturbances (frequent premature ventricular beats, transient episodes of atrial fibrillation, first-degree atrioventricular block or sinoatrial block), and systolic blood pressure increase. Autonomic features not included in the ICHD-3 criteria include nausea, phonophobia, photophobia, and osmophobia.

Once a cluster period begins, individual headaches can be triggered or precipitated by alcohol (in particular red wine) and other vasodilators (i.e. nitroglycerin or histamine). When in remission, alcohol rarely precipitates an attack. The use of alcohol and cigarettes is higher in patients with CH compared to controls or patients with other primary headaches (66–95% in CH vs. 17–33% in other primary headaches) [30].

3.1.3.2 Paroxysmal Hemicrania

Paroxysmal hemicranias (PH) is a rare headache condition with an estimated 1-year prevalence of 0.5 per 1000 or less [31]. PH attacks are excruciating, occurring several times a day, with a mean of 11 and median length of 19 min. Pain tends to affect men and women equally. Bouts are

Table 3.12 Diagnostic criteria of paroxysmal hemicrania [3]

A. At least 20 attacks fulfilling criteria B–E
B. Severe unilateral orbital, supraorbital, and/or temporal pain lasting 2–30 min
C. Either or both of the following
1. At least one of the following symptoms or signs, ipsilateral to the headache
(a) Conjunctival injection and/or lacrimation
(b) Nasal congestion and/or rhinorrhoea
(c) Eyelid oedema
(d) Forehead and facial sweating
(e) Miosis and/or ptosis
2. A sense of restlessness or agitation
D. Occurring with a frequency of >5 per day
E. Prevented absolutely by therapeutic doses of indomethacin
F. Not better accounted for by another ICHD-3 diagnosis

Table 3.13 Diagnostic criteria of short-lasting unilateral neuralgiform headache attacks [3]

A. At least 20 attacks fulfilling criteria B–D
B. Moderate or severe unilateral head pain, with orbital, supraorbital, temporal, and/or other trigeminal distributions, lasting for 1–600 s and occurring as single stabs or series of stabs or in a saw-tooth pattern
C. At least one of the following five cranial autonomic symptoms or signs, ipsilateral to the pain
1. Conjunctival injection and/or lacrimation
2. Nasal congestion and/or rhinorrhoea
3. Eyelid oedema
4. Forehead and facial sweating
5. Miosis and/or ptosis
D. Occurring with a frequency of at least one a day
E. Not better accounted for by another ICHD-3 diagnosis

strictly unilateral, rarely can shift sides between attacks, most commonly affect the first division of the trigeminal nerve, and are associated with unilateral cranial autonomic symptoms [3, 32] (Table 3.12). In contrast to CH, there is no circadian or circannual element to the timing of headache. Using the same criteria as for CH, PH is classified as either episodic (20–35%) or chronic (65–80%). Roughly, two-thirds of patients with PH will have accompanying photophobia and phonophobia, most characteristically lateralized to the same side as the pain. Additionally, such as CH, agitation and restlessness are common during attacks, in contrast to migraine [33]. While most attacks in PH arise spontaneously, about 10% are triggered mechanically; in particular the C2–C3 region of the neck is particularly sensitive [32]. An absolute response to indomethacin is diagnostic.

3.1.4 SUNCT/SUNA

SUNCT and SUNA occur at a similar frequency as PH [31, 34]. SUNCT is characterized by still shorter and more frequent attacks than PH. These are, per definition, accompanied by conjunctival injection, lacrimation, and other cranial autonomic symptoms and last 1–600 s, occurring up to 100 times a day (Table 3.13). Attacks can be triggered by mechanical stimuli to the skin and can also occur as repetitive stabs. In contrast to trigeminal neuralgia, a refractory period subsequent to an attack is not typical [35]. Pain distribution is typically orbital or periorbital, and the character can be electric or shock-like, hence the name neuralgiform. Between attacks, most patients are completely pain-free, and only seldom do attacks occur at night. In SUNA, there may be any number of the previously described cranial autonomic features, but only one or neither of conjunctival injection and tearing.

3.1.4.1 Hemicrania Continua

HC is considered rare but is likely underreported. Pain is typically mild to moderate and not as severe as with the other TACs, but it never remits completely, waxing and waning throughout the day. During exacerbations pain is severe or very severe, and photophobia, phonophobia, nausea, and autonomic symptoms ipsilateral to the pain are prominent (Table 3.14). As with the other TACs, pain is unilateral, and in contrast to migraine, the patient may become restless and agitated during exacerbations [36]. HC is more commonly found in women and exists in two forms, remitting and unremitting, with the latter being the most common. Like PH, HC responds absolutely to indomethacin.

Table 3.14 Diagnostic criteria of hemicrania continua [3]

A. Unilateral headache fulfilling criteria B–D
B. Present for >3 months, with exacerbations of moderate or greater intensity
C. Either or both of the following
1. At least one of the following symptoms or signs, ipsilateral to the headache
(a) Conjunctival injection and/or lacrimation
(b) Nasal congestion and/or rhinorrhoea
(c) Eyelid oedema
(d) Forehead and facial sweating
(e) Miosis and/or ptosis
2. A sense of restlessness or agitation or aggravation of the pain by movement
D. Responds absolutely to therapeutic doses of indomethacin
E. Not better accounted for by another ICHD-3 diagnosis

3.1.5 Other Primary Headache Disorders

The *other primary headaches* (Table 3.1) include clinically heterogeneous disorders with poorly understood pathogenesis and treatment based on anecdotal reports or uncontrolled trials. These entities are a challenging diagnostic problem as can be primary or secondary; in fact, headaches with similar characteristics to several of these disorders can be symptomatic of other causes, also life-threatening. It is mandatory, when they first present, to carefully evaluate the patient with prompt imaging or other appropriate tests.

3.1.5.1 Primary Cough Headache

The lifetime prevalence of cough headache is reported to be 1%. Age of onset tends to be more than 40 years with a male predominance. The head pain is sudden onset, bilateral, and *precipitated* (rather than aggravated, as occurs in migraine) by coughing, straining, or Valsalva manoeuvre. The duration ranges from 1 s to 120 min. Typically pain arises moments after coughing, reaches a peak almost instantaneously, and then subsides over several seconds or minutes. Most patients are pain-free between attacks but some may have a dull headache afterwards which persists for hours. Typically, migrainous features such as photophobia and phonophobia are uncommon. Associated symptoms such as vertigo, nausea, and sleep abnormality have been reported by up to two-thirds of patients. The syndrome of cough headache is symptomatic in about 40% of cases, and the majority of patients in whom this is so have Arnold-Chiari malformation type I.

3.1.6 Primary Exercise Headache

Prevalence ranges between 12 and 30% [37]. In contrast to primary cough headache, the disorder is more prevalent in younger individuals (generally below the age of 50) with a personal or family history of migraine. It occurs particularly during hot weather or at high altitude. Unlike primary cough headache, which can be triggered by short-lasting trains of efforts (i.e. Valsalva-like manoeuvres), primary exercise headache is a headache brought on by, and occurring only during or after, prolonged physical exercise. Pain can be prevented by avoidance of physical exertion; it can be of thunderclap or gradual onset, bilateral and less commonly unilateral, pulsating in quality, and with or without migrainous features. Symptoms persist less than 48 h.

3.1.7 Primary Headache Associated with Sexual Activity

The estimated prevalence of headache related to sexual activity is 1% [38]. There is a male preponderance. The mean age of onset is in the fourth decade, and up to 40% of all cases run a chronic course over more than a year. Pain increases in intensity with increasing of sexual excitement and has an abrupt explosive intensity just before or with orgasm. Headache is bilateral in two-thirds of cases, occipitally localized in 80% of cases. It has pressing, pulsating, or "exploding" quality and lasts from 1 min to 24 h with severe intensity and up to 72 h with mild intensity [3]. Primary sexual headache occurs independently of the type of sexual activity and is not accompanied by autonomic or vegetative symptoms in most cases.

3.1.8 Primary Thunderclap Headache

Thunderclap headache (TCH) is a severe headache of the explosive type that appears suddenly, like a "clap of thunder", with pain peak intensity occurring at onset (usually within 30 s). Thunderclap headache is a rare type of headache with an incidence of 43 cases per 100,000 adults per year. Primary TCH closely mimics secondary forms of TCH, and therefore appropriate instrumental investigations are absolutely mandatory to rule out possible organic causes. Thunderclap headache is a sudden onset severe headache, which reaches maximum severity within a minute, and lasts for more than 5 min [3]. The total duration is variable, but generally it persists several hours and then gradually decreases and sometimes persists for a few weeks. Nausea and vomiting may occur from the onset. Headache is often occipitally localized, although it may be widespread. In some patients recurrent episodes can be triggered by modest physical efforts and in others then can occur at rest for periods ranging from 7–10 days up to a year. Other primary headaches, such as cough, exercise, and sexual headache, can sometimes occur with the features of thunderclap headache.

3.1.9 Other Primary Headache Disorders

Among other primary headaches, the IHS classifies *cold-stimulus headache*, *external-pressure headache*, *primary stabbing headache*, *nummular headache*, *hypnic headache*, and *new daily persistent headache (NDPH)* (Table 3.1) (IHS).

Cold-stimulus headache is caused by a cold stimulus applied externally to the head or ingested or inhaled. Patients develop intense, short-lasting, stabbing headache frontally or temporally, and pain resolves in 10–30 min after removal of the cold stimulus.

External-pressure headache results from sustained compression of or traction on pericranial soft tissues, for example, with a tight band around the head, hat or helmet, or diving mask.

Primary stabbing headache consists in transient and localized stabs of pain in the head that occur spontaneously in the absence of organic disease [3]. The prevalence of primary stabbing headache varies from 2 to 35%; this discrepancy in part is likely to be related to the populations studied [39]. In more than 50% of cases, the disorder is associated with other primary headaches, in particular in 40% of migraineurs and 30% of cluster headache sufferers. Patients describe pain as needle-, nail-, or pinprick-like. Head pain occurs as a single jab or a series of jabs. In the majority of patients, jabs last 1–2 s at a time, at most for 10 s. Although pain is reported to be predominantly in the distribution of the first division of the trigeminal nerve, in patient cohorts it is frequently experienced in the distribution of C2 [40]. Pain can be unifocal or multifocal in site. Attacks occur with irregular frequency, from once to many times a day. Pain is usually spontaneous and without additional features. However, in patients who also have migraine, jabs can be associated with migraine attacks or occur independently.

Nummular headache (NH) is a rare well-defined primary clinical condition characterized by local pain that occurs in a small (typically 1–6 cm in diameter), rounded, or elliptical area of the head [3, 41]. NH is characterized by circumscribed areas of mild to moderate head pain which is usually chronic and continuous but can also be remitting and relapsing. Superimposed on the continuous pain may be associated lancinating jabs of pain that may vary from seconds to hours. The affected area may also have paraesthesias, dysesthesias, and allodynia even during periods of remission. The most characteristic feature of NH is its precise localization over a localized area over the scalp. The most common area described is the parietal area, although other areas as well as bilateral and multifocal involvement have been described. Only a limited number of patients have been described worldwide. NH has also been described in patients with intracranial lesions.

Hypnic headache is a rare pathology. Attacks develop only during sleep, cause wakening, and last for up to 4 h, usually without characteristic-associated symptoms [3]. The pain is typically moderately severe, generalized, dull, and featureless. Attacks usually last 15–240 min and can occur up to six times per night, with the mean number of one per night [42]. Pain can be unilateral, throbbing, with nausea and only uncommonly presents with autonomic features, photophobia, and phonophobia.

New daily persistent headache (NDPH) is a persistent headache, daily from its onset, and lasts more than 3 months [3]. Eighty percent of patients remember the exact date of headache onset. From a cohort of 56 patients, 30% associated onset with an infection, 12% with extracranial surgery, and 12% a stressful life event [43]. Thirty-eight percent had a prior history of episodic headache, most commonly migraine. None had a prior history of chronic headache. NDPH may have features suggestive of either migraine or tension-type headache, also in their chronic form. NDPH has a self-limiting form that typically resolves within several months without therapy and a refractory form that is resistant to aggressive treatment regimens. Accompanying phenomena are also frequent (nausea 68%, photophobia 66%, phonophobia 61%, throbbing pain 54%, and visual aura 9%).

3.2 Secondary Headaches

There are only four main types of primary headaches; in contrast, the causes of secondary or symptomatic headaches are numerous (Table 3.2). Quite often secondary headaches have the same characteristics as migraine or tension-type headache; therefore, it is sometimes difficult to determine whether the pain is secondary or primary. The IHS classification chooses a close temporal relationship as the decisive factor. If a headache occurs for the first time in close temporal proximity to an organic disorder, it is coded as a secondary headache. If it occurs a long time after the organic disorder, it is not accepted as a secondary headache.

In the initial evaluation, whenever faced with a primary headache that presents in atypical fashion or when the IHS criteria are not fulfilled, it is important to exclude a secondary form. In the

Table 3.15 Headache "red flags"

1. Acute or sudden onset headache or first or worst headache
2. New-onset headache
3. Headache with neurologic symptoms or signs
4. Headache onset after age 50
5. Progressive or worsening headache
6. Headache with change in pattern
7. Headache during exertion, with coughing, with sneezing, related to sexual activity or with Valsalva manoeuvre
8. Headache with postural link
9. Headache with systemic symptoms (fever, weight loss, cough)
10. Headache in a setting of malignancy or diabetes mellitus or retroviral disease
11. Headache with a history of head or neck injury

same way, the experienced physician must look for "headache alarms" or "red flags" (Table 3.15) that suggest the possibility of a secondary headache disorder; in these cases it is imperative to investigate and rule out an underlying secondary condition that can sometimes be life-threatening.

Careful history taking and physical examination remain the most important part of the assessment of the headache patient [44]. A thorough history should investigate the onset of headache, the quality, the location and irradiation of pain, associated symptoms experienced before and during the headache, concomitant medical conditions, medication use, recent trauma, or interventions. The examination should then target areas identified as abnormal during the headache history. Blood testing and dosage of inflammation indexes should be performed in all headache patients especially when an infective or inflammatory condition is suspected. In the emergency department, non-contrast computed tomography (CT) is the preferred imaging study and is used to rule out haemorrhage, while most patients should perform a magnetic resonance imaging (MRI) brain scan followed by CT/MRI angiography if brain vessel disease is suspected (such as cervical artery dissection, aneurysms, and cerebral venous thrombosis). Lumbar puncture may help to diagnose subarachnoid haemorrhage (SAH), infection, tumours, and disorders related to CSF hypertension or hypotension.

We report the clinical features of the main secondary life-threatening headaches that can be found in the emergency department and that may occur, at least in the initial phase, only with headache: subarachnoid haemorrhage, intracerebral haemorrhage, cerebral venous thrombosis, cervical artery dissection, brain tumours, and intracranial infections.

3.2.1 Subarachnoid Haemorrhage

Subarachnoid haemorrhage (SAH) is a serious condition, related to high mortality and disability rates. The most common causes of SAH are a ruptured saccular aneurysm or angioma (the ratio of aneurysm to angioma varies from 5:1 to 25:1), a head injury, or an intracerebral haemorrhage. Less commonly, bleeding may be a result of blood dyscrasias, cerebral tumour, or some form of arteritis. A sudden headache that has never been previously experienced and that is accompanied by depressed consciousness and neck stiffness is the hallmark of SAH. Patients describe pain as "worst ever", "tremendous", exploding", "bursting", and "unbearable". IHS classifies SAH as pain with sudden or thunderclap onset [3]. Although headache is initially focal and lateralized, pain rapidly generalizes and radiates into the occipitonuchal region. When blood seeps into the spinal subarachnoid space, back pain, meningism, and radicular symptoms follow. The duration of SAH-related headache varies, with the minor haemorrhage, from 2 to 3 days and up to several days with large haemorrhages. The excruciating headache that usually drives the patient to seek medical care lasts 1–2 h. Neurologic symptoms and signs accompanying SAH are neck stiffness, disorientation, nausea, vomiting, altered mentation, focal neurologic deficits, seizures, and unconsciousness.

One or more brief severe headaches may precede SAH by several months. Such "sentinel" headaches have been reported from 10% up to 43% of patients who later developed SAH [45]. These headaches are usually bioccipital, bifrontal, or unilateral and are unlike anything the patient has never experienced before. They may be associated with vomiting and neck stiffness, suggesting that they are caused by a small preliminary leak.

3.2.2 Intracerebral Haemorrhage

Headache accompanies intracerebral haemorrhage in about 60% of cases and is more common in cerebellar and lobar haemorrhage than in thalamic, caudate, capsuloputaminal, or brainstem haemorrhage. Headache is a presenting feature in those patients with signs of meningeal irritation or CT evidence of intraventricular or subarachnoid bleeding, hydrocephalus, transtentorial herniation, or midline shift. In most patients, the headache is overshadowed by the rapid onset of a devastating neurologic deficit, drowsiness, or vomiting. Headache associated with intracerebral haemorrhage is often unilateral and of mild or moderate severity; nausea, vomiting, and severe hypertension are often associated features. On the contrary, headache associated with cerebellar haemorrhage is often acute and can be maximal at onset and severe, mimicking SAH; occipital location and associated neck stiffness are common [46]. Although cerebellar haemorrhage often progresses to brainstem compression within hours, it is unpredictable and can occur in days. Brainstem compression is related to impaired level of consciousness and neurologic focal deficits.

3.2.3 Cerebral Venous Thrombosis

The estimated incidence of cerebral venous thrombosis (CVT) is 5–8/100,000 per year; there is a female preponderance, with mean age of onset in the third and fourth decade [47]. Headache can be due to the causes or the consequences of the venous occlusion. Causes of CTV can be focal (such as head trauma, intracranial tumour, cerebral abscess, meningitis, or cranial infections) or general (primary or secondary polycythaemia or any systemic infection). Headache as a consequence of venous occlusion is due to intracranial hypertension secondary to impaired cerebrospinal fluid absorption or from chronic raised venous pressure. Headache is the most frequent symptom of CVT, presenting in 80–90% of cases, and it is often the initial symptom [47]. It has no specific characteristics; it is most often diffuse, progressive, and severe, but can be unilateral and sudden (as thunderclap), or mild, and sometimes mimics other primary headaches. Pain is usually constant, but it can be intermittent, particularly initially, and can never occur in attacks. In 95% of cases, it is associated with neurologic signs that point to an organic intracranial disorder.

3.2.4 Cervical Artery Dissection

Cervical dissections are important causes of ischemic stroke. They affect the internal carotid artery (ICA) more frequently than the vertebral artery (VA) and are more common extracranially than intracranially. The incidence is 2–3/100,000 per year for ICA and 1/100,000 for VA [48]. Cephalic pain is the most frequent symptom (55–100%) and the most frequent inaugural symptom (33–86% of cases). The mode of onset is variable, it may be gradual, over a few hours or days in 85% of ICA dissection and in 72% of VA dissection, or it may be sudden. There are no specific characteristics of cephalic pain in ICA/VA dissections. Headache is usually ipsilateral to the dissection; however bilateral and diffuse pain can occur, even when the dissection is unilateral. In ICA dissections, pain is more frequently localized in the upper lateral cervical regions, with ipsilateral mandible, eye or ear irradiation. With VA dissections, pain is usually located in the occiput and posterior neck and more frequently felt medially than laterally, even when dissection is unilateral [49]. Headache is severe in 75% of cases, described excruciating or as thunderclap, but it can also be very mild and ignored. It is as frequently aching, pressing or sharp in quality, and throbbing [49]. In over 90% of cases, headache resolves in less than 10 days. Head pain is rarely the only sign of dissection; in most cases neurologic signs occur immediately (70%) or after 3–15 days (30%) [48]. Cervical artery dissection may be associated with intracranial artery dissection, which is a potential cause of SAH.

3.2.5 Brain Tumours

Headaches are initially present in 20% of patients with brain tumour and rise to about 60% during the disease [50], without differences in frequency between primary and metastatic neoplasms. Unless an intracranial neoplasm or other space-occupying lesion affects a strategic position along the line of the drainage pathways of the cerebral ventricles, it is able to reach a considerable size before causing headache. Since intracranial vessels have to be pushed aside before pain is registered, infiltrating tumours, such as gliomas, may extend throughout one hemisphere without causing headache, because the position of vessels may remain undisturbed until the last stages of the disease. The incidence of headache in primary brain tumours is related to the rate of growth and location. Slow-growing, low-grade supratentorial tumours are more likely to cause seizures than to cause headaches, whereas the faster-growing malignant neoplasms cause headaches in about half of patients. Tumours that obstruct cerebrospinal fluid pathways are commonly associated with headache.

The cephalic pain may mimic primary headaches, such as tension-type headache (77%) or migraine (9%) [51]. Pain is usually intermittent and tends to develop and resolve over several hours. It occurs more frequently at night and sometimes awakes the patient from sleep; it worsens with bending and with the Valsalva manoeuvre [52]. The most common headache location is frontal or frontotemporal, particularly in patients with a supratentorial tumour; however, occipital and diffuse headaches also commonly occur. Neck and occipital pain accompanies headache in patients with infratentorial tumours or increased intracranial hypertension. The intensity is commonly moderate, and it becomes severe, constant, associated with nausea and vomiting, and not relieved by common analgesics when increased intracranial hypertension occurs [51]. Brain-tumour headache without other symptoms is uncommon (8%); only few brain-tumour headaches last more than 10 weeks without other symptoms developing [49, 53].

3.2.6   Intracranial Infections

Headache is common in intracranial infections, including meningitis, encephalitis, brain abscess, and subdural empyema.

Bursting headache is the initial symptom of acute bacterial *meningitis*, rapidly increasing in severity over minutes, generalized or frontal, with radiation down the neck and into the spinal region, and associated with photophobia, nausea, neck stiffness, fever, and general malaise. Patients adopt a flexed posture with head retraction. Neurologic signs and cognitive functions vary according to the stage and progress of the disease [54]. Other subacute clinical patterns depend on other factors, such as the responsible microorganism, age of patients, and immunosuppression. In these cases, headache, fever, muscle weakness, and behavioural disorders may be the only symptoms lasting from weeks to months and may increase in severity due to meningeal irritation, worsening of intracranial pressure, and hydrocephalus.

In acute *encephalitis*, abrupt and severe headache may occur early and is associated with confusion, delirium, coma, and focal neurologic deficit. Occasionally, a prodrome of less severe but constant headache associated with malaise, mild fever, and myalgia may precede the onset of the neurologic deficit by several days. The clinical pictures may be mild up to catastrophic, depending on the type of microorganism.

Brain abscess occurs with an incidence of about 1 per 100,000. Causes of brain abscess are skull fracture, neurosurgical procedure, and penetrating injury (10%); infections of the paranasal sinus, middle ear, or mastoid (40%); pulmonary infections (10%); infective endocarditis (20%); and no identifiable source (20%). Headache is usually the first manifestation. Fever is often absent. In acute abscess, headache is persistent and severe; in the chronic form, headache is paroxysmal and gradually worsens. Nausea, vomiting, focal neurologic signs, and depressed level of consciousness follow the headache, more rapidly in the acute forms [55].

Subdural empyema is an intracranial infection between the inner surface of the dura and the outer portion of the arachnoid that usually arises in the frontal or ethmoid sinuses. Less common sites of origin include the sphenoid and maxillary sinuses, the middle ear, and the mastoids. The infection usually enters the subdural space by direct extension through the bone and dura or by thrombophlebitis of the venous sinuses. Patients initially report an exacerbation of local pain due to chronic sinusitis or mastoiditis; fever, meningism, focal neurologic deficits, and alteration in the level of consciousness occur within 1–2 weeks [56].

References

1. Rasmussen BK, Jensen R, Schroll M, Olesen J. Epidemiology of headache in a general population-a prevalence study. J Clin Epidemiol. 1991;44(11):1147–57.
2. Göbel H, Petersen-Braun M, Soyka D. The epidemiology of headache in Germany: a nationwide survey of a representative sample on the basis of the headache classification of the International Headache Society. Cephalalgia. 1994;14(2): 97–106.
3. Headache Classification Committee of the International Headache Society (IHS). The international classification of headache disorders, 3rd edition. Cephalalgia. 2018;38(1):1–211.
4. Rasmussen BK. Epidemiology of migraine. In: Olesen J, Goadsby PJ, et al., editors. The headaches. 3rd ed. Philadelphia: Lippincott Williams & Wilkins; 2006. p. 235–42.
5. Quintela E, Castillo J, Muñoz P, Pascual J. Premonitory and resolution symptoms in migraine: a prospective study in 100 unselected patients. Cephalalgia. 2006;26(9):1051–60.
6. Pavlovic JM, Buse DC, Sollars CM, Haut S, Lipton RB. Trigger factors and premonitory features of migraine attacks: summary of studies. Headache. 2014;54(10):1670–9.
7. Eriksen MK, Thomsen LL, Olesen J. New international classification of migraine with aura (ICHD-2) applied to 362 migraine patients. Eur J Neurol. 2004;11(9):583–91.
8. Viana M, Sances G, Linde M, Ghiotto N, Guaschino E, Allena M, Terrazzino S, Nappi G, Goadsby PJ, Tassorelli C. Clinical features of migraine aura: results from a prospective diary-aided study. Cephalalgia. 2017;37(10):979–89.
9. Airy H. On a distinct form of transient hemiopsia. Philos Trans R Soc Lond Ser B Biol Sci. 1870;160:247–64.
10. Jolly F. Über flimmerskotom und migräne. Berlin Klin Wschr. 1902;42:973–6.

11. Russell MB, Olesen J. A nosographic analysis of the migraine aura in a general population. Brain. 1996;119(Pt 2):355–61.

12. Bradshaw P, Parsons M. Hemiplegic migraine, a clinical study. Q J Med. 1965;34:65–85.

13. Heyck H. Varieties of hemiplegic migraine. Headache. 1973;12(4):135–42.

14. Alstadhaug KB, Bekkelund S, Salvesen R. Circannual periodicity of migraine? Eur J Neurol. 2007;14(9):983–8.

15. Campbell JK. Manifestations of migraine. Neurol Clin. 1990;8(4):841–55.

16. Kelman L. Pain characteristics of the acute migraine attack. Headache. 2006;46(6):942–53.

17. Kelman L. The premonitory symptoms (prodrome): a tertiary care study of 893 migraineurs. Headache. 2004;44(9):865–72.

18. Drummond PD. Pupil diameter in migraine and tension headache. J Neurol Neurosurg Psychiatry. 1987;50(2):228–30.

19. Russell MB. Genetics of tension-type headache. J Headache Pain. 2007;8(2):71–6.

20. Rasmussen BK, Jensen R, Olesen J. A population-based analysis of the diagnostic criteria of the International Headache Society. Cephalalgia. 1991;11(3):129–34.

21. Russell MB, Levi N, Saltyte-Benth J, Fenger K. Tension-type headache in adolescents and adults: a population based study of 33,764 twins. Eur J Epidemiol. 2006;21(2):153–60.

22. Schwartz BS, Stewart WF, Simon D, Lipton RB. Epidemiology of tension-type headache. JAMA. 1998;279(5):381–3.

23. Hatch JP, Prihoda TJ, Moore PJ, Cyr-Provost M, Borcherding S, Boutros NN, Seleshi E. A naturalistic study of the relationships among electromyographic activity, psychological stress, and pain in ambulatory tension-type headache patients and headache-free controls. Psychosom Med. 1991;53(5):576–84.

24. Puca F, Genco S, Prudenzano MP, Savarese M, Bussone G, D'Amico D, Cerbo R, Gala C, Coppola MT, Gallai V, Firenze C, Sarchielli P, Guazzelli M, Guidetti V, Manzoni G, Granella F, Muratorio A, Bonuccelli U, Nuti A, Nappi G, Sandrini G, Verri AP, Sicuteri F, Marabini S. Psychiatric comorbidity and psychosocial stress in patients with tension-type headache from headache centers in Italy. The Italian Collaborative Group for the Study of Psychopathological Factors in Primary Headaches. Cephalalgia. 1999;19(3):159–64.

25. Drummond PD. Autonomic disturbance in cluster headache. Brain. 1988;111:1199–209.

26. Newman LC. Trigeminal autonomic cephalalgias. Contin Lifelong Learn Neurol. 2015;21:1041–57.

27. Dodick DW, Rozen TD, Goadsby PJ, Silberstein SD. Cluster headache. Cephalalgia. 2000;20(9):787–803.

28. Swanson JW, Yanagihara T, Stang PE, O'Fallon WM, Beard CM, Melton LJ 3rd, Guess HA. Incidence of cluster headaches: a population-based study in Olmsted County, Minnesota. Neurology. 1994;44(3 Pt 1):433–7.

29. Fischera M, Marziniak M, Gralow I, Evers S. The incidence and prevalence of cluster headache: a meta-analysis of population-based studies. Cephalalgia. 2008;28(6):614–8.

30. Mannix LK, Frame JR, Solomon GD. Alcohol, smoking, and caffeine use among headache patients. Headache. 1997;37(9):572–6.

31. Sjaastad O, Bakketeig LS. Cluster headache prevalence. Vågå study of headache epidemiology. Cephalalgia. 2003;23(7):528–33.

32. Cittadini E, Matharu MS, Goadsby PJ. Paroxysmal hemicrania: a prospective clinical study of 31 cases. Brain. 2008;131(Pt 4):1142–55.

33. Irimia P, Cittadini E, Paemeleire K, Cohen AS, Goadsby PJ. Unilateral photophobia or phonophobia in migraine compared with trigeminal autonomic cephalalgias. Cephalalgia. 2008;28(6):626–30.

34. Sjaastad O, Bakketeig LS. The rare, unilateral headaches. Vaga study of headache epidemiology. J Headache Pain. 2007;8:19–27.

35. Cohen AS, Matharu MS, Goadsby PJ. Short-lasting unilateral neuralgiform headache attacks with conjunctival injection and tearing (SUNCT) or cranial autonomic features (SUNA)—a prospective clinical study of SUNCT and SUNA. Brain. 2006;129:2746–60.

36. Cittadini E, Goadsby PJ. Hemicrania Continua: a clinical study of 39 patients with diagnostic implications. Brain. 2010;133:1973–86.

37. Chen SP, Fuh JL, Lu SR, Wang SJ. Exertional headache--a survey of 1963 adolescents. Cephalalgia. 2009;29(4):401–7.

38. Frese A, Eikermann A, Frese K, Schwaag S, Husstedt IW, Evers S. Headache associated with sexual activity: demography, clinical features, and comorbidity. Neurology. 2003;61(6):796–800.

39. Sjaastad O, Pettersen H, Bakketeig LS. The Vågå study; epidemiology of headache I: the prevalence of ultrashort paroxysms. Cephalalgia. 2001;21(3):207–15.

40. Shin JH, Song HK, Lee JH, Kim WK, Chu MK. Paroxysmal stabbing headache in the multiple dermatomes of the head and neck: a variant of primary stabbing headache or occipital neuralgia? Cephalalgia. 2007;27(10):1101–8.

41. Guerrero AL, Cortijo E, Herrero-Velázquez S, Mulero P, Miranda S, Peñas ML, Pedraza MI, Fernández R. Nummular headache with and without exacerbations: comparative characteristics in a series of 72 patients. Cephalalgia. 2012;32(8):649–53.

42. Evers S, Goadsby PJ. Hypnic headache: clinical features, pathophysiology, and treatment. Neurology. 2003;60(6):905–9.

43. Li D, Rozen TD. The clinical characteristics of new daily persistent headache. Cephalalgia. 2002;22(1):66–9.

44. Locker TE, Thompson C, Rylance J, Mason SM. The utility of clinical features in patients presenting with nontraumatic headache: an investigation of

adult patients attending an emergency department. Headache. 2006;46(6):954–61.

45. Polmear A. Sentinel headaches in aneurysmal sub-arachnoid haemorrhage: what is the true incidence? A systematic review. Cephalalgia. 2003;23(10):935–41.

46. Melo TP, Pinto AN, Ferro JM. Headache in intracerebral hematomas. Neurology. 1996;47(2):494–500.

47. Stam J. Thrombosis of the cerebral veins and sinuses. N Engl J Med. 2005;352(17):1791–8.

48. Schievink WI. Spontaneous dissection of the carotid and vertebral arteries. N Engl J Med. 2001;344(12):898–906.

49. Silbert PL, Mokri B, Schievink WI. Headache and neck pain in spontaneous internal carotid and vertebral artery dissections. Neurology. 1995;45(8):1517–22.

50. Jaeckle KA. Causes and management of headaches in cancer patients. Oncology (Williston Park). 1993;7(4):27–31.

51. Forsyth PA, Posner JB. Headaches in patients with brain tumors: a study of 111 patients. Neurology. 1993;43(9):1678–83.

52. Suwanwela N, Phanthumchinda K, Kaoropthum S. Headache in brain tumor: a cross-sectional study. Headache. 1994;34(7):435–8.

53. Vázquez-Barquero A, Ibáñez FJ, Herrera S, Izquierdo JM, Berciano J, Pascual J. Isolated headache as the presenting clinical manifestation of intracranial tumors: a prospective study. Cephalalgia. 1994;14(4):270–2.

54. Van de Beek D, de Gans J, Spanjaard L, et al. Clinical features and prognostic factors in adults with bacterial meningitis. N Engl J Med. 2004;351:1849–59.

55. Brouwer MC, Tunkel AR, McKhann GM 2nd, van de Beek D. Brain abscess. N Engl J Med. 2014;371(5):447–56.

56. Brennan MR. Subdural empiema. Am Fam Physician. 1995;51(1):157–62.

Imaging of Headache

Maja Ukmar, Roberta Pozzi Mucelli,
Irene Zorzenon, and Maria Assunta Cova

4.1 Introduction

Headache is one of the most frequent reported symptoms in neurological clinical practice. Nevertheless only a relatively small group of patients needs neuroimaging in order to confirm the diagnosis. Mainly the cause and the diagnosis are based on the clinical history and neurological examination and are focused on symptoms or signs which prompt further diagnostic testing. Neuroimaging usually is not required in the setting of primary headaches, although it can show same pathological features, but it is important in the evaluation of the secondary ones in order to exclude potentially curable headaches [1].

Electronic Supplementary Material The online version of this chapter (https://doi.org/10.1007/978-3-319-99822-0_4) contains supplementary material, which is available to authorized users.

M. Ukmar (✉)
SC (UCO) Radiologia Diagnostica e Interventistica, Azienda Sanitaria Universitaria Integrata di Trieste (ASUITS), Trieste, Italy
e-mail: maja.ukmar@asuits.sanita.fvg.it

R. Pozzi Mucelli · I. Zorzenon · M. A. Cova
University of Trieste, Department of Radiology, Cattinara Hospital, Trieste, Italy
e-mail: m.cova@fmc.units.it

4.2 Imaging Modalities

Imaging modalities in the diagnostic algorithm of headache are computed tomography (CT), magnetic resonance (MR), and angiography.

CT is the preferred technique in the emergency setting, usually to rule out an intracranial mass or hemorrhage. Evaluation with bone windows is useful to exclude bone lesions or infectious disease of paranasal sinuses. In addition, in the presence of hemorrhage, it could be useful to perform a CT angiography (CTA) to evaluate the presence of aneurysms or vascular malformations. A CT scan after contrast media administration, in venous phase, could also rule out venous cerebral thrombosis. More recently CT perfusion, performed during contrast media administration and dynamic continuous scan acquisition of a brain volume (whole brain with newest CT), is applied in many centers in the evaluation of patients with acute onset of neurological deficit in suspected acute stroke. CT perfusion may help in the differentiation between acute stroke and migrainous aura.

MR is the technique of choice in the evaluation of patients with headache. The technique varies depending on different clinical issues. Whereas in the study of primary headache contrast media administration is not needed, contrarily it is useful in the evaluation of secondary headaches. In primary headache the examination consists mainly of T1, T2, and FLAIR imaging. A MR angiography (MRA) without contrast media could be added to exclude aneurysms. In case of suspected intracranial occlusion or stenosis or in the presence of coils, an MRA with contrast media is more accurate. Considering secondary headaches, several sequences could be added to the standard protocol, including GE T2 or SWI sequences and diffusion-weighted (DWI) sequences, and in most of the cases, contrast media should be administrated. In particular the administration of contrast media is mandatory if there is a suspect of meningeal pathology, in case of neoplasms or, in skull base, orbital and rhinogenic causes of headache. In case of hydrocephalus, a phase-contrast sequence could be applied to evaluate cerebrospinal fluid dynamics.

Digital subtraction angiography (DSA) is of value in vascular pathology both as a diagnostic and therapeutic tool.

4.3 Imaging Findings

4.3.1 Primary Headaches

Primary headaches are those where there is no underlying cause identifiable and where the diagnosis is arrived at through detailed history and pattern recognition. Approximately 90% of headaches are of the primary type. Such headaches mainly include tension headache, cluster headache, trigeminal autonomic cephalgias, and migraine.

4.3.1.1 Migraine
Migraine is a common neurological disorder, characterized by paroxysmal attacks of typically unilateral throbbing headache accompanied by nausea, photophobia, and phonophobia that occur with or without aura [2]. Around 25% of people with migraine present transient and reversible neurological symptoms that resolve before the onset of headache (migraine aura). Once the aura is resolved, headache might be mild or even absent. The most frequent type of aura is characterized by visual symptoms with fortification spectra or scintillating scotoma. A subset of migraine attacks may manifest with acute neurologic symptoms that can also be

found in acute stroke. Sensory aura is less prevalent and almost always accompanied by visual symptoms [3]. The incidence of migraine attacks varies considerably between individuals; some have several attacks a month, but others have less than a month. In particular attacks of migraine with aura present with a lower frequency, ranging from one to two episodes in a year to one or more attacks in a month [4].

The diagnosis of migraine is based on anamnestic and clinical data; however, substantial problems may arise in the acute phase because accurate information is often incomplete or difficult to obtain [5], especially in those patients that clinically mimic an ischemic stroke. Distinguishing between migrainous aura, cerebral ischemia, and Todd paralysis following a seizure may be difficult, but accurate differential diagnosis is mandatory for a correct treatment.

The role of imaging and specifically of conventional MRI is still debated. The association of migraine phenomena with neuroimaging abnormalities, as demonstrated by CT and MRI, has been the subject of much debate [6].

Possible MRI findings, especially in patients with migraine with aura (MA), are supratentorial, but also subcortical deep white matter lesions (Fig. 4.1), silent posterior circulation territory infarcts, and infratentorial T2-hyperintense lesions [7] (Fig. 4.2). Lesions most frequently described in migraine patients are silent infarct-like lesions with the aspect of white matter T2 or FLAIR hyperintensities at MRI [8], but white matter hyperintensities can also be seen in apparently healthy people [9]. In the most important recent study, the CAMERA analysis (Cerebral Abnormalities in Migraine, an Epidemiological Risk Analysis), that analyzed a total of 295 patients, 161 affected by MA, the authors detected a significant incidence of silent brain infarction in the posterior territory, the majority located in cerebellum and more pronounced in patients with MA (8%). Females with migraine also presented deep white matter lesions, with a higher incidence in patients with higher attack frequency [10].

In the study of Uggetti et al., their results are in opposition with all previous studies, as they

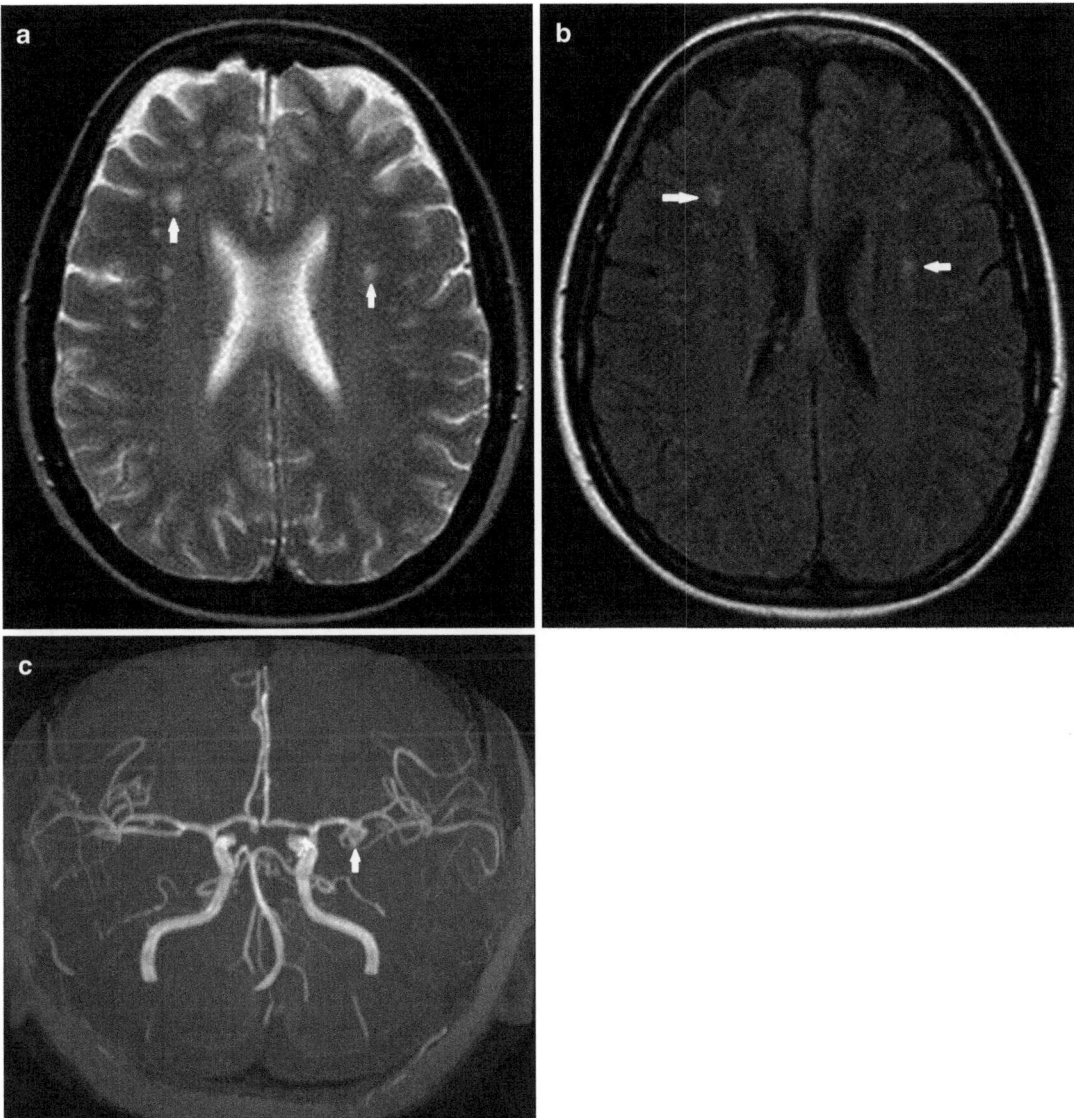

Fig. 4.1 Patient with migraine and aura. Axial SE T2-weighted (**a**) and FLAIR (**b**) sequences show supratentorial white matter hyperintensities. Incidental aneurysms were found on MRA (**c**) at the middle cerebral artery bifurcation and anterior communicating artery

did not find a statistically significant difference in incidence of white matter hyperintensities between patients with MA and controls [11].

Some authors report reversible splenial lesions of the corpus callosum in patients with migraine with aura [12].

Functional neuroimaging of patients with headache is useful to study the pathophysiology rather than for diagnostic purposes. To understand the functional imaging possibilities in headaches, it is necessary to remember how pain structures participate in painful conditions other than headache. In migraine with aura the primary event occurs in the cortex and, including hypothalamus and thalamus, it finishes in the cortex, manifesting pain. In migraine without aura, brain stem findings suggest a dysfunctional pain system [13].

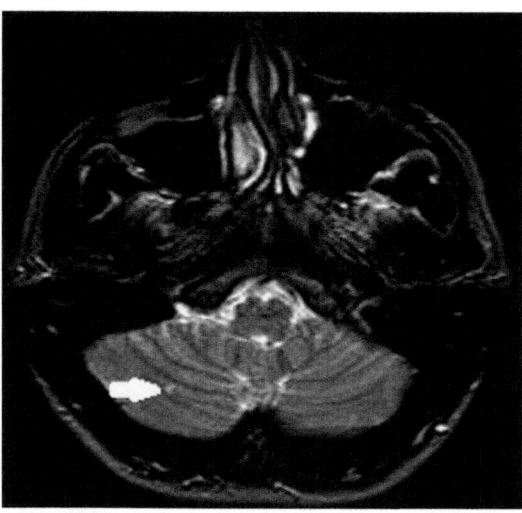

Fig. 4.2 Patient with migraine and aura. Axial SE T2-weighted image: hyperintense specific lesion in the right cerebellum

MR imaging has demonstrated that migrainous aura may be associated with perfusion abnormalities (CBF measurements). Usually, there is hypoperfusion in more than one vascular territory during the migrainous aura, lasting for a few hours (~4), which holds the greatest potential to differentiate migraine from stroke, where hypoperfusion is usually limited to a single vascular territory. A possible differential diagnosis for this pattern of hypoperfusion is severe stenosis of the extracranial vessels; however, this can be assessed by MRA of the extracranial vessels. Some published studies report hyperperfusion; however, this mainly occurs during the headache stage, 6–24 h after the onset of symptoms [14–19]. In literature an occipital predominance of vasoconstriction during the aura is reported [20].

Cerebral perfusion changes during migraine with aura have been described also by BOLD functional MRI studies. In the typical visual aura of migraine, functional MRI has revealed multiple neurovascular events in the occipital cortex, resuming the cortical spreading depression (CSD):

1. An initial hyperemia lasting 3.0–4.5 min, spreading at a rate of 3.5 mm per min.

2. Followed by mild hypoperfusion lasting 1–2 h.
3. An attenuated response to visual activation.
4. Like CSD, in migraine aura, the first affected area is the first to recover [13].

Resnick et al. [21] described reversible changes located in the right parieto-occipital cortex on DWI images in a patient with acute onset of headache. The presence of positive DWI images, with the absence of low apparent diffusion coefficient value, could be in accordance with focal prolonged hyperperfusion associated with vasogenic leakage.

Cerebral perfusion abnormalities may be studied also with CT perfusion; early studies of migraine with aura reveal regional CBF changes of focal hyperemia and spreading oligemia from posterior brain regions. The pathophysiology of the CBF during the acute migraine aura phase and into the period post-headache remains unclear. In the work of Shah et al. [22], they describe the transition from the initial phase of stroke-like symptoms (aura) to an asymptomatic stage, using noninvasive perfusion techniques. There is initial hypoperfusion of the entire left cerebral hemisphere, and the resolution of stroke-like symptoms in 72 h correlates with hyperperfusion and corresponds to decreased MTT and elevated CBF. It is proposed that a "metabolic burnout" leads to possible vasodilation, as there is a gradual increase in CBF (hyperperfusion) seen within the entire left hemisphere. Prior studies from case reports reveal cortical hyperperfusion on the day of migraine aura that carries on until as late as day 14 [23]. There was no documentation of initial hypoperfusion that then resulted in hyperperfusion in any prior case [23]. Perhaps the prolonged and severe symptoms of their case indicate a higher chance of CBF changes occurring as a two-phase process, or possibly other studies have missed the critical moments when such a two-phase process can be imaged. Despite the findings in the literature, in some of our cases (unpublished data) no perfusion defects could be demonstrated.

Noninvasive perfusion techniques allow identifying areas of acute cerebral ischemia and infarction to assist in determination of the need for thrombolysis with tissue plasminogen activator (tPA). Advanced imaging techniques can be expected to show differentiation between migraine and stroke.

Hemiplegic Migraine

Familial (FHM) and sporadic hemiplegic migraine (SHM) are subtypes of migraine characterized by transient motor weakness during the aura phase and caused by mutations in CACNA1A, ATP1A2, or SCN1A. Its incidence is of 0.01% [24], with the familial and sporadic types occurring with equal frequency.

The pathogenesis of hemiplegic migraine is not well established; however, it is hypothesized that it arises from a wave of neuronal excitation in the gray matter that spreads across the cerebral cortex [25].

The diagnosis of hemiplegic migraine is made clinically in accordance with international guidelines [2]. Hallmark symptoms are intermittent episodes of motor weakness that spontaneously settle over time ranging from hours to weeks.

Neuroimaging in acute attacks of hemiplegic migraine is often normal. However, imaging may reveal cerebral cortical hyperintensity and edema [26, 27] contralateral to the hemiparesis. These abnormalities seen on imaging often resolve within weeks to months after an attack.

Repeated ictal and postictal neuroimaging revealed cytotoxic edema during attacks leading to brain atrophy which halted after cessation of severe HM attacks [28]. A complication of this type of migraine is a migrainous infarction (Fig. 4.3).

Retinal Migraine

Retinal migraine is a rare entity characterized by headache associated with transient monocular visual disturbances. While fully reversible monocular phenomena and normal ophthalmological examination between the attacks are the hallmark of retinal migraine according to the International Headache Society (IHS) classification [2], an association with persistent monocular visual loss and abnormal ophthalmological findings has been reported. Recurrent attacks of retinal migraine may weaken the optic nerve, with a final migraine attack that provokes a permanent visual loss, caused by a threshold rupture of the reduced functional reserve. Vasoconstriction as a potential cause for permanent defects in migraine may be supported by MRI angiography.

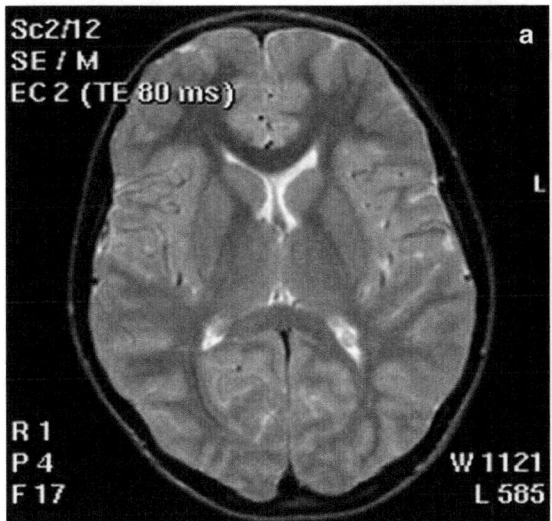
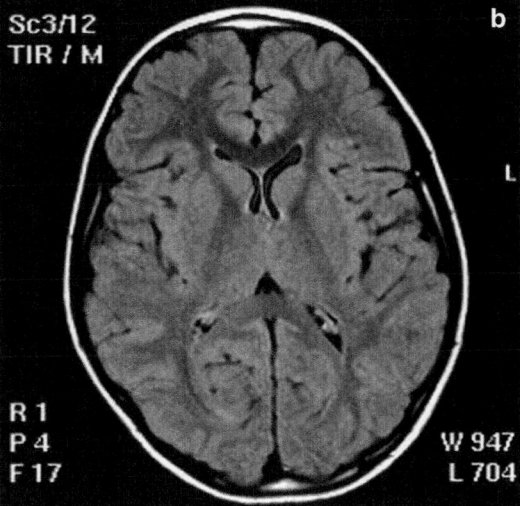
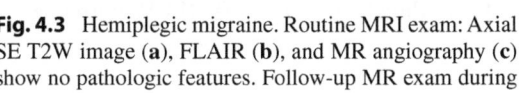

Fig. 4.3 Hemiplegic migraine. Routine MRI exam: Axial SE T2W image (**a**), FLAIR (**b**), and MR angiography (**c**) show no pathologic features. Follow-up MR exam during prolonged left hemiplegia: SE T2W image (**d**), FLAIR (**e**), and DWI (**f**) show acute ischemic stroke in the right thalamus and posterior arm of internal capsule

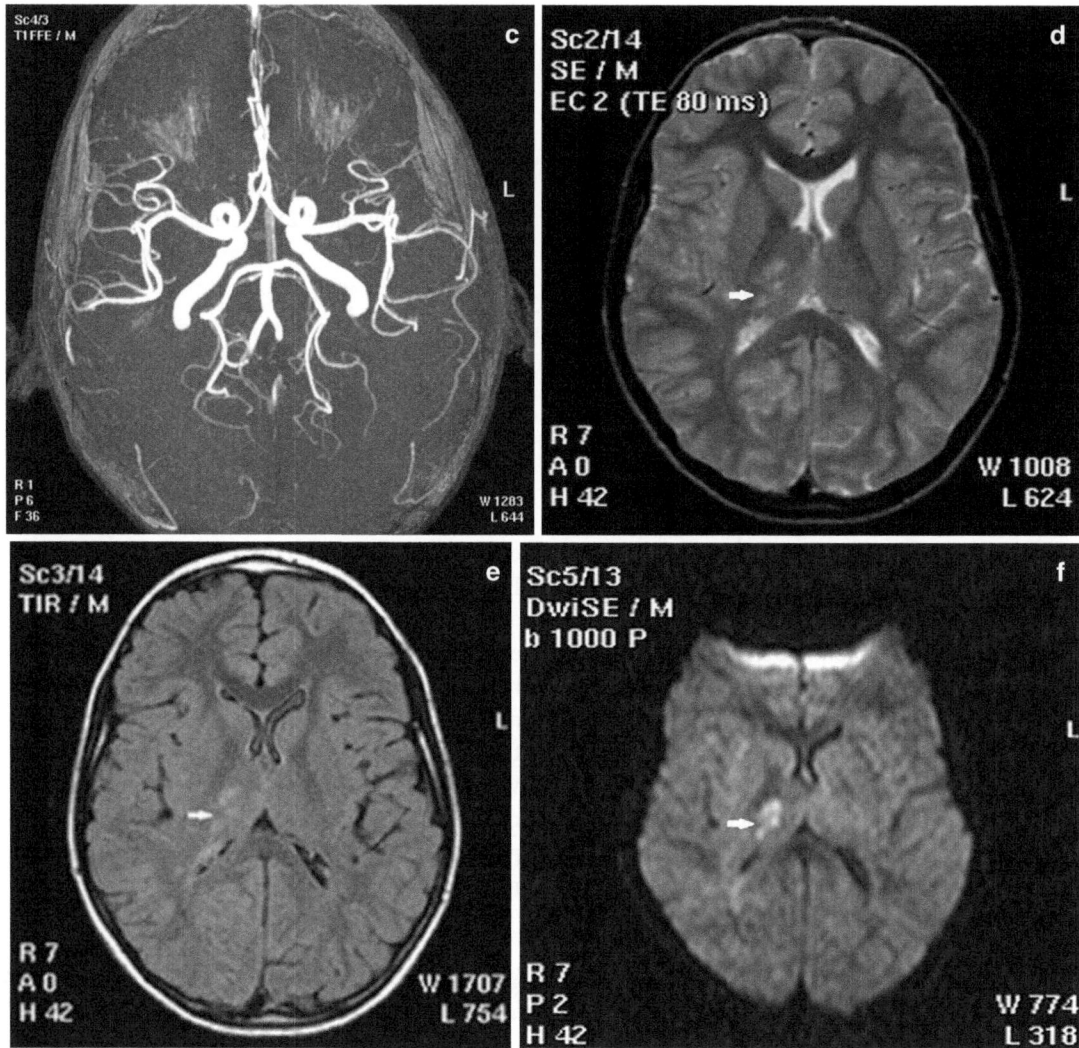

Fig. 4.3 (continued)

MRI, through STIR T2 sequences, may also prove signal alteration of the optic nerve involved, associated with slight bilateral distension of the perioptic subarachnoid spaces. Also at 6 days and 2 months follow-up, a slight pallor and minimal atrophy of the optic disk involved compared to the ipsilateral may be identified [29].

Chronic Migraine

Chronic migraine (CM) usually evolves slowly from episodic migraine (EM) and approximately 2.5% of episodic migraineurs transition to CM each year [30]. Risk factors for chronification include high headache frequency and overuse of acute headache medications among others such as obesity, low educational level, or female sex [31].

The conventional MR patterns are the same as those in episodic migraine. Moreover CM patients show alterations in gray matter volume (GMV) compared to matched healthy controls when analyzed with voxel-based morphometry (VBM). In whole brain analysis testing at a significant threshold of $p < 0.05$ (FEW-corrected), a cluster of GMV increase has been observed with a peak maximum in the amygdala and an

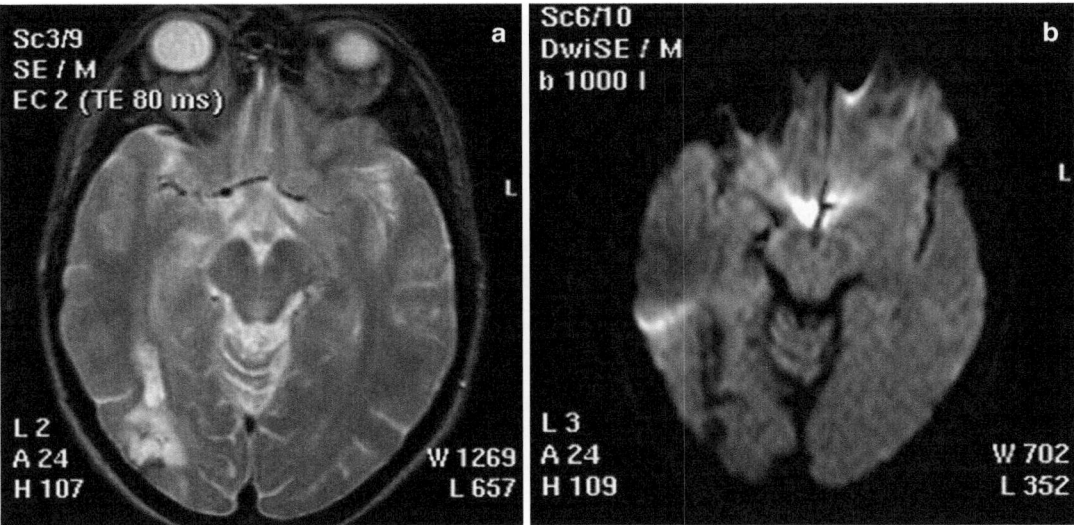

Fig. 4.4 Migrainous infarction. Axial SE T2-weighted image (**a**) and DWI (**b**). Chronic ischemic stroke in right temporal-occipital lobe in a patient with migraine

extension into the putamen [32], which are regions involved in pain perception and processing, but also in affective and cognitive aspects of pain. GMV increase may reflect a remodeling of the central nervous system due to repetitive headache attacks leading to chronic sensitization and a continuous ictal-like state of the brain in chronic migraineurs.

Migrainous Infarction

According to the IHS criteria, migrainous infarction is a typical attack of migrainous aura in a patient with previous history of MA and evidence of cerebral ischemia proven by neuroimaging.

Migrainous infarction is considered a rare complication of migraine. Epidemiologic studies have shown that 0.5–1.5% of all ischemic strokes are migrainous infarctions [33, 34]. Among younger patients with unusual etiology, migrainous infarction was reported to account for 13% of first-ever ischemic strokes [35].

Transient neurologic symptoms are typical for MA, but differentiation among MA, transient ischemic attacks, and migrainous infarction can be very difficult or even impossible on clinical grounds alone. Brain imaging (CT and MRI) is essential for diagnosis of migrainous infarction according to the criteria of the International Headache Society (IHS) [2]. Silent infarctions were detected predominantly in the posterior circulation territory, especially thanks to T2-weighted and FLAIR images [36, 37] (Fig. 4.4). Compared to CT, MRI has proven to be more efficient, especially in acute onsets, since differentiation between migrainous aura and cerebral ischemia can be difficult in the first hours using clinical criteria alone. In these cases DWI provides relevant additional information substantially influencing further management. Given the high sensitivity to detect acute ischemic lesions including even small lacunar or punctuate cortical infarcts, DWI is extremely valuable in the hyperacute phase for positive stroke diagnosis and exclusion of stroke mimics such as migrainous aura symptoms [38–40] and should therefore be preferred in the acute setting.

4.3.1.2 Tension-Type Headache (TTH)

TTH has a high prevalence in general population ranging between 30 and 78% in several studies, and according to ICHD-3 beta [2] and the EHF committee [41], patients with TTH do not exhibit structural brain abnormalities on routine MRI scans. Therefore when clinical features fulfill the diagnostic criteria for TTH, further neuroimaging investigation is not needed, unless three first-line preventive treatments fail [41]. The pathogenesis of TTH remains incompletely understood. Peripheral pain mechanisms are most likely to predominate in TTH, whereas involvement of central pain mechanisms remains to be determined. Only one study values the functional abnormalities in patients with TTH using fMRI and regional homogeneity (ReHo). Their results suggest that TTH patients exhibit reduced synchronization of neuronal activity in several areas involved in the integration and processing of pain [42]. According to Chen et al. [43], several areas such as primary somatosensory cortex, anterior cingulated cortex, and anterior insula undergo gray matter density dynamic and reversible changes in episodic TTH patients between pain and pain-free phases, valuated with voxel-based morphometry (VBM) analysis.

4.3.1.3 Trigeminal Autonomic Cephalalgias (TACs)

The trigeminal autonomic cephalalgias are a group of primary headache disorders relatively rare in comparison with migraine or TTH. TACs are characterized by pain with a unilateral trigeminal distribution that occurs in association with ipsilateral cranial autonomic features and with typical periodicity or cycling of the attacks and bouts. The group includes cluster headache, paroxysmal hemicrania, hemicrania continua, short-lasting unilateral neuralgiform headache attacks with conjunctival injection and tearing (SUNCT), and short-lasting unilateral neuralgiform headache attacks with cranial autonomic symptoms (SUNA). They differ in attack duration, frequency, and response to therapy. Due to the characteristic presentation, diagnosis is mainly clinical. However the EHF committee recommends for all TACs a brain MRI with detailed study of the pituitary area and cavernous sinus, in order to exclude secondary causes [41, 44]. A recent review reports several structural lesions causing symptoms that are indistinguishable from those of idiopathic TACs: tumors, mainly pituitary adenomas, carotid dissection, cerebral infarctions, trigeminal nerve

compression by vascular structures, and multiple sclerosis plaques [45].

In recent times neuroimaging has made substantial contributions to understanding of this syndrome [46]. Iacovelli et al. reviewed several studies which used PET, SPECT, fMRI, MRS, and VBM to better understand the pathophysiology of TACs [47]. All the abnormalities shown by these imaging techniques can be summarized in three major observations: posterior hypothalamic activation during the attacks, involvement of the pain matrix, and involvement of the central opioid system. DTI study results on functional connectivity anomalies in TACs, especially cluster headache, are very diverse and partly contradictory on superficial examination, showing very widespread alterations all over the brain, underlining a complex pain network rather than a single defected structure [48].

4.3.2 Secondary Headaches

Here are several types of headache due to other primary causes and could be classified as follows, according to ICHD-3b secondary headaches (Table 4.1).

The choice of the neuroimaging modality depends on the characteristics of headache: patients with sudden onset and peak intensity of headache should perform an emergent CT

Table 4.1 Causes of secondary headaches according to ICHD-3b

| 1. Headache attributed to trauma or injury to the head and/or neck |
| 2. Headache attributed to cranial or cervical vascular disorder |
| 3. Headache attributed to nonvascular intracranial disorder |
| 4. Headache attributed to a substance or its withdrawal |
| 5. Headache attributed to infection |
| 6. Headache attributed to disorder of homoeostasis |
| 7. Headache or facial pain attributed to disorder of the cranium, neck, eyes, ears, nose, sinuses, teeth, mouth, or other facial or cervical structure |
| 8. Painful cranial neuropathies and other facial pains |

without contrast to rule out intracranial hemorrhage. Additional imaging may be needed depending on the cause of headache at initial findings of CT. Brain MRI is better compared to CT to evaluate the posterior fossa, acute infarcts, and mass lesions. Contrast enhancement should be administrated in suspicion of meningitis, neoplasm, demyelination, and low CSF pressure conditions [49].

4.3.2.1 Headache Attributed to Trauma or Injury to the Head and/or Neck

It is among the most common secondary headache disorders. When a headache occurs for the first time in close temporal relation to trauma or injury to the head and/or neck, it is coded as a secondary headache attributed to the trauma or injury. It has to develop within 7 days of trauma or injury or within 7 days after regaining consciousness and/or the ability to sense and report pain when these have been lost following trauma or injury. Although this 7-day interval is somewhat arbitrary, and although some experts argue that headache may develop after a longer interval in a minority of patients, there is not enough evidence at this time to change this requirement. During the first 3 months from onset, they are considered acute; if they continue beyond that period, they are designated as persistent [2].

Neuroimaging is indicated if there is skull fracture, focal neurologic deficit, or progression of symptoms (Fig. 4.5). With acute head trauma, noncontrast head CT is the primary imaging procedure of choice. MRI with GRE, FLAIR, and SVI and imaging with diffusion-weighted sequence are reserved for severe acute head trauma and in cases in which the patient is much worse on clinical examination than can be explained by CT results. MRI is the primary imaging modality for evaluating delayed effects of brain injury. Furthermore, if MRI and CT are negative but neuropsychological evaluation identifies impairment of mood, executive function, or cognitive endurance, then diffusion tensor imaging might be useful to support the clinical diagnosis [1].

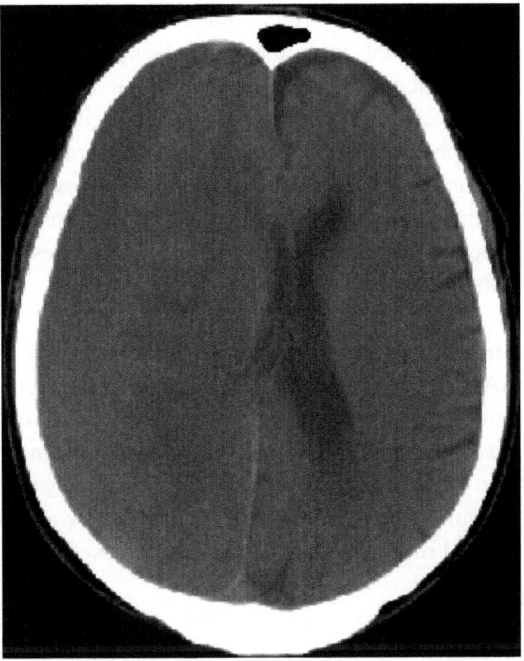

Fig. 4.5 Subdural hematoma; history of trauma in patient with mild left hemiparesis and headache. Axial CT scan: right subdural hematoma with mass effect and median line shift

4.3.2.2 Headache Attributed to Cranial or Cervical Vascular Disorder

Ischemic Stroke

In patients with cerebrovascular event symptoms such as paresis, ataxia and loss of speech are the predominant clinical features. Nonetheless headache has been frequently reported in several studies, with a range of 8–34% [50]. Stroke-related headache can be a sentinel headache (before stroke onset), an onset headache, or a late-onset headache [51], and the characteristic is more similar to the criteria of tension-type headache than migraine [52]. In a lesion mapping study, Seifert et al. found that ischemic strokes that involve the insular cortex, in particular the anterior part, are highly associated with the development of headache. Similar to the insula, the somatosensory cortex has also been demonstrated to be also involved in pain processing during ischemic stroke [50]. Moreover, Chen et al. reported that strokes that arise in the cerebellum, medulla, or posterior cerebral artery cortex are more likely to be associated with onset headache compared with other cerebral territories [51]. Recently, Seifert et al. found a correlation between headache phenotype and specific lesion patterns: pulsating headache occurred with widespread cortical and subcortical strokes, while tension-type headache was not related to specific lesion pattern [53].

Subarachnoid Hemorrhage (SAH)

SAH is the most common cause of persistent, intense, and incapacitating headache of abrupt onset (thunderclap headache) with a high mortality rate (nearly 50%) and a high disability rate (about 50%) [2]. SAH may be caused by aneurysmal rupture or non-aneurysmal causes [54]:

- Arteriovenous malformation
- Dural arteriovenous fistula
- Cavernous angioma
- Vertebral dissection
- Vasculitis
- Amyloid angiopathy
- Cerebral venous thrombosis
- Reversible cerebral vasoconstriction syndrome
- Perimesencephalic SAH

Unenhanced CT performed within 6 h of symptom onset has 100% sensitivity in detecting SAH as hyperdensity within the subarachnoid spaces. Within 24 h, sensitivity is approximately 93%, falling to 50% at 4 days, with the majority of examinations normal at 10 days, as the aging hemorrhage becomes more isodense to water over time, making it harder to detect in the subacute and chronic phases [54]. A minor bleed may be missed on the initial CT so, if the clinical suspicion remains high, a LP revealing high opening pressure and elevated RBC count should be performed [55]. Although CT remains the exam of choice in the acute setting, MRI can be very sensitive for detection of SAH: T2* sequences have shown sensitivity of 94% in the acute phase (within 4 days) and 100% in the subacute phase (after 4 days), while FLAIR sequences have sensitivity of 81% acutely and 87% in the subacute phase. On T2* sequences SAH is seen

as low signal intensity while on FLAIR sequences is seen as hyperintensity in the subarachnoid spaces; however, it should be kept in mind that there are other multiple causes of subarachnoid hyperintensity [49, 54].

After detecting SAH, other imaging investigation should be undertaken to determine the etiology: a ruptured aneurysm account for 80% of non-traumatic SAH. DSA remains the gold standard for the detection of aneurysms, but in the emergency setting, CTA is performed: CTA has 100% sensitivity and specificity for the detection of aneurysms >3 mm; it might be less sensitive and accurate than DSA for aneurysms <3 mm [55]. MRA is a possible alternative to CTA or DSA for aneurysm detection: 3D TOF MRA at high magnetic field (3.0 T) can safely replace DSA in the diagnostic work-up of patients with small aneurysm with a sensitivity of more than 95% [56]. Sacciform aneurysms usually develop at vessel bifurcation or branching points, and most of them occur at typical locations within or near the circle of Willis: the most common locations are the middle cerebral artery bifurcation and along the anterior communicating artery, followed by the origin of posterior communicating artery and ophthalmic artery, while in the posterior circulation, the tip of the basilar artery and the origins of the posterior inferior cerebellar arteries are the most common locations [54]. Hemorrhage localized to the basal cisterns are indicators of aneurysmal SAH, and patterns of hemorrhage help to predict site of aneurysm, particularly ruptured middle cerebral artery or anterior communicating artery aneurysms; parenchymal hematoma is an excellent predictor of the site of a ruptured aneurysm [54]. If the initial angiogram is negative, a second DSA should be performed in the first 2 weeks. The indications for a second DSA include heavy blood load, small aneurysm size, and vasospasm, hematoma, or thrombosis within the aneurysm [49]. In case of negative imaging, in particular DSA, "sine causa" SAH should be considered (Fig. 4.6).

Other Intracranial Hemorrhages

While subdural and epidural hematomas are often related to head trauma, intraparenchymal cerebral hemorrhage (ICH) may underlie several different pathologies (Table 4.2).

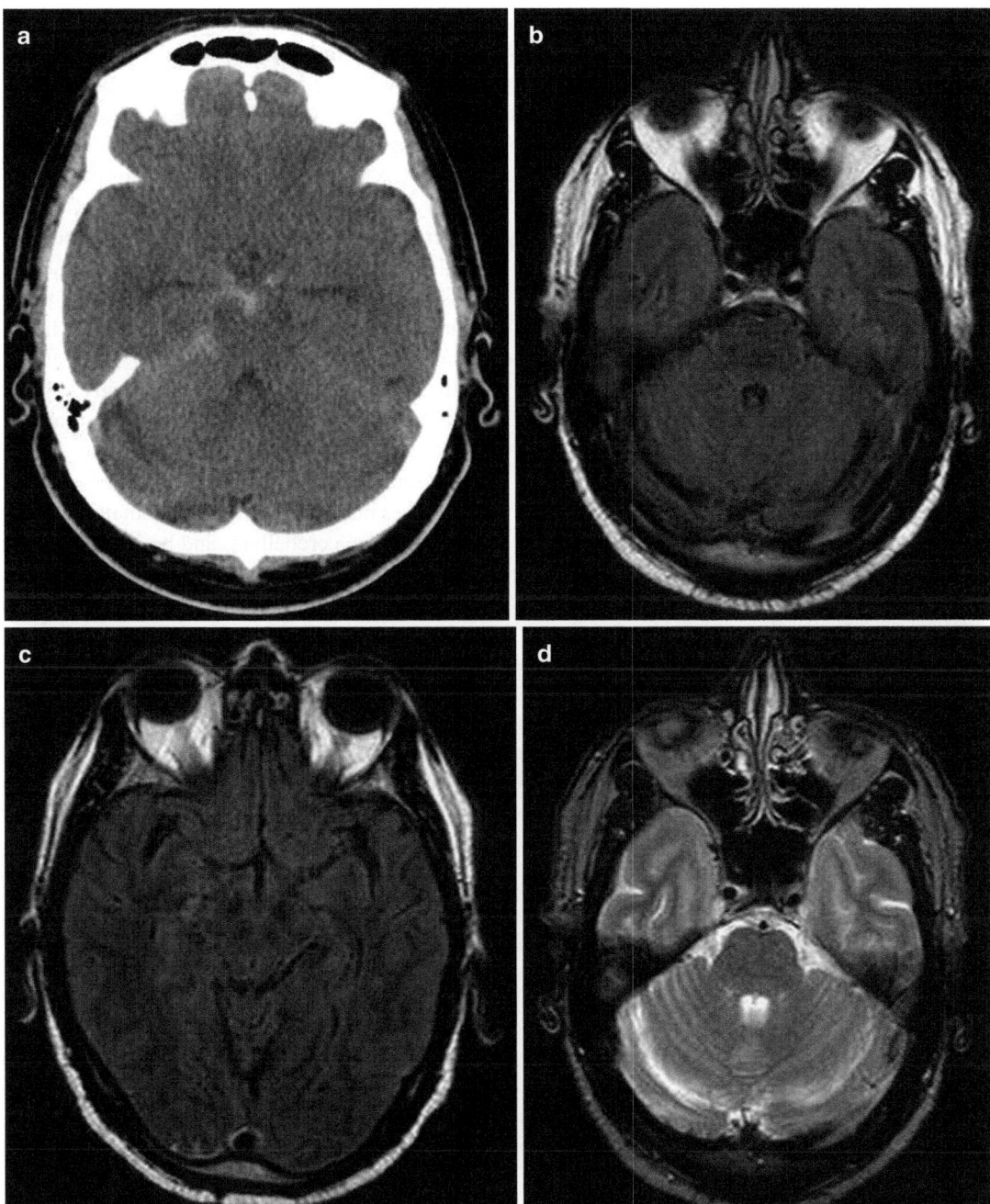

Fig. 4.6 SAH: Patient with thunderclap headache. Axial CT scan (**a**) detects SAH as hyperdensity within the perimesencephalic cistern. On axial FLAIR images (**b, c**) mild hyperintense signal is detected in prepontine cistern and temporo-occipital sulci. On T2W image (**d**) only slight linear hypointensity is shown in prepontine cistern

ICH due to hypertension typically affects patients of 60–70 years old and has a 30–50% mortality rate. On CT exam acute ICH due to hypertension classically presents as an intra-axial hyperdense region of hemorrhage centered within the basal ganglia, cerebellum, or occipital lobes. The hemorrhage may vary in size from a relatively small hematoma without significant mass effect to very large hematomas with significant local mass effect and brain herniation that need emergent surgical decompression or evacuation [57]. Acute ICH in nonclassical intra-axial location or acute ICH in patient younger than 50 should prompt consideration of other causes of bleeding, and additional diagnostic information may be obtained by CTA and/or MRI [57].

Table 4.2 Causes of solitary or multiple intraparenchymal cerebral hemorrhage (ICH)

Solitary ICH	Multiple ICHs
Hypertension	Cavernous malformation
Cerebral amyloid angiopathy	Chronic hypertension
Primary and secondary neoplasms	Cerebral amyloid angiopathy
Cerebral aneurysms	Hemorrhagic metastases
Cerebral arteriovenous malformations	Coagulopathy
Dural arteriovenous fistulae	Cerebral venous thrombosis
Cerebral venous thrombosis	
Coagulopathy	

In cerebral amyloid angiopathy (CAA), the deposition of amyloid-b peptide within cerebral arterial walls results in cerebral microhemorrhages, sulcal SAH, or larger ICH. There are several imaging characteristics to differentiate ICH due to CAA rather than hypertension: ICH secondary to CAA is firstly identified by CT as a hyperdense intra-axial hemorrhage in the subcortical region sparing the basal ganglia, posterior fossa, and brain stem. There may be diffuse white matter hypoattenuation in both cerebral hemispheres that represents underlying microangiopathic changes. MRI may more strongly suggest the diagnosis of CAA by the presence of numerous small microhemorrhages presenting as foci of susceptibility blooming on GRE or SWI sequences in the subcortical white matter sparing basal ganglia, cerebellum, and brain stem. Other typical MRI findings are ICHs at different ages and hyperintensity focal or confluent white matter areas on T2/FLAIR sequences representing microangiopathy [57] (Fig. 4.7).

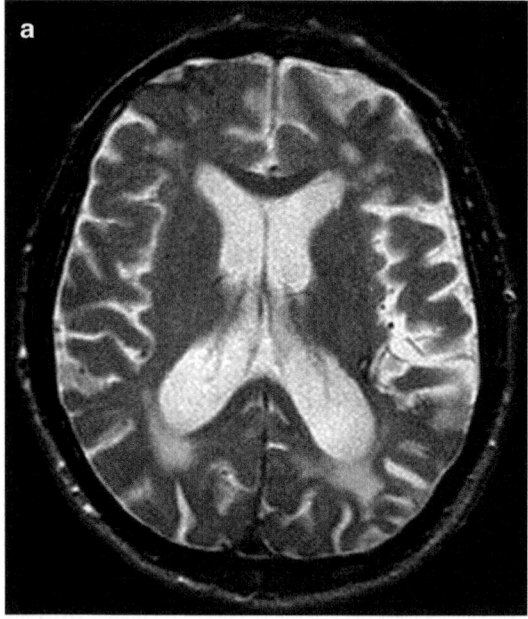
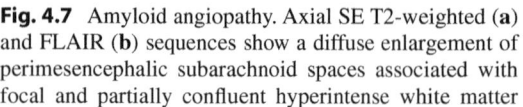
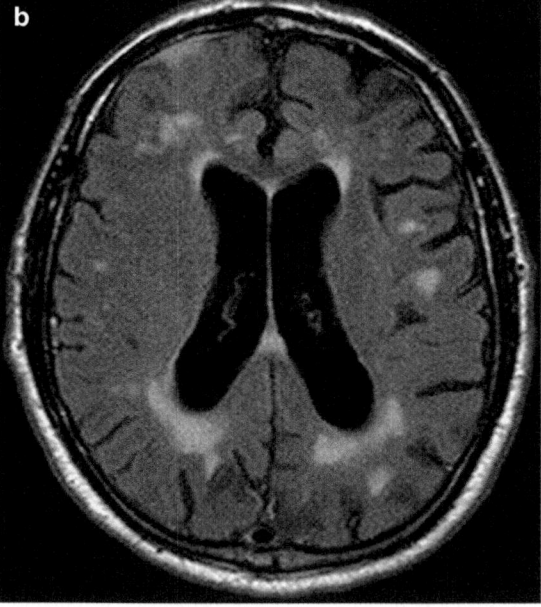

Fig. 4.7 Amyloid angiopathy. Axial SE T2-weighted (**a**) and FLAIR (**b**) sequences show a diffuse enlargement of perimesencephalic subarachnoid spaces associated with focal and partially confluent hyperintense white matter subcortical and periventricular areas. GRE T2* sequence (**c**) allows the identification of cortical, subcortical, and subarachnoid hemosiderin deposition

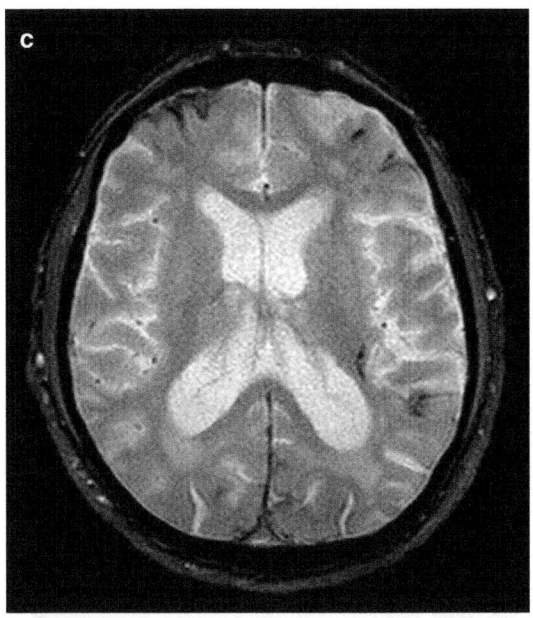

Fig. 4.7 (continued)

Another frequent cause of ICH is cerebrovascular disease which includes aneurysms, arteriovenous malformations (AVMs) (Fig. 4.8), cavernous malformation (Fig. 4.9), dural arteriovenous fistulae (DAVF), hemorrhagic conversion of ischemic stroke, vasculitis, and cortical venous or venous sinus thrombosis.

AVMs are ten times less common than aneurysms and generally affect young patients. They tend to be solitary, and they are composed of a nidus of vessels through which arteriovenous shunting occurs. Their rupture can result with either acute ICH, SAH, or intraventricular hemorrhage (IVH) presenting in the acute setting on CT as hyperdensity within these compartments. AVMs may be identified by CTA, MRA, or DSA. DSA is the gold standard showing a tightly packed mass of enlarged feeding arteries that supply a central nidus; one or more dilated veins drain the nidus, and the abnormal opacification of

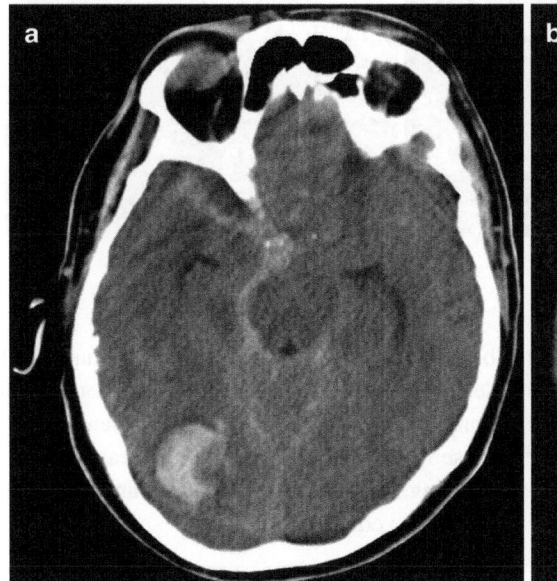

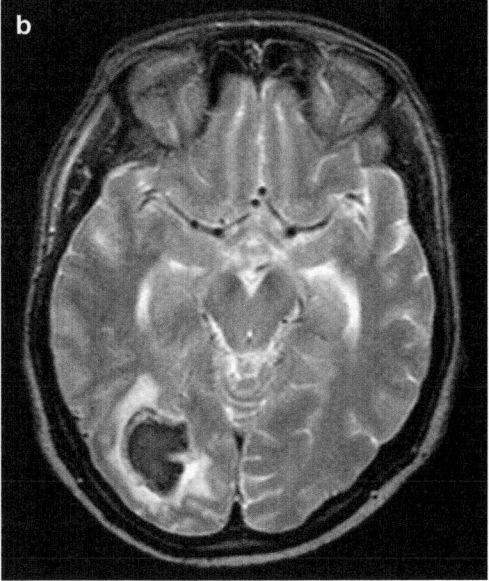

Fig. 4.8 ICH caused by ruptured AVM. On axial CT scan (**a**) a right temporo-occipital ICH, associated with subarachnoid and perimesencephalic hemorrhage, was found. Axial SE T2w (**b**), coronal SE T2w (**c**), and axial SE T1w (**d**) sequences show the early subacute ICH with small vessels along transverse sinus. MRA (**e**) and further DSA (**f**) demonstrate the presence of an underlying AVM associated with dural fistula

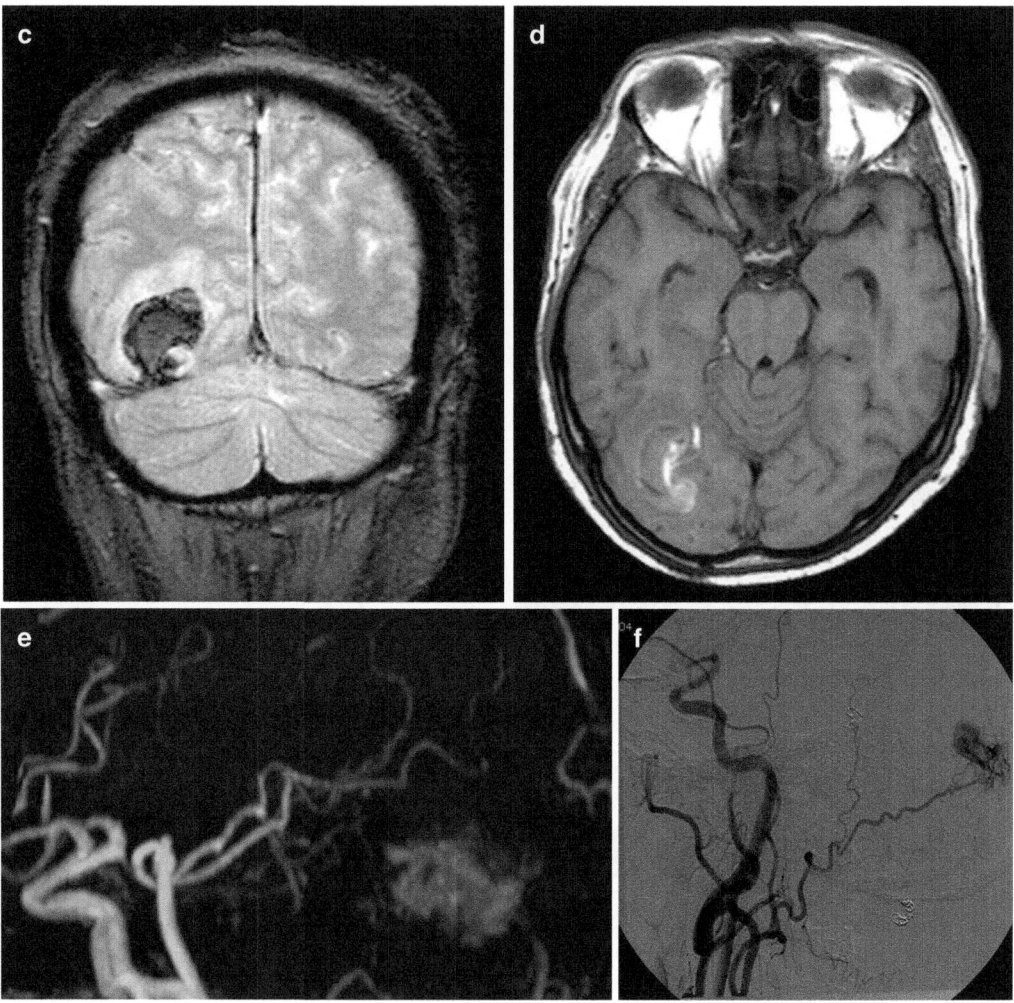

Fig. 4.8 (continued)

veins occurs in the arterial phase, representing shunting. DSA should be performed in every patient presenting with a ruptured cerebral AVM to determine whether the presence of a nidal or perinidal aneurysm may require emergent endovascular or surgical treatment [57, 58].

Headache commonly represents a consequence of ICH or seizures which are the two main manifestations of cavernous malformations [2] (Fig. 4.9): on CT these lesions can be seen as a focal hyperdensity. MRI is the modality of choice demonstrating a typical popcorn appearance with a rim of signal loss due to hemosiderin; the T1 and T2 signal intensity depends on the age of the blood products and fluid-fluid levels may

be evident. GRE or SWI sequences have higher sensitivity in detecting small cavernous malformations than conventional SE sequences. When these lesions bleed, they may increase in size on imaging, showing acute ICH and associated vasogenic edema [58].

Cervical Carotid or Vertebral Artery Dissection

Cranial cervical dissection is one of the most frequent causes of stroke in young patients. Headache with or without neck pain can be the only manifestation of cervical artery dissection (Fig. 4.10). It is the most frequent symptom, usually unilateral, severe, and persistent; it can

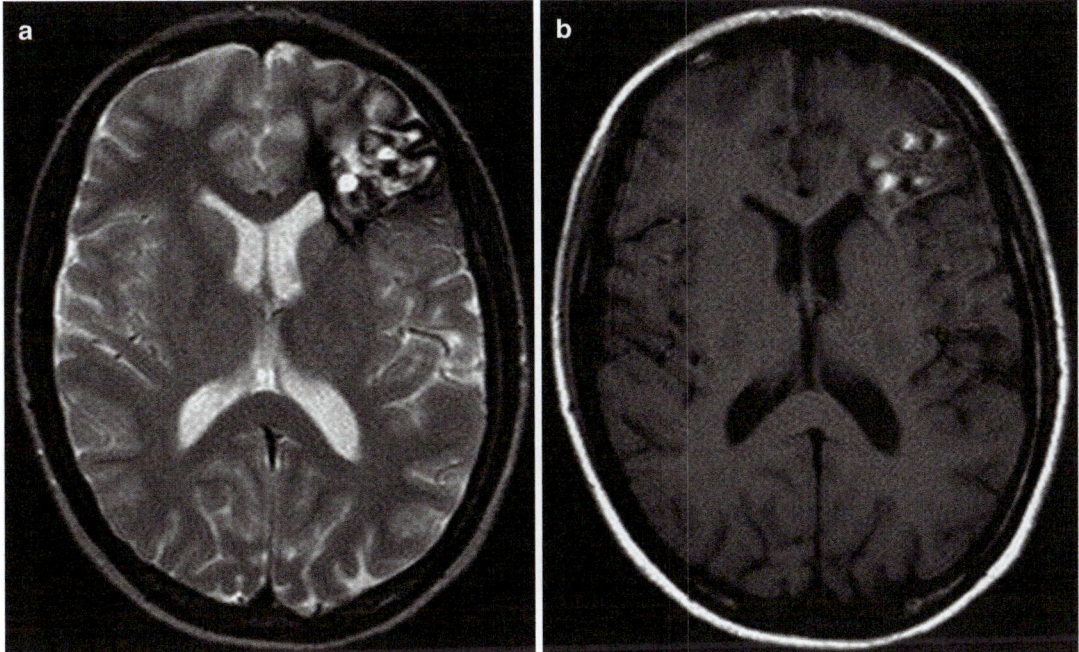

Fig. 4.9 Cavernous malformation in patient with headache. Axial SE T2w (**a**) and SE T1w (**b**) sequences show a large cavernoma in left frontal lobe with subacute bleeding

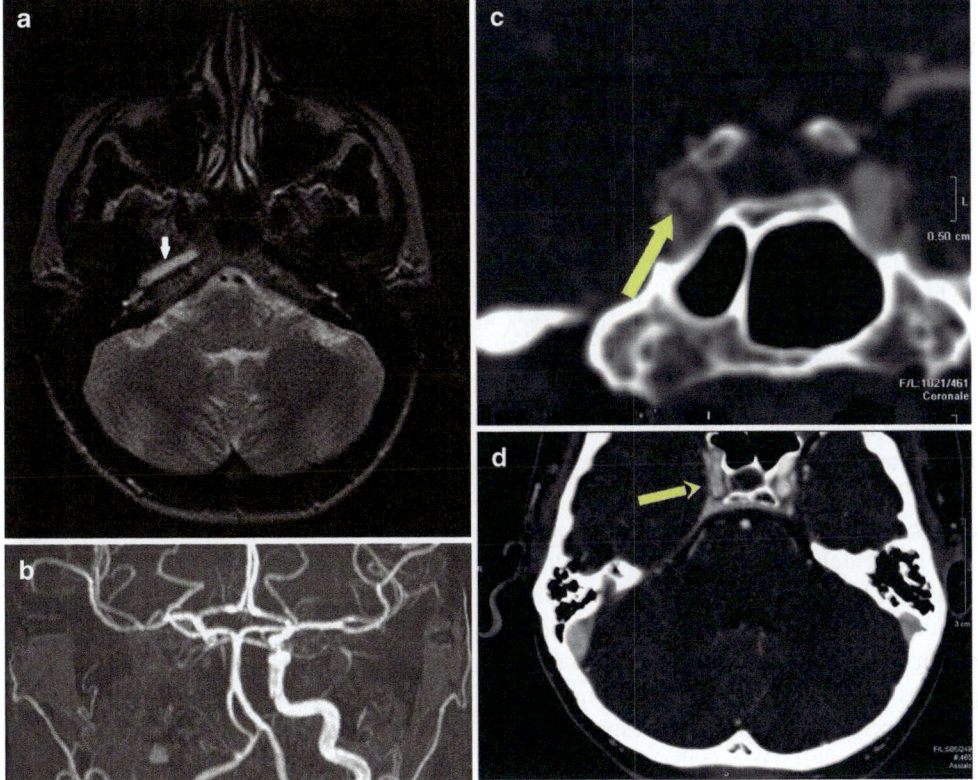

Fig. 4.10 Carotid artery dissection in patient with headache. An hyperintense right carotid artery signal was found on axial SE T2w images (**a**); the lack of visualization of the right carotid artery signal was confirmed on MRA sequences (**b**). A further CTA scan on coronal and axial plane (**c**, **d**) confirmed the presence of a carotid artery dissection flap

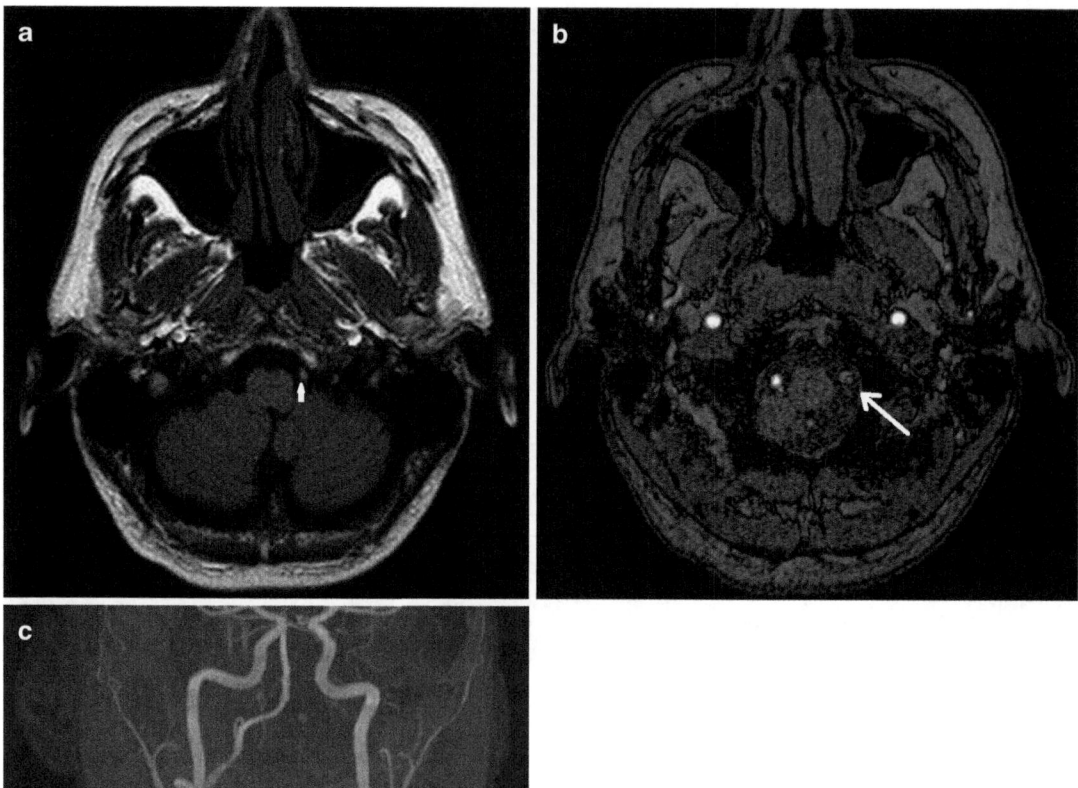

Fig. 4.11 Vertebral artery dissection in patient with acute cervical pain and headache. Axial SE T1w image (**a**) shows a focal hyperintensity in the lumen of the left verte- bral artery. MRA source image (**b**) shows the intimal flap within the vessel (arrow), and MIP reconstruction (**c**) con- firms the absence of flow signal in the left vertebral artery

remain isolated or precede signs of cerebral or retinal ischemic stroke. Cervical artery dissection may be associated with intracranial artery dissec- tion, which is a potential cause of SAH [2]. The first diagnostic imaging modalities include CTA and MRA. Reported sensitivity and specificity of CTA and MRA for diagnosis of craniocervical arterial dissection are relatively similar, although sensitivity for vertebral arterial dissection may be less [59]; however, a contrast-enhanced MRA may show signal loss within the vertebral artery (Fig. 4.11). Acutely, it is difficult to visualize a dissection on T1-weighted images with fat satu- ration due to obscuration from the surrounding tissue. In the subacute stage, the dissection appears as a crescent-shaped hyperintensity around an eccentric flow void corresponding to the vessel lumen [49]. DSA is the gold standard, and the angiographic features include luminal

narrowing, vessel irregularity, wall thickening/ hematoma, pseudoaneurysm formation, and inti- mal flap [54].

Cerebral Venous Sinus Thrombosis (CVST)

In 80–90% of cases, CVST presents with head- ache which can be an isolated symptom and may present as thunderclap or progressive headache. Headache may be associated also with focal signs (neurological deficits or seizures) and/or signs of subacute encephalopathy, intracranial hyperten- sion, or cavernous sinus syndrome [2].

Although cerebral angiography is considered the gold standard for the evaluation of CVST, nowadays, CT is usually the first exam performed [60]. Unenhanced CT is often abnormal in patients with neurological signs: a fresh clot is visible as a hyperdensity in cortical veins or dural venous sinuses. This should be confirmed by

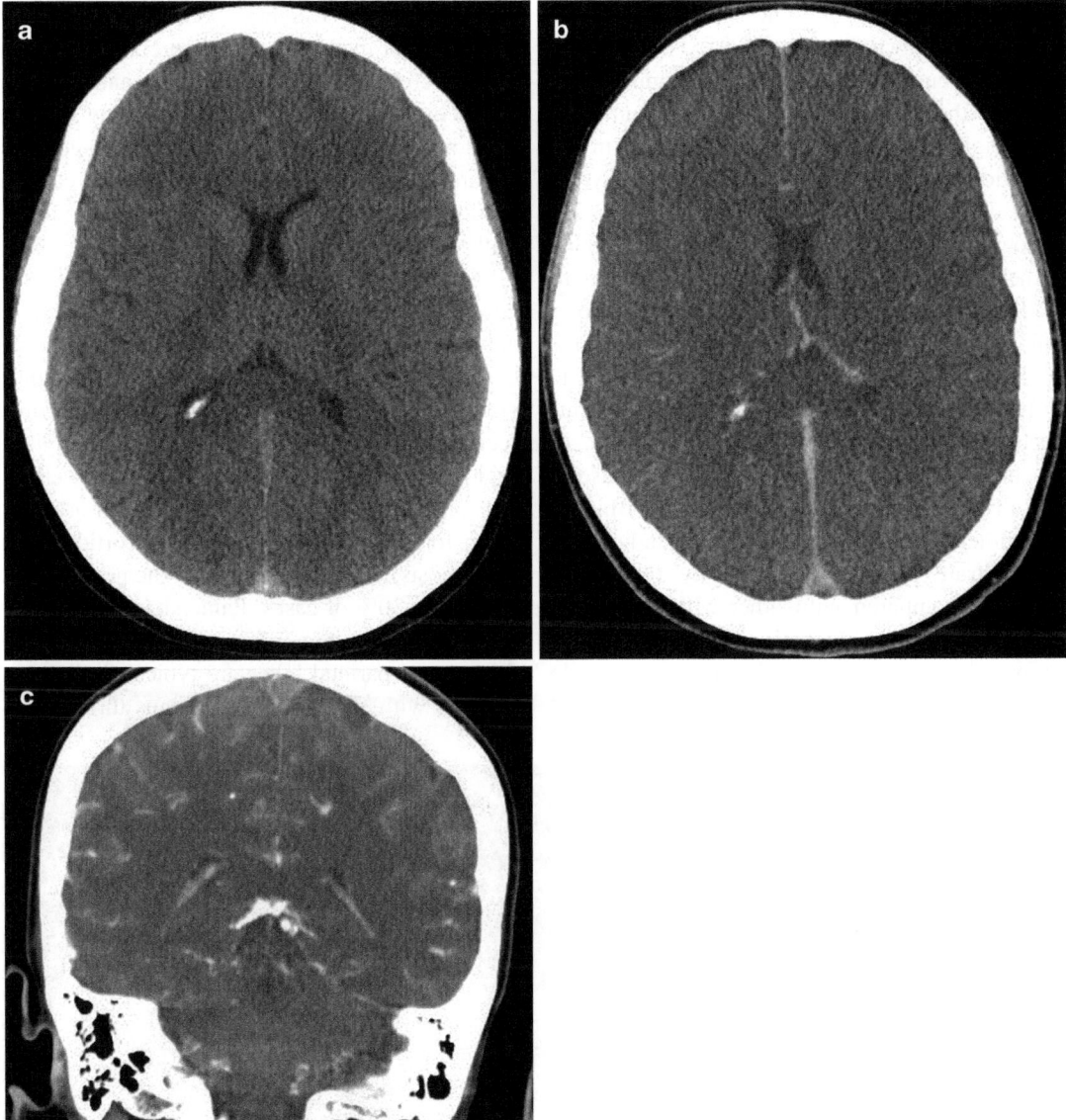

Fig. 4.12 Cerebral venous thrombosis in intractable headache. Axial unenhanced CT scan (**a**) shows hyperdensity in the lumen of the superior sagittal sinus. Axial and coronal contrast-enhanced CT scans (**b, c**) confirm the presence of an empty delta sign, representing lack of contrast media filling in venous fresh clot

contrast-enhanced CT (venography CT) showing the hallmark empty delta sign [54] (Fig. 4.12).

On conventional MRI the absence of a flow void and the presence of altered signal intensity in the sinus are primary findings of sinus thrombosis; slow or turbulent flow may also cause altered sinus signal intensity. The signal intensity on T1- and T2-weighted sequences depends on the age of the thrombus: isointense signal on T1-weighted sequences and hypointense signal on T2-weighted sequences in early acute stages (1–5 days), hyperintensity signal on both T1- and T2-weighted sequences from 5 to 15 days, and isointense signal on T1-weighted sequence and hyperintensity on T2-weighted sequences at later stages [49]. T2* sequences may be an important diagnostic aid: the presence of paramagnetic blood breakdown products (deoxyhemoglobin and metahemoglobin) produces blooming artifacts in the thrombosed venous segment [54]. PD-weighted sequences could also help in the detection of thrombus which appears as a hyperintense defect (Fig. 4.7). Magnetic resonance venography (MRV) with phase-contrast imaging is helpful for the diagnosis and follow-up of CVST. However, MRV may not detect the thrombus, showing only absence of signal in the occluded vein; sometimes it may be difficult to differentiate it from normal anatomic variants such as sinus hypoplasia, flow asymmetry, or arachnoid granulation [49]. Therefore the use of 3D T1-weighted GRE CE sequences is highly recommended as shown by recent studies that demonstrate its highest sensitivity for CVST detection compared with other MRI sequences [60, 61] (Fig. 4.13). Recently, ASL-PWI has been proposed as a further MRI sequence to help identify CVST presenting a bright sinus signal

intensity [62]. Cerebral venous thrombosis results in an increased venous pressure that can lower cerebral perfusion pressure and induces parenchymal changes due to vasogenic edema, cytotoxic edema, intracranial hemorrhage, and subarachnoid hemorrhage [62]. Edema can be predominantly cytotoxic or vasogenic, hence with mixed DWI signal alterations (Fig. 4.8). CVST leads to venous infarction in about 50% of cases, but distribution of venous drainage areas is subject to variation. However, there are some characteristics that may guide to proper diagnosis: bilaterally involvement of deep structures (cerebral deep vein thrombosis) or parasagittal regions (sagittal sinus thrombosis), as well as uni- and bilateral changes in peripheral areas of brain lobes or the temporal lobe (cortical vein thrombosis) [54]. Parenchymal hemorrhage is present in 30% of cases: flame-shaped, irregular zones of lobar hemorrhage in the parasagittal frontal and parietal lobes are typical findings in patients with superior sagittal sinus thrombosis,

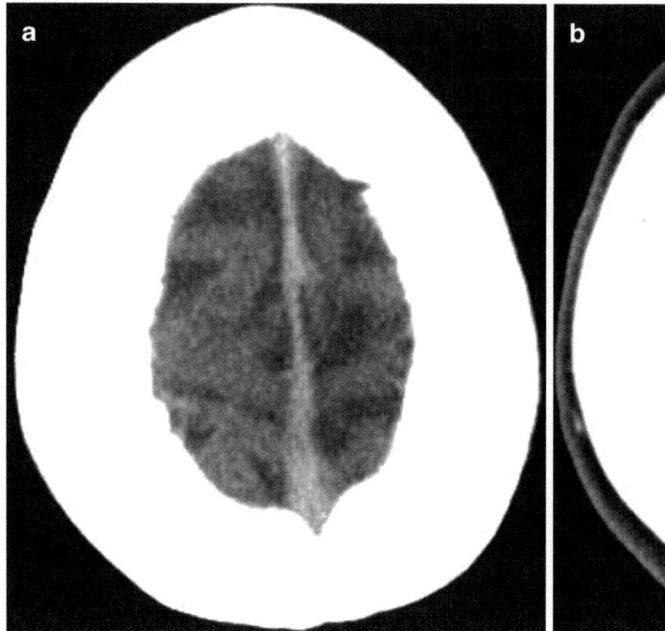
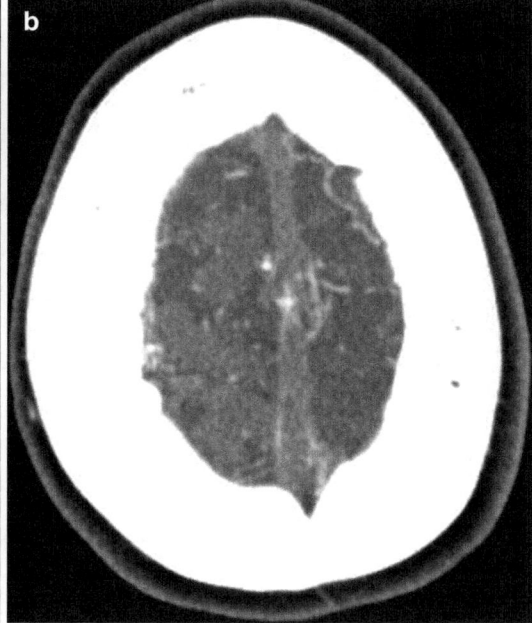

Fig. 4.13 Cerebral venous thrombosis in patient with headache. Unenhanced CT scan (**a**) shows hyperdensity in superior sagittal sinus (SSS) with empty delta sign on enhanced CT (**b**). MRI shows hyperintense signal at the level of frontoparietal sulci on FLAIR image (**c**); it confirmed the presence of a subacute thrombus in SSS and

cortical veins on T1 w image (**d**) and lack of opacification after contrast media (**e, f**). Follow-up scan demonstrated resolution of the thrombosis with disappearance of hyperintensity on FLAIR image (**g**), thrombus on T1w image (**h**), and complete opacification of SSS (**i, j**)

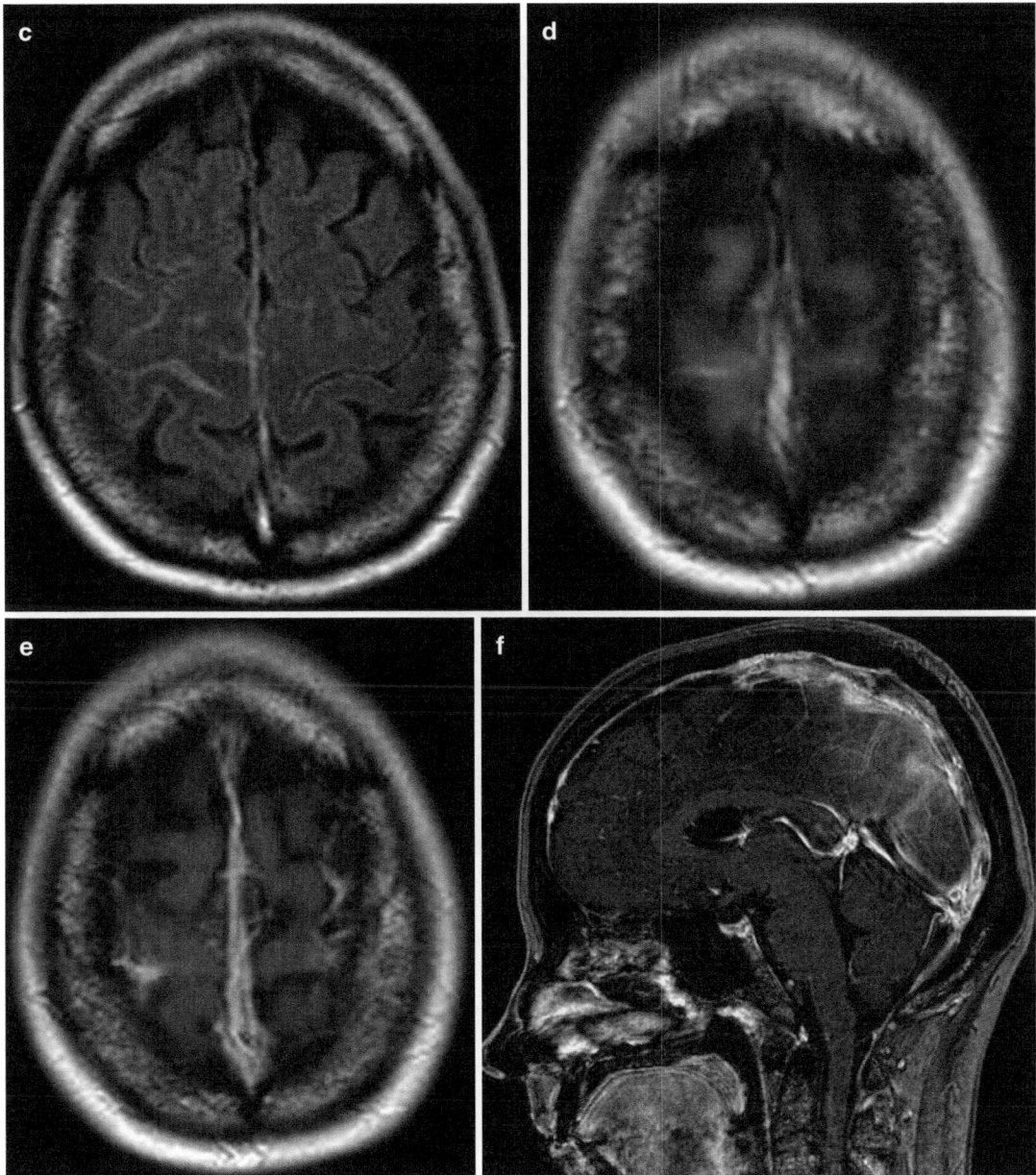

Fig. 4.13 (continued)

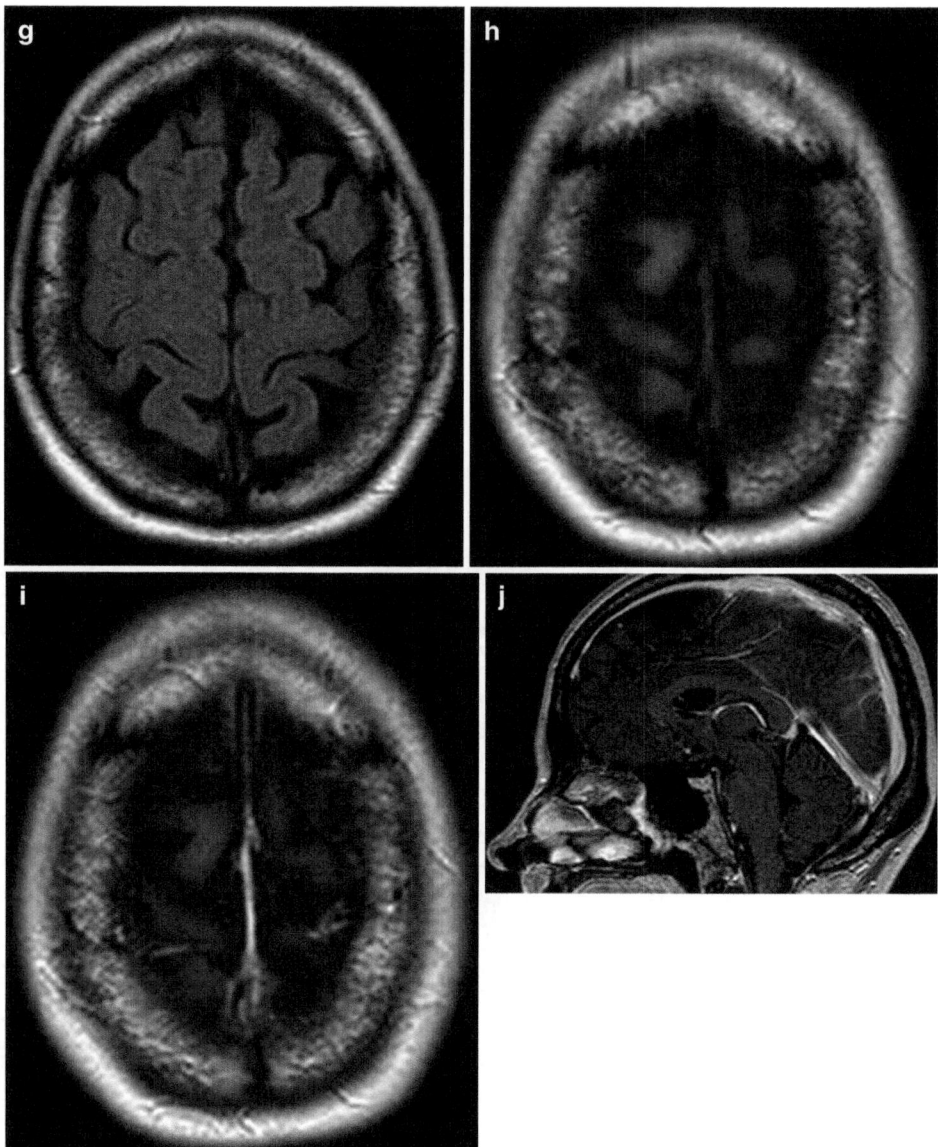

Fig. 4.13 (continued)

whether hemorrhage in the temporal and occipital lobes is more typical of transverse sinus thrombosis. T2* sequences have high sensitivity in the depiction of parenchymal hemorrhage. Rarely CVST may be associated also with SAH [54]. Recent studies evaluated the usefulness of ASL-PWI sequences to determine the hypoperfusion of brain parenchyma drained by the thrombosed sinus, showing a decreased CBF in the affected area [62].

Reversible Vasoconstriction Syndrome (RCVS)

RCVS is a term used to group reversible angiopathies that present with a sudden thunderclap headache with or without focal neurological deficits and/or seizures, recurrent in 1 month and triggered by several factors such as sexual activity, exertion, and Valsalva maneuver. Typically RCVS presents with multifocal arterial vasoconstriction. During the first week after clinical onset, neuroimaging investigation can be normal [2]. Abnormal findings may develop later, revealing cortical SAH over the convexities of the cerebral hemispheres, intracerebral hemorrhage (ICH), infarction in a watershed zone, or brain edema [49]. Ischemic stroke is the most common, followed by isolated convexity SAH and isolated ICH. Brain infarcts and hemorrhages are typically located in watershed zones, usually in posterior regions, in a pattern which can be similar to that of an atypical posterior reversible leukoencephalopathy syndrome (PRES) (there is a 10% overlap with this condition) [54] (Figs. 4.14 and 4.15).

MRI may be more sensitive than CT for detecting subtle cortical SAH, cerebral edema, infarction, and leukoencephalopathy. The gold standard for diagnosis is DSA which detects the typical alternating areas of arterial constriction and dilatation, often called "beading," in multiple vascular beds [63]. These alterations are usually bilateral and multiple and affect all intracerebral arteries and their branches, while the extracranial segments of the internal carotid and vertebral arteries are rarely involved. These changes usually resolve within 3 months [54, 64]. CT angiography and MRA are alternative and less invasive methods for identifying the arterial changes [63]. Furthermore, the ASL MRI perfusion maps may reveal hypoperfusion of several cerebral areas as reported by Komatsu et al. [65].

Cerebral Autosomal Dominant Arteriopathy with Subcortical Infarcts and Leukoencephalopathy (CADASIL)

CADASIL is the most common monogenetic cause of adult onset progressive cerebrovascular disease. It is an autosomal dominant arteriopathy characterized by migraine usually with aura presenting in early adulthood (at a mean age of 30), recurrent ischemic events, mood disturbances, progressive cognitive impairment mostly affecting executive function, and acute encephalopathy [49, 66]. Onset of radiologic manifestations closely mirrors the onset of migraine with mean age of imaging abnormalities starting at 30 years. By the age of 35, essentially all patients with CADASIL have abnormal MRI findings [66]. MRI is the most clinically relevant imaging modality. In early stages nonspecific periventricular and subcortical hyperintensities on T2/FLAIR sequences may be seen. The typical radiologic findings of advanced stages of CADASIL are confluent, large, symmetrical white matter changes on T2/FLAIR sequences, particularly in the anterior temporal poles, external capsula, and superior frontal gyrus [66]. Anterior temporal pole alterations have a high sensitivity and specificity for this disease (approximatively 90% for each) (Fig. 4.16). DWI sequences may show acute and subacute ischemic events. GRE sequences may show in a variable number of cases (30–70%) cerebral micro-bleeds most commonly affecting the thalami, basal ganglia, and brain stem [66, 67]. The MRI findings that are most strongly related to clinical deficit are number and volume of lacunes, brain atrophy, and white matter disease [68]. Recently DTI has been used to characterize tissue damage in CADASIL: DTI helps demonstrating the extensive microstructural changes involving intra- and interhemispheric cerebral, thalamocortical, and cerebro-cerebellar connections; moreover the severity of microstructural changes correlates with extension of T2/FLAIR hyperintensities [69].

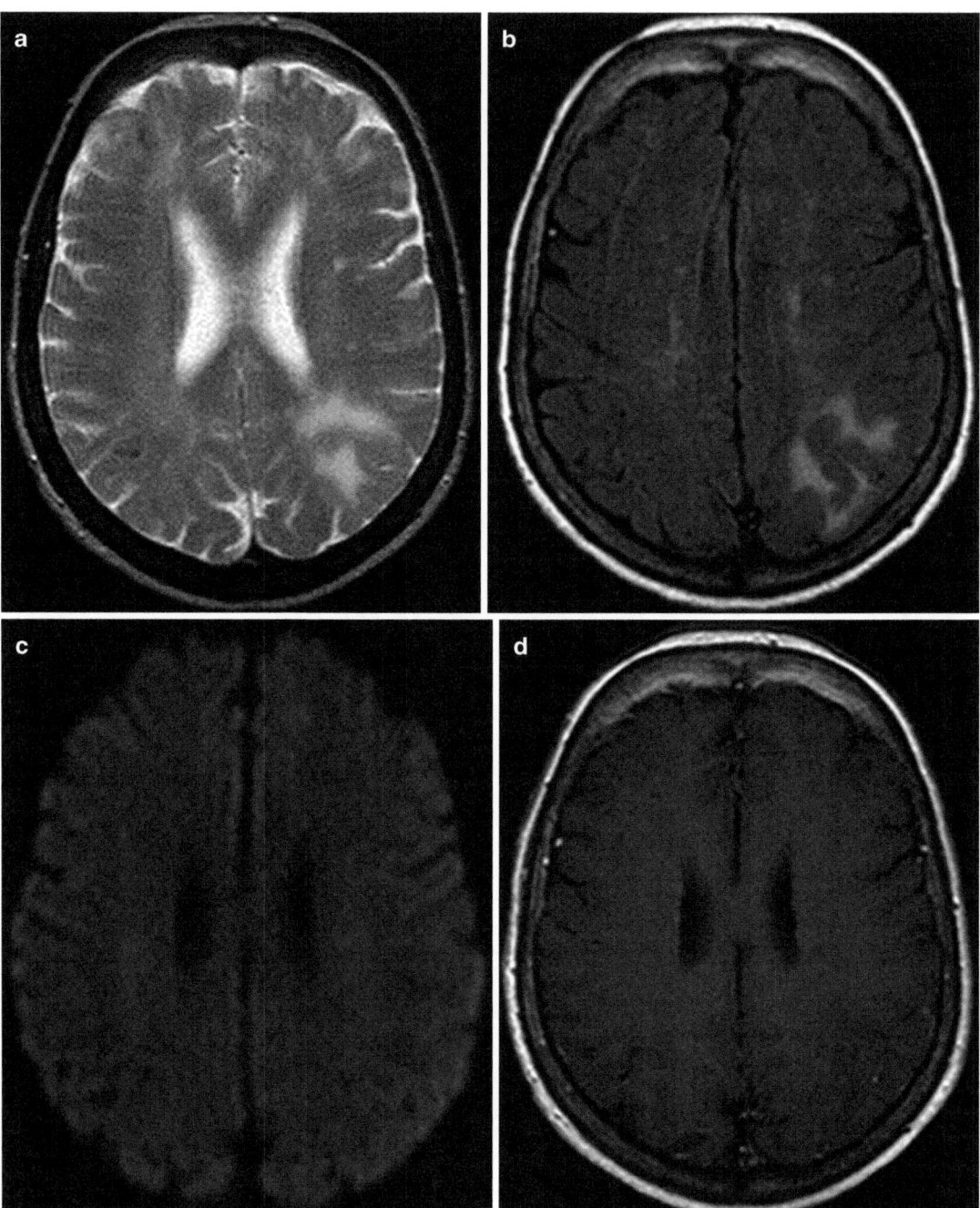

Fig. 4.14 RCVS in patient with thunderclap headache and seizures. Axial SE T2w (**a**) and FLAIR (**b**) sequences show a left parietal subcortical white matter hyperintensity, sparing the cerebral cortex, with no significant alterations on DWI (**c**) and SE T1w + Gd (**d**) sequences. The GRE T2*w sequence helps identify parietal and frontal SAH (**e**)

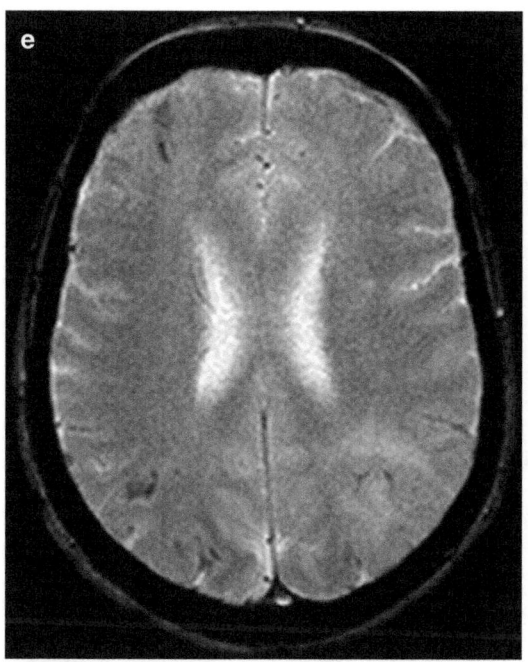

Fig. 4.14 (continued)

4.3.2.3 Headache Attributed to Nonvascular Intracranial Disorders

Spontaneous Intracranial Hypotension

Spontaneous intracranial hypotension (IH) occurs as a result of spinal cerebral fluid leak due to iatrogenic, traumatic, or spontaneous causes. Typically IH presents with orthostatic headaches associated with other symptoms such as neck pain, tinnitus, change in hearing, photophobia, and nausea. Some patients however do not present classical symptoms, but show atypical clinical presentation with non-orthostatic headaches or absence of headaches [70]. CT has little diagnostic value although subdural fluid collections or increased tentorial enhancement may be detected [49]. MRI with gadolinium administration has an important role in diagnosis of IH, particularly in atypical clinical presentation. Typical MRI findings of

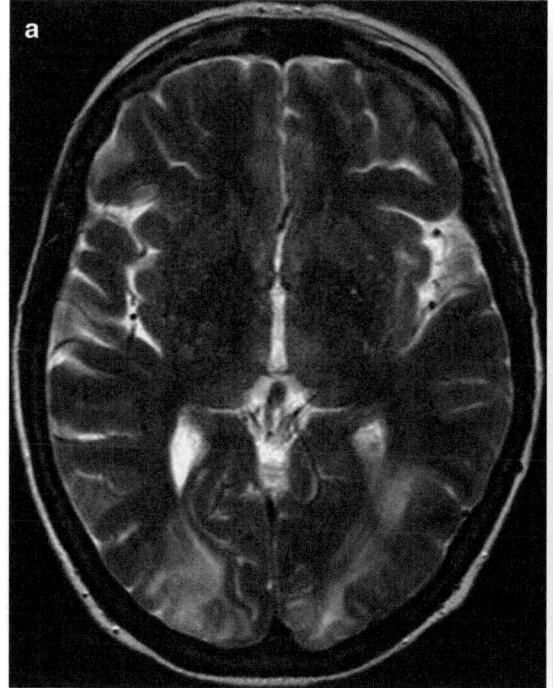

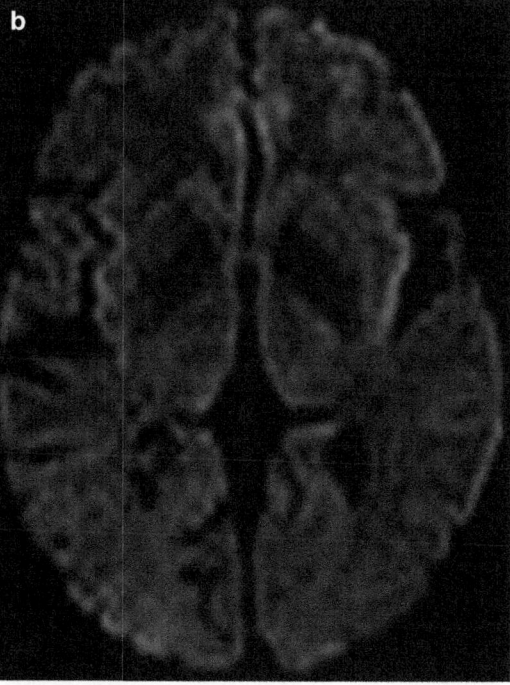

Fig. 4.15 Patient with prolonged severe hypertension and headache—PRESS. Bilateral parieto-occipital cortical-subcortical focal hyperintensities on axial SE T2w images (**a**) with no signal restriction on DWI (**b**). MRI control after 3 weeks (**c**, **d**) shows no focal alterations with complete resolution of the previous findings

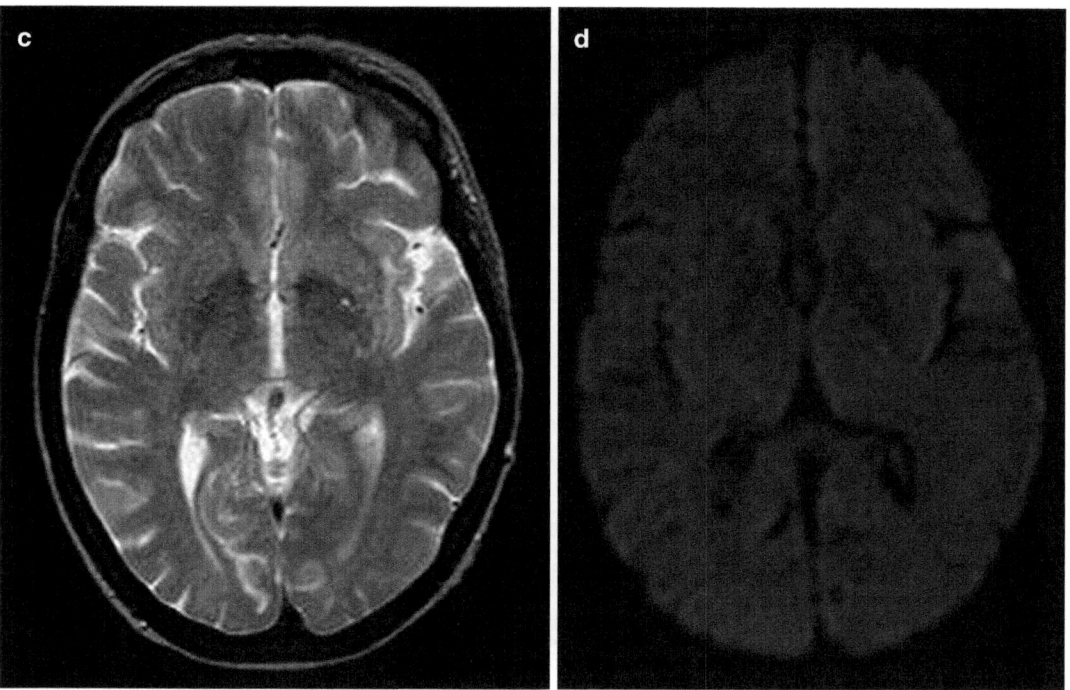

Fig. 4.15 (continued)

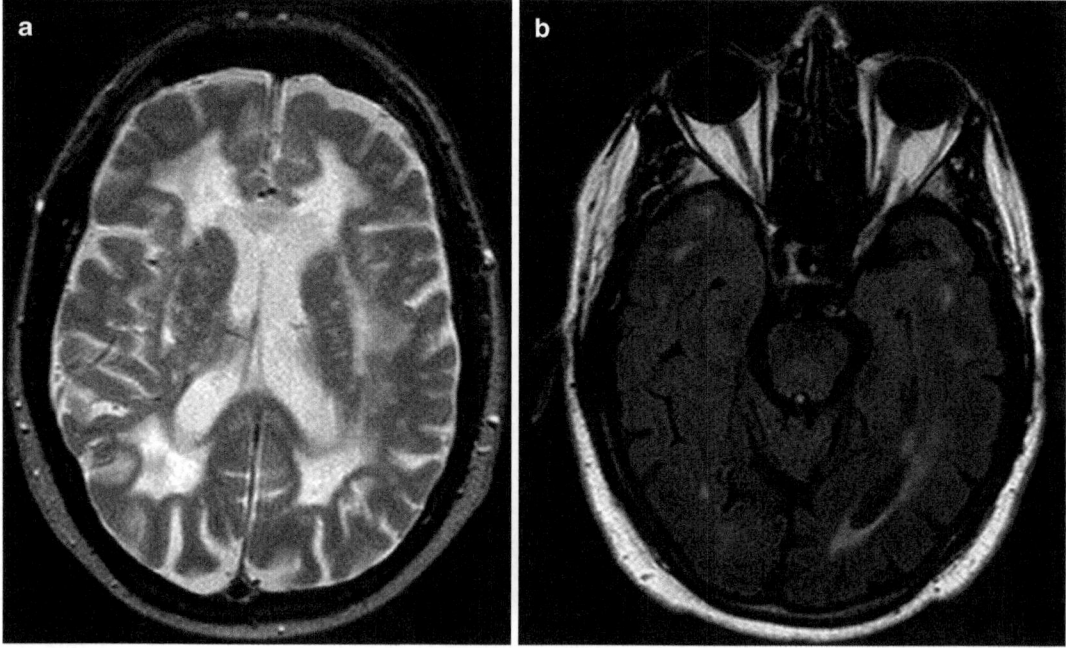

Fig. 4.16 Recurrent headache and stroke episodes in patients with CADASIL. Large, confluent, symmetrical subcortical white matter hyperintensities on SE T2w (**a**) and FLAIR (**b**) sequences, with involvement of the external capsule and the anterior temporal poles

IH include diffuse, non-nodular, pachymeningeal enhancement, engorgement and enhancement of cerebral venous sinuses, and pituitary gland enlargement. Coronal and sagittal images may show downward displacement of the brain, tonsillar herniation, flattening of the pons and optic chiasm, and decreased size of subarachnoid cisterns [49, 70]. Subdural fluid collections may be present as a late finding of untreated IH; when moderate or large in size, there can be secondary hemorrhage causing subdural hematomas because of stretching and rupture of bridging veins [70]. Spine abnormalities associated with IH can be detected with MRI, and they include extra-arachnoid fluid collections, spinal meningeal enhancement, engorgement of epidural venous plexus, and intradural spinal veins [70, 71]. A coronal MR myelography has been recommended for detecting the leakage of CSF as a first-choice modality, followed by axial MRI and if necessary CT myelography [70] (Fig. 4.17).

Increased Cerebrospinal Fluid Pressure

CSF circulatory dysfunction can likewise be a source of headache. A particular form of this is the cerebral pseudotumor, which can arise as a primary disorder (idiopathic intracranial hypertension) or from secondary causes such as exogenous agents or venous sinus thrombosis [49].

The most common diagnostic sign is papilledema on the fundoscopic exam. Visual acuity and visual fields using perimetry need to be documented on these patients because of the potential for visual loss. A lumbar puncture opening pressure of at least 259 mm supports the diagnosis of pseudotumor cerebri syndrome [49].

CT or MRI of the brain is required prior to performing the diagnostic lumbar puncture to rule out a space-occupying lesion. CT should be normal and without evidence of intracranial mass or hydrocephalus.

MRI is the examination of choice to help support the diagnosis. Typical imaging findings are flattening of the papilla in axial T2w images as well

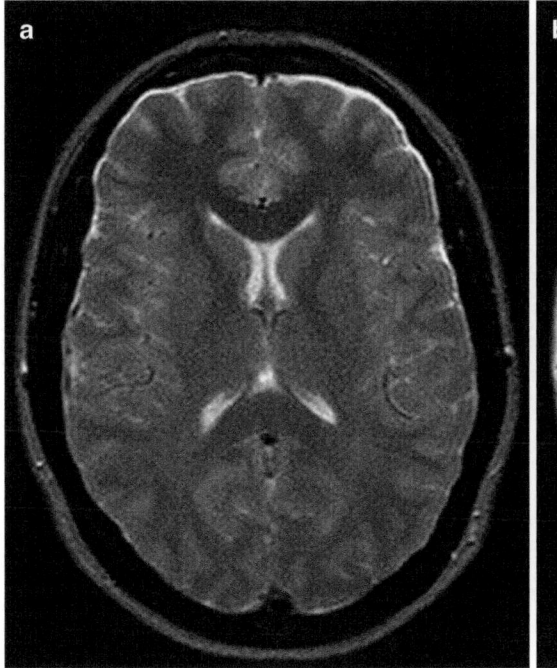
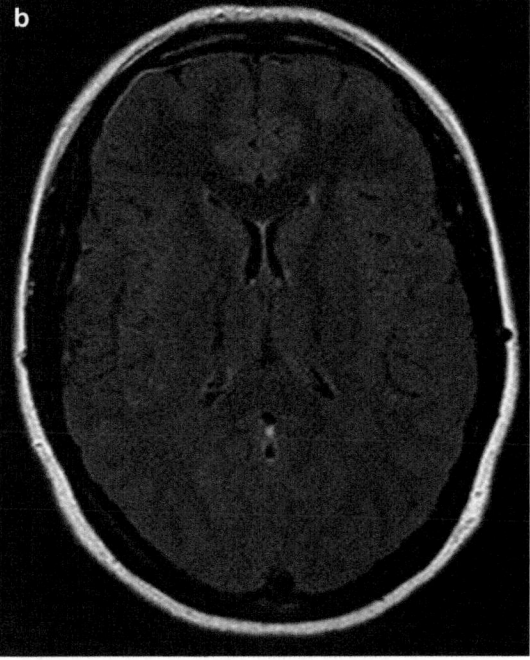
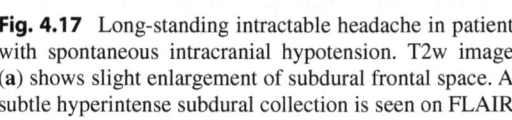

Fig. 4.17 Long-standing intractable headache in patient with spontaneous intracranial hypotension. T2w image (**a**) shows slight enlargement of subdural frontal space. A subtle hyperintense subdural collection is seen on FLAIR image (**b**) and diffuse thickening and pachymeningeal enhancement is seen on T1w image after contrast media (**c**). Myelo-RM (**d**, **e**) well demonstrates spontaneous CSF leakage at the level of C2–C3

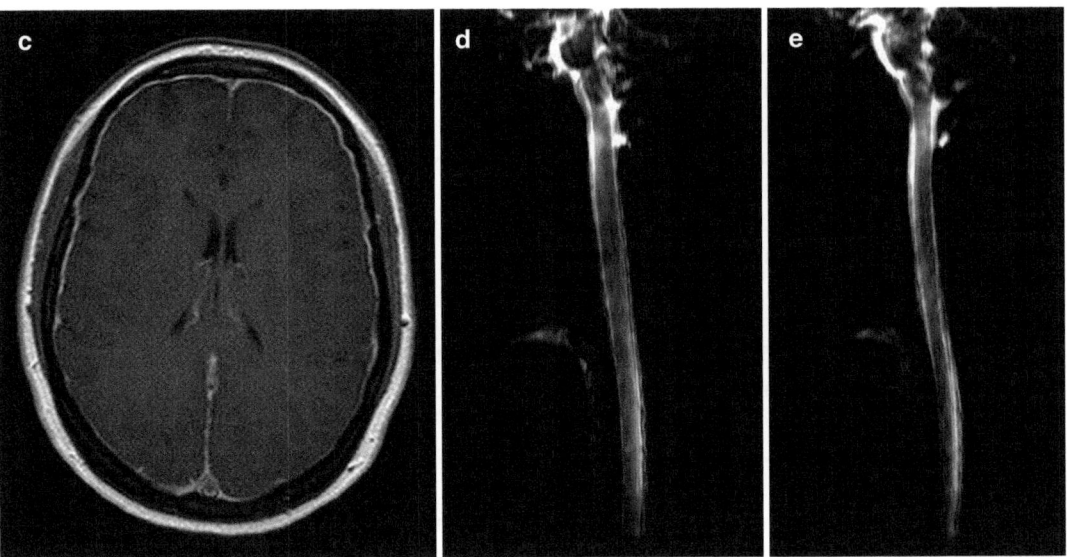

Fig. 4.17 (continued)

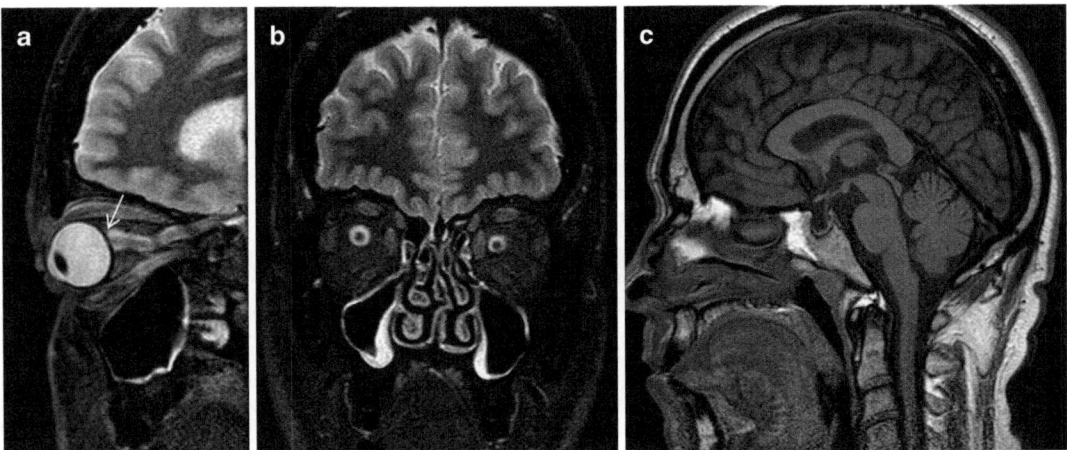

Fig. 4.18 Intracranial hypertension and headache. Sagittal (**a**) and coronal (**b**) STIR images and sagittal SE T1-weighted image (**c**) show flattened posterior sclera (arrow) (**a**), prominent subarachnoid space around the optic nerve (**b**), and partial empty sella (**c**)

as a gyrose optic nerve. Coronal images reveal an enhancement of the optic nerve sheath; this phenomenon can be easily assessed using T2w images with fat saturation. Additionally, sagittal views frequently reveal that the pituitary gland is flattened (so-called empty sella syndrome) or tonsillar descent (Fig. 4.18). Venous angiography frequently reveals stenosis in the transverse sinus [72].

Intracranial Neoplasia

Headaches caused by brain tumors have been classically described as severe, early morning, or nocturnal headaches associated with nausea and vomiting. In these types of patients, headache has developed in temporal relation to the intracranial neoplasia or let to its discovery. It usually significantly worsens in parallel with worsening of the intracranial neoplasia and may significantly improve in temporal relation to the successful treatment of the neoplasia [2]. However, several studies have shown that headaches arising from brain tumors can present with the same phenotype as primary headache disorders such as migraine or tension-type headaches. Most patients have atypical features, and only 17% of patients fit the classic brain tumor headache descriptions [73].

Imaging, both CT and MRI, rules out space-occupying lesions or hydrocephalus. MRI, however, is more sensible than CT for the detection and evaluation of the extension of the tumor. This is particularly true for some brain regions (such as sellar, auditory canal, etc.) or meningeal pathology (Fig. 4.19). A particular case of tumor, which causes headache, is the *colloid cyst*. This is a protein-rich cyst of the roof of the third ventricle emanating from the endoderm [74]. Colloid cysts can be an incidental finding in cranial imaging or can manifest themselves with headaches. Headaches arising from a colloid cyst of the third ventricle are often thunderclap and recurrent. Headaches

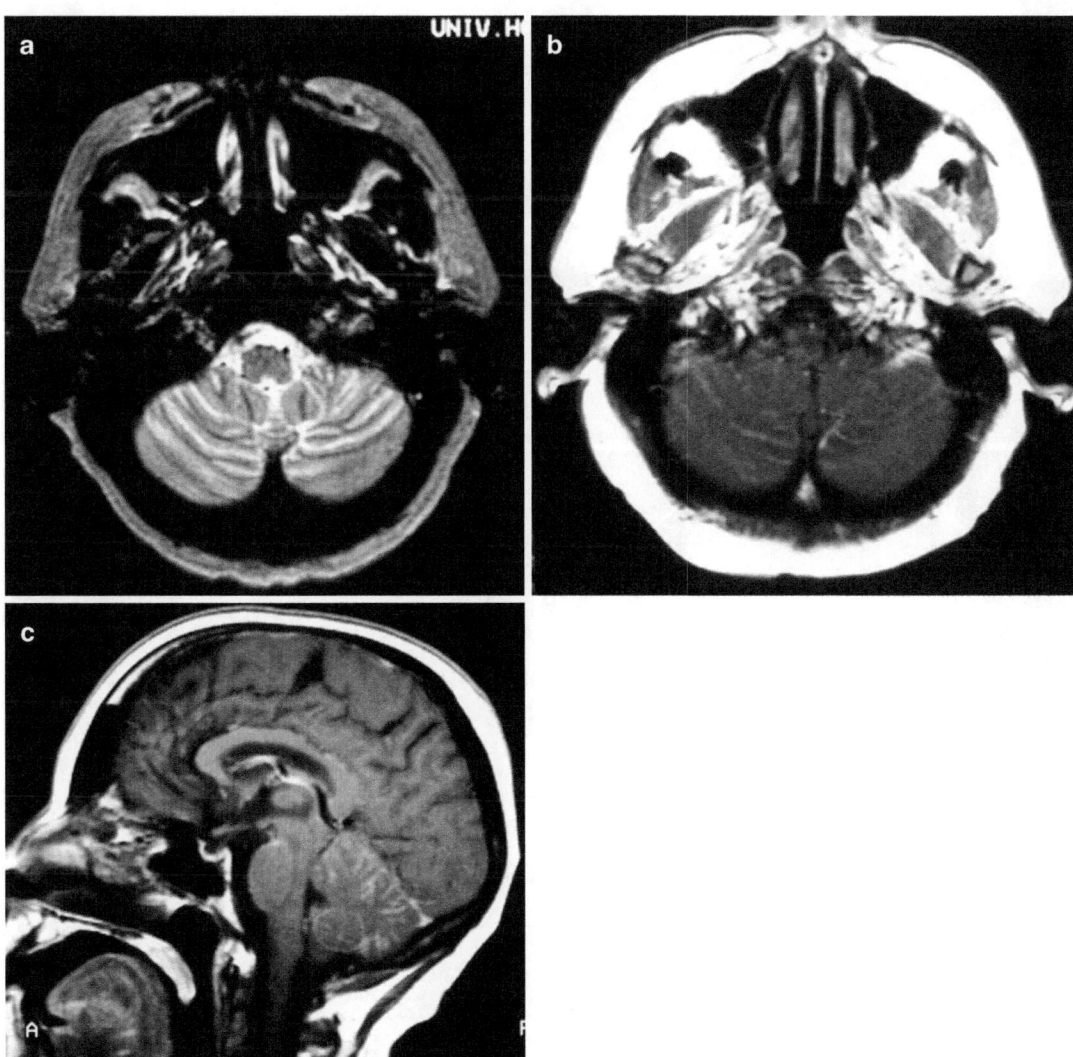

Fig. 4.19 Carcinomatous meningitis—intractable headache in patient with previous breast cancer. Axial SE T2w image (**a**), axial and sagittal SE T1w image after Gd (**b, c**): mild enlargement of the cerebellar sulci on T2W images (**a**) and diffuse leptomeningeal enhancement on T1W images after CM (**b, c**)

may improve in the supine position and are often located in the bilateral frontoparietal or fronto-occipital regions. The cyst may cause obstructive hydrocephalus as it is located close to the foramen of Monro. There are no restricted diffusion and hyperintensity seen on FLAIR sequences. On T1-weighted images, the central portion of the mass is hyperintense, whereas the periphery is isointense. The central portion is markedly hypointense, while the peripheral portion is isointense in T2-weighted images [75] (Fig. 4.20).

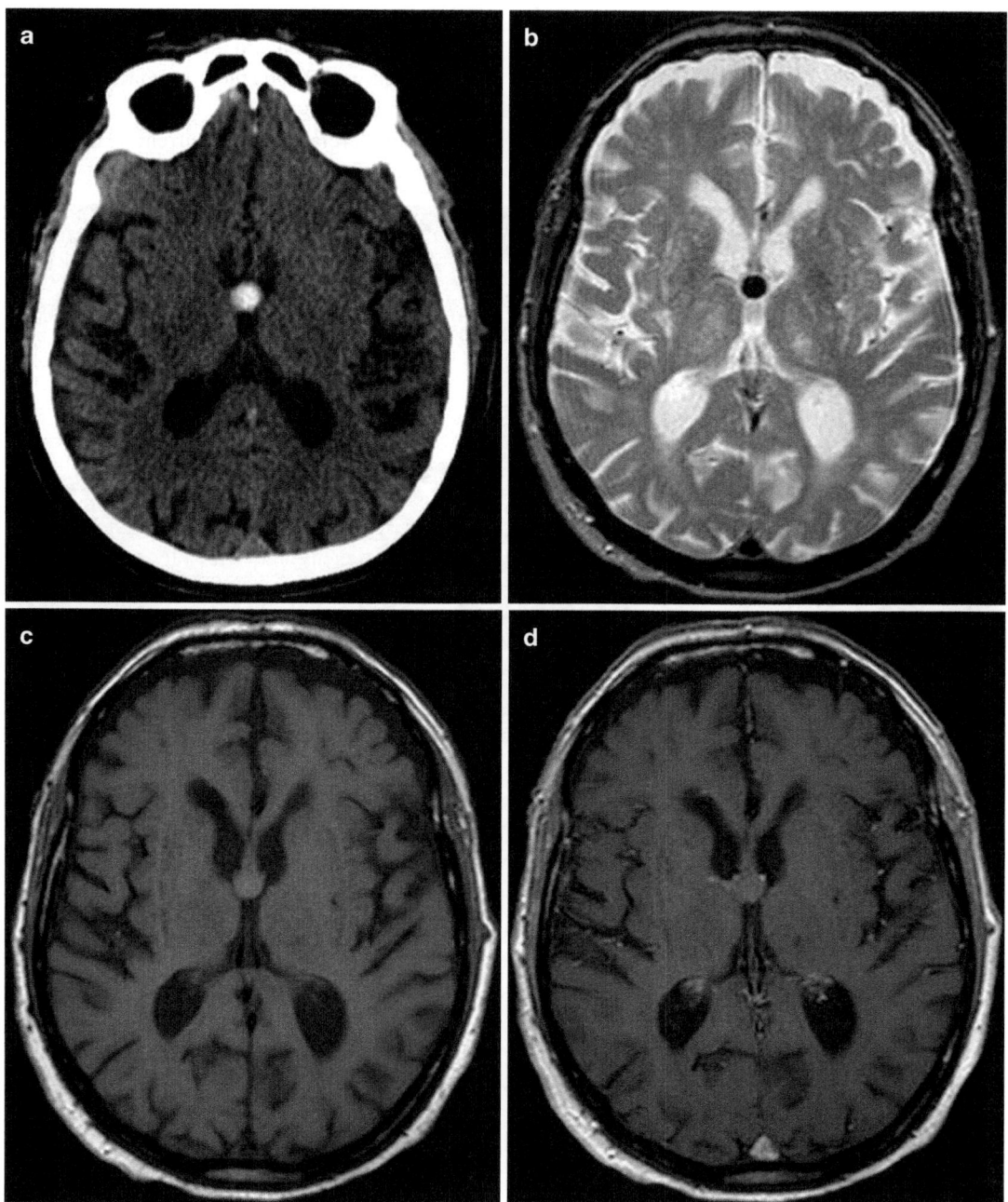

Fig. 4.20 Colloid cyst in patient with positional headache. Hyperdense cyst in the third ventricle at the level of Monro foramen is visible on axial CT scan (**a**). It appears hypointense on axial SE T2w sequence (**b**) and hyperintense on axial SE T1w sequence (**c**) and does not enhance after Gd administration on SE T1 sequences (**d**)

Chiari Malformation Type I

Chiari malformation type I (CM1) headaches are often precipitated by cough or Valsalva maneuver. There may be associated symptoms of brain stem, cerebellar, or cervical dysfunction. The associated headaches are occipital or suboccipital and generally last longer than primary cough headaches which last several seconds to a few minutes (although some patients experience mild to moderate headache for 2 h) [2]. MRI is required for the diagnosis to obtain detailed sagittal images. Brain MRI shows at least 5 mm of caudal descent of the cerebellar tonsils which appear "peglike" and pointed. Other MRI findings include crowding of subarachnoid space at craniocervical junction and kinking of the medullary cervical junction and brain stem [76]. Tonsillar herniation of less than 5 mm does not exclude the diagnosis, if other features on brain MRI are present and patient is symptomatic. Asymptomatic tonsillar ectopia may be differentiated from symptomatic CM1 using CSF flow studies. An abnormal CSF flow pattern is seen in CM1 [77]. A spinal MRI is necessary to look for syringomyelia which may be seen in 40% of the patients, commonly located between the C4 and C6 levels [78]. Tonsillar ectopia may also be caused by disorders producing high and low CSF pressure, including mass lesions, which are distinct from a true Chiari malformation (Fig. 4.21).

4.3.2.4 Headache Attributed to Intracranial Infection

In cases of cerebral infections, these can be focal (i.e., abscess) or diffuse. In the latter situation, a distinction can be made between inflammation of the cerebral parenchyma (encephalitis) and cerebral membranes (meningitis).

The guiding symptoms of intracranial infection are headache and fever. Depending on the site and extent of the infection, additional neurological symptoms, including death, may occur.

Particular attention, however, should be paid to immune system-compromised and HIV-positive patients [79]. Intracranial pathology is found in cases of new-onset headache in up to 82% of these patients [80, 81]. Therefore cerebral imaging should be performed after new-onset

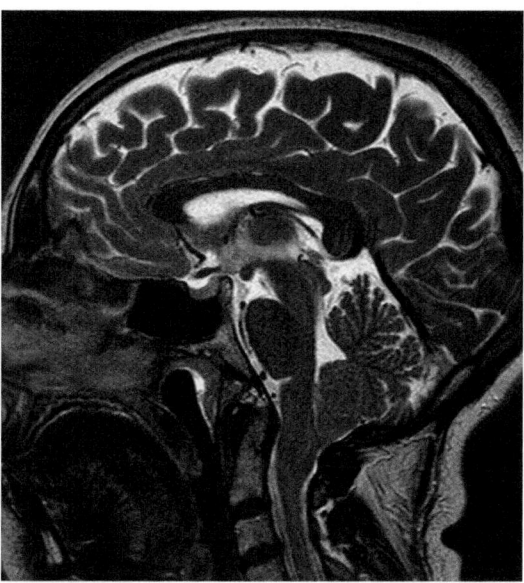

Fig. 4.21 Arnold-Chiari type I and headache. Sagittal T2w image: caudal descent of cerebellar tonsils. Narrowing of subarachnoid space at craniocervical junction

headache or if existing symptoms change in type or intensity.

Meningitis is a clinical diagnosis supported by testing cerebrospinal fluid. The use of imaging therefore is to exclude contraindications for a lumbar puncture [82]. Performing non-enhanced CT is sufficient here. In cases of bacterial meningitis and in those with unfavorable progression of the disease, CT or MRI with contrast media should be performed (Fig. 4.22).

If encephalitis is suspected, an MRI should be performed. Inflammatory changes appear as hyperintense signal alterations in FLAIR images and in diffusion-weighted images can be distinguished earlier as hyperintense signal alteration. Administration of contrast agent is required, and contrast-enhanced images should be acquired on at least two planes.

4.3.2.5 Painful Cranial Neuropathies and Other Facial Pains

Glossopharyngeal Neuralgia

Glossopharyngeal neuralgia (GN) is an uncommon facial pain syndrome and is often misdiagnosed as trigeminal neuralgia. Generally, GN is

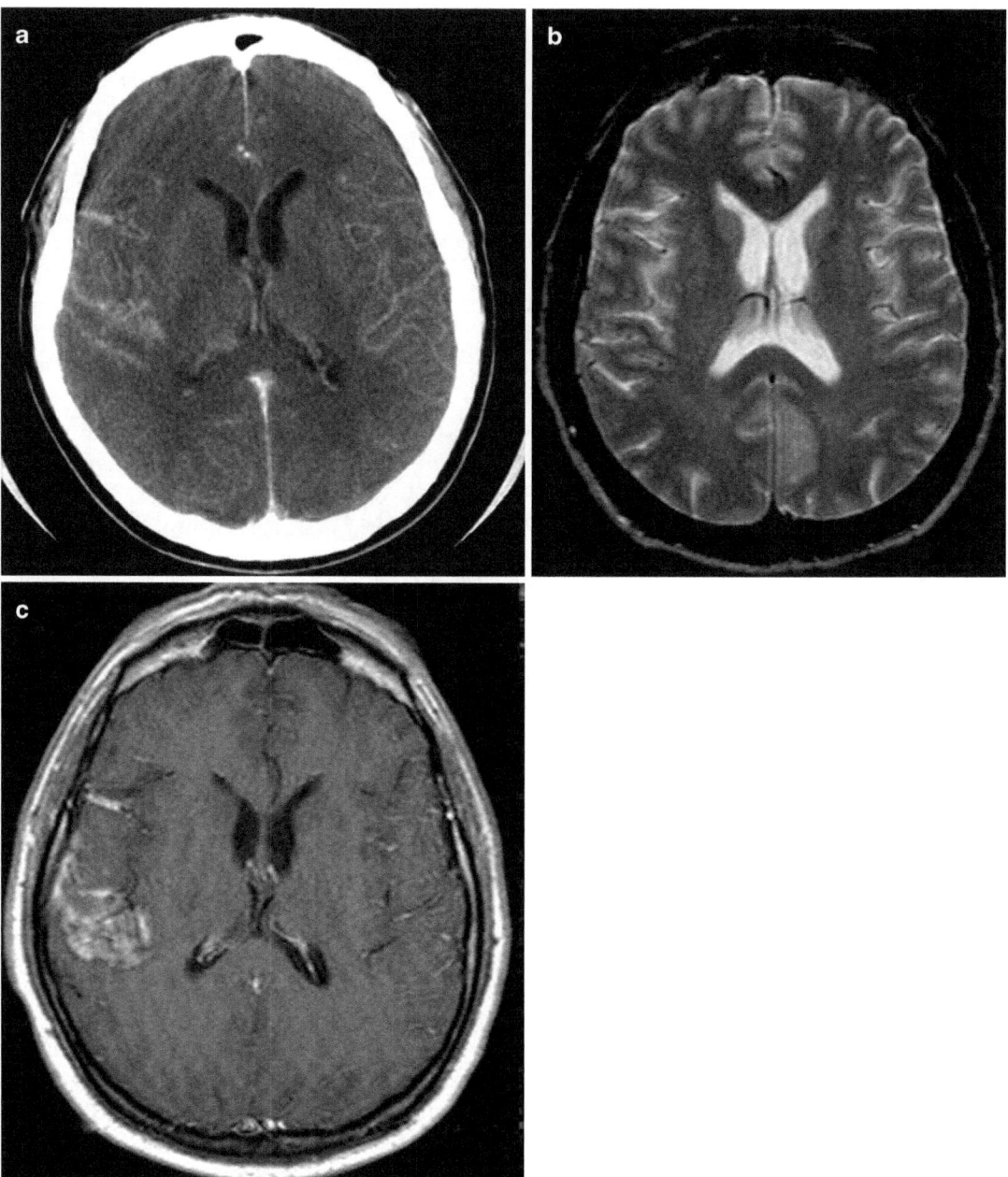

Fig. 4.22 TBC meningitis in patient with headache and subtle left hemiparesis. CT scan after CM (**a**), SE T2-weighted image (**b**), SE T1w image after CM (**c**). Meningeal thickening and enhancement at the level of right insula is demonstrated both in CT (**a**) and T1W image after contrast media administration (**c**). No clear pathologic sign is shown on T2w image (**b**)

caused by neurovascular compression, while trauma, neoplasms, infection, or an elongated styloid process represent only a minor percentage. Imaging of the neck is necessary to exclude a neoplasm of the hypopharynx, larynx, or piriform sinus or an elongated styloid process (Fig. 4.23). MRI is the exam of choice to rule out the presence of a neurovascular compression: the

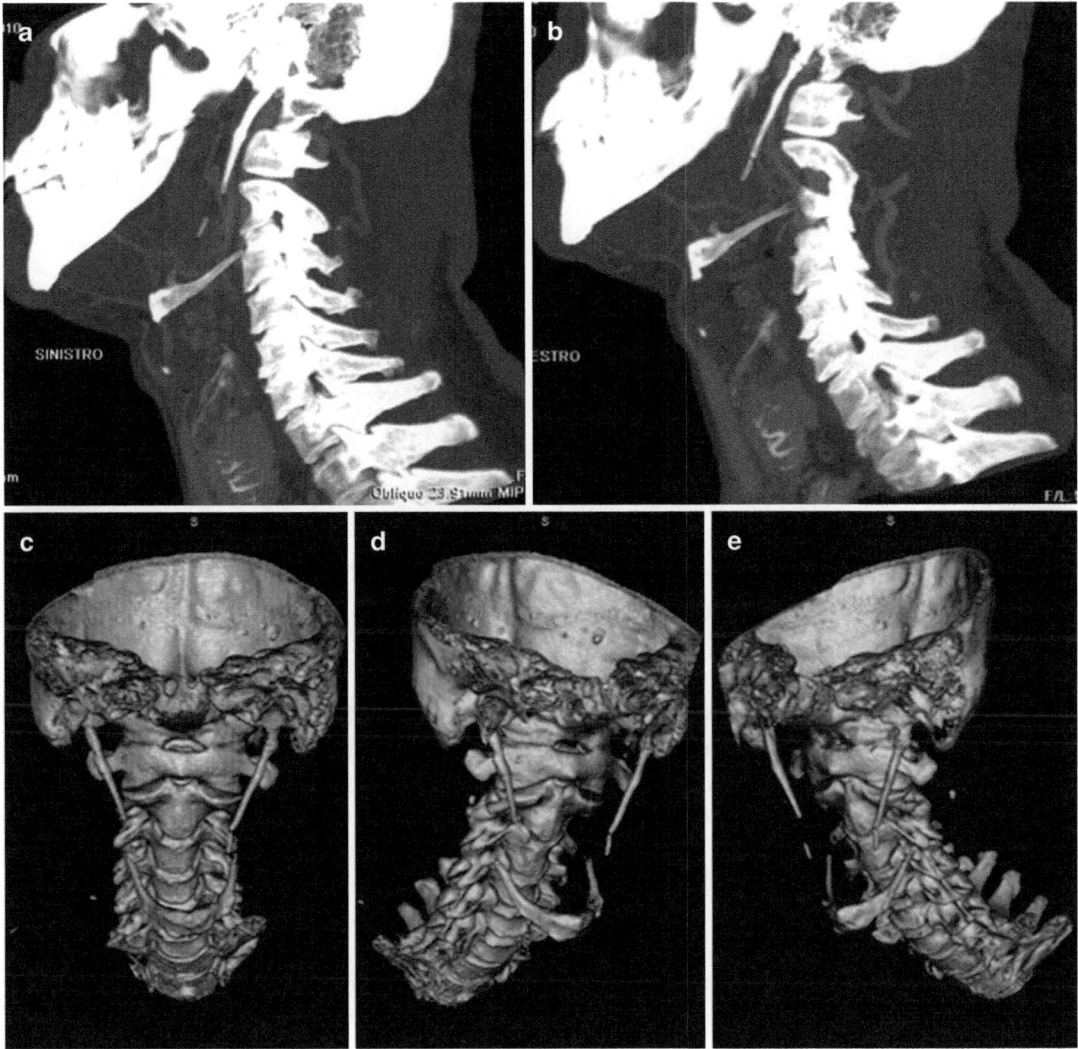

Fig. 4.23 Eagle syndrome in patient with parapharyngeal chronic pain. CT MIP sagittal (**a, b**) and 3D reconstruction (**c–e**) show an elongated styloid process on the left associated with calcification of stylohyoid ligament

combination of high-resolution 3D T2-weighted imaging with 3D time-of-flight angiography and 3D T1-weighted gadolinium-enhanced sequences is considered the standard of reference for the detection of neurovascular compression and can successfully guide neurosurgical treatment [83]. MRI allows precise assessment of the relationship between the IX nerve and the conflicting artery in the supraolivary fossette, which is the site of origin of the IX nerve; the posterior inferior cerebellar artery and less frequently the anterior inferior cerebellar artery are responsible for nerve compression [83, 84] (Fig. 4.24).

Tolosa-Hunt Syndrome

Tolosa-Hunt syndrome (THS) is a very rare disorder characterized by unilateral orbital pain associated with paresis of one or more of the third, fourth, and/or fifth cranial nerves. It is a benign condition caused by granulomatous inflammation in the cavernous sinus, superior orbital fissure, or both which resolve promptly after corticosteroid treatment [2, 85]. MRI is important to rule out other pathologies of the cavernous sinus such as neoplasms, infections, vascular abnormalities, and venous thrombosis as

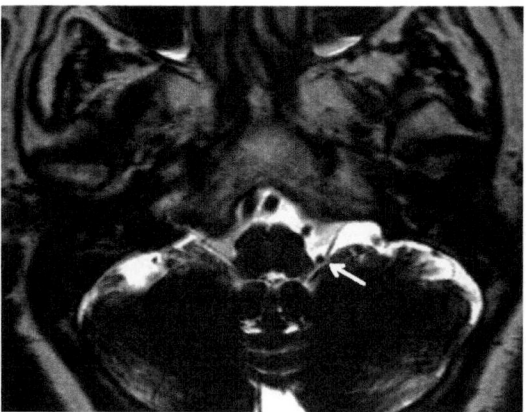

Fig. 4.24 Glossopharyngeal neuralgia—left pharyngeal pain. 3D TSE T2-weighted image: left glossopharyngeal nerve in contact with left PICA at supraolivary fossette (arrow)

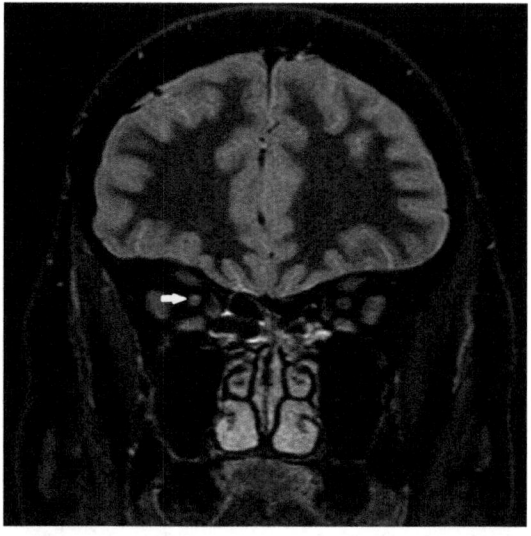

Fig. 4.25 Optic neuritis in patient with visual lost and orbital pain. Coronal STIR demonstrates hyperintensity of the right optic nerve

the cause of symptoms. Typical MRI findings in THS include enlargement of the cavernous sinus due to soft tissue extending through the superior orbital fissure into the orbital apex. The soft tissue lesion shows isointense signal intensity on T1w and iso-hypointense signal intensity on T2w sequences with enhancement after contrast media injection. The follow-up MRI after corticosteroid therapy shows resolution of radiological findings which supports the diagnosis and also identifies the relapse early [85–87].

Optic Neuritis

Optic neuritis (ON) is characterized by unilateral or bilateral pain localized in retro-orbital, orbital, frontal, and/or temporal regions, aggravated by eye movement and accompanied by impairment of central vision [2]. The optic nerve is not well characterized on conventional brain MRI sequences because of its small size and surrounding orbital fat; therefore an orbital MRI protocol is used, with T1 and T2 sequences obtained before and after gadolinium injection and with fat suppression sequences since the orbital portion of the optic nerve is surrounded by fat (Fig. 4.25). ON is a common presentation of multiple sclerosis (MS) in approximately 20% of patients: common imaging features in MS-ON are a short involvement of the optic nerves, often unilaterally [88, 89]. Otherwise, a

unilateral or bilateral long involvement of the posterior aspects of the nerve and/or chiasma may suggest the presence of a neuromyelitis optica spectrum disorder (NMOSD), in accordance to other clinical, serological, and neuroimaging features [89]. A diagnosis of NMOSD should be kept in mind in more severe ON, usually involving optic nerves bilaterally, with positivity of serum anti-aquaporin 4 autoantibody (anti-AQP4 Ab) and in patients with associated acute transverse myelitis, mostly longitudinally extended (with three or more vertebral segments involved), with central cord involvement, cord expansion, and T1 hypointensity during the acute phase [89].

References

1. Douglas AC, Wippold FJ, Broderick DF, Aiken AH, Amin-Hanjani S, Brown DC, et al. ACR appropriateness criteria headache. J Am Coll Radiol. 2014;11(7):657–67.
2. Olesen J. The international classification of headache disorders, 3rd edition. Cephalagia. 2013;33(9):629–808.
3. Vetvik KG, MacGregor EA. Sex differences in the epidemiology, clinical features, and pathophysiology of migraine. Lancet Neurol. 2017;16(1):76–87.

4. Blau J. Migraine: clinical and research aspects. Baltimore: Johns Hopkins University Press; 1987. p. 695.

5. Schoenen J, Sándor PS. Headache with focal neurological signs or symptoms: a complicated differential diagnosis. Lancet Neurol. 2004;3(4):237–45.

6. Cooney BS, Grossman RI, Farber RE, Goin JE, Galetta SL. Frequency of magnetic resonance imaging abnormalities in patients with migraine. Headache. 1996;36(10):616–21.

7. Kamson DO, Illés Z, Aradi M, Orsi G, Perlaki G, Leél-Ssy E, et al. Volumetric comparisons of supratentorial white matter hyperintensities on FLAIR MRI in patients with migraine and multiple sclerosis. J Clin Neurosci. 2012;19(5):696–701.

8. Sher A, Gudmundsson L, Sigurdsson S, Ghambaryan A, Aspelund T, Eiriksdottir G, et al. Migraine headache in middle age and late-life brain infarcts: the age gene/environment susceptibility—Reykjavik study. JAMA. 2009;301(24):2563–70.

9. Kurth T, Mohamed S, Maillard P, Zhu Y-C, Chabriat H, Mazoyer B, et al. Headache, migraine, and structural brain lesions and function: population based epidemiology of vascular ageing-MRI study. BMJ. 2011;342:c7357.

10. Kruit MC, Van Buchem MA, Launer LJ, Terwindt GM, Ferrari MD. Migraine is associated with an increased risk of deep white matter lesions, subclinical posterior circulation infarcts and brain iron accumulation: the population-based MRI CAMERA study. Cephalalgia. 2010;30(2):129–36.

11. Uggetti C, Squarza S, Longaretti F, Galli A, Di Fiore P, Reganati PF, et al. Migraine with aura and white matter lesions: an MRI study. Neurol Sci. 2017;38:11–3.

12. Lin FY, Yang CY. Reversible splenial lesion of the corpus callosum in migraine with aura. Neurologist. 2011;17(3):157–9.

13. Sanchez Del Rio M, Bakker D, Wu O, Agosti R, Mitsikostas DD, Østergaard L, et al. Perfusion weighted imaging during migraine: spontaneous visual aura and headache. Cephalalgia. 1999;19(8):701–7.

14. Baron J. Stroke: imaging and differential diagnosis. J Neural Transm Suppl. 2002;63:19–36.

15. Cheng M, Wu Y, Tang S. Cerebral perfusion changes in hemiplegic migraine: illustrated by Tc-99m ECD brain perfusion scan. Clin Nucl Med. 2010;35(6):456–8.

16. Linn J, Freilinger T, Morhard D, Brückmann H, Straube A. Aphasic migraineous aura with left parietal hypoperfusion: a case report. Cephalalgia. 2007;27(7):850–3.

17. Relja G, Granato A, Ukmar M, Ferretti G, Antonello RM, Zorzon M. Persistent aura without infarction: description of the first case studied with both brain SPECT and perfusion MRI. Cephalalgia. 2005;25(1):56–9.

18. Yamada K, Harada M, Inoue N, Yoshida S, Morioka M, Kuratsu JI. Concurrent hemichorea and migrainous aura—a perfusion study on the basal ganglia using xenon-computed tomography. Mov Disord. 2008;23(3):425–9.

19. Kato Y, Araki N, Matsuda H, Ito Y, Suzuki C. Arterial spin-labeled MRI study of migraine attacks treated with rizatriptan. J Headache Pain. 2010;11(3):255–8.

20. Floery D, Vosko MR, Fellner FA, Fellner C, Ginthoer C, Gruber F, et al. Acute-onset migrainous aura mimicking acute stroke: MR perfusion imaging features. AJNR Am J Neuroradiol. 2012;33(8):1546–52.

21. Resnick S, Reyes-Iglesias Y, Carreras R, Villalobos E. Migraine with aura associated with reversible MRI abnormalities. Neurology. 2006;66(6):946–7.

22. Shah L, Rana S, Valeriano J, Scott TF. Reversible CT perfusion abnormalities in patient with migraine variant: a two phase process. Clin Neurol Neurosurg. 2013;115(6):830–2.

23. Hansen JM, Schytz HW, Larsen VA, Iversen HK, Ashina M. Hemiplegic migraine aura begins with cerebral hypoperfusion: imaging in the acute phase. Headache. 2011;51(8):1289–96.

24. Lykke Thomsen L, Kirchmann Eriksen M, Faerch Romer S, Andersen I, Ostergaard E, Keiding N, et al. An epidemiological survey of hemiplegic migraine. Cephalalgia. 2002;22:361–75.

25. Welch KM. Contemporary concepts of migraine pathogenesis. Neurology. 2003;61(8 Suppl 4):S2–8.

26. Cha YH, Millett D, Kane M, Jen J, Baloh R. Adult-onset hemiplegic migraine with cortical enhancement and oedema. Cephalalgia. 2007;27(10):1166–70.

27. Dreier JP, Jurkat-Rott K, Petzold GG, Tomkins O, Klingebiel R, Kopp UA, et al. Opening of the blood-brain barrier preceding cortical edema in a severe attack of FHM type II. Neurology. 2005;64(12):2145–7.

28. Pelzer N, Hoogeveen ES, Ferrari MD, Poll-The BT, Kruit MC, Terwindt GM. Brain atrophy following hemiplegic migraine attacks. Cephalalgia. 2017;38:1199.

29. Codeluppi L, Bonifacio G, Chiari A, Ariatti A, Nichelli PF. Optic nerve involvement in retinal migraine. Headache. 2015;55(4):562–4.

30. Bigal ME, Serrano D, Buse D, Scher A, Stewart WF, Lipton RB. Acute migraine medications and evolution from episodic to chronic migraine: a longitudinal population-based study. Headache. 2008;48(8):1157–68.

31. Scher AI, Stewart WF, Ricci JA, Lipton RB. Factors associated with the onset and remission of chronic daily headache in a population-based study. Pain. 2003;106(1-2):81–9.

32. Neeb L, Bastian K, Villringer K, Israel H, Reuter U, Fiebach JB. Structural gray matter alterations in chronic migraine: implications for a progressive disease? Headache. 2017;57(3):400–16.

33. Kittner SJ, Stern BJ, Wozniak M, Buchholz DW, Earley CJ, Feeser BR, et al. Cerebral infarction in young adults: the Baltimore-Washington Cooperative Young Stroke Study. Neurology. 1998;50:890–4.

34. Sacquegna T, Baldrati A, Lamieri C, Guttmann S, De Carolis P, Lugaresi E, et al. Ischemic stroke in young adults: the relevance of migrainous infarction. Cephalalgia. 1989;9(4):255–8.

35. Arboix A, Massons J, García-Eroles L, Oliveres M, Balcells M, Targa C. Migrainous cerebral infarction in the Sagrat Cor Hospital of Barcelona stroke registry. Cephalalgia. 2003;23(5):389–94.
36. Swartz RH, Kern RZ. Migraine is associated with magnetic resonance imaging white matter abnormalities: a meta-analysis. Arch Neurol. 2004;61(9):1366–8.
37. Kruit MC. Migraine as a risk factor for subclinical brain lesions. JAMA. 2004;291(4):427.
38. Gass A, Ay H, Szabo K, Koroshetz WJ. Diffusion-weighted MRI for the "small stuff": the details of acute cerebral ischaemia. Lancet Neurol. 2004;3(1):39–45.
39. Fiebach J, Jansen O, Schellinger P, Knauth M, Hartmann M, Heiland S, et al. Comparison of CT with diffusion-weighted MRI in patients with hyperacute stroke. Neuroradiology. 2001;43(8):628–32.
40. Ay H, Buonanno FS, Rordorf G, Schaefer PW, Schwamm LH, Wu O, et al. Normal diffusion-weighted MRI during stroke-like deficits. Neurology. 1999;52(9):1784–92.
41. Mitsikostas DD, Ashina M, Craven A, Diener HC, Goadsby PJ, Ferrari MD, et al. European headache federation consensus on technical investigation for primary headache disorders. J Headache Pain. 2015;17(1):5.
42. Wang P, Du H, Chen N, Guo J, Gong Q, Zhang J, et al. Regional homogeneity abnormalities in patients with tensiontype headache: a resting-state fMRI study. Neurosci Bull. 2014;30(6):949–55.
43. Chen B, He Y, Xia L, Guo L-L, Zheng J-L. Cortical plasticity between the pain and pain-free phases in patients with episodic tension-type headache. J Headache Pain. 2016;17(1):105.
44. Holle D, Obermann M. The role of neuroimaging in the diagnosis of headache disorders. Ther Adv Neurol Disord. 2013;6:369–74.
45. de Coo IF, Wilbrink LA, Haan J. Symptomatic trigeminal autonomic cephalalgias. Curr Pain Headache Rep. 2015;19(8):39.
46. May A. New insights into headache: an update on functional and structural imaging findings. Nat Rev Neurol. 2009;5(4):199–209.
47. Iacovelli E, Coppola G, Tinelli E, Pierelli F, Bianco F. Neuroimaging in cluster headache and other trigeminal autonomic cephalalgias. J Headache Pain. 2012;13(1):11–20.
48. Naegel S, Holle D, Obermann M. Structural imaging in cluster headache. Curr Pain Headache Rep. 2014;18(5):415.
49. Chaudhry P, Friedman DI. Neuroimaging in secondary headache disorders. Curr Pain Headache Rep. 2015;19(7):1–11.
50. Seifert CL, Schönbach EM, Magon S, Gross E, Zimmer C, Förschler A, et al. Headache in acute ischaemic stroke: a lesion mapping study. Brain. 2016;139(1):217–26.
51. Chen PK, Chiu PY, Tsai IJ, Tseng HP, Chen JR, Yeh SJ, et al. Onset headache predicts good outcome in patients with first-ever ischemic stroke. Stroke. 2013;44(7):1852–8.
52. Verdelho A, Madureira S, Ferro JM, Basile AM, Chabriat H, Erkinjuntti T, et al. Differential impact of cerebral white matter changes, diabetes, hypertension and stroke on cognitive performance among non-disabled elderly. The LADIS study. J Neurol Neurosurg Psychiatry. 2007;78(12):1325–30.
53. Seifert CL, Schönbach EM, Zimmer C, Förschler A, Tölle TR, Feurer R, et al. Association of clinical headache features with stroke location: an MRI voxel-based symptom lesion mapping study. Cephalalgia. 2016;38:283.
54. Mortimer AM, Bradley MD, Stoodley NG, Renowden SA. Thunderclap headache: diagnostic considerations and neuroimaging features. Clin Radiol. 2013;68(3):101–13.
55. De Oliveira Manoel AL, Mansur A, Murphy A, Turkel-Parrella D, Macdonald M, Macdonald RL, et al. Aneurysmal subarachnoid haemorrhage from a neuroimaging perspective. Crit Care. 2014;18(6):557.
56. Li M-H, Li Y, Gu B, Cheng Y, Wang W, Tan H, et al. Accurate diagnosis of small cerebral aneurysms ≤5 mm in diameter with 3.0-T MR angiography. Radiology. 2014;271(2):553–60.
57. Heit JJ, Iv M, Wintermark M. Imaging of intracranial hemorrhage. J Stroke. 2017;19(1):11–27.
58. Lester MS, Liu BP. Imaging in the evaluation of headache. Med Clin North Am. 2013;97(2):243–65.
59. Provenzale JM, Sarikaya B. Comparison of test performance characteristics of MRI, MR angiography, and CT angiography in the diagnosis of carotid and vertebral artery dissection: a review of the medical literature. AJR Am J Roentgenol. 2009;193(4):1167–74.
60. Sadigh G, Mullins ME, Saindane AM. Diagnostic performance of MRI sequences for evaluation of dural venous sinus thrombosis. Am J Roentgenol. 2016;206(6):1298–306.
61. Sari S, Verim S, Hamcan S, Battal B, Akgun V, Akgun H, et al. MRI diagnosis of dural sinus - cortical venous thrombosis: immediate post-contrast 3D GRE T1-weighted imaging versus unenhanced MR venography and conventional MR sequences. Clin Neurol Neurosurg. 2015;134:44–54.
62. Kang JH, Yun TJ, Yoo RE, Yoon BW, Lee AL, Kang KM, et al. Bright sinus appearance on arterial spin labeling MR imaging AIDS to identify cerebral venous thrombosis. Medicine (Baltimore). 2017;96(41):e8244.
63. Velez A, McKinney JS. Reversible cerebral vasoconstriction syndrome: a review of recent research. Curr Neurol Neurosci Rep. 2013;13(1):319.
64. Ioannidis I, Nasis N, Agianniotaki E, Katsouda E, Andreou A. Reversible cerebral vasoconstriction syndrome: treatment with multiple sessions of intra-arterial nimodipine and angioplasty. Interv Neuroradiol. 2012;18(3):297–302.
65. Komatsu T, Kimura T, Yagishita A, Takahashi K, Koide R. A case of reversible cerebral vasoconstriction syndrome presenting with recurrent neurological deficits: evaluation using noninvasive arterial spin labeling MRI. Clin Neurol Neurosurg. 2014;126:96–8.

66. Di Donato I, Bianchi S, De Stefano N, Dichgans M, Dotti MT, Duering M, et al. Cerebral Autosomal Dominant Arteriopathy with Subcortical Infarcts and Leukoencephalopathy (CADASIL) as a model of small vessel disease: update on clinical, diagnostic, and management aspects. BMC Med. 2017;15(1):41.

67. Zhu S, Nahas SJ. CADASIL: imaging characteristics and clinical correlation. Curr Pain Headache Rep. 2016;20(10):57.

68. Viswanathan A, Godin O, Jouvent E, O'Sullivan M, Gschwendtner A, Peters N, et al. Impact of MRI markers in subcortical vascular dementia: a multimodal analysis in CADASIL. Neurobiol Aging. 2010;31(9):1629–36.

69. Mascalchi M, Pantoni L, Giannelli M, Valenti R, Bianchi A, Pracucci G, et al. Diffusion tensor imaging to map brain microstructural changes in CADASIL. J Neuroimaging. 2017;27(1):85–91.

70. Aslan K, Gunbey HP, Tomak L, Ozmen Z, Incesu L. Magnetic resonance imaging of intracranial hypotension. J Comput Assist Tomogr. 2017;0(0):1.

71. Haritanti A, Karacostas D, Drevelengas A, Kanellopoulos V, Paraskevopoulou E, Lefkopoulos A, et al. Spontaneous intracranial hypotension. Clinical and neuroimaging findings in six cases with literature review. Eur J Radiol. 2009;69(2):253–9. https://doi.org/10.1016/j.ejrad.2007.10.013.

72. Langner S, Kirsch M. Radiological diagnosis and differential diagnosis of headache. RöFo. 2015;187(10):879–91.

73. Schankin CJ, Ferrari U, Reinisch VM, Birnbaum T, Goldbrunner R, Straube A. Characteristics of brain tumour-associated headache. Cephalalgia. 2007;27(8):904–11.

74. Osborn AG, Preece MT. Intracranial cysts: radiologic-pathologic correlation and imaging approach. Radiology. 2006;239(3):650–64.

75. Urso JA, Ross GJ, Parker RK, Patrizi JD, Stewart B. Colloid cyst of the third ventricle: radiologic-pathologic correlation. J Comput Assist Tomogr. 1998;22(4):524–7.

76. Amer TA, El-Shmam OM. Chiari malformation type I: a new MRI classification. Magn Reson Imaging. 1997;15(4):397–403.

77. Hofkes SK, Iskandar BJ, Turski PA, Gentry LR, McCue JB, Haughton VM. Differentiation between symptomatic Chiari I malformation and asymptomatic tonsilar ectopia by using cerebrospinal fluid flow imaging: initial estimate of imaging accuracy. Radiology. 2007;245(2):532–40.

78. Elster AD, Chen MY. Chiari I malformations: clinical and radiologic reappraisal. Radiology. 1992;183(2):347–53.

79. Krope K, Speil A, Pantazis G, Nägele T, Horger M. Wertigkeit der MRT in der Diagnostik primärer und sekundärer zerebraler Infektionen. RöFo. 2013;185(6):539–45.

80. Edlow JA, Panagos PD, Godwin SA, Thomas TL, Decker WW. Clinical policy: critical issues in the evaluation and management of adult patients presenting to the emergency department with acute headache. Ann Emerg Med. 2008;52(4):407–36.

81. Joshi SG, Cho TA. Pathophysiological mechanisms of headache in patients with HIV. Headache. 2014;54(5):946–50.

82. van Crevel H, Hijdra A, de Gans J. Lumbar puncture and the risk of herniation: when should we first perform CT? J Neurol. 2002;249(2):129–37.

83. Haller S, Etienne L, Kövari E, Varoquaux AD, Urbach H, Becker M. Imaging of neurovascular compression syndromes: trigeminal neuralgia, hemifacial spasm, vestibular paroxysmia, and glossopharyngeal neuralgia. AJNR Am J Neuroradiol. 2016;37(8):1384–92.

84. Singh P, Trikha A, Kaur M. An uncommonly common: glossopharyngeal neuralgia. Ann Indian Acad Neurol. 2013;16(1):1.

85. Arshad A, Nabi S, Panhwar MS, Rahil A. Tolosa-Hunt syndrome: an arcane pathology of cavernous venous sinus. BMJ Case Rep. 2015;2015:bcr2015210646.

86. Sánchez Vallejo R, Lopez-Rueda A, Olarte AM, San Roman L. MRI findings in Tolosa-Hunt syndrome (THS). BMJ Case Rep. 2014;2014:bcr2014206629.

87. Wani NA, Jehangir M, Lone PA. Tolosa-Hunt syndrome demonstrated by constructive interference steady state magnetic resonance imaging. J Ophthalmic Vis Res. 2017;12(1):106–9.

88. Zabad R, Stewart R, Healey K. Pattern recognition of the multiple sclerosis syndrome. Brain Sci. 2017;7(11):138.

89. Whittam D, Wilson M, Hamid S, Keir G, Bhojak M, Jacob A. What's new in neuromyelitis optica? A short review for the clinical neurologist. J Neurol. 2017;264(11):2330–44.

Trigeminal Nerve: Clinical Features

5

Paolo Manganotti and Antonio Granato

5.1 Introduction

Trigeminal neuralgia (TN) is a distinct, painful disorder of the face that is easily evoked by trivial stimuli and undergoes a relapsing, remitting course. It is also called as trifacial neuralgia, Fothergill's disease, and tic douloureux. The International Headache Society defines TN as "recurrent unilateral brief electric shock-like pains, abrupt in onset and termination, limited to the distribution of one or more divisions of the trigeminal nerve and triggered by innocuous stimuli" [1]. The best indication about the prevalence of TN comes from a study by Penman [2], who in 1969 reported rates of 107.5/1,000,000 in men and 200.2/1,000,000 in women. The annual incidence rates for men and women were 4.67 and 7.15, respectively. The peak TN incidence occurs in the fifth to seventh decade, with 90% of cases beginning after age of 40 and progressively increases with increasing age: from 17.5/100,000/year between 60 and 69 years of age up to 25.6/100,000/year after 70 [3]. The *female-to-male ratio* was 1.74:1 in the Katusic et al. study [3] and 3:2 in another study by Ashkenazi and Levin [4]. Familial cases of TN are very rare but have been reported [3, 5–8]. In these familial cases TN presented earlier in each successive generation.

5.2 Pathophysiology

Although multiple mechanisms involve peripheral pathologies at root (compression or traction), and dysfunctions of brain stem, basal ganglion, and cortical pain modulatory mechanisms could have a role, neurovascular conflict is the most accepted theory [9]. Artery or vein is usually compressing the trigeminal nerve near the pons injuring myelin sheath and causing erratic hyperactive functioning of the nerve [10].

Although it has been generally assumed that vascular contact at the root entry zone (REZ) causes TN, conflict anywhere on the root at central or peripheral myelin, in the region of REZ, or at transition zone between central and peripheral myelin can cause TN [11]. REZ and transition zone between central and peripheral myelin are distinct sites and that these terms should never be used interchangeably. Peripheral myelin is more resistant to compression as compared to central myelin or transition zone [12]. The normal pulsation of artery may not be traumatic [12] enough to produce TN; strokes due to unbending of artery

P. Manganotti (✉)
SC (UCO) Clinica Neurologica, Dipartimento di Scienze Mediche, Chirurgiche e della Salute—Università degli Studi di Trieste, Azienda Sanitaria Universitaria Integrata di Trieste (ASUITS), Trieste, Italy
e-mail: pmanganotti@units.it

A. Granato
SC (UCO) Clinica Neurologica, Azienda Sanitaria Universitaria Integrata di Trieste (ASUITS), Trieste, Italy
e-mail: antonio.granato@asuits.sanita.fvg.it

© Springer Nature Switzerland AG 2019
M. A. Cova, F. Stacul (eds.), *Pain Imaging*, https://doi.org/10.1007/978-3-319-99822-0_5

loop usually cause pathological changes in root [13]. Although displacement or grooving of the nerves has been observed in normal individuals [14], more severe root indentation or distortion in proximal root is likely to produce TN. Arterial compression is commonly seen; venous conflict alone or in combination to arterial compression has been observed in some patients as a cause of TN [15]. Persistent primitive trigeminal artery, its aneurysm, and vertebrobasilar dolichoectasia may cause TN. Sharper trigeminal-pontine angle and smaller cerebellopontine angle cisterns can facilitate the neurovascular compression.

Focal arachnoid thickening, angulation, adhesion, traction, tethering or torsion, fibrous ring around the root, cerebellopontine angle tumors, brain stem infarction, aneurism, and arteriovenous malformation can also cause TN [16].

Central causes of the disease have also been proposed for TN; reduced basal ganglia μ-opioid receptor [17] and altered gray matter in sensory and motor cortex have been implicated [18]. The dysfunction of multiple modulatory mechanisms probably plays a key role in the pathophysiology.

Demyelination, dysmyelination giving increases to electrical hyperexcitability, spontaneous and triggered ectopic impulse, and cross excitation among neighboring afferents have been proposed in ignition hypothesis [19]. According to the bioresonance hypothesis, trigeminal nerve fibers are damaged when the vibration frequency of nerve and surrounding structure becomes close to each other [20]. The brain sagging/arterial elongation hypothesis is also believed to cause nerve compression.

Predisposition to pain of the fifth cranial nerve could be related to familial TN; in particular, genetic influence on vascular growth patterns, membrane stability, and anatomic constraints (narrower middle and anterior cranial fossae) may be involved [8].

Exact pathophysiology of TN remains controversial. Chronic nerve compression results in demyelination, with progressive axonal degeneration in small unmyelinated and thinly myelinated fibers. Demyelination can lead to ephaptic transmission; reentry mechanism causes an amplification of sensory inputs. Ultrastructural and biochemical changes in axon and myelin are not only seen in root but also in Gasserian ganglion or in both the structures [21]. Atrophy of the trigeminal nerve is also seen [22, 23]. The gray matter volume reduction in the primary and secondary somatosensory cortex, orbitofrontal areas, thalamus, insula, anterior cingulate cortex, cerebellum, and dorsolateral prefrontal cortex has been observed [24, 25]. Lower axial kurtosis and higher axial diffusivity in corticospinal tract, superior longitudinal fasciculus, anterior thalamic radiation, inferior longitudinal fasciculus, inferior fronto-occipital fasciculus, cingulated gyrus, forceps major, and uncinate fasciculus were observed. There was complex functional connectivity density reorganization of hippocampus, striatum, thalamus, precentral gyrus, precuneus, prefrontal cortex, and inferior parietal lobule [26]. It is difficult to say whether the changes in cortical and subcortical areas are cause or effect in TN.

5.3 Clinical Features

The current International Classification of Headache Disorders distinguishes the pain attributed to a lesion or disease of the trigeminal nerve in two subforms: *trigeminal neuralgia* (*classical trigeminal neuralgia*, *secondary trigeminal neuralgia*, and *idiopathic trigeminal neuralgia*) and *painful trigeminal neuropathy* (Table 5.1) [1]. The characteristics of TN are neuralgic pain, and they are the same in all three subforms (Table 5.2); on the contrary, characteristics of painful trigeminal neuropathy fulfill criteria for neuropathic pain [1]. Clinical predictors for secondary TN and painful trigeminal neuropathy are shown in Table 5.3 [9].

5.3.1 Trigeminal Neuralgia

Trigeminal neuralgia is characterized by episodes of spontaneous pain or a triggered intense facial pain that last for short duration. Symptoms begin with a modest and occasional neuralgic pain. When the attacks are located at the dental arch,

Table 5.1 Classification of pain attributed to a lesion or disease of the trigeminal nerve (adapted from the International Classification of Headache Disorders 3rd edition) [1]

Trigeminal neuralgia
Classical trigeminal neuralgia
Classical trigeminal neuralgia, purely paroxysmal
Classical trigeminal neuralgia with concomitant continuous pain
Secondary trigeminal neuralgia
Trigeminal neuralgia attributed to multiple sclerosis
Trigeminal neuralgia attributed to space-occupying lesion
Trigeminal neuralgia attributed to other cause
Idiopathic trigeminal neuralgia
Idiopathic trigeminal neuralgia, purely paroxysmal
Idiopathic trigeminal neuralgia with concomitant continuous pain
Painful trigeminal neuropathy
Painful trigeminal neuropathy attributed to herpes zoster
Trigeminal postherpetic neuralgia
Painful post-traumatic trigeminal neuropathy
Painful trigeminal neuropathy attributed to other disorder
Idiopathic painful trigeminal neuropathy

Table 5.2 diagnostic criteria of trigeminal neuralgia (IHS 2018)

A. Recurrent paroxysms of unilateral facial pain in the distribution(s) of one or more divisions of the trigeminal nerve, with no radiation beyond, and fulfilling criteria B and C
B. Pain has all of the following characteristics
1. Lasting from a fraction of a second to 2 min
2. Severe intensity
3. Electric shock-like, shooting, stabbing, or sharp in quality
C. Precipitated by innocuous stimuli within the affected trigeminal distribution
D. Not better accounted for by another ICHD-3 diagnosis

Table 5.3 Clinical predictors for secondary trigeminal neuralgia and painful trigeminal neuropathy

Trigeminal sensory deficits
Bilateral involvement of the trigeminal nerves
Younger age
Predominant continuous pain and rare superimposed brief pain paroxysms
Absence of refractory periods
Unresponsiveness to treatment
Abnormal trigeminal reflexes

they are almost constantly attributed to local pathology, and often this belief leads to unnecessary extractions or dental care. In the first years, the temporal trend is that of remission periods alternating with recrudescence. Quite typically spring and autumn coincide with the upsurge. Over the years, the periods with neuralgic pain become longer and longer, until no more remissions occur.

The pain strictly occurs in one or more division of the trigeminal nerve, with no radiation beyond the trigeminal distribution. Patients have 61% right-sided attacks and 36% left-sided attacks. Most individuals experience pain in the maxillary and mandibular divisions. It occurs much less frequently in the ophthalmic divisions (Table 5.2). Only 4% of trigeminal neuralgia cases are bilateral, and most of these individuals have multiple sclerosis. TN never spreads across the midline, and bilateral cases are never synchronous [27].

The pain comes in repetitive flashes, which may be like stabbing, electric shocks, burning, pressing, crushing, exploding, shooting, boring, shock-like sensations, piercing, prickling, or a combination, lasting from a fraction of a second to 2 min. Between clusters of pain, the patient is usually pain-free (*TN purely paroxysmal*), but a continuous dull aching pain of moderate intensity in the affected area may persist (*TN with concomitant continuous pain*). The patient lives in dread of the future pain. Although a subset of patients can progress from the *purely paroxysmal* to the *continuous pain* form over time, their pathological and prognostic profiles nevertheless resembled those of the *purely paroxysmal* form. Proponents of progressive change in character of pain theory think that the TN, atypical neuralgia, and trigeminal neuropathic pain may represent a continuous spectrum rather than discrete pathology, whereas others believe that *purely paroxysmal* to the *continuous pain* TN represents distinct entities [28]. Pain usually does not occur when the person is asleep.

Trigger zones are very frequent (91%) and can be small as 1–2 mm in diameter. These zones are areas innervated by the trigeminal nerve that when stimulated by non-noxious stimuli cause the onset of flashes of pain. They are usually in the central part of the face around the nose and lips. Daily activities such as eating, talking, yawning, sneezing, coughing, washing the face, and cleaning the teeth can precipitate the electric shocks. Light touch and vibratory stimuli are more effective in eliciting the pain than a pinch or pinprick. The pain intensity is independent of the trigger zone size. In most patients, the pain starts within the trigger zone, but in 5–9% of patients, it occurs outside of it.

Following a painful paroxysm, there is usually a refractory period. Patients find that after a paroxysmal of pain there is a period of time that can last up to several minutes during which stimulation of the trigger zone will not elicit a paroxysmal of pain. The duration of the relative refractory period is usually proportional to the length and severity of prior painful attack.

When very severe, the pain often evokes contraction of the muscle of the face on the affected side (tic douloureux) [29]. Mild autonomic symptoms such as lacrimation and/or redness of the eye may be present. A patient experiencing a TN attack typically freezes in place with the hands slowly rising to the area of pain on the face but not touching it. The patient then grimaces or quirks the face with the tic douloureux and then remains in this position or cries out in pain.

There are no certain data regarding the prognosis of the disease, but common experience suggests that the disorder tends to aggravate and that it responds less and less to the various therapeutic attempts over time.

5.3.2 Classical Trigeminal Neuralgia

The International Headache Society defines classical trigeminal neuralgia as pain fulfilling criteria for TN (Table 5.2) [1], with demonstration on MRI or during surgery of neurovascular compression with morphologic changes in the trigeminal nerve root. Morphologic changes consist in atrophy or displacement. Atrophic changes may include demyelination, neuronal loss, and changes in microvasculature. The simply contact on the root is not sufficient to cause TN. Between paroxysms, most patients are asymptomatic (*classical trigeminal neuralgia, purely paroxysmal*), or less frequently a prolonged background pain in the affected area may persist (*classical trigeminal neuralgia with concomitant continuous pain*).

5.3.3 Secondary Trigeminal Neuralgia

Secondary trigeminal neuralgia is caused by an underlying disease except for neurovascular compression that is able to cause and explain the neuralgia (multiple sclerosis, tumor in the cerebellopontine angle, arteriovenous malformation). Characteristics of pain fulfill criteria for TN (Table 5.2) [1]. Clinical examination shows sensory changes in a significant proportion of patients. Trigeminal neuralgia attributed to *multiple sclerosis* occurs in 2–5% of patients with multiple sclerosis, sometimes bilaterally. In these patients, MRI or appropriate electrophysiological studies demonstrate a plaque at the trigeminal root entry zone or in the pons affecting the intrapontine primary afferents. The space-occupying lesions cause TN by contact with the affected trigeminal nerve. Patients may or may not have clinically detectable sensory signs, but trigeminal brain stem reflexes are almost always abnormal.

5.3.4 Idiopathic Trigeminal Neuralgia

In idiopathic trigeminal neuralgia, the pain fulfills criteria for TN (Table 5.2) [1], and neither electrophysiological tests nor MRI shows significant abnormalities. A contact between a blood vessel and the trigeminal nerve and/or nerve root may be found, but without evidence of morphological changes. Two subforms of idiopathic trigeminal neuralgia are identified: a *purely paroxysmal* and *with concomitant continuous pain* form.

5.3.5 Painful Trigeminal Neuropathy

Painful trigeminal neuropathy is defined by the International Headache Society as "head and/or facial pain in the distribution of one or more branches of the trigeminal nerve caused by another disorder and indicative of neural damage" [1].

Subforms of painful trigeminal neuropathy are *painful trigeminal neuropathy attributed to herpes zoster, trigeminal post-herpetic neuralgia, painful post-traumatic trigeminal neuropathy, painful trigeminal neuropathy attributed to other disorder*, and *idiopathic painful trigeminal neuropathy* (Table 5.1), depending on their etiology. Unlike trigeminal neuralgia, the main pain is usually continuous or near-continuous, commonly described as burning or squeezing, or likened to pins and needles. There are also superimposed brief pain paroxysms, but these are not absolutely the predominant pain type. Clinically evident positive (hyperalgesia, allodynia) and/or negative (hypesthesia, hypalgesia) signs of trigeminal nerve dysfunction affecting the trigeminal branches are constant.

In *painful trigeminal neuropathy attributed to herpes zoster*, pain is distributed in one or more trigeminal branches and lasts less than 3 months. The onset of acute herpes zoster usually is heralded by pain that precedes the vesicular eruption by a few days. No practical method has been found to establish the diagnosis while pain is the only feature. Vesicles dry out within about 1 week and heal within about 1 month. The main complication is postherpetic neuralgia, which ensues in about 10–15% of patients [30].

Trigeminal postherpetic neuralgia is more likely in the elderly, and up to 50% or more suffer pain lasting more than a year. The pathology involves atrophy of the dorsal horn and cell loss, axon loss, and demyelination with fibrosis in the dorsal root ganglion. Pain persists more than 3 months, characterized by constant burning and aching with superimposed jabs of shooting or lancinating pain. Patients show a clear sensory deficit and brush-evoked mechanical allodynia in the trigeminal distribution involved. At 2 years, 53% of patients have a poor outcome despite therapy, 22% benefit from therapy, and 25% have a good outcome without treatment [31].

Painful post-traumatic trigeminal neuropathy is caused by traumatic event (mechanical, chemical, thermal, radiation) to the trigeminal nerve. Pain is localized to the distribution of the trigeminal branch affected by trauma; it has mixed qualities (from paroxysmal to constant) and develops within 6 months after the traumatic event. It may occur after neuroablative procedures for trigeminal neuralgia.

Painful trigeminal neuropathy attributed to other disorder may develop secondary to multiple sclerosis, space-occupying lesion, or systemic disease. The pain is localized to the distribution of the trigeminal nerve(s) and may be bilateral. Signs of trigeminal nerve dysfunction are evident, and trigeminal reflexes are invariably delayed or absent.

In the *idiopathic painful trigeminal neuropathy*, the pain is indicative of neural damage; it is unilaterally or bilaterally distributed in one or more trigeminal branches, but no cause has been identified.

References

1. Arnold M. Headache Classification Committee of the International Headache Society (IHS). The international classification of headache disorders. Cephalalgia. 2018;38(1):1–211.
2. Penman J. Trigeminal neuralgia. In: Vinken PJ, Bryn GW, editors. Handbook of clinical neurology, vol. 5. Amsterdam: North Holland; 1968. p. 296–322.
3. Katusic S, Beard M, Bergstralh E, Kurland LT. Incidence and clinical features of trigeminal neuralgia, Rochester, Minnesota, 1945–1984. Ann Neurol. 1990;27:89–95.
4. Ashkenazi A, Levin M. Three common neuralgias. How to manage trigeminal, occipital, and postherpetic pain. Postgrad Med. 2004;116:16–32.
5. Harris W. An analysis of 1,433 cases of paroxysmal trigeminal neuralgia and the end results of gasserian alcohol injection. Brain. 1940;43:209–44.
6. Yoshimasu F, Kurland LT, Elveback LR. Tic douloureux in Rochester, Minnesota, 1945–1969. Neurology. 1972;22(9):952–6.
7. Pollack IF, Jannetta PJ, Bissonette DJ. Bilateral trigeminal neuralgia: a 14-year experience with microvascular decompression. J Neurosurg. 1988;68(4):559–65.
8. Smyth P, Greenough G, Stommel E. Familial trigeminal neuralgia: case reports and review of the literature. Headache. 2003;43(8):910–5.

9. Cruccu G, Gronseth G, Alksne J, Argoff C, Brainin M, Burchiel K, et al. AAN-EFNS guidelines on trigeminal neuralgia management. Eur J Neurol. 2008;15:1013–28.
10. Thomas KL, Vilensky JA. The anatomy of vascular compression in trigeminal neuralgia. Clin Anat. 2014;27:89–93.
11. De Ridder D, Møller A, Verlooy J, Cornelissen M, De Ridder L. Is the root entry/exit zone important in microvascular compression syndromes? Neurosurgery. 2002;51:427–33.
12. Adamczyk M, Bulski T, Sowinska J, Furmanek A, Bekiesinska-Figatowska M. Trigeminal nerve—artery contact in people without trigeminal neuralgia – MR study. Med Sci Monit. 2007;13(Suppl 1):38–43.
13. Baliazina EV. Topographic anatomical relationship between the trigeminal nerve trunk and superior cerebellar artery in patients with trigeminal neuralgia. Morfologiia. 2009;136:27–31.
14. Ramesh VG, Premkumar G. An anatomical study of the neurovascular relationships at the trigeminal root entry zone. J Clin Neurosci. 2009;16:934–6.
15. Miller JP, Acar F, Hamilton BE, Burchiel KJ. Radiographic evaluation of trigeminal neurovascular compression in patients with and without trigeminal neuralgia. J Neurosurg. 2009;110:627–32.
16. Sindou M, Howeidy T, Acevedo G. Anatomical observations during microvascular decompression for idiopathic trigeminal neuralgia (with correlations between topography of pain and site of the neurovascular conflict). Prospective study in a series of 579 patients. Acta Neurochir. 2002;144(1):12.
17. DosSantos MF, Martikainen IK, Nascimento TD, Love TM, Deboer MD, Maslowski EC, et al. Reduced basal ganglia μ-opioid receptor availability in trigeminal neuropathic pain: A pilot study. Mol Pain. 2012;8:74.
18. DeSouza DD, Moayedi M, Chen DQ, Davis KD, Hodaie M. Sensorimotor and pain modulation brain abnormalities in trigeminal neuralgia: A paroxysmal, sensory-triggered neuropathic pain. PLoS One. 2013;8:e66340.
19. Devor M, Govrin-Lippmann R, Rappaport ZH. Mechanism of trigeminal neuralgia: An ultrastructural analysis of trigeminal root specimens obtained during microvascular decompression surgery. J Neurosurg. 2002;96:532–43.
20. Jia DZ, Li G. Bioresonance hypothesis: a new mechanism on the pathogenesis of trigeminal neuralgia. Med Hypotheses. 2010;74:505–7.
21. Marinkovic S, Gibo H, Todorovic V, Antic B, Kovacevic D, Milisavljevic M, et al. Ultrastructure and immunohistochemistry of the trigeminal peripheral myelinated axons in patients with neuralgia. Clin Neurol Neurosurg. 2009;111:795–800.
22. Park SH, Hwang SK, Lee SH, Park J, Hwang JH, Hamm IS. Nerve atrophy and a small cerebellopontine angle cistern in patients with trigeminal neuralgia. J Neurosurg. 2009;110:633–7.
23. Wang Y, Li D, Bao F, Guo C, Ma S, Zhang M. Microstructural abnormalities of the trigeminal nerve correlate with pain severity and concomitant emotional dysfunctions in idiopathic trigeminal neuralgia: a randomized, prospective, double-blind study. Magn Reson Imaging. 2016;34:609–16.
24. Obermann M, Rodriguez-Raecke R, Naegel S, Holle D, Mueller D, Yoon MS, et al. Gray matter volume reduction reflects chronic pain in trigeminal neuralgia. NeuroImage. 2013;74:352–8.
25. DeSouza DD, Hodaie M, Davis KD. Structural magnetic resonance imaging can identify trigeminal system abnormalities in classical trigeminal neuralgia. Front Neuroanat. 2016;10:95.
26. Tian T, Guo L, Xu J, Zhang S, Shi J, Liu C, et al. Brain white matter plasticity and functional reorganization underlying the central pathogenesis of trigeminal neuralgia. Sci Rep. 2016;6:36030.
27. Oliveira CM, Baaklini LG, Issy AM, Sakata RK. Bilateral trigeminal neuralgia: case report. Rev Bras Anestesiol. 2009;59:476–80.
28. Miller JP, Acar F, Burchiel KJ. Classification of trigeminal neuralgia: Clinical, therapeutic, and prognostic implications in a series of 144 patients undergoing microvascular decompression. J Neurosurg. 2009;111:1231–4.
29. Mittal P, Mittal G. Painful tic convulsif syndrome due to vertebrobasilar dolichoectasia. J Neurosci Rural Pract. 2011;2:71–3.
30. Feller L, Khammissa RAG, Fourie J, Bouckaert M, Lemmer J. Postherpetic neuralgia and trigeminal neuralgia. Pain Res Treat. 2017;2017:1681765. doi: 10.1155/2017/1681765. Epub 2017 Dec 5.
31. Watson CP, Watt VR, Chipman M, Birkett N, Evans RJ. The prognosis with postherpetic neuralgia. Pain. 1991;46(2):195–9.

Imaging of Trigeminal Neuralgia

L. Pasquini and A. Bozzao

6.1 Radiological Anatomy and Physiology

The trigeminal nerve is a mixed sensory-motor nerve which presents a general sensory afferent and a special visceral efferent (motor) component. The first part collects somatic sensory from the skin and mucous membranes of the face, forehead, anterior scalp, nasal and oral cavities, conjunctiva, paranasal sinuses, teeth, anterior two thirds of the tongue, part of the external surface of the tympanic membrane, and the dura of anterior and middle cranial fossae. The motor component comprehends all the efferent branches deputed to innerve the muscles of mastication.

The sensory and motor trigeminal nerve roots leave together the mid-lateral surface of the pons, enter the subarachnoid space in the cerebellopontine angle cistern, and pierce the dura mater at the petrous apex to enter the Meckel's cave, which encloses the trigeminal ganglion and the three division branches of the trigeminal nerve: ophthalmic (V1), maxillary (V2), and mandibular (V3) branches. The three division branches follow different paths: V1 and V2 elapse within the dura mater which forms the lateral wall of the cavernous sinus; at this point V1 passes through the superior orbital fissure, while V2 crosses the foramen rotundum, both going toward the orbit. The ophthalmic nerve (V1) carries sensory information from the scalp and forehead, the upper eyelid, the conjunctiva and cornea of the eye, the nose (including the tip of the nose, except alae nasi), the nasal mucosa, the frontal sinuses, and parts of the meninges (Fig. 6.1). The maxillary nerve (V2) carries sensory information from the lower eyelid and cheek; the nares and upper lip; the upper teeth and gums; the nasal mucosa; the palate and roof of the pharynx; the maxillary, ethmoid, and sphenoid sinuses; and parts of the meninges (Fig. 6.1).

The last division branch of the trigeminal nerve, the mandibular branch (V3), doesn't join the other two roots in the cavernous sinus but rather deviates its course at the level of the Meckel's cave, going down through the foramen ovale toward the mandibular and infratemporal regions. The mandibular nerve (V3) carries sensory information from the lower lip, the lower teeth and gums, the chin and jaw (except the angle of the jaw, which is supplied by C2–C3), parts of the external ear, and parts of the meninges. The mandibular nerve carries touch-position and pain-temperature sensations from the mouth, and one of its branches—the lingual nerve—carries sensation from the tongue (apart from taste) [1] (Fig. 6.1).

Electronic Supplementary Material The online version of this chapter (https://doi.org/10.1007/978-3-319-99822-0_6) contains supplementary material, which is available to authorized users.

L. Pasquini (✉) · A. Bozzao
Neuroradiology Unit, NESMOS (Neuroscience, Mental Health and Sensory Organs) Department, Sant'Andrea Hospital, La Sapienza University, Rome, Italy

M. A. Cova, F. Stacul (eds.), *Pain Imaging*, https://doi.org/10.1007/978-3-319-99822-0_6

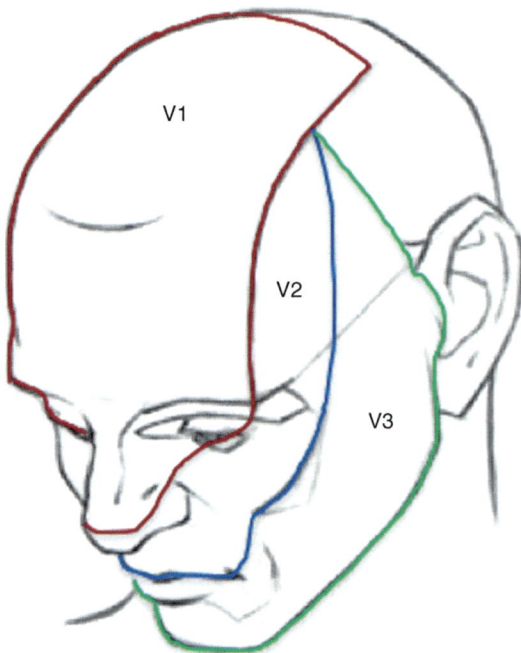

Fig. 6.1 Innervation territories of the peripheral trigeminal branches, V1 (ophthalmic, red), V2 (maxillary, blue), and V3 (mandibular, green)

Keeping in mind this course, the trigeminal nerve can be divided anatomically into five segments: brainstem, cisternal, Meckel's cave, cavernous sinus, and extracranial segments. This division allows an anatomy-based classification of trigeminal nerve pathology, which improves our imaging interpretation skills [2].

6.1.1 Central Segment

This segment lays inside the brainstem and houses the motor and sensory nuclei, which constitute the central component of the trigeminal nerve (Fig. 6.2).

The sensory nucleus can be subdivided into three smaller nuclei: the major sensory nucleus, which lays in the pontine tegmentum, ventral and lateral to the IV ventricle, and its superior (mesencephalic) and inferior (spinal) extension.

The major sensory nucleus carries tactile sensation from the face; the mesencephalic nucleus carries proprioceptive information from the muscles of mastication. The spinal trigeminal nucleus extends caudally until C2 = second cervical vertebra, where

it merges with the substantia gelatinosa and receives inputs from VII, IX, and X cranial nerves, carrying pain, temperature, and crude touch.

The motor nucleus is far smaller than the major sensory nucleus and is localized in the midpons, anterior and medial to the sensory one, providing motor innervation to the muscles of mastication.

6.1.2 Cisternal Segment

The passage between central and cisternal segments of cranial nerves is known anatomically as the root detachment point [3–5]. This site corresponds approximately to the apparent origin of the nerve, where it can be visualized surrounded by CSF (Fig. 6.2). The apparent origin of the trigeminal nerve is at the ventrolateral aspect of the belly of the pons, where it emerges as two different roots: a larger sensory root and a smaller motor root.

Some authors demonstrated a somatotopic organization of the trigeminal sensory root, displaying a rostral component which contains the V1 fibers, a medial component related to the fibers of V2, and a caudolateral part, which gives rise to the mandibular branch (V3) [6].

The two roots form a main trunk which passes through the prepontine cistern, travelling anterior and laterally, and enters the dura mater of the middle cranial fossa trough the porus trigeminus.

As most of the other cranial nerves, the trigeminus is enrolled in a mixed myelin cover, with a proximal oligodendrocyte-myelinated component and a distal Schwann cell-myelinated component. The zone of transition between these two different myelinated parts of the nerve is called the transitional zone (TZ) (also called Obersteiner-Redlich zone), which is located approximately 1 mm or less from the AO for the motor root and on average 3 mm for the sensory root [3, 7, 8]. At visual neurosurgical inspection, the TZ looks like a thinning of the trigeminal myelin sheath where the pia mater can be seen covering the centrally myelinated component [3, 8].

At the level of the porus trigeminus, both dura mater and arachnoid meninges form a CSF-filled sinus situated at the posterolateral aspect of the

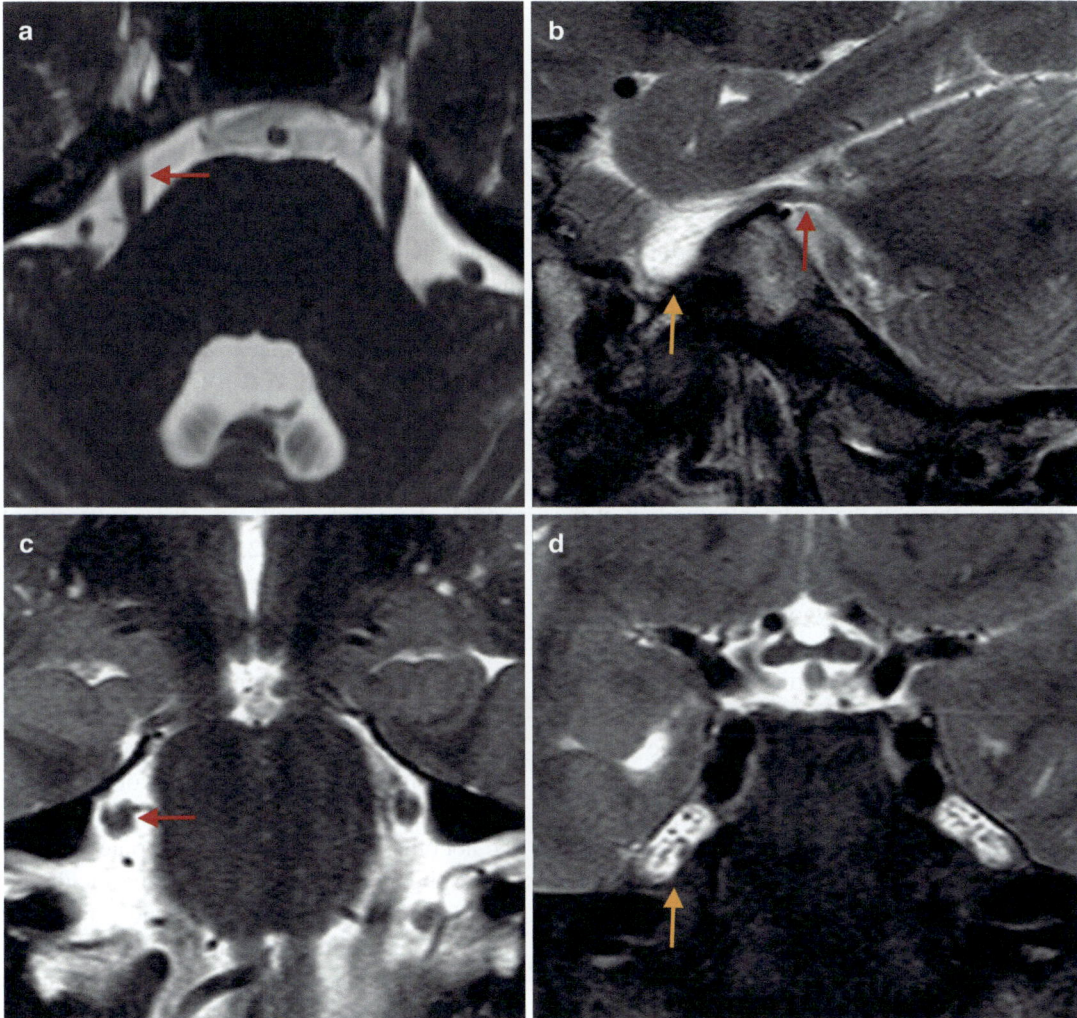

Fig. 6.2 Normal radiological anatomy of the trigeminal nerve. On the left, T2-weighted images displaying the cisternal portion of the nerve on axial (**a**, red arrow) and coronal (**b**, red arrow) plane. On the right, T2-weighted images displaying the trigeminal nerve at the level of the Meckel's cave (yellow arrow) on sagittal (**c**, red arrow) and coronal (**d**) plane

cavernous sinus on either side of the sphenoid bone, which hosts the trigeminal nerve and the gasserian or semilunar ganglion: the Meckel's cave (Fig. 6.2). The location where a cranial nerve exits the subarachnoid space and is no longer surrounded by CSF is called the subarachnoid angle. In the case of the trigeminal nerve, this hallmark is located distal to the posterior margin of the gasserian ganglion, at the distal portion of the Meckel's cave.

The sensory root enters the ganglion and splits into three branches: ophthalmic (V1), maxillary (V2), and mandibular (V3).

Differently, the motor root oversteps the ganglion and turns inferiorly to exit the skull base through the foramen ovale together with the mandibular division of the sensory root (V3) and enters the nasopharyngeal masticator space.

6.1.3 Cavernous Segment

V1 and V2 divisions of the sensory root extend along the lateral wall of the cavernous sinus, together and below cranial nerve IV and lateral to cranial nerve VI, which lays inside the cavernous sinus near the internal carotid artery (ICA, cavernous tract—C4), surrounded by the cavernous venous plexus [3].

6.1.4 Peripheral Branches

The ophthalmic division (V1) leaves the anterior portion of the cavernous sinus through the superior orbital fissure, giving off three major collateral branches (frontal nerve, lacrimal nerve, and nasociliary nerve) and a terminal branch, the supraorbital nerve, which enters the supraorbital foramen and leaves the orbit.

The maxillary division (V2) exits the central skull base through the foramen rotundum at the inferior surface of the cavernous sinus, where it is surrounded by a perineural vascular plexus [3, 9]. Then it enters the pterygopalatine fossa, giving off some collateral branches (meningeal, zygomatic, pterygopalatine, and posterior-superior alveolar nerves). The terminal branch of the nerve enters the orbit through the inferior orbital fissure and becomes the infraorbital nerve, which travels within the infraorbital canal toward the infraorbital foramen.

The mandibular division (V3) is the largest peripheral branch of trigeminal nerve.

It exits the skull base through the foramen ovale, where it is surrounded by a perineural vascular plexus [3] together with the motor root, and enters the masticator space, where it splits in four sensory branches: buccal, auriculotemporal, lingual, and inferior alveolar nerves. The main trunk then proceeds as the inferior alveolar nerve, enters the mandibular foramen at the lingual aspect of the mandibular ramus, and travels along the body of the mandible within the inferior alveolar canal toward the mental foramen in the parasymphyseal region, where it terminates as mental nerve.

After exiting the foramen ovale, the motor root divides into two major branches: the masticator nerve which supplies motor innervation to the temporal, masseter, and pterygoid muscles, and the mylohyoid branch, which supplies the mylohyoid and the anterior belly of the digastric muscle.

6.2 Imaging the Trigeminal Nerve

MRI represents the gold standard for trigeminal nerve evaluation and has almost entirely overcome CT. In patients with contraindications for MR imaging, a complete CT protocol should include helical or volume acquisition scans from the orbital roof to the mandibular symphysis after intravenous administration of iodinated contrast material, keeping the slice thickness below 3 mm, without interslice gap. Axial, coronal, and sagittal plane reconstructions, on both soft tissue and bony algorithms, should be performed [2, 10].

CT angiography of the posterior circulation should be performed in the suspect of neurovascular conflicts [2, 10].

A correct MR imaging protocol for the evaluation of trigeminal nerve should be targeted to the affected segment. 3T (or new 1.5T scanners with digital transmission of signal) shows higher clarity and signal-to-noise ratio compared to lower field intensities, especially in the detection of fine findings such as perineural spread of neoplastic disease [11], and should be preferred if available and not otherwise deemed inappropriate.

Despite a complete brain evaluation with volumetric Fat-suppressed FLAIR and volumetric T1 after gadolinium injection, T2W fast spin-echo (FSE) images of the brainstem and upper cervical cord (until C4 at least) are useful in most of the pathologies affecting the central segment of the nerve.

A complete evaluation of the cisternal segment requires the use of heavily T2-weighted (T2W) sequences to enhance the contrast between CSF and thin neurovascular structures which cross the cisterns. In this case, 3D sequences have demonstrated a significant advantage compared with 2D-FSE T2 [3].

High-resolution steady-state free precession (SSFP) sequences are 3D sequences with a mixed T1/T2 weight which allow for a heavily T2W appearance of the cisternal compartment together with the possibility of injecting contrast medium. Contrast-enhanced SSFP sequences combine the possibility of highlighting the enhancement of pathological processes to the heavy T2 contrast.

Segment	Most common Diagnoses	Key Images
Brainstem	• Multiple Sclerosis (MS) and mimickers inflammatory/infectious conditions • Vascular lesions: Stroke (most commonly as Wallemberg syndrome), AVMs, Cavernous venous malformations • Tumors: Gliomas, Metastatic disease • Others	• MS: High quality T2-weighted images including cervical spinal cord), post Gd T1-weighted images • DWI and ADC sequences (stroke), T2*/SWI sequences (cavernous malformations), 3D-TOF and CE Angio-MR, post-Gd 3D-TOF (AVMs)
Cisternal/Meckel's cave	• Neuro-vascular conflict (NVC) • Cisternal masses: tumors (meningiomas, chondromas, chordomas, schwannomas, metastasis), non-neoplastic masses (epidermoid cyst, dermoid cyst, lipoma inflammatory pseudotumor) • Non-tumoral nerve enhancement (NTNE): autoimmune, infectious, idiopathic • Others	• NVC: Pre and post-Gd SSFP, 3D-TOF (arteries), post-Gd 3D-T1 (veins). Fusion images • T2-weighted images (chordomas), DWI (epidermoid cyst), T1 DIXON (dermoid cyst)
Cavernous sinus	• Non-encasing lesions (type I): interdural tumors (nerve sheet tumors, melanocytoma), epidermoid cyst, chordoma • Encasing and narrowing lesions (type II): intracavernous tumors (meningioma, hemangiopericytoma) • Encasing non-narrowing lesions (type III): pituitary macroadenomas, epidermoid cyst • Infectious/inflammatory diseases: infections, Tolosa-Hunt syndrome (may resemble type II lesions), others	• Cavernous sinus masses: 3D-TOF Angio-MR (narrowing of the ICA), T2-weighted images (chordomas), DWI (epidermoid cyst), post-Gd SSFP, 3D-T1 with fat saturation, dynamic contrast imaging for pituitary macroadenomas • Paranasal sinuses CT imaging
Peripheral branches	• Communal conditions: perineural spread, trauma, inflammatory pseudotumor, others • V1: orbital masses, spread of infection • V2: spread of infection, masses • V3: dental pathologies, masticatory space lesions	• CT for trauma • High-resolution T1WI and post-Gd fat-suppressed T1WI (obliteration of fat pads) • Pre-Gd T2 DIXON, post-Gd T1 DIXON (orbital imaging) • DentaScan CT

Fig. 6.3 The table shows the main diseases affecting the segments of the trigeminal nerve. Some useful imaging techniques and sequences are indicated in the last column on the right

Moreover, contrast injection enhances the nerve segments surrounded by a vascular plexus, providing a high-definition evaluation of the cavernous segment and the foraminal tracts of the peripheral branches [3, 12, 13]. The gasserian ganglion also demonstrates a physiological enhancement on post-contrast imaging.

Thin section spin-echo (SE) T1-weighted (T1W) images in the axial and coronal planes or multiplanar gradient echo T1W sequences (SPGR, GRASS, or MPRAGE), with post-gadolinium fat suppression, allow for a better anatomic depiction of the nerve [2, 9, 14]. Other authors suggested to obtain the T1 weighting with volumetric interpolated breath-hold examination (VIBE) sequence, which is a type of T1W gradient-recalled echo sequence [15].

High-resolution TOF (3D FISP or FLASH) and contrast-enhanced magnetic resonance angiography (MRA) should be used to rule out neuro-vascular conflicts [2, 9, 14].

Diffusion tensor imaging (DTI) has also been used to track trigeminal fibers in the brainstem, cisternal, and extraforaminal segments.

One study demonstrated the feasibility of DTI tractography of cranial nerves in the head and neck region, using parallel imaging, fat-saturation techniques, and a 3T scanner [16] (Fig. 6.3).

6.3 Radiological Pathology of the Trigeminal Nerve

According to the International Headache Society (International Classification of Headache Disorders, ICDH 3 beta), TN includes two main categories: classical type and secondary TN (painful trigeminal neuropathy) [17].

Classical TN is defined as a specific category of TN in which MRI demonstrates vascular compression with morphologic changes of the trigeminal nerve root. This category is furthermore divided in purely paroxysmal (trigeminal neuralgia without persistent background facial pain) and trigeminal neuralgia with persistent background facial pain (atypical TN or TN type 2) [17].

Patients who suffer from secondary trigeminal neuralgia must have a major neurologic disease that causes their condition, which can be either acute herpes virus infection or postherpetic neuralgia, posttraumatic neuropathy, multiple sclerosis, space-occupying lesion (benign or malignant), and other conditions.

Idiopathic TN occurs without apparent cause.

According to many authors, an anatomy-based approach to the trigeminal nerve differential diagnoses represents the best way to handle the subject. After investigating the patient's clinical symptoms, the imaging study should be targeted at a precise segment, based on clinical suspicion.

In this perspective, the following paragraphs have been structured by dividing the trigeminal nerve in its main segments and listing the most frequent causes of trigeminal neuralgia for each one of them.

6.3.1 Central Segment

Theoretically, any process that has an impact on the adjacent brain parenchyma can have an impact on cranial nerve (CN) nuclei. Therefore, either stroke, inflammatory processes, infections, tumors, or other brainstem affections can result in nuclear-based trigeminal neuropathies.

The neural structures of the brainstem show high compaction, limiting the trigeminal nerve exclusive affection to a rare event, almost confined to demyelinating plaques, segmental strokes in the PICA territory, cavernous malformations, and small metastatic deposits [2].

MR is the modality of choice for central segment imaging.

6.3.1.1 Inflammatory and Infectious Lesions

Multiple sclerosis (MS) is by far the most common causative of central trigeminal neuropathy, especially in patients under the age of 50 and in case of bilateral affection [18, 19]. The prevalence of TN in patients with MS ranges from 1.9% to 4.9% [20], and some patients may show a single demyelinating plaque at the location of the trigeminal nuclei as presenting symptom [21]. Recent studies support the hypothesis of a double crush mechanism in the development of MS-related TN, by the concurrence of demyelinating plaques and vascular compression [20].

The most frequent location of the plaque is the root entry zone (REZ), but also the trigeminal nuclei can be involved, and the plaque may extend to the cisternal segment of the nerve [18, 21, 22]. Imaging features depend on the phase of the plaque. In the acute phase, lesions may show high signal intensity on long TR sequences (T2W and FLAIR), low to intermediate signal intensity on T1W images, and enhancement after intravenous administration of gadolinium. In the chronic phase, lesions show hyperintense signal on long TR sequences, hypointense signal on T1W ("black hole" appearance), and no contrast enhancement after gadolinium injection. The suspect of an inflammatory lesion of the brainstem requires further investigations to confirm a diagnosis of MS (Fig. 6.4).

Regarding the imaging protocol, the examination should extend from the brain to the upper spinal cord until the level of C4 at least, with thin-section FSE T2W images. The use of 3D T2W sequences may improve the diagnostic quality [18], as well as 3D FLAIR with fat saturation.

Many other inflammatory and infectious diseases may develop similar brainstem lesions to those of MS. A partial list may include acute disseminated encephalomyelitis (ADEM), progressive multifocal leukoencephalopathy (PML), HIV encephalitis, Behcet's disease, Lyme disease, neurosarcoidosis, Whipple's disease, Bickerstaff's brainstem encephalitis, and rhombencephalitis sustained by different etiologies.

Rhombencephalitis refers to the involvement of the brainstem in an inflammatory process, which often occurs secondary to herpes simplex and rhinocerebral fungal infections, mostly due to *Mucor* or *Aspergillus* species [2, 23, 24].

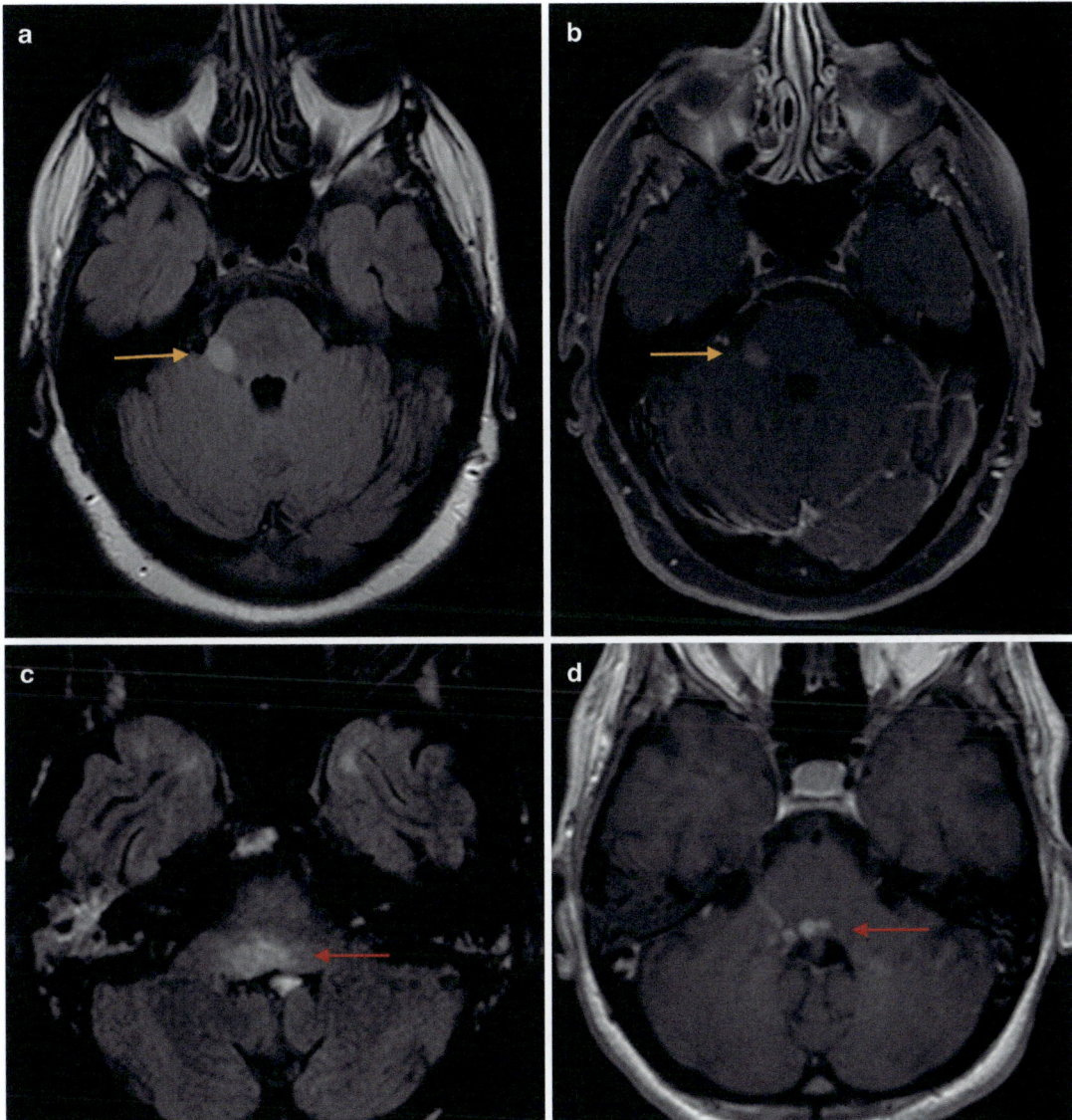

Fig. 6.4 Multiple sclerosis (MS) is the most frequent cause of trigeminal neuralgia in the brainstem. On MR, this condition presents as patchy T2/FLAIR hyperintense lesions involving the trigeminal pontine nuclei (**a**), with post-Gd enhancement in the case of active demyelination (**c**). Other inflammatory or infectious conditions may mimic MS findings on both T1- and T2-weighted images, as for Listeria rhombencephalitis (**b**, **d**)

Listeria rhombencephalitis may cause TN in specific endemic contexts, also in otherwise healthy subjects [24] (Fig. 6.4).

Postherpetic trigeminal neuralgia has also been related to the presence of T2 hyperintense brainstem lesions [25].

In patients with trigeminal neuralgia, the presence of linear hyperintense bands along the intrapontine trigeminal fibers has been suggested to be a sign of herpes zoster-related trigeminal neuropathy [26]. The etiopathogenesis of this sign is related to a centripetal migration of varicella zoster virus (VZV) from the gasserian ganglion to the pontine sensory fibers [27].

DTI performed at the level of the REZ and trigeminal nucleus showed a reduction of fractional anisotropy in the affected side compared to the unaffected one [26].

6.3.1.2 Vascular Lesions

The trigeminal sensory nuclei are located within the tegmentum of the pons, extending cranially toward the midbrain and caudally to the medulla and cervical spinal cord.

In the upper midbrain, the mesencephalic trigeminal nucleus lays in the anteromedial region and is supplied by groups of perforators which arise from the interpeduncular fossa. In the lower midbrain, the mesencephalic nucleus is localized in the posterior vascular territory, which is supplied by a dense vascular plexus over the colliculi, formed from a posterior group of mesencephalic arteries, mainly coming from the superior cerebellar artery (SCA), and secondarily from the collicular artery and posteromedial choroidal artery [28, 29].

At the level of the upper pons, the trigeminal complex (mainly still constituted by the mesence-phalic nucleus) is located within the posterior vascular territory, which is supplied by posterior pontine perforators arising from the SCA. Differently, the low pons houses the trigeminal nuclei in the lateral vascular territory, supplied by lateral pontine perforators directly from the basilar artery (BA), from the anteroinferior cerebellar artery (AICA), or from the SCA. Particularly, the superior lateral pontine artery arises directly from the BA to penetrate the lateral pons in the region of the exit zone of CN 5 [28, 29].

The spinal extension of the trigeminal sensory nucleus is localized in the lateral vascular territory of the medulla. This region is supplied by perforator branches of the PICA, by minor branches of the vertebral artery (VA) medially, and by the BA and AICA superiorly [28, 29].

Approximately 25% of acute strokes develop in the brainstem and may affect the trigeminal complex [24] (Fig. 6.5).

The most typical symptom is loss of function, such as hemifacial hypoesthesia or motor deficits.

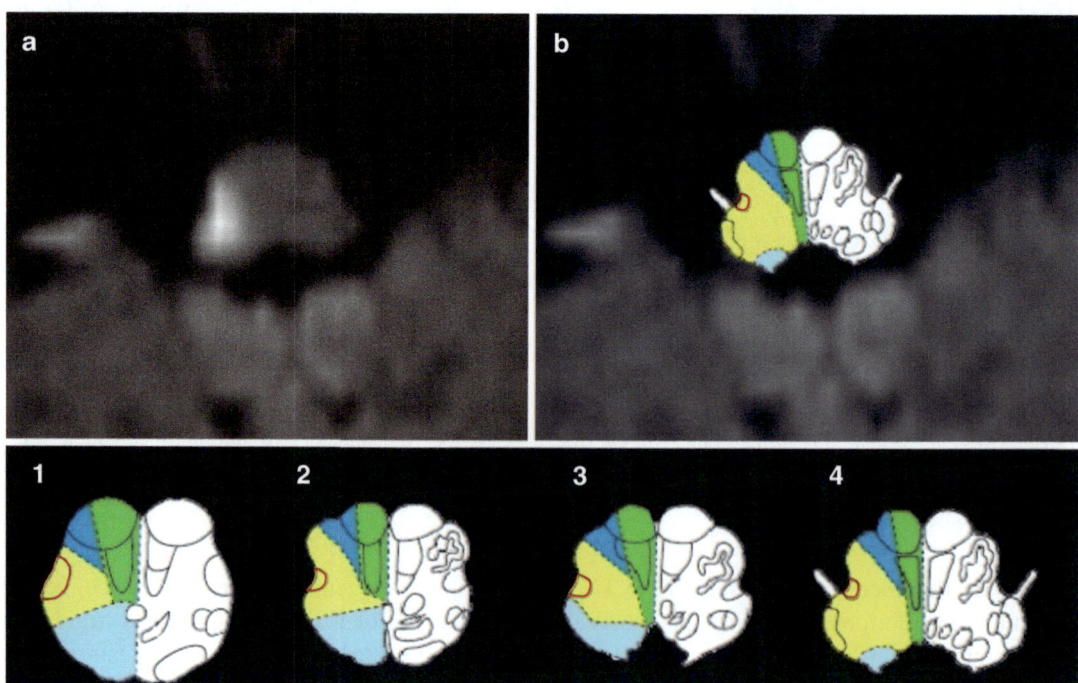

Fig. 6.5 The DWI image on the left displays a lateral medullar signal hyperintensity, which refers to acute infarction, often seen in the context of the Wallenberg's syndrome (**a**). The left DWI image shows the involvement of the trigeminal nuclei (highlighted in red) at the level of the lateral vascular territory of the medulla (**b**, yellow). The medullar vascular territories are displayed below (*1–4*): lateral territory (yellow), anterior territory (green), antero-lateral territory (dark blue), and posterior territory (light blue)

Rarely, TN can be a consequence of brainstem stroke involving the PICA vascular territory in the lateral medulla. In these cases, the trigeminal neuralgia takes part of a wide spectrum of symptoms which depend on the damaged structures. The most common clinical presentation of medullary infarcts is lateral medullary or Wallenberg syndrome, characterized by the triad of ipsilateral Horner's syndrome (ptosis, miosis, and anhydrosis), ipsilateral ataxia, and contralateral hemisensory findings. Wallenberg's syndrome is commonly associated with ipsilateral facial pain, which may start just at the stroke onset or present a latency between 2 weeks and 6 months. In some cases, the pain associated with Wallenberg's syndrome takes the attributes of symptomatic TN, showing specific characteristics: ophthalmic branch involvement, coexisting sensory deficits, absence of triggers, rapid evolvement, and remission [30, 31].

Pons infarcts have also been reported among the causes of TN, mainly due to lateral ischemic lesions, at the root entry zone of the trigeminal nerve (occlusion of pontine branches of the basilar artery) [32–36].

The mechanism underlying TN in postischemic lesions of the brainstem is still debated. A suggested mechanism is demyelination of the central trigeminal pathways which may promote an ephaptic transmission, as for MS.

Acute-stage infarcts present with subtle T2 and FLAIR prolongation and restriction to water diffusion on diffusion-weighted imaging (DWI), which is a mandatory sequence in the suspect of vascular pathogenesis.

Intracranial vertebral artery dissection has been reported as an extremely rare cause of isolated facial pain that mimics TN. In this case, the symptoms can develop with no evidence of brainstem infarction on MR images, and MRA may experience a progressive narrowing of the vertebral artery [37].

Hemorrhagic lesions involving the brainstem may cause trigeminal neuropathy, as in the case of hypertensive bleedings (typical hemorrhage), cavernous venous malformations (CM), arterovenous malformations (AVMs), or trauma [24].

CM are benign vascular hamartomas which contain masses of closely apposed immature blood vessels ("caverns"), with no neural tissue. They manifest as locules of variable size with blood at different stages of evolution and a classical "popcorn" shape. On MR, they show heterogeneous signal intensity on both T1W and T2W images, with complete hypointense hemosiderin rim on T2 and markedly hypointense signal with a "blooming" effect on T2*. Contrast enhancement after gadolinium administration is unlikely, unless when associated with a developmental venous anomaly [38]. CM of the trigeminal nerve with trigeminal neuralgia has been reported in few cases in the literature, with almost one half involving the brainstem, and the others situated either in the gasserian ganglion or the cisternal segment [39] (Fig. 6.6, Video 6.1).

Brainstem AVMs can be divided into pial lesions and parenchymal lesions. Pial AVMs are restricted to the pial surface, typically receive arterial inflow from the SCA or the AICA and drain into the prepontine or petrosal sinuses.

Parenchymal AVMs are located inside the brainstem, merged with neural tissue, and receive arterial supply from brainstem perforating vessels and drainage from the petrosal sinus and vein of Galen [24] (Fig. 6.7).

In the case of hemorrhagic lesions, the imaging protocol should include T2* or susceptibility-weighted sequences (SWI), to highlight the "blooming" effect of the hematic component.

6.3.1.3 Brainstem Tumors

Isolated trigeminal nerve deficits may represent the debut symptom of a brainstem tumor which involves the trigeminal nuclei. Nevertheless, such an eventuality is quite rare since the involvement of trigeminal nuclei generally comes with other adjacent structures and is usually associated to complex neurological syndromes including long fiber tract and other cranial nerves dysfunction [2, 23].

Tumors presenting with isolated TN are often infiltrative gliomas.

These gliomas are more frequently seen in the pediatric population and appear as expansive,

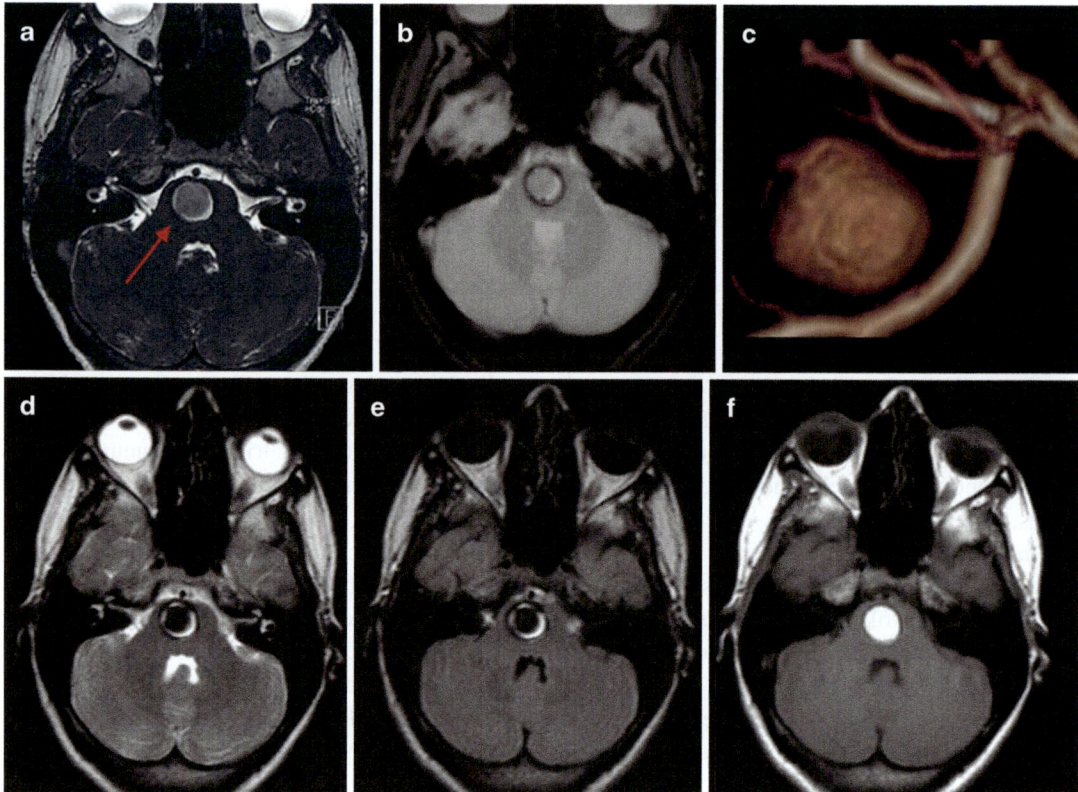

Fig. 6.6 Cavernous venous malformations of the brain may rarely cause trigeminal neuralgia when situated within the pons (**a**, red arrow). The symptoms onset usually depends on hemorrhagic complication, showing hyperintense signal on T1WI (**f**) and hypointense signal on T2/ FLAIR-WI (**a**, **d**, **e**). The presence of hemosiderin peripheral ring on T2*WI is highly typical (**b**). TOF angio-MR may show low performance in these cases, because of the blood susceptibility artifact which can mimic aneurysms or other arterial hemorrhagic diseases (**c**)

infiltrative processes with low-to-normal signal intensity on T1W images and heterogeneous high signal intensity on T2W and FLAIR images, with or without contrast enhancement [40] (Fig. 6.8, Video 6.2a–f).

Lymphoma has been reported as an extremely rare cause of CN V dysfunction [2, 23]. Typical features include an intense and homogeneous enhancement in immunocompetent patients and hyperdensity on CT. In immunocompromised patients, hemorrhage or necrosis may be seen quite frequently. On advanced imaging, lymphomas show restricted diffusion on DWI and apparent diffusion coefficient (ADC) maps and low relative cerebral blood volume (rCBV) values on perfusion-weighted imaging (PWI), with a classical appearance of the perfusion curve, characterized by the overstep of the basal line during the post-capillary phase [41, 42]. The classical intracranial location of primitive lymphoma is within the basal ganglia or periventricular white matter, with 60–80% being supratentorial, and often involves the corpus callosum [38].

Metastasis has also been related to TN, with the most frequent metastatic brain tumors being bronchogenic carcinoma and breast carcinoma [24].

6.3.1.4 Others

As the spinal trigeminal nucleus extends at least to C2 and sometimes to C4, involvement of the upper cervical cord may also lead to trigeminal neuropathy.

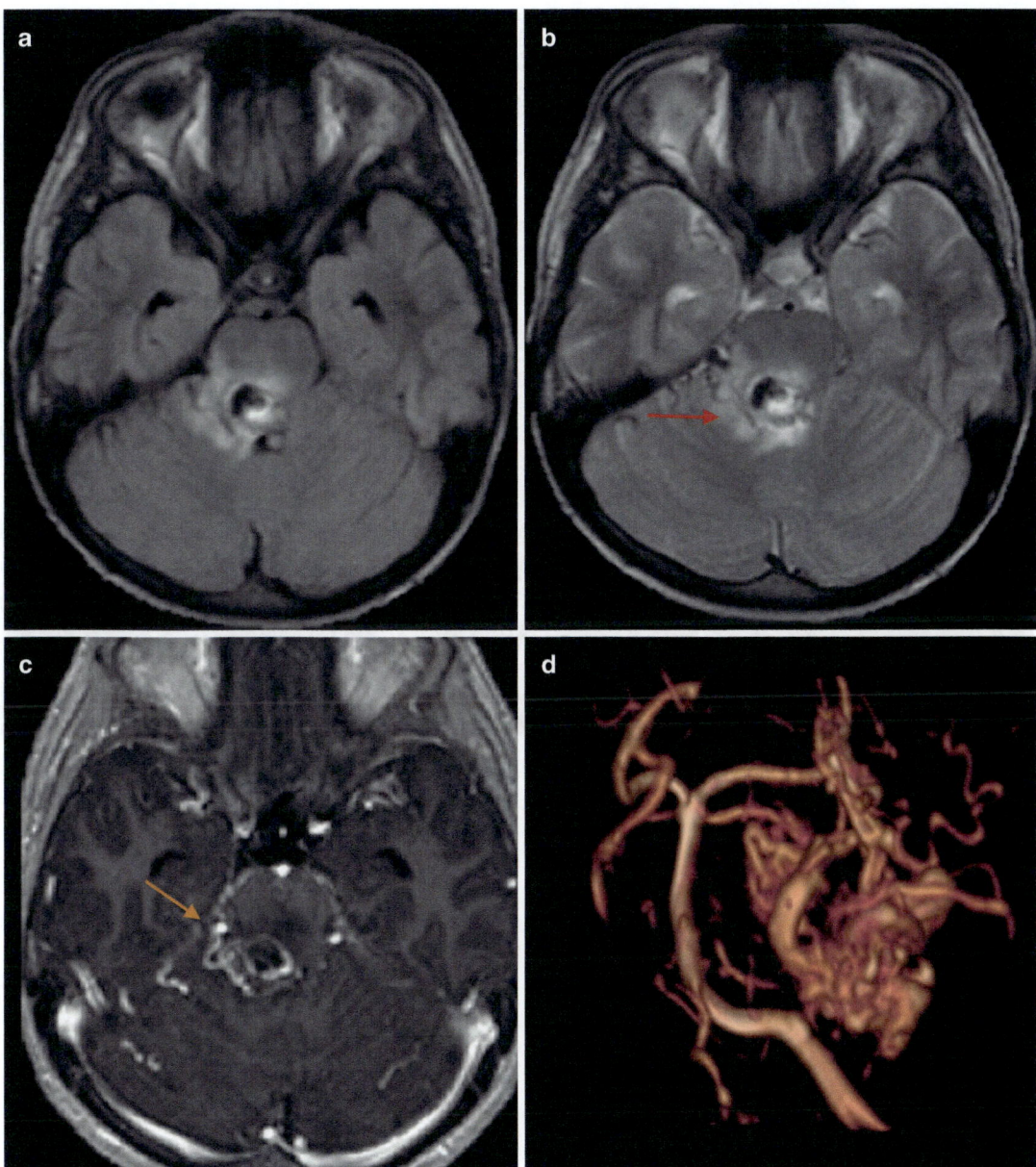

Fig. 6.7 AVM of the brainstem on axial FLAIR (**a**), T2 (**b**) and post-mdc T1-MPRAGE (**c**) images. The finding is characterized by arterial feeders from the posterior circu-lation (**c**, yellow arrow), as displayed by the 3D-TOF angio-MR (**d**). The surrounding brain parenchyma shows high T2 signal intensity due to brain edema (**b**, red arrow)

The conditions affecting this region include some of the abovementioned etiologies (demyelination, tumors, vascular lesions) and others, such as trauma, disc herniations, and syrinx formation [23].

Hydromyelia constitutes a possible cause of trigeminal neuralgia in children with Chiari I malformation due the spinal trigeminal nucleus compression [43].

Dandy et al. reported posterior fossa malformations as possible causatives or predisposing factors for trigeminal neuralgia. Cystic malformations of the posterior fossa, such as Dandy-Walker

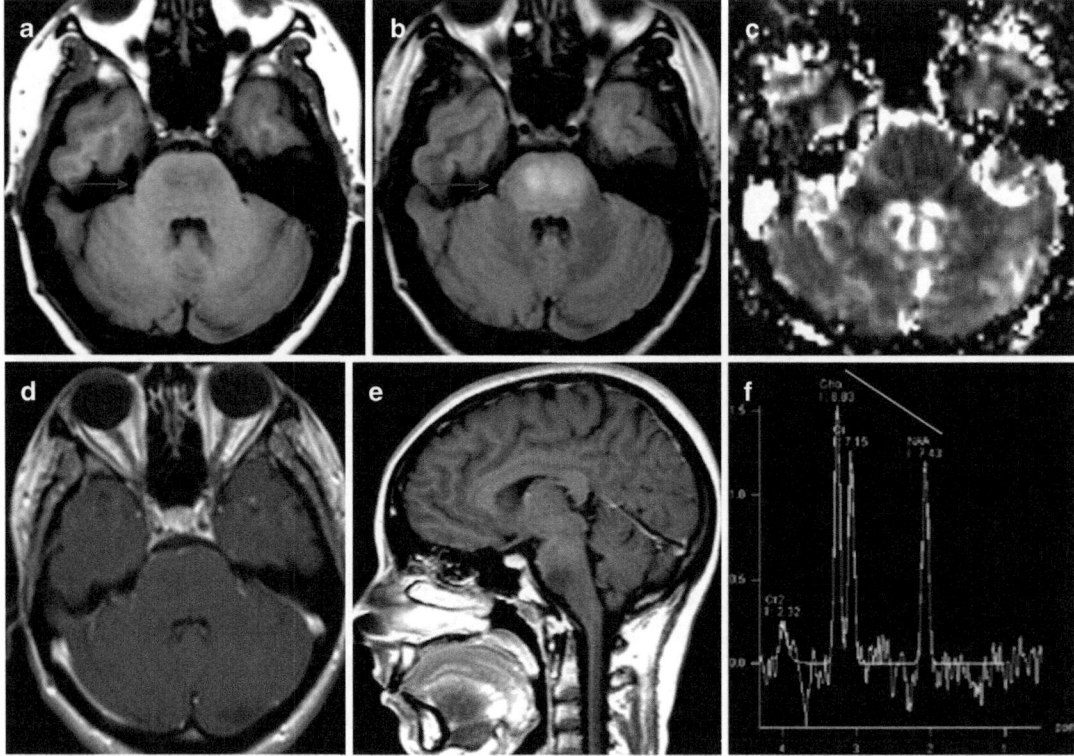

Fig. 6.8 Diffuse infiltrating pontine glioma (**a**, **b**, red arrows) showing low-grade features such as lack of contrast enhancement (**d**, **e**) and no restricted diffusion (**c**, ADC map). On MR spectroscopy, the lesion shows the typical inversion of the NAA and Cho peaks (**f**, yellow line)

malformation, Blake's pouch, and arachnoid cysts, may compress the brainstem or induce anatomic variations which can approach the trigeminus and surrounding vascular structures [44].

6.3.2 Cisternal Segment and Meckel's Cave

6.3.2.1 Neurovascular Conflict

There is strong evidence that the classical form of trigeminal neuralgia is caused by a focal injury of the nerve due to vascular compression, a condition known as neurovascular conflict (NVC).

It is estimated that this condition accounts for up to 90% of classical TN [24], being accountable to the high rates of pain relief after microvascular decompression (MVD) in drug-resistant cases.

The concept of neurovascular conflict as a cause of TN was first proposed by Dandy in 1934, but only in 2005, Jannetta et al. confirmed that classical TN was a painful condition caused by an abnormal vascular compression at the REZ and promoted MVD as a surgical procedure for its treatment [45]. According to the neurovascular compression theory, the trigeminal nerve should be damaged by an offending vessel which focally contacts the nerve and provokes a local demyelination in the region of compression [17–19].

This process should result in the generation of ectopic sensory impulses which spread to adjacent fibers and increase the spontaneous activity of the nerve, leading to chronic modifications of the trigeminal system, with hyperactivity of the nuclei and development of neuralgia [18, 19, 46].

The offending vessel is usually the SCA, normally located above the trigeminus, or the AICA coming from below [7, 47, 48]. Less frequently, the trigeminal nerve may be compressed by the basilar and vertebral arteries, [2] saccular aneurysms of the posterior communicating artery [49], a persistent trigeminal artery [7, 50], arterio-venous malformations [51], or veins [52].

A small cerebellopontine angle cistern appears to predispose to NVC [7].

Nevertheless, the vascular compression alone doesn't constitute a sufficient criterion to establish a diagnosis of classical trigeminal neuralgia due to neurovascular conflict, because of its relative frequency in healthy subjects, ranging from 25% to 74% of the cases [53]. The radiological find of a vascular compression should rise in the context of a well-defined clinical background, with respect to the diagnostic criteria for classical trigeminal neuralgia, and should be accompanied by other imaging features which increase the specificity of the diagnosis.

The most suggestive imaging features for the radiological diagnosis of trigeminal neuralgia include:

– Contact at the level of the transitional zone between central and peripheral myelination of the trigeminal nerve
– Modifications of the nerve, which include displacement and atrophy
– An artery as offending vessel
– Perpendicular contact [2]

TN is more frequent in proximal (<3 mm) than in distal cisternal portion of the trigeminus [7, 53, 54], where the transitional zone is supposed to be located. According to most of the studies, the transitional zone of myelination lays in the proximal cisternal part of the trigeminus: Peker et al. reported a distance of <2.5 mm away from the brainstem, while Guclu et al. identified the TZ at 4.19 ± 0.81 mm.

Keeping in mind these subtle discrepancies, Haller et al. proposed a cutoff of 3 mm for the location of the TZ with respect to the root exit zone, as a compromise to help the radiological evaluation of the compression [7].

Neurovascular conflict (NVC) can be classified into three grades on MRI: grade I when the vessel simply contacts the nerve, grade II when the vessel displaces and/or distorts the nerve root, and grade III when the vessel indents the nerve root, resulting in nerve atrophy [55].

A recent meta-analysis showed an impressive increment of the MRI specificity and positive predictive value in detecting a symptomatic nerve, by combining the findings of a vascular contact in the REZ and nerve atrophy [53].

These evidences confirm the impression that trigeminal neurovascular contact within the REZ is likely to be symptomatic when it is associated with anatomical nerve changes and should be reported with confidence only in cases of grade III NVC within the appropriate clinical context [53] (Fig. 6.9).

The event of an offending vein causing trigeminal pain has been described, but it represents a seldom finding, mainly involving the transverse pontine vein at the level of the Meckel's cave or the cerebellopontine fissure veins, ponto-trigeminal veins, middle cerebellar peduncle, and lateral mesencephalic veins [52, 55].

Aneurysms located in the proximity of the trigeminal nerve may produce neuralgia by direct compression, with the internal carotid, posterior communicating artery, AICA, and SCA as the most involved vessels [55–57]. A persistent trigeminal artery may compress the trigeminal nerve and lead to the development of classic neuralgia [55, 58].

Yoshino et al. investigated the relationship between the site of compression at the root entry zone and the type of neuralgic manifestation, finding a somatotopic organization of the nerve fibers at the REZ. Accordingly, patients with maxillary symptoms had neurovascular conflicts at the medial side of the trigeminal root, while patients with mandibular symptoms showed an involvement of the lateral side [2, 59].

In the case of suspected neurovascular compression, the standard of reference for

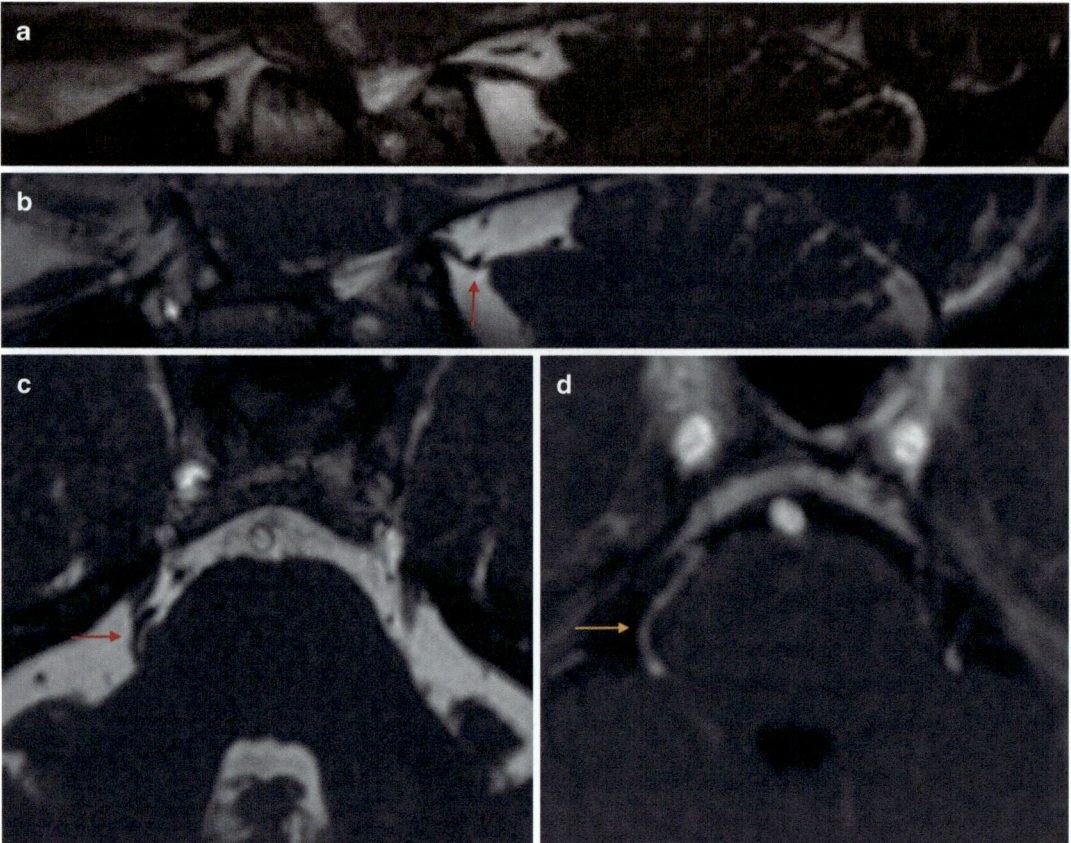

Fig. 6.9 Neurovascular conflict between the right trigeminal nerve and the right superior cerebellar artery. Figure "(**a**)" displays the normal relationship between the trigeminal nerve and the SCA, while images "(**b**)" and "(**c**)" show the abnormal contact between the two structures, with nerve indentation, displacement and atrophy (**b, c**, red arrow). Post-Gd T1WI shows the vessel enhancement (**d**, yellow arrow)

imaging protocol include a combination of high-resolution SSFP 3D sequences with 3D time-of-flight (TOF) angiography and 3D T1W gadolinium-enhanced sequences, which help in discriminating venous structures and micro-AVM unseen on 3D TOF technique [7, 55] (Fig. 6.10).

More recently, DTI with tractography has been investigated as a marker of disease activity and treatment response [7].

Desouza et al. demonstrated that the affected trigeminal nerve may present lower fractional anisotropy (FA) and higher radial diffusivity (RD), axial diffusivity (AD), and mean diffusivity (MD) compared to controls [19]. The reversibility of the FA reduction after successful microvascular decompression has also been reported but necessitates further support [24, 60].

6.3.2.2 Cisternal Masses

Many neoplastic lesions have been associated with TN. More frequently, an extrinsic tumor may cause trigeminal dysfunction by compressing or distorting the cisternal segment, but also an intrinsic tumor of the trigeminal nerve may manifest with pain due to the anatomo-physiological alterations of the nerve fibers. The most common benign extrinsic tumors, which can compress the cisternal segment of the trigeminal nerve, include meningioma, vestibular schwannoma, and chondromas, while the most frequent intrinsic tumor is the trigeminal schwannoma.

Meningiomas of the Meckel's cave or posterior fossa are possible secondary causes of TN [27, 61].

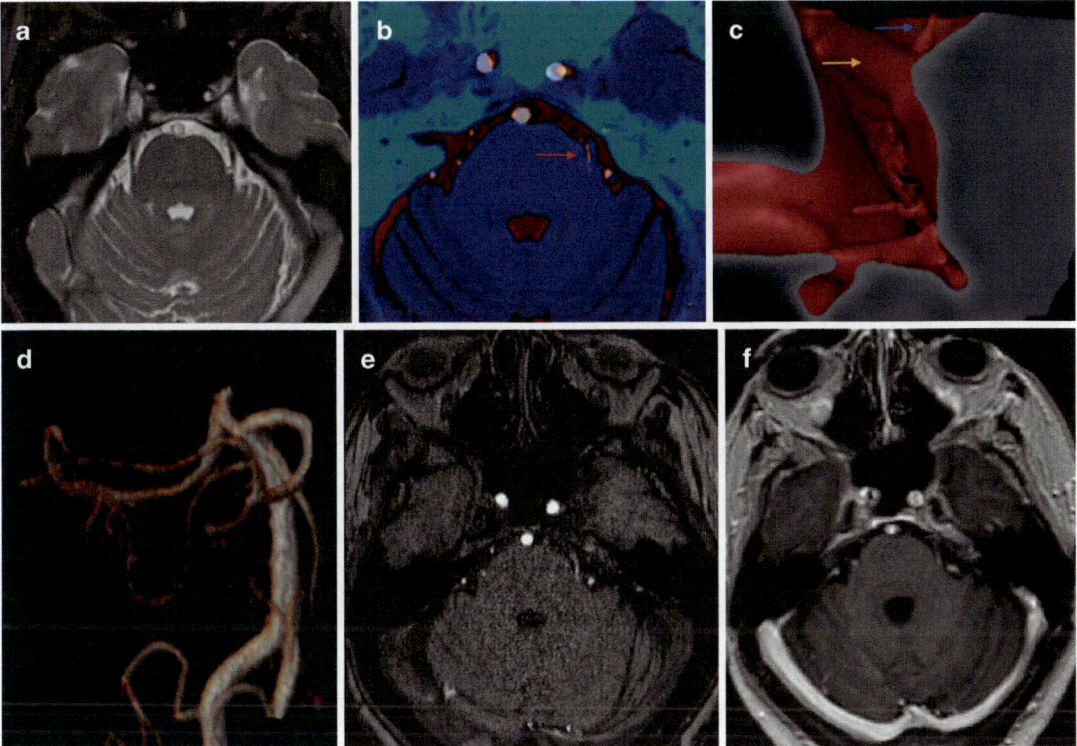

Fig. 6.10 Neurovascular conflict between the left trigeminal nerve and the left superior cerebellar artery. The relationship between the vessel and the nerve is slightly visible in T2WI (**a**) but is well highlighted in fusion images (**b**, red arrow) and 3D VR reconstructions (**c**, trigeminal nerve,yellow arrow; artery, blue arrow). The vessel is well depicted in TOF images (**d**, **e**) and post-Gd T1WI (**f**)

Petroclival meningiomas comprise 20% of all intracranial meningiomas [2, 62] and may compress the trigeminal nerve when growing anteriorly into the prepontine cistern. As extra-axial tumors, meningiomas show the distinctive characteristic of a dural implant, in this case involving the posterior surface of the petrous bone and a dome-shaped medial surface, with frequent calcifications on CT. On MR, they often appear isointense to gray matter on T1W images and iso- to slightly hyperintense on T2W images, with variable hypointense components due to calcifications. Intense and homogeneous contrast enhancement is highly characteristic, and the presence of adjacent dural enhancement, the "dural tail" sign, is frequent [2, 62] (Fig. 6.11).

Chondromas of the skull base are extremely rare benign cartilaginous tumors which arise from embryonal remnants of chondrocytic cells more often within the petro-occipital synchondrosis and may compress adjacent segments of the trigeminal nerve at the level of the Meckel's cave or cavernous sinus, thus leading to trigeminal neuralgia [63, 64]. On CT they often show calcifications (Fig. 6.11).

Trigeminal schwannoma is the most common intrinsic tumor of the trigeminus and may present with pain, paresthesia, and numbness along the course of the nerve divisions [2, 65, 66].

Depending on the tumoral epicenter, trigeminal schwannomas can be divided into four subgroups:

Type I lesions, the most common, arise from the trigeminal ganglion in the Meckellesions.

Type II lesions originate from the cisternal segment.

Type III tumors, the second most common, arise in between the prepontine cistern and the Meckel's cave, separated by a thin waist at the

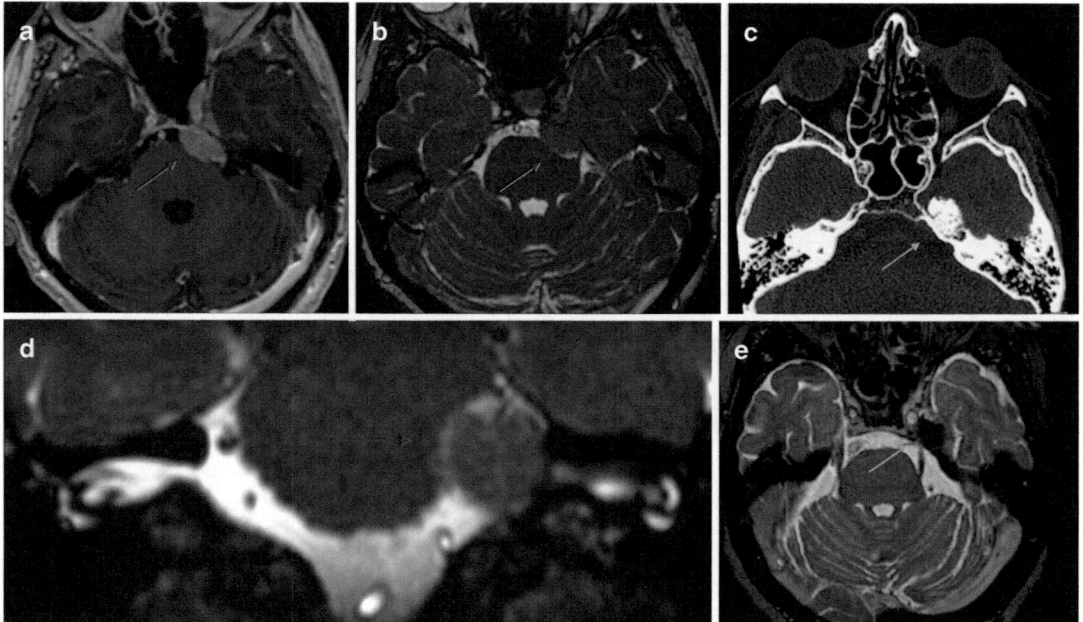

Fig. 6.11 Tumoral masses of the prepontine cistern and Meckel's cave. The most common neoplasm affecting this area is petroclival meningioma, which often shows the typical dumbbell shape (**a**, **b**, **d**, red arrows). Chondromas of the skull base are extremely rare benign cartilaginous tumors, which often show calcifications in CT (**c**, yellow arrow) and extremely low signal intensity on T2WI (**e**, yellow arrow), due to calcium deposit

level of the porus trigeminus and characterized by a typical dumbbell shape.

Type IV lesions comprise all the extracranial tumors which originate from the peripheral branches of the trigeminal nerve [2, 24].

A peculiar characteristic of schwannomas is the oblong shape, due to the tumoral growth pattern which follows the long axis of the nerve, with the evidence of constrictions at the level of dural openings or skull base neural foramina. However, meningiomas can also grow along neurovascular foramina and follow the course of cranial nerves, mimicking schwannomas [2].

Denervation atrophy of the muscles of mastication when the motor root is involved may also aid the diagnosis.

Larger schwannomas may present heterogeneous texture, with cystic components and rarely necrosis and internal hemorrhage [38], which could rise the suspicion of malignancy.

Malignant neural sheath tumors should be suspected whenever there is rapid growth or aggressive bone destructive changes [22].

Multiple schwannomatosis is typical of neurofibromatosis, especially in subtype 2 where it is often associated with meningiomas and ependymomas [67].

CT may depict bone remodeling or erosion along the canals and skull base neurovascular foramina, adding important diagnostic information. MR best depicts the tumoral texture and is much more sensitive in highlighting small tumors that would otherwise be missed, through gadolinium-enhanced T1W images.

Metastatic lesions and tumoral leptomeningeal spread may cause trigeminal neuropathy, although more often associated with other cranial nerve deficits, in a wide spectrum of neurological symptoms [2, 23].

Moreover, nonneoplastic masses may cause trigeminal dysfunction by compressing or distorting the cisternal portion of the trigeminal nerve, acting as extrinsic tumors. These lesions include cerebellopontine angle or Meckel's cave epidermoid cyst, dermoid cyst, and lipoma (Fig. 6.12).

Epidermoid cysts are soft congenital lesions composed of desquamated cellular debris,

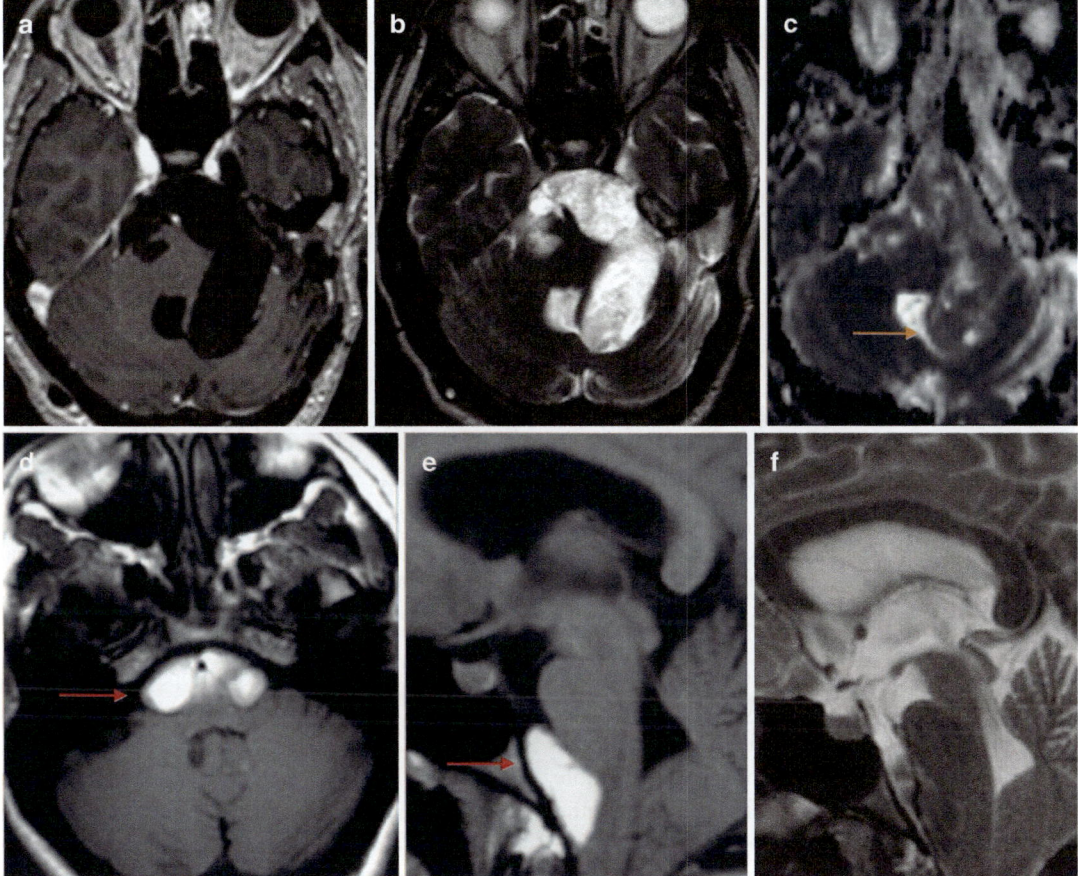

Fig. 6.12 Nonneoplastic cisternal masses. Epidermoid cyst (**a–c**) shows characteristic CSF-like signal on T1- and T2WI (**a, b**) and restricted diffusion on ADC maps (**c**, yellow arrow). The images below show a typical dermoid cysts (**d–f**) with fat-like signal intensity on unenhanced T1WI (**d, e**, red arrows)

keratin, lipids, and cholesterol, lined by a single layer of squamous epithelium. They present a "plastic" behavior, with the tendency to encase and stretch the adjacent structures, without significant displacement [2, 68]. The most common localization is the cerebellopontine angle cistern and prepontine cistern, but they can also arise from the Meckel's cave, being associated with TN [27, 69].

On MR, epidermoid cysts show a CSF-like signal in T1 and T2 and present a characteristic restricted diffusion on DWI, which is essential to confirm the diagnosis (Fig. 6.12).

Lipomas have also been associated with cranial nerves compression, accounting for <1% of cerebellopontine angle masses. They usually originate from a failure in the normal embryo-

logic development of the meninx: during the fetal life, the meninx primitiva embraces the developing brain and is reabsorbed between the 8 and the 10 weeks of gestational age, leading to the development of subarachnoid cisterns. If the reabsorption is incomplete, the meninx primitiva persists and degenerates into fat [67, 70]. The presence of congenital lipomas, especially when situated along the midline, may be a spy of an underlying genetic syndrome.

Inflammatory pseudotumor (IPT) is an extremely rare cause of trigeminal neuralgia. This condition, also known as the "great mimicker," is a benign inflammatory lesion of unknown pathogenesis, which can present as an isolated finding or as multiple masses affecting every region of the body. This lesion is

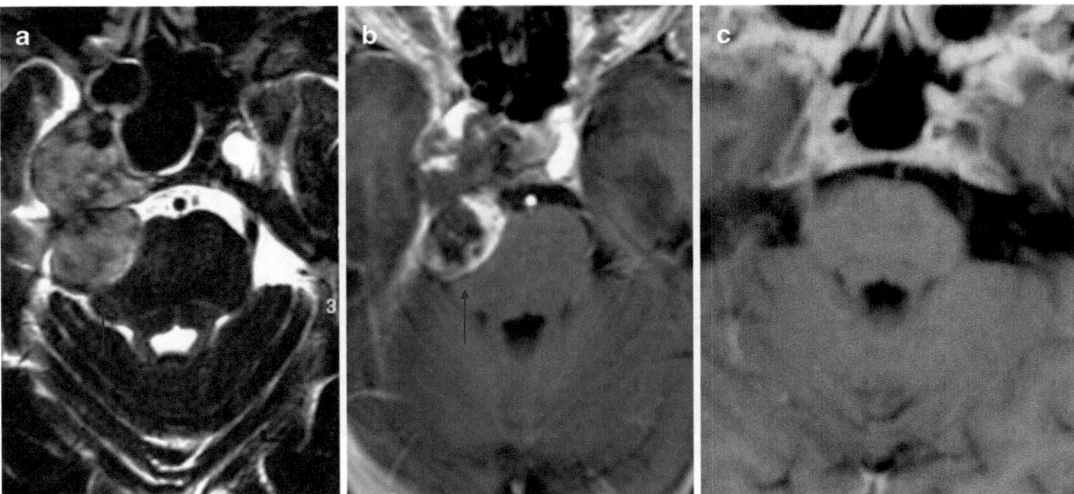

Fig. 6.13 Inflammatory pseudotumor is a rare entity which may develop in the prepontine cistern and Meckel's cave involving the trigeminal cisternal segment (**a**, **b**, red arrows). The imaging features may challenge the diagnosis, for they typically show tumor-like inhomogeneous contrast enhancement (**b**) and T2 signal iso-hyperintensity (**a**). After corticosteroid treatment, the mass usually disappears (**c**)

characterized by the presence of myofibroblastic spindle cells admixed with lymphoplasmacytic infiltrate against a myxoedematous, hypercellular, or sclerotic background, presenting variable amounts of fibrosis and necrosis. The intracranial location is an unusual presentation of IPT, which may involve the trigeminal nerve when developing at the level of the cerebellopontine angle cistern. In these cases, the differential diagnosis with petroclival meningiomas and other neoplastic lesions may be difficult, even more so because IPT often presents unspecific imaging features [71, 72].

On MR images, IPT shows different behaviors depending on the grade of fibrosis and necrosis. It usually shows low signal intensity on both T1- and T2-weighted images, reflecting a prominent fibrotic component and may present homogeneous or heterogeneous contrast enhancement [71] (Fig. 6.13).

Corticosteroid treatment usually provides a complete remission of the lesion.

6.3.2.3 Non-tumoral Nerve Enhancement (NTNE)

NTNE refers to the trigeminal enhancement of non-tumoral origin, which may manifest in the context of a wide spectrum of pathologic conditions, including autoimmune, infectious diseases, and some cases of idiopathic trigeminal neuralgia, in which no underlying disease can be identified [24].

Such a finding, especially if apparently isolated, requires a meticulous clinical framing to help the diagnosis.

Many infectious diseases are associated with cranial nerve enhancement, either in the context of a widespread leptomeningitis or as an isolated finding, more frequently in viral infections.

Enhancement of the preganglionic segment of the trigeminal nerve may depend on granulomatous neuritis and is seen in granulomatous diseases such as sarcoidosis, tuberculosis, Wegener, and syphilis. A transient enhancement of the cisternal segment may be seen in fungal and bacterial infections, with or without enlargement of the nerve [24, 73, 74].

Cranial neuritis secondary to Lyme neuroborreliosis may manifest with cranial nerve impairments, including trigeminal neuralgia [75].

Nerve inflammation secondary to petrous apicitis may also occur in Gradenigo's syndrome which is defined by the triad of facial pain in the distribution of the trigeminal nerve, convergent strabismus due to CN VI palsy, and suppurative otitis media. The infection starts in the mastoid and spreads to the petrous apex, involving the dural coverings of the Meckel's cave, in which lays the gasserian ganglion of the trigeminal nerve.

Viral infections can manifest in association with variable degree of enhancement. Herpes simplex and varicella zoster are the most reported pathogens in post-viral neuritis of the trigeminal nerve and may cause nerve inflammation as an isolated finding or as part of the Ramsay Hunt syndrome (herpes zoster cephalicus) [27].

HIV can be rarely associated with trigeminal neuralgia, showing bilateral enhancement of the nerve [76].

Trigeminal nerve enhancement has been described in multiple sclerosis, more often bilaterally and in younger patients [77], and in other chronic inflammatory neuropathies, including Charcot-Marie-Tooth disease, which is part of the hereditary motor and sensory neuropathy (HMSN) disorders, a group of genetically based diseases characterized by progressive motor weakness, decreased nerve conduction velocities, and nerve root enlargement [78].

Gq1b antibody-related disorders (Guillain-Barré syndrome, Miller Fisher syndrome, and Bickerstaff's encephalitis) usually manifest with polyneuropathies which can involve the V cranial nerve, showing a complex and ill-defined spectrum of symptoms, including facial dysesthesia.

Pathologic enhancement of the trigeminal nerve together with severe headache has been reported as a sign of intracranial hypotension [79].

6.3.2.4 Other Conditions

The pseudotumor cerebri syndrome (PTCS) consists in a perplexing syndrome of increased intracranial pressure without the presence of a space-occupant lesion, whose incidence peaks in young women between 20 and 40 years who weigh 20% or more than their ideal body weight [80]. This condition may manifest with cranial nerve abnormalities, including trigeminal neuralgia [81] and may be associated with several risk factors including medications (growth hormone, vitamin A, tetracycline), endocrine disorders (Addison, hypoparathyroidism, obesity), and infections or develop without a secondary cause (idiopathic intracranial hypertension). Several studies indicate that many people with pseudotumor cerebri have an obstruction to venous drainage due to dural sinus stenosis, more frequently involving both the transverse sinuses.

The clinical presentation of the syndrome includes headache, visual deficits (transient visual obscurations, visual loss, diplopia), and pulsatile tinnitus. In the case of a PTCS-suggestive clinical history, an MR examination should be performed to rule out the presence of an intracranial mass and other possible causatives of raised intracranial pressure. The diagnostic criteria for the typical form of PTCS include papilledema, normal neurologic examination except for cranial nerve abnormalities, normal CSF composition, elevated lumbar puncture opening pressure (>250 mm CSF in adults and >280 mm CSF in children), and the exclusion of a space occupant lesion on neuroimaging. Moreover, other MR signs are considered suggestive of pseudotumor cerebri, such as empty sella, flattening of the posterior aspect of the globe and prominence of the papilla, distention of the perioptic subarachnoid space with or without a tortuous optic nerve, and transverse venous sinus stenosis on MR venography [80].

Another possible cause of trigeminal neuralgia in the cisternal space is the presence of arachnoid adherences and strands which may compress and distort the nerve. Arachnoid cysts have been reported as possible compressing lesions at this level and may exceptionally develop after microvascular decompression leading to TN recurrence [82].

6.3.3 Cavernous Sinus

The cavernous sinus is a bilateral symmetric parasellar cavity housed in a dural fold, formed by two walls: the lateral wall and the medial wall (endosteal layer of the dura).

This cavity contains the cavernous venous plexus, the cavernous tract (C4) of the internal carotid artery (ICA), and some nervous structures and should be considered a venous dural sinus rather than a venous plexus, for they share similar structure [83].

The lateral dural wall of the sinus is composed of two layers, the outer dural layer (dura propria) and the inner membranous layer, which can be easily separated. The dura propria is thicker and more resistant, while the inner layer is a membranous lamina formed by the sheaths of the III and IV cranial nerves, V1 and V2 trigeminal branches, and a membranous lattice extending between these sheaths. The venous channels of the cavernous plexus lay medially to the inner layer, between this lamina and the endosteal layer of the dura mater (medial wall). The intracavernous nerves can be considered as part of the lateral wall of the sinus, except for the VI which is located within the venous plexus, nearby the ICA.

Most of the pathologic processes involving the cisternal segment of the trigeminal nerve may also affect the cavernous segment, due to its proximity.

In theory, every mass originating nearby the cavernous sinus can determine trigeminal compression and rarely lead to trigeminal neuralgia. However, only a part of these entities has been reported in the literature as TN causative.

Primitive cavernous sinus neoplasms are described as interdural or intracavernous, depending on whether they origin from between the two layers of the lateral wall or from inside the sinus, respectively [83, 84].

Nerve sheath tumors (schwannomas and malignant nerve sheath tumors) more frequently originate from the interdural compartment, where the IV CN and the trigeminal peripheral branches are contained. Other frequently interdural tumors are melanocytomas, while meningiomas and hemangiopericytomas more often belong to the intracavernous compartment.

Epidermoid cysts can be either interdural or intracavernous lesions [85, 86] (Fig. 6.14).

Moreover, neoplasms originating nearby the cavernous sinus, like pituitary macroadenomas and skull base tumors, may involve the sinus and affect the trigeminal nerve [2, 87].

To better address the differential diagnosis, an imaging-based classification of the neoplasms originating nearby or properly from inside the cavernous sinus is provided.

Depending on the relationship with the internal carotid artery (ICA), cavernous sinus masses can be divided into three groups:

- Displacing lesions: the ICA is more displaced than surrounded by the mass (type I).

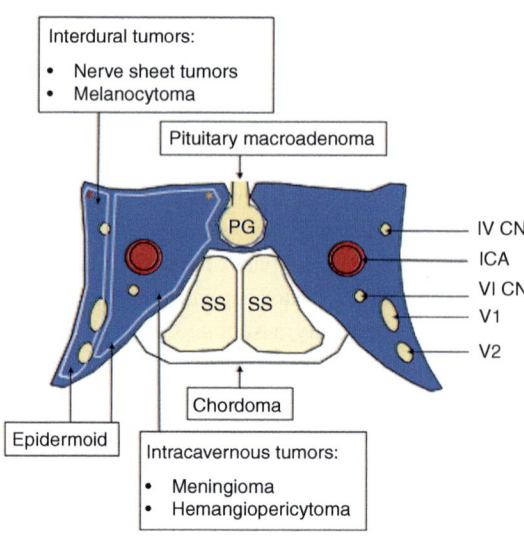

Fig. 6.14 The figure shows the most frequent lesions of the cavernous sinus area, displayed according to their site of origin. The cavernous sinus can be divided in interdural compartment (red asterisk) and intracavernous compartment (yellow asterisk). *CN* cranial nerve, *ICA* internal carotid artery, *SS* sphenoidal sinus, *PG* pituitary gland

- Encasing and narrowing lesions: the ICA is embraced by the mass, which constricts the vessel as it grows, resulting in a reduction of the ICA lumen (type II).
- Encasing-without-narrowing lesions: the mass surrounds the ICA, which keeps its own diameter (type III).

Type I lesions tend to displace the internal carotid artery without encasement or narrowing. The main actors in this category are the interdural tumors (schwannomas, malignant nerve sheath tumors, melanocytomas).

Meningeal melanocytomas are rare benign primary melanocytic tumors of the central nervous system derived from leptomeningeal melanocytes and characterized by different content of melanin, which affect the macroscopic as well as the radiologic appearance [88, 89].

Posterior fossa, Meckel's cave and cavernous sinus constitute frequent intracranial sites of origin, although they mainly arise from the spinal meninges.

The tumoral epicenter location in the Meckel's cave is frequently associated with a nevus of Ota, a dermal melanocytic nevus with benign behavior which involves the ophthalmic and maxillary branches of the trigeminal nerve [90].

The MRI appearance depends on the content of melanin which typically shows hyperintense signal on T1 and blooming effect on T2* or SWI sequences. The major differential comes from other melanocytic lesions, which include melanocytic meningiomas and metastasis of melanoma. Hemorrhagic lesions should also be ruled out.

Chordomas of the skull base may involve the cavernous sinus and displace the internal carotid artery, with no encasement, due to their origin from outside the sinus (Fig. 6.15). In some cases, the ICA lumen may be distorted by the displacement [91].

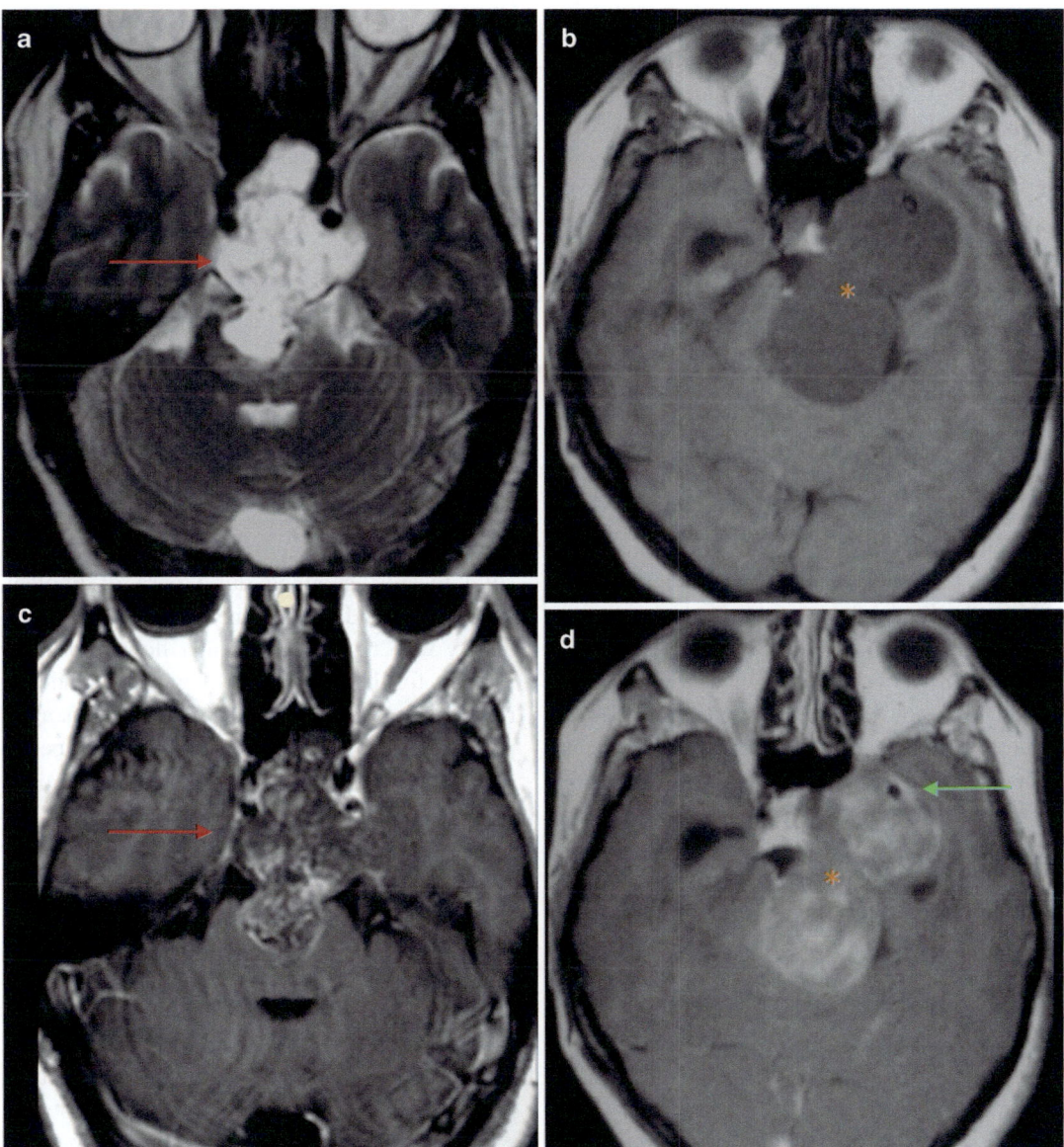

Fig. 6.15 Chordomas typically present high signal intensity on T2WI (**a**, red arrow) and inhomogeneous CE (**c**, red arrow). They can behave like type II lesions (encasing and narrowing the ICA). A T2 signal intensity higher than CSF may suggest a chondroid subtype. Trigeminal schwannomas (**b**, **d**, yellow asterisks) tend to displace the ICA (green arrow), without narrowing its lumen

These malignant tumors originate from notochord remnants and are typically located in the midline, at the level of the clivus. More than one-third of these tumors arise in this area because the notochord terminates at the level of the basisphenoid, just inferior to the sella turcica [92].

Chordomas usually present as midline lesions with both bone destruction and soft tissue mass on CT, without intratumoral calcifications. On MR they show a polilobular surface with hypo-isointensity on T1WI, hyperintensity on T2WI, and inhomogeneous contrast enhancement (Fig. 6.15). Cystic areas containing hemorrhagic or mucoid material are frequently present [2, 92].

Chordomas are aggressive tumors with a poor prognosis, and their imaging findings often overlap with those of chondrosarcomas which represent completely different skull-base neoplasms, showing low progression rate and good outcome.

Both pathologies may be associated with trigeminal neuropathy and neuralgia due to the involvement of the cavernous sinus or the gasserian ganglion [64, 93].

Skull-base chondrosarcomas are more often located off-midline, arising either from the synchondroses that remain after ossification replaces the embryonic chondroid basal plate, more often involving the petro-occipital synchondrosis [2, 91]. Another possible location is the junction between nasal septum and rostrum of the sphenoid bone. Less frequently, these tumors may arise from the midline in the basisphenoid synchondrosis.

Chondrosarcomas present well-/moderately differentiated chondrocytes surrounded by an extracellular matrix, which characterizes two main histologic types: hyaline and myxoid. The hyaline matrix can mineralize, leading to the development of characteristic ringlet calcifications, which can be appreciated on CT. Moreover, due to its chondroid nature, chondrosarcoma shows a typical appearance on MR T2WI, characterized by strong high signal intensity, which can be even brighter than CSF, and usually enhances more homogeneously than chordomas.

The term "chondroid chordoma" refers to a peculiar variant of chordoma, characterized by an extracellular matrix which resembles the chondroid matrix of chondrosarcoma. This entity should be considered more a histologic mimic of chondrosarcoma than a "bridge entity" between the two different neoplasms and shares similar prognosis to chordoma.

Chondrosarcomas are usually single neoplasms but can arise in consequence of malignant degeneration of chondromas in the Ollier (multiple enchondromatosis) and Maffucci syndromes (multiple enchondromas associated with subcutaneous hemangiomas).

Type II lesions are more frequently represented by meningiomas and hemangiopericytomas. These neoplasms often encase the ICA and shrink its lumen (Fig. 6.16).

Hemangiopericytomas are WHO grade II or III tumors which account for less than 1% of all intracranial neoplasms. In the past, these tumors have been classified as angioblastic subtype meningiomas or rather lesions of the smooth muscle perivascular pericytes, while the 2016 WHO classification considers them in the spectrum of the solitary fibrous tumors of the dura, which originate from dural fibroblasts [89].

Imaging features may overlap with those of meningiomas, for they often occur as extra-axial solid masses, showing dural base of implant, dural tale, vivid enhancement, and T2/T1 isointensity with numerous vascular flow voids. Key features for the differential diagnosis include the relationship with the adjacent bone: hemangiopericytoma erodes the bone and has no hyperostosis associated [94, 95].

The presence of metastasis is far more frequent in hemangiopericytoma (up to 20% of the cases), involving the lungs, the liver, and the bones.

Meningioma is characterized by the spoke wheel sign, which refers to the pattern of vessels coursing in cross section, where the feeder arterial branches show a radial arrangement, resembling a spoke wheel on T2-weighted or post-contrast images.

Advanced MR imaging techniques may aid some information to the differential diagnosis. Perfusion-weighted images (PWI) show the typical "mother-in-law" appearance for

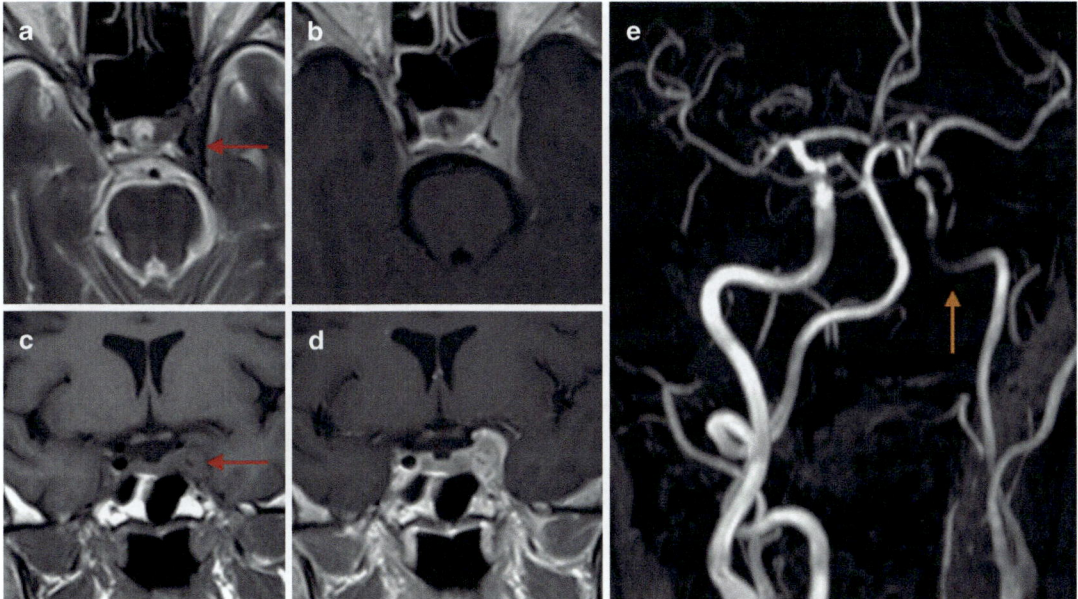

Fig. 6.16 The most frequent encasing with ICA-narrowing lesion (type II) of the cavernous sinus is meningioma. The figure displays a left cavernous sinus meningioma, with hypointense T2 signal of the affected sinus (**a**, red arrow) and isointense signal on unenhanced T1WI (**c**, red arrow). After Gd administration, the lesion displays homogeneous CE on T1WI (**b**, axial plane, **d**, coronal plane). TOF Angio-MR shows a clear reduction of the ICA caliber (**e**, yellow arrow)

meningiomas, characterized by an early enhancement during the arterial phase which remains stable after the venous phase. MR spectroscopy (MRS) display an augmented alanine peak in meningiomas, which is absent in hemangiopericytomas [38, 96].

Pituitary macroadenomas may invade the cavernous sinus and surround the ICA. Generally, these tumors progressively encase the ICA without narrowing its lumen (type III) [83, 97] (Fig. 6.17).

Macroadenomas are the most common suprasellar masses in adults, twice as common as microadenomas. They are defined as pituitary gland adenomas greater than 10 mm in size and typically show isointense signal on both T1 and T2 images and may present cystic components, with moderate to bright enhancement of the solid portion, and micro- or macrohemorrhages (apoplectic component).

Cavernous sinus invasion represents a relative frequent event and has been classified by Knosp et al., taking in count the relationship with the ICA.

The grading system is defined by the relation between the limits of macroadenoma invasion and three carotid lines. These lines, named medial, median, and lateral carotid lines, pass through the supra- and intracavernous parts of the ICA in coronal view [98, 99] (Fig. 6.17).

- Grade 0: adenoma does not reach the medial carotid line.
- Grade 1: adenoma oversteps the medial line, without reaching the median line.
- Grade 2: tumor extends between the median and lateral line.
- Grade 3: tumor extends beyond the lateral line. This group has been furtherly divided into two subgroups by Micko et al. in 2015:
  - 3A: tumor invades the superior CS compartment.
  - 3B: tumor invades the inferior CS compartment.
- Grade 4: tumor surrounds the intracavernous carotid artery.

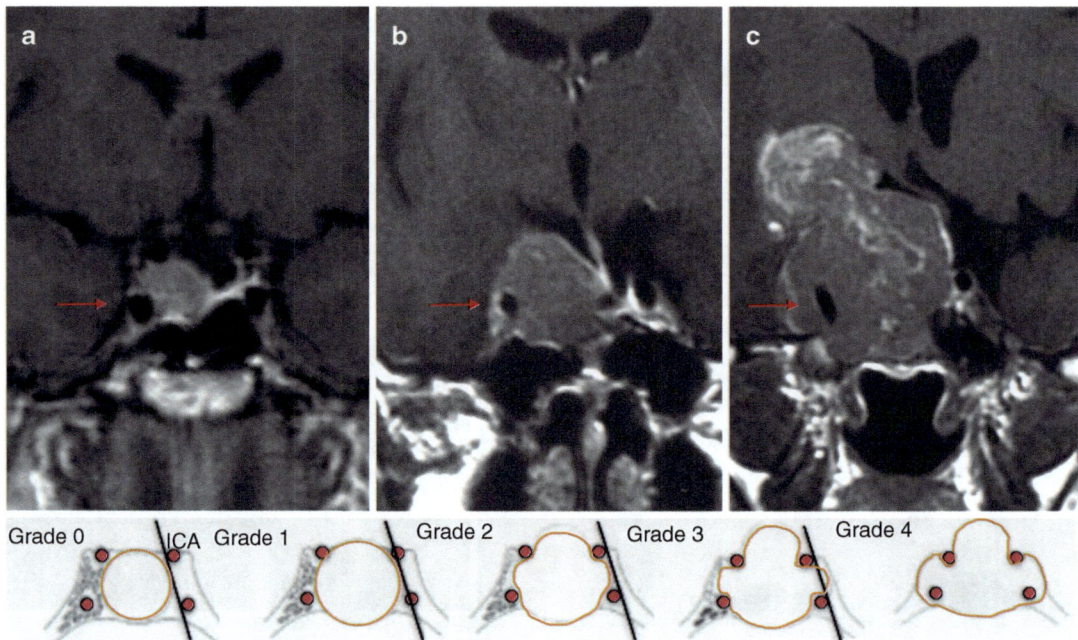

Fig. 6.17 Examples of pituitary macroadenomas classified according to Knosp classification (grade 0–4): grade 2 (**a**, red arrow), grade 3 (**b**, red arrow), grade 4 (**c**, red arrow). Pituitary macroadenomas typically encase the ICA without narrowing its lumen (type III lesions)

Epidermoid cysts may act either as type I or type III lesions and be located both in interdural and intracavernous compartments of the cavernous sinus.

Rarely, metastasis or other tumors spreading from adjacent territories may involve the cavernous sinus, thus leading to a wide amount in clinical manifestations, including TN [24].

6.3.3.1 Infectious and Inflammatory Diseases

Trigeminal neuralgia can result from peripheral infections which reach the cavernous sinus spreading along nerves and vessels (angiocentric growth). This growth pattern is typical of invasive fungal infections, almost exclusively seen in immunocompromised patients and often originating from the paranasal sinuses. *Aspergillus* or *Mucor* species are the most frequent etiologies [2, 100].

A frequent complication of infectious involvement of the cavernous sinus is thrombophlebitis.

The inflammation which accompanies these aggressive infections usually shows T1 hypointensity and T2 hyperintensity on MR, with variable enhancement depending on the degree of avascular necrosis and suppuration. Due to these features, MR angiography may add some important information to the diagnosis, showing the integrity of major vessels. CT may also help the diagnosis by displaying bone erosion, especially regarding the involvement of paranasal sinuses as site of origin. Fungal mycelia and hypha have a characteristic aspect on MR imaging because of the presence of manganese, which has paramagnetic properties and shows low signal intensity on both T1W and T2W images, with major post-contrast enhancement [101].

DWI clearly shows restricted diffusivity in case of suppuration.

In diabetic patients, malignant otitis externa by *Pseudomonas aeruginosa* may extend to the middle ear and spread inside the skull [2].

Tolosa-Hunt syndrome is an inflammatory noninfectious infiltration of the dura of the cavernous sinus and orbital apex, which leads to painful ophthalmoplegia [38].

The predominant cellular population in the infiltrate is mononuclear inflammatory cells of unknown etiology.

The inflammatory tissue shows T1W and T2W hypointense signal, for the lymphocytic predominance of the inflammatory infiltrate, together with abnormal thickening and enhancement of the dura (Fig. 6.18). A differential diagnosis with neoplasm, including lymphoma, is mandatory. The cavernous portion of the internal carotid artery is often narrowed, resembling type II tumors of the cavernous sinus [24, 102, 103].

6.3.3.2 Vascular

Giant aneurysms of the cavernous tract of the ICA may compress V1–V2 trigeminal branches

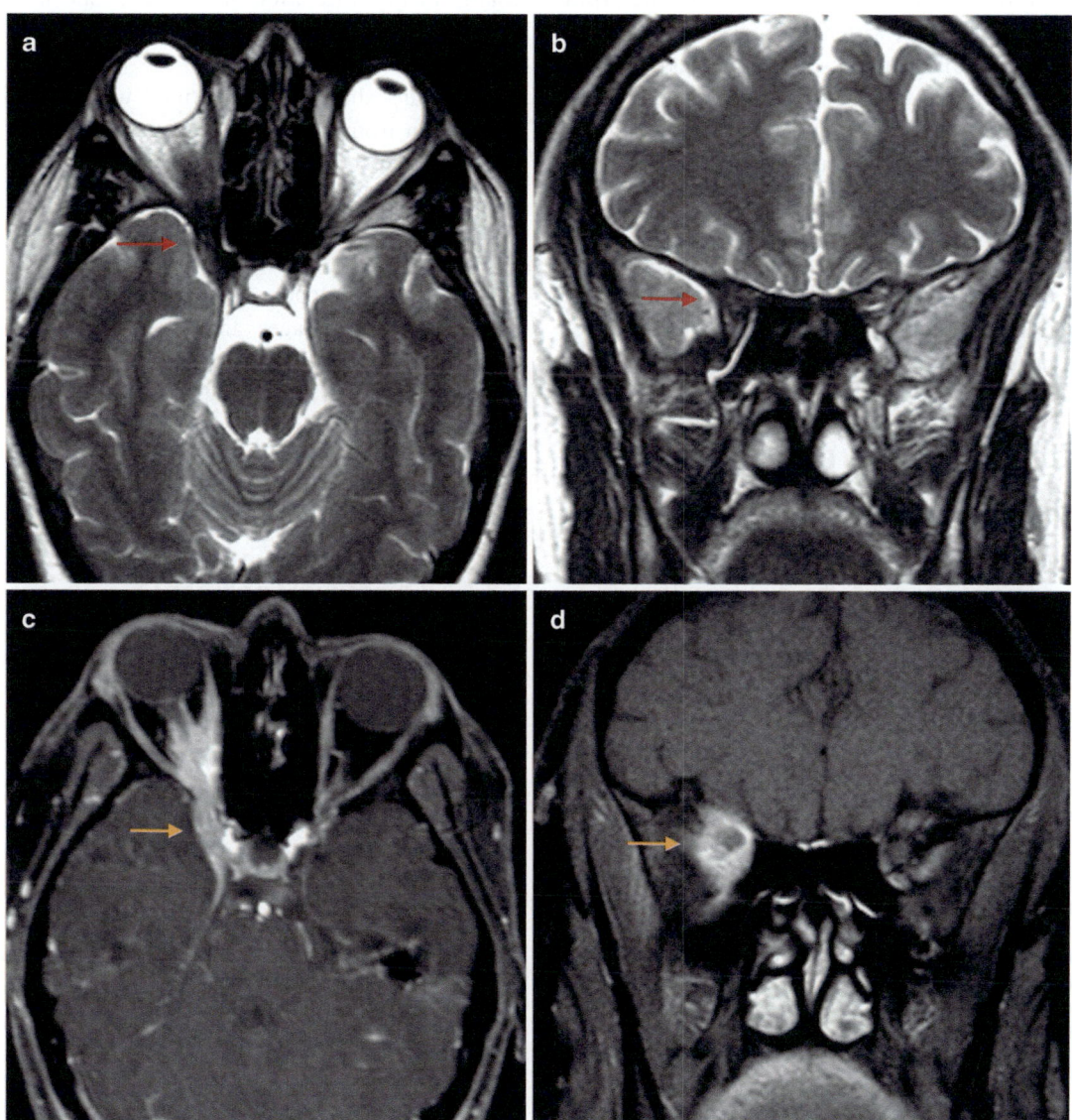

Fig. 6.18 The Tolosa-Hunt syndrome is an inflammatory noninfectious infiltration of the dura of the cavernous sinus and orbital apex, characterized by T2 hypointense signal (**a**, **b**, red arrows), for the lymphocytic predominance of the inflammatory infiltrate, together with abnormal thickening and enhancement of the dura on post-Gd T1WI with fat suppression (**c**, **d**, yellow arrows)

and promote a secondary neuralgia [104]. Cavernous-carotid fistulas, more often resulting from head trauma, may also provoke a trigeminal neuropathy [24].

The differential diagnosis of these lesions requires an adequate study of the intracranial vasculature. Giant aneurysms show a prominent flow void on T2 images, which differentiates these lesions from other masses. Angio-MR with TOF technique can sharply delineate the profile of the aneurysm, with 3D reconstructions. A possible sign of cavernous-carotid fistulas is the arterialization of the cavernous sinus, due to abnormally augmented flux coming from the pathological communication between arterial and venous vascular district. Such a finding is clearly displayed on contrast-enhanced images, as early post-contrast opacification of the cavernous sinus, during the arterial phase. Similarly, a bright cavernous sinus on arterial angio-MR TOF may suggest the presence of a fistula [105].

6.3.4 Peripheral Branches

CT and MR often play a complementary role in the imaging of trigeminal peripheral branches.

In fact, many of the diseases affecting the peripheral segments show key features in both imaging techniques: the relationship between the lesion and the adjacent bone, as well as the involvement of soft tissues, often represents pivotal information to provide a surgical roadmap of the disease extension and to distinguish benign-behaving from aggressive-behaving lesions.

CT images are mandatory in the case of trauma patients, primary bone and fibro-osseous conditions. The relationship between the lesion and the adjacent bone characterizes its behavior: bone remodeling, periosteal reaction, and bone erosion or invasion can address the differential diagnosis and are useful in head and neck tumor grading. Moreover, the involvement of the skull base requires CT scans to image the neurovascular foramina [2].

MR is more sensible to image the soft tissue components of the lesion, in terms of anatomic relationship with intracranial contents and extracranial tissues. MR is the technique of choice to depict perineural spread, which represents the most common condition affecting the peripheral branches of the trigeminal nerve and should be carefully investigated in tumoral grading [2, 106, 107]. In these cases, MR may also highlight secondary signs of tumoral spread, such as denervation-related muscle changes and obliteration of fat pads, especially in the orbit, pterygopalatine fossa and neurovascular foramina [2].

CT scans should be performed with helical acquisition from the orbital roof to the jaw and reconstructed in the axial, coronal, and sagittal planes, on both soft tissue and bony algorithms, with slice thickness below 3 mm and no interslice gap [2].

The MR protocol should include high-resolution T1W images and post-contrast fat-suppressed T1W images to better outline the lesions near the fat containing spaces [2].

For the fact that tumoral spread may affect the entire course of the trigeminal nerve, often presenting skip lesions, MR images should be performed from the brainstem to the periphery.

6.3.4.1 Communal Conditions

These groups of pathologic conditions affect all the trigeminal branches, with some possible predilections.

Perineural Spread

Perineural tumor spread (PNS) of head and neck cancers consists in a form of metastatic dissemination with peripheral migration along the endoneurium or perineurium of cranial nerves (Fig. 6.19). The diagnosis of PNS is often delayed because of the silent course of the disease until advanced stages. For this reason, such a pattern of growth has a poor prognosis and requires aggressive treatment.

Perineural spread of head and neck malignancies represents the most common lesion affecting the peripheral trigeminal nerve, and trigeminal neuralgia is an uncommon presentation. PNS more often involves the maxillary and mandibular trigeminal branches [106, 107].

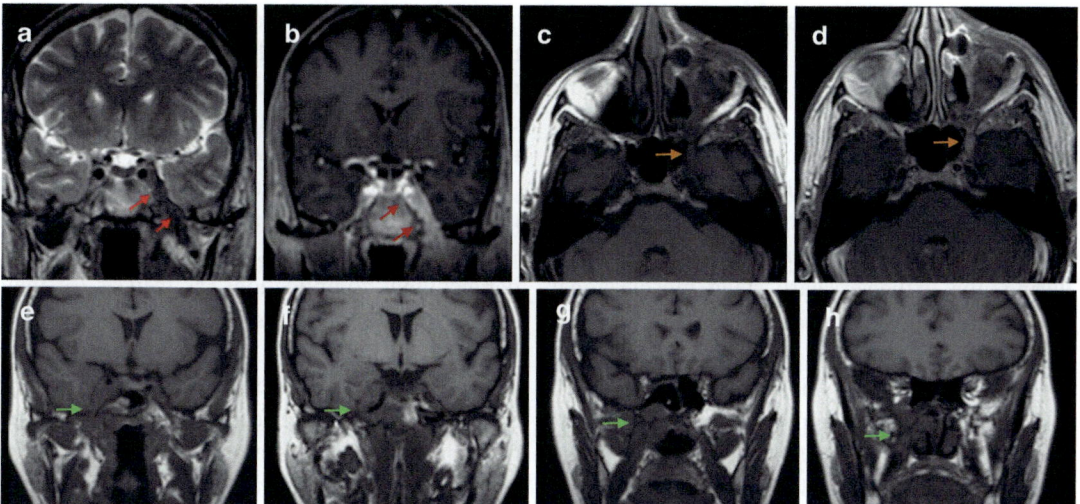

Fig. 6.19 Different patterns of perineural spread along the trigeminal nerve. Images "(**a**)" and "(**b**)" show perineural spread along the left V3 on T2WI (**a**, red arrow) and CE T1WI (**b**, red arrow). Images "(**c**)" and "(**d**)" display the involvement of the left V1 on unenhanced T1WI (**c**, yellow arrow) and CE T1WI (**d**, yellow arrow). Unenhanced T1WI highlight the obliteration of fat pads, as shown in this case of perineural spread along the right V3 trigeminal branch (**e–h**, green arrows)

Several types of head and neck tumors may present this pattern of growth, including squamous cell carcinoma, adenoid cystic and mucoepidermoid carcinomas of salivatory glands, lymphoma, and melanoma. The most common neoplasms associated with PNS are primary salivary malignancies; however, the most frequent finding is squamous cell carcinoma, due to its increased prevalence [2]. The close relationship of the auriculotemporal division of the mandibular nerve to the parotid gland allows PNS by tumors arising from the parotid gland, such as adenoid cystic carcinomas.

As general rule, the location of the primary tumor affects the pattern of PNS: tumors of the orbit or forehead usually follow the ophthalmic division; tumors of the midface and pterygopalatine fossa tend to follow the maxillary division; and tumors of the nasopharynx, squamous cell carcinoma, and, among all, tumors of the masticator space or external auditory canal more often spread through the mandibular branch [106, 107].

The pterygopalatine fossa affection represents a crucial element in tumoral grading, because it behaves as common hub for the main head and neck spaces, thanks to its multiple connections.

The pterygopalatine fossa is a bilateral cone-shaped deep depression of the infratemporal fossa, between the maxilla and the sphenoid, which communicate medially with the nasal cavity via the sphenopalatine foramen, laterally with the masticator space via the pterygomaxillary fissure, anteriorly with the orbit via the inferior orbital fissure, postero-superiorly with the Meckel's cave and cavernous sinus via the foramen rotundum, postero-inferiorly with the middle cranial fossa via the vidian canal, postero-medially with the nasopharynx via the palatovaginal canal, and inferiorly with the palate via the palatine canals [108].

Perineural spread of cancer can occur in both retrograde or anterograde directions and often presents skip lesions, in which apparently unaffected segments of the nerve are interposed to metastatic tracts, so that clear surgical margins do not guarantee the absence of perineural spread and imaging should include the trigeminal nerve to its all length [106, 107].

Imaging features of trigeminal PNS include smooth thickening of a trigeminal branch, with enhancement after Gd administration, best seen on T1 fat-suppressed images; obliteration of juxta-foraminal fat pads, especially at the level of the foramen ovale, best seen on T1 images without fat suppression; replacement of the normal T2 hyperintensity of the trigeminal cisterns by an isointense mass; lateral bulging of the cavernous sinus dural; and atrophy of the masticatory muscles [70, 106] (Fig. 6.19).

Denervation-related muscle changes vary during time. In the very early stage, muscle signal may be normal on either T1W or T2W images. The typical change in the acute stage is an increase in T2 signal which is best displayed on STIR or other fat-suppressed T2W images; contrast enhancement may be present. Chronic changes are characterized by muscle atrophy and fat infiltration, which result in augmented signal on T1W images [109, 110].

Nasopharyngeal carcinoma accounts for nearly 70% of all primary malignancies of the nasopharynx. The typical site of origin is the Rosenmüller fossa of the nasopharynx, which is a bilateral invagination of the pharyngeal mucosa located superior and posterior to the torus tubarius (the internal orifice of the Eustachian tube).

Clinical presentation is often late, and the prognosis is poor, for it is generally detected when invasion of the adjacent structures and metastasis are already prominent. Clinical presentation includes epistaxis and conductive hearing loss due to eustachian tube obstruction. The presence of fluid in the middle ear is often a precocious sign of the disease, which can be detected either on CT or MR images [38, 111].

Trauma

Peripheral trigeminal neuropathy may result from a head trauma involving specific districts.

The supraorbital nerve may be injured in orbital roof fractures and superior orbital rim fractures, while the involvement of the superior orbital fissure leads to dysfunction of the entire V1 branch.

Fractures extending through the foramen rotundum, the inferior orbital rim or the pterygoid plates affect the maxillary nerve.

Fractures of the central skull base may involve the foramen ovale and the mandibular nerve. V3 may be also injured from mandibular fractures extending to the mandibular canal which contains the inferior alveolar nerve.

CT scans are the imaging of choice in head trauma due to their high sensibility in depicting subtle bone fractures and possible major parenchymal complications, as well as for their rapid use in emergencies [2, 24].

Other Communal Lesions

Some primitive bone affections such as the group of fibro-osseous diseases may involve the trigeminal nerve by shrinking its neural foramina. Fibrous dysplasia and Paget's disease are included among these disorders.

The main foramina crossed by the trigeminal divisions are superior orbital fissure (V1, entire branch), superior orbital foramen (supraorbital nerve from V1), foramen rotundum (V2, entire branch), inferior orbital fissure and infraorbital foramen (infraorbital nerve from V2), pterygo-palatine fossa (pterygopalatine ganglion of V2 and divisions), greater and lesser palatine foramen (palatine nerves from V2), foramen ovale (V3 entire branch), mandibular foramen (inferior alveolar nerve, from V3), and mental foramen (mental nerve, from V3) [1, 106].

Inflammatory pseudotumor (IPT) is a rare cause of peripheral trigeminal neuralgia, which can manifest as an intra-orbital mass or involve the paranasal sinuses. This condition has already been discussed in the chapter of the trigeminal cisternal segment [71].

6.3.4.2 Specific Alterations of the Trigeminal Branches

Ophthalmic Division (V1)

Orbital masses can compress, distort, or invade the trigeminal ophthalmic division, leading to a painful neuropathy. V1 is more frequently affected by primitive neoplasms, which usually are neural sheath tumors, such as schwannoma and plexiform neurofibroma, both typically encountered in NF1 [67].

Rarely, invasive bacterial or fungal sinusitis may cross the bony sinus wall and extend to the orbit. In those cases, V1 affection depends on the involvement of the supraorbital fissure [24].

Maxillary Division (V2)

Due to the proximity of the maxillary branch to the paranasal sinuses, the spread of aggressive bacterial or fungal infections starting from the paranasal sinuses may involve this trigeminal division [24, 112].

Juvenile angiofibroma (JAF) is a benign, nonencapsulated fibrovascular neoplasm, more often affecting young adults. The site of origin usually involves the superolateral wall of the choana or the vomer.

JAF shows a typical pattern of spread, characterized by submucosal extension, often involving the sphenopalatine foramen and pterygopalatine fossa, and occasionally causing V2 neuropathy. The classical clinical manifestation of this tumor is recurrent epistaxis [67].

Mandibular Division (V3)

A clear causative relation between dental procedures and trigeminal neuralgia has never been reported, partially due to the high prevalence of patients affected by an undiagnosed otherwise-caused trigeminal neuralgia who undergo unnecessary dental procedures.

Odontogenic infection of the maxillary molars and lower second and third molars may produce abscesses in the masticator space, whereas infection of the lower first molar and premolar teeth tends to involve the sublingual space. Myositis and abscess formation within the pterygoid muscles may involve the proximal part of V3 at the masticator space entrance, resulting in V3 painful neuropathy. Acute and chronic osteomyelitis may progress to involve the mandibular canal and, therefore, the inferior alveolar nerve, causing intense pain and numbness of the chin and lips [113].

Osteoradionecrosis of the mandible typically occurs months or years after high-dose irradiation of oral cavity or oropharyngeal tumors. Because of the inferior alveolar nerve impairment, patients may present with paresthesia or pain.

CT may show multiple, ill-defined radiolucent areas, cortical disruption, sequestrate, areas of sclerosis, and periosteal reactions, while MR displays typical inflammatory changes either in infectious or radio-induced osteomyelitis [114, 115].

High-resolution evaluation of the mandible canal and its relations with the radices of the tooth, the integrity of bone cortex, and the morphology and structure of the bone trabecula represent key features in the report and are best depicted by DentaScan (GE Healthcare, Princeton, New Jersey) software with 2D curved reconstructions along the mandibular canal.

Lesions originating from the masticator space may affect the mandibular branch and its divisions. The masticator space contains mainly muscles, lymphatic tissue, and the ascending branch of the mandible, so that nonneural neoplasms arising from this site include rhabdomyosarcoma, lymphoma, and mandibular tumors, such as ameloblastoma, osteosarcoma, and chondrosarcoma. Rhabdomyosarcoma is one of the most common soft tissue sarcomas and originates from mesenchymal tissue. It represents the most common malignant tumor of the head and neck in the pediatric population [67] and goes differential with nasopharyngeal carcinoma, which is less common in this age and often comes with a prominent involvement of the adjacent lymph nodes.

When head/neck cancer is suspected, the radiologic investigation should be performed with a field of view (FOV) extending from the orbit roof to the base of the neck, due to possible dissemination, perineural spread, and metastatic lymph nodes.

6.3.5 Imaging-Silent Trigeminal Neuralgia

Clinical and laboratory analysis play a central role in addressing the diagnosis in case of imaging-silent trigeminal neuralgia.

With a negative imaging, laboratory tests should be performed to exclude neuralgia caused by infectious agents or connective tissue diseases and vasculitis. Among connectivopathies, mixed connective tissue disease and rheumatoid arthritis have more often been reported in association with trigeminal pain [116, 117]. Lupus eritematosus sistemicus (LES) has also been related to trigeminal neuralgia without any specific imaging finding [118].

The mechanism underlying the neural pain seen in connective tissue diseases is not well understood. Chronic compression of the nerve from fibrosis or aberrant blood vessels, as well as vasculitis of the vasa vasorum, may lead to demyelination of the nerve fibers [116].

Paraneoplastic involvement of the trigeminus has been reported in association with anti-Hu antibodies, from small lung cell carcinoma or ovarian cancer. In these cases, the trigeminal neuropathy is more often part of a brainstem encephalitis rather than an isolated finding [119].

After excluding every other cause of painful neuropathy, idiopathic trigeminal neuralgia can be diagnosed.

6.3.6 Posttreatment Imaging

The current guidelines for TN management have been published by the American Academy of Neurology (AAN) and the European Federation of Neurological Societies (EFNS) [120, 121]. According to these guidelines, in a patient with classical trigeminal neuralgia, the treatment approach should begin with medical therapy, consisting in two main drugs (carbamazepine and oxcarbazepine), which can be interchangeably used. If the patient is a non-responder to either of these two drugs, or cannot take them because of specific counter indications or cannot reach the therapeutic dosage because of excessive adverse effects, the diagnosis of "refractory trigeminal neuralgia" can be made [122].

In the case of refractory neuralgia, the most effective approach is surgical microvascular decompression, which aims to separate the offending vessel from the trigeminal nerve at the level of the neurovascular conflict, interposing a Teflon pledge or a decompression sling to maintain them apart.

For patients who do not accept surgery, lamotrigine as add-on or botulinum toxin injections should be tried [122].

Other possible alternative treatments to posterior fossa microvascular decompression are Gasserian ganglion percutaneous techniques and Gamma Knife radiosurgery targeting the affected trigeminal root [121].

6.3.6.1 Imaging Microvascular Decompression (MVD)

The role of imaging in postsurgical course of trigeminal neuralgia comprehends the assessment of early-onset and delayed complications.

Early-onset complications are related to the surgical procedure itself, including bleeding and infections.

MR imaging is also used to evaluate the results of the procedure. The pledget or pad is typically hypointense on CISS sequences, does not enhance, and may occasionally become displaced. Delayed complications include Teflon granuloma, which forms as a foreign body reaction to the pledget, resulting in mass effect on CN V, and commonly shows enhancement or calcifications [27] (Fig. 6.20). The presence of a Teflon granuloma, as well as arachnoid adhesions and recurrent vascular conflict, may require additional surgery [123].

6.3.6.2 Other Posttreatment Imaging Findings

Gamma Knife radiosurgery (GKR) may produce a persistent enhancement of the treated trigeminal segment, which may be associated with less satisfactory pain control and more frequently detected facial sensory loss [124].

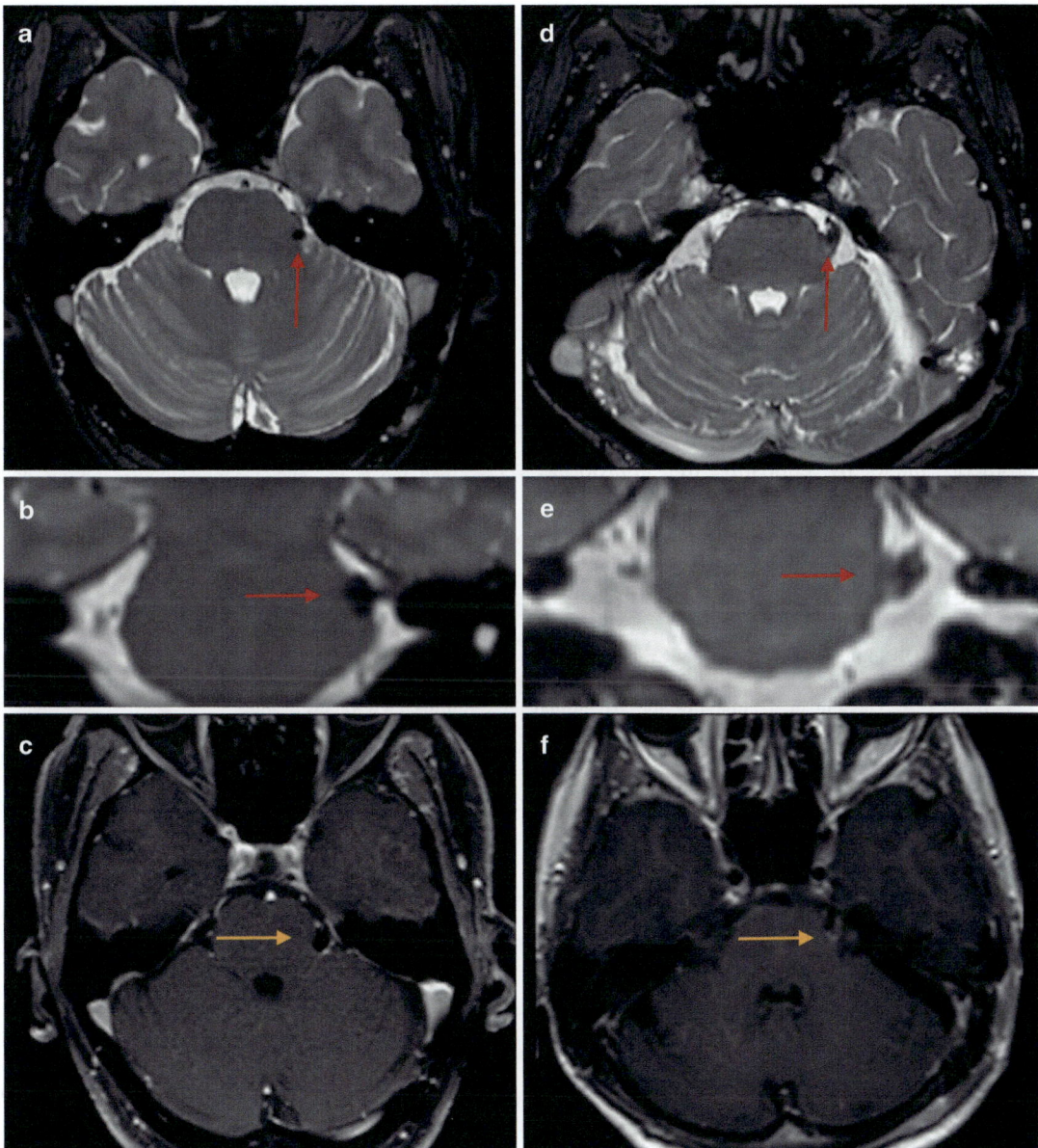

Fig. 6.20 Posttreatment imaging after MVD showing the normal appearance of the Teflon pledget which separates the trigeminal nerve from the offending vessel (**a–c**), characterized by low T2 signal intensity (**a**, **b**, red arrows) and no CE on post-Gd T1WI (**c**, yellow arrow). Teflon granuloma is a possible complication of MVD. In this case, the pledget is surrounded by inflammatory tissue and shows higher T2 signal intensity (**d**, **e**, red arrows) and CE on post-Gd T1WI (**f**, yellow arrow)

6.4 Conclusions

Trigeminal neuralgia is a communal manifestation of several possible etiologies. Classical type is defined as sudden, usually unilateral, severe, brief, stabbing recurrent episodes of pain in the distribution of one or more branches of the trigeminal nerve, with no cause other than a neurovascular compression. In these cases, a medical therapy should be offered, while MVD showed optimal results in refractory neuralgias. An anatomy-based imaging approach should be used to investigate neurovascular conflict, as well as possible causes of secondary TN, with a target-suited protocol, made by choosing the appropriate sequences and parameters.

References

1. Binder D, Sonne D, Fischbein N. Cranial nerves. New York: Thieme; 2010.
2. Borges A, Casselman J. Imaging the trigeminal nerve. Eur J Radiol. 2010;74:323–40.
3. Blitz A, Choudhri A, Chonka Z, Ilica A, Macedo L, Chhabra A, et al. Anatomic considerations, nomenclature, and advanced cross-sectional imaging techniques for visualization of the cranial nerve segments by MR imaging. Neuroimaging Clin N Am. 2014;24:1–15.
4. Tomii M, Onoue H, Yasue M, Tokudome S, Abe T. Microscopic measurement of the facial nerve root exit zone from central glial myelin to peripheral Schwann cell myelin. J Neurosurg. 2003;99:121–4.
5. Campos-Benitez M, Kaufmann A. Neurovascular compression findings in hemifacial spasm. J Neurosurg. 2008;109:416–20.
6. Gudmundsson K, Rhoton A, Rushton J. Detailed anatomy of the intracranial portion of the trigeminal nerve. J Neurosurg. 1971;35:592–600.
7. Haller S, Etienne L, Ko vari E, Varoquaux A, Urbach H, Becker M. Imaging of neurovascular compression syndromes: trigeminal neuralgia, hemifacial spasm, vestibular paroxysmia, and glossopharyngeal neuralgia. Am J Neuroradiol. 2016;37:1384–92.
8. Lang J. Clinical anatomy of the head. Berlin: Springer-Verlag; 1983.
9. Williams LS, Schmalfuss IM, Sistrom CL, Inoue T, Tanaka R, Seoane ER, et al. MR imaging of the trigeminal ganglion, nerve, and the perineural vascular plexus: normal appearance and variants with correlation to cadaver specimens. Am J Neuroradiol. 2003;24:1317–23.
10. Borges A, Casselman J. Imaging the cranial nerves part I: methodology, infectious and inflammatory, traumatic and congenital lesions. Eur Radiol. 2007;175:2112–25.
11. Penn R, Abemayor E, Nabili V, Bhuta S, Kirsch C. Perineural invasion detected by high-field 3.0-T magnetic resonance imaging. Am J Otolaryngol. 2010;31:482–4.
12. Casselman J, Kuhweide R, Deimling M, Ampe W, Dehaene I, Meeus L. Constructive interference in steady state-3DFT MR imaging of the inner ear and cerebellopontine angle. Am J Neuroradiol. 1993;14:47–57.
13. Sheth S, Branstetter BF IV, Escott EJ. Appearance of normal cranial nerves on steady-state free precession MR images1. RadioGraphics. 2009;29:1045–55.
14. Casselman J, Mermuys K, Delanote J, Ghekiere J, Coenegrachts K. MRI of the cranial nerves—more than meets the eye: technical considerations and advanced anatomy. Neuroimaging Clin N Am. 2008;18:197–231.
15. Seeburg D, Northcutt B, Aygun N, Blitz A. The role of imaging for trigeminal neuralgia. Neurosurgery Clin N Am. 2016;27:315–26.
16. The International Classification of Headache Disorders. 3rd ed. (Beta version) [Internet]. ICHD3b. 2017 [cited 22 November 2017]. Available from: https://www.ichd-3.org/.
17. Akter M, Hirai T, Minoda R, Murakami R, Saiki S, Okuaki T, et al. Diffusion tensor tractography in the head-and-neck region using a clinical 3-T MR scanner. Acad Radiol. 2009;16:858–65.
18. Mazhari A. Multiple sclerosis-related pain syndromes: an imaging update. Curr Pain Headache Rep. 2016;20:63.
19. Tekkok I, Sumer M. Bilateral trigeminal neuralgia and Charcot-Marie-Tooth disease: diagnosis and successful microsurgical treatment of bilateral neurovascular compression. Zentralbl Neurochir – Cent Eur Neurosurg. 2008;69:148–51.
20. Truini A, Prosperini L, Calistri V, Fiorelli M, Pozzilli C, Millefiorini E, et al. A dual concurrent mechanism explains trigeminal neuralgia in patients with multiple sclerosis. Neurology. 2016;86:2094–9.
21. Gass A, Kitchen N, MacManus D, Moseley I, Hennerici M, Miller D. Trigeminal neuralgia in patients with multiple sclerosis: lesion localization with magnetic resonance imaging. Neurology. 1997;49:1142–4.
22. Mills R, Young C, Smith E. Central trigeminal involvement in multiple sclerosis using high-resolution MRI at 3 T. Br J Radiol. 2010;83:493–8.
23. Bathla G, Hegde A. The trigeminal nerve: an illustrated review of its imaging anatomy and pathology. Clin Radiol. 2013;68:203–13.
24. Becker M, Kohler R, Vargas M, Viallon M, Delavelle J. Pathology of the trigeminal nerve. Neuroimaging Clin N Am. 2008;18:283–307.

25. Haanpaa M, Dastidar P, Weinberg A, Levin M, Miettinen A, Lapinlampi A, et al. CSF and MRI findings in patients with acute herpes zoster. Neurology. 1998;51:1405–11.

26. D'Amico A, Russo C, Ugga L, Mazio F, Capone E, D'Arco F, et al. Can pontine trigeminal T2-hyperintensity suggest herpetic etiology of trigeminal neuralgia? Quant Imaging Med Surg. 2016;6:490–5.

27. Dueland A, Ranneberg-Nilsen T, Degré M. Detection of latent varicella zoster virus DNA and human gene sequences in human trigeminal ganglia by in situ amplification combined with in situ hybridization. Arch Virol. 1995;140:2055–66.

28. Burger K, Tuhrim S, Naidich T. Brainstem vascular stroke anatomy. Neuroimaging Clin N Am. 2005;15:297–324.

29. Tatu L, Moulin T, Vuillier F, Bogousslavsky J. Arterial territories of the human brain. Front Neurol Neurosci. 2012;30:99–110.

30. Fitzek S, Baumgartner U, Marx J, Joachimski F, Axer H, Witte OW, et al. Pain and itch in Wallenberg's syndrome: anatomical-functional correlations. Suppl Clin Neurophysiol. 2006;58:187–94.

31. Ordás C, Cuadrado M, Simal P, Barahona R, Casas J, Matías-Guiu Antem J, et al. Wallenberg's syndrome and symptomatic trigeminal neuralgia. J Headache Pain. 2011;12:377–80.

32. Balestrino M, Leandri M. Trigeminal neuralgia in pontine ischaemia. J Neurol Neurosurg Psychiatry. 1997;62:297–8.

33. Golby A, Norbash A, Silverberg G. Trigeminal neuralgia resulting from infarction of the root entry zone of the trigeminal nerve: case report. Neurosurgery. 1998;43:620–3.

34. Kim J, Kang J, Lee M. Trigeminal neuralgia after pontine infarction. Neurology. 1998;51:1511–2.

35. Peker S, Akansel G, Sun I, Pamir N. Trigeminal neuralgia due to pontine infarction. Headache J Head Face Pain. 2004;44:1043–5.

36. Katsuno M, Teramoto A. Secondary trigeminal neuropathy and neuralgia resulting from pontine infarction. J Stroke Cerebrovasc Dis. 2010;19:251–2.

37. Nakamizo T, Koide T, Miyazaki H. Progressive intracranial vertebral artery dissection presenting with isolated trigeminal neuralgia-like facial pain. Case Rep Neurol Med. 2015;2015:1–4.

38. Osborn A, Salzman K, Jhaveri M. Diagnostic imaging. Philadelphia: Elsevier; 2016.

39. Adachi K, Hasegawa M, Hayashi T, Nagahisa S, Hirose Y. A review of cavernous malformations with trigeminal neuralgia. Clin Neurol Neurosurg. 2014;125:151–4.

40. Barkovich A. Diagnostic imaging: pediatric neuroradiology. 2nd ed. Philadelphia: Elsevier Health Sciences; 2014.

41. Hartmann M, Heiland S, Harting I, Tronnier VM, Sommer C, Ludwig R, et al. Distinguishing of primary cerebral lymphoma from high-grade glioma with perfusion-weighted magnetic resonance imaging. Neurosci Lett. 2003;338:119–22.

42. Haldorsen I, Espeland A, Larsson E. Central nervous system lymphoma: characteristic findings on traditional and advanced imaging. Am J Neuroradiol. 2010;32:984–92.

43. Liu J, Yuan Y, Zhang L, Fang Y, Liu H, Yu Y. Hemifacial spasm and trigeminal neuralgia in Chiari's I malformation with hydrocephalus: case report and literature review. Clin Neurol Neurosurg. 2014;122:64–7.

44. Zhang W, Chen M, Zhang W. Trigeminal neuralgia due to dandy-walker syndrome. J Craniofac Surg. 2013;24:1457–9.

45. Jannetta P, Mclaughlin M, Casey K. Technique of microvascular decompression. Neurosurg Focus. 2005;18:1–5.

46. Love S. Trigeminal neuralgia: pathology and pathogenesis. Brain. 2001;124:2347–60.

47. Guclu B, Sindou M, Meyronet D, Streichenberger N, Simon E, Mertens P. Cranial nerve vascular compression syndromes of the trigeminal, facial and vagoglossopharyngeal nerves: comparative anatomical study of the central myelin portion and transitional zone; correlations with incidences of corresponding hyperactive dysfunctional syndromes. Acta Neurochir. 2011;153:2365–75.

48. Sindou M, Howeidy T, Acevedo G. Anatomical observations during microvascular decompression for idiopathic trigeminal neuralgia (with correlations between topography of pain and site of the neurovascular conflict). Prospective study in a series of 579 patients. Acta Neurochir. 2002;144:1–13.

49. Ros de San Pedro J. Posterior communicating artery aneurysms causing facial pain: a comprehensive review. Clin Neurol Neurosurg. 2017;160:59–68.

50. de Bondt B, Stokroos R, Casselman J. Persistent trigeminal artery associated with trigeminal neuralgia: hypothesis of neurovascular compression. Neuroradiology. 2006;49:23–6.

51. García-Pastor C, López-González F, Revuelta R, Nathal E. Trigeminal neuralgia secondary to arteriovenous malformations of the posterior fossa. Surg Neurol. 2006;66:207–11.

52. Matsushima T, Huynh-Le P, Miyazono M. Trigeminal neuralgia caused by venous compression. Neurosurgery. 2004;55:334–7.

53. Antonini G, Di Pasquale A, Cruccu G, Truini A, Morino S, Saltelli G, et al. Magnetic resonance imaging contribution for diagnosing symptomatic neurovascular contact in classical trigeminal neuralgia: a blinded case-control study and meta-analysis. Pain. 2014;155:1464–71.

54. Suzuki M, Yoshino N, Shimada M, Tetsumura A, Matsumura T, Fukayama H, et al. Trigeminal neuralgia: differences in magnetic resonance imaging characteristics of neurovascular compression between

symptomatic and asymptomatic nerves. Oral Surg Oral Med Oral Pathol Oral Radiol. 2015;119:113–8.

55. Harsha K, Kesavadas C, Chinchure S, Thomas B, Jagtap S. Imaging of vascular causes of trigeminal neuralgia. J Neuroradiol. 2012;39:281–9.

56. İldan F, Göçer A, Bağdatoğlu H, Uzuneyüpoğlu Z, Tuna M, Çetinalp E. Isolated trigeminal neuralgia secondary to distal anterior inferior cerebellar artery aneurysm. Neurosurg Rev. 1996;19:43–6.

57. Peluso J, van Rooij W, Sluzewski M, Beute G. Superior cerebellar artery aneurysms: incidence, clinical presentation and midterm outcome of endovascular treatment. Neuroradiology. 2007;49:747–51.

58. Pereira L, Nepomuceno L, Coimbra P, Oliveira Neto S, Natal M. Persistent trigeminal artery: angiotomography and angio-magnetic resonance finding. Arq Neuro-Psiquiatr. 2009;67:882–5.

59. Yoshino N, Akimoto H, Yamada I, Nagaoka T, Tetsumura A, Kurabayashi T, et al. Trigeminal neuralgia: evaluation of neuralgic manifestation and site of neurovascular compression with 3D CISS MR imaging and MR angiography. Radiology. 2003;228:539–45.

60. Herweh C, Kress B, Rasche D, Tronnier V, Troger J, Sartor K, et al. Loss of anisotropy in trigeminal neuralgia revealed by diffusion tensor imaging. Neurology. 2007;68:776–8.

61. Delfini R, Innocenzi G, Ciappetta P, Domenicucci M, Cantore G. Meningiomas of Meckel's cave. Neurosurgery. 1992;31:1000–7.

62. Carvalho G, Matthies C, Tatagiba M, Eghbal R, Samii M. Impact of computed tomographic and magnetic resonance imaging findings on surgical outcome in petroclival meningiomas. Neurosurgery. 2000;47:1287–95.

63. Narro-Donate J, Huete-Allut A, Velasco-Albendea F, Escribano-Mesa J, Mendez-Román P, Masegosa-González J. Condroma adyacente al cavum de Meckel simulando un neurinoma del quinto par craneal. A propósito de un caso. Neurocirugía. 2016;27:144–8.

64. Leclercq D, Thiebaut J, Héran F. Trigeminal neuralgia. Diagn Interv Imaging. 2013;94:993–1001.

65. Zakrzewska JM. Trigeminal neuralgia. Clin Evid. 2002;7:1221–31.

66. Larrier D, Lee A. Anatomy of headache and facial pain. Otolaryngol Clin N Am. 2003;36:1041–53.

67. Tortori-Donati P, Rossi A, Biancheri R. Pediatric neuroradiology. Berlin: Springer; 2005.

68. Muzammil S, Leong K. A case of cerebellopontine angle epidermoid cyst presenting as trigeminal neuropathy. South Med J. 2009;102:534–6.

69. Furtado S, Hegde A. Trigeminal neuralgia due to a small Meckel's cave epidermoid tumor: surgery using an extradural corridor. Skull Base. 2009;19:353–7.

70. Majoie C, Verbeeten B, Dol J, Peeters F. Trigeminal neuropathy: evaluation with MR imaging. RadioGraphics. 1995;15:795–811.

71. Patnana M, Sevrukov A, Elsayes K, Viswanathan C, Lubner M, Menias C. Inflammatory pseudotumor: the great mimicker. Am J Roentgenol. 2012;198:W217–27.

72. Lui P, Fan Y, Wong S, Chan A, Wong G, Chau T, et al. Inflammatory pseudotumors of the central nervous system. Hum Pathol. 2009;40:1611–7.

73. Bangiyev L, Kornacki S, Mikolaenko I. Rare isolated trigeminal nerve sarcoidosis mimicking schwannoma. Clin Imaging. 2015;39:133–5.

74. Seidel E, Hansen C, Urban P, Vogt T, Muller-Forell W, Hopf H. Idiopathic trigeminal sensory neuropathy with gadolinium enhancement in the cisternal segment. Neurology. 2000;54:1191–2.

75. Fritz C, Rösler A, Heyden B, Braune H. Trigeminal neuralgia as a clinical manifestation of Lyme neuroborreliosis. J Neurol. 1996;243:367–8.

76. Hashmi M, Guha G, Saha B. Trigeminal neuralgia in an HIV patient. J Global Infect Dis. 2010;2:65.

77. Pichiecchio A, Bergamaschi R, Tavazzi E, Romani A, Todeschini A, Bastianello S. Bilateral trigeminal enhancement on magnetic resonance imaging in a patient with multiple sclerosis and trigeminal neuralgia. Mult Scler J. 2007;13:814–6.

78. Bird TD, Ott J, Giblett ER. Evidence for linkage of Charcot-Marie-Tooth neuropathy to the Duffy locus on chromosome 1. Am J Hum Genet. 1982;34:388–94.

79. Albayram S, Asik M, Hasiloglu Z, Dikici A, Erdemli H, Altintas A. Pathological contrast enhancement of the oculomotor and trigeminal nerves caused by intracranial hypotension syndrome. Headache J Head Face Pain. 2011;51:804–8.

80. Friedman D. The pseudotumor cerebri syndrome. Neurol Clin. 2014;32:363–96.

81. Davenport R, Will R, Galloway P. Isolated intracranial hypertension presenting with trigeminal neuropathy. J Neurol Neurosurg Psychiatry. 1994;57:381.

82. Kouyialis A, Stranjalis G, Boviatsis E, Ziaka D, Bouras T, Sakas D. Recurrence of trigeminal neuralgia due to an acquired arachnoid cyst. J Clin Neurosci. 2008;15:1409–11.

83. Larson J, van Loveren H, Balko M, Tew J. Evidence of meningioma infiltration into cranial nerves: clinical implications for cavernous sinus meningiomas. J Neurosurg. 1995;83:596–9.

84. El-Kalliny M, van Loveren H, Keller J, Tew J. Tumors of the lateral wall of the cavernous sinus. J Neurosurg. 1992;77:508–14.

85. Wang M, Li G, Jia D, Shen J. Clinical characteristics and surgical outcomes of patients with interdural epidermoid cyst of the cavernous sinus. J Clin Neurosci. 2013;20:53–6.

86. Korchi A, Cuvinciuc V, Caetano J, Becker M, Lovblad K, Vargas M. Imaging of the cavernous sinus lesions. Diagn Interv Imaging. 2014;95:849–59.

87. Gazioğlu N, Tanriöver N, Tüzgen S. Pituitary tumour presenting with trigeminal neuralgia as an isolated symptom. Br J Neurosurg. 2000;14:579.

88. Faro S, Koenlgsberg R, Turtz A, Croul S. Melanocytoma of the cavernous sinus: CT and MR findings. Am J Neuroradiol. 1996;17:1087–90.

89. Louis D, Perry A, Reifenberger G, von Deimling A, Figarella-Branger D, Cavenee W, et al. The 2016 World Health Organization classification of tumors of the central nervous system: a summary. Acta Neuropathol. 2016;131:803–20.

90. Pan H, Wang H, Fan Y. Intracranial meningeal melanocytoma associated with nevus of Ota. J Clin Neurosci. 2011;18:1548–50.

91. Goel A. Chordoma and chondrosarcoma: Relationship to the internal carotid artery. Acta Neurochir. 1995;133:30–5.

92. Som P, Curtin H. Head and neck imaging. St. Louis: Mosby; 2003.

93. Almefty K, Pravdenkova S, Colli B, Al-Mefty O, Gokden M. Chordoma and chondrosarcoma: similar, but quite different, skull base tumors. Cancer. 2007;110:2467–77.

94. Smith A, Horkanyne-Szakaly I, Schroeder J, Rushing E. From the radiologic pathology archives: mass lesions of the dura: beyond meningioma—radiologic-pathologic correlation. RadioGraphics. 2014;34:295–312.

95. Starr C, Cha S. Meningioma mimics: five key imaging features to differentiate them from meningiomas. Clin Radiol. 2017;72:722–8.

96. Hakyemez B, Yildirim N, Erdoğan C, Kocaeli H, Korfali E, Parlak M. Meningiomas with conventional MRI findings resembling intraaxial tumors: can perfusion-weighted MRI be helpful in differentiation? Neuroradiology. 2006;48:695–702.

97. Vieira J, Cukiert A, Liberman B. Evaluation of magnetic resonance imaging criteria for cavernous sinus invasion in patients with pituitary adenomas: logistic regression analysis and correlation with surgical findings. Surg Neurol. 2006;65:130–5.

98. Knosp E, Steiner E, Kitz K, Matula C. Pituitary adenomas with invasion of the cavernous sinus space. Neurosurgery. 1993;33:610–8.

99. Micko A, Wöhrer A, Wolfsberger S, Knosp E. Invasion of the cavernous sinus space in pituitary adenomas: endoscopic verification and its correlation with an MRI-based classification. J Neurosurg. 2015;122:803–11.

100. Maschio M, Mengarelli A, Girmenia C, Vidiri A, Kayal R, Gallo M, et al. Trigeminal neuralgia as unusual isolated symptom of fungal paranasal sinusitis in patients with haematological malignancies. Neurol Sci. 2011;33:647–52.

101. Zinreich S, Kennedy D, Malat J, Curtin H, Epstein J, Huff L, et al. Fungal sinusitis: diagnosis with CT and MR imaging. Radiology. 1988;169:439–44.

102. Schuknecht B, Sturm V, Huisman T, Landau K. Tolosa-Hunt syndrome: MR imaging features in 15 patients with 20 episodes of painful ophthalmoplegia. Eur J Radiol. 2009;69:445–53.

103. Yousem D, Atlas S, Grossman R, Sergott R, Savino P, Bosley T. MR imaging of Tolosa-Hunt syndrome. Am J Roentgenol. 1990;154:167–70.

104. Hahn C, Nicolle D, Lownie S, Drake C. Giant cavernous carotid aneurysms. J Neuro-Ophthalmol. 2001;20:253–8.

105. Tsai Y, Chen L, Su C, Lu T, Wu C, Kuo C. Utility of source images of three-dimensional time-of-flight magnetic resonance angiography in the diagnosis of indirect carotid-cavernous sinus fistulas. J Neuro-Ophthalmol. 2004;24:285–9.

106. Bartiromo F, Cirillo L, Caranci F, Elefante A, D'Amico A, Tortora F, et al. Trigeminal perineural spread of head and neck tumors. Neuroradiol J. 2007;20:116–23.

107. Maroldi R, Farina D, Borghesi A, Marconi A, Gatti E. Perineural tumor spread. Neuroimaging Clin N Am. 2008;18:413–29.

108. Tashi S, Purohit B, Becker M, Mundada P. The pterygopalatine fossa: imaging anatomy, communications, and pathology revisited. Insights Imaging. 2016;7:589–99.

109. Russo CP, Smoker WR, Weissman JL. MR appearance of trigeminal and hypoglossal motor denervation. Am J Neuroradiol. 1997;18:1375–83.

110. Davis SB, Mathews VP, Williams DW. Masticator muscle enhancement in subacute denervation atrophy. Am J Neuroradiol. 1995;16:1292–4.

111. Razek A, King A. MRI and CT of nasopharyngeal carcinoma. Am J Roentgenol. 2012;198:11–8.

112. Chun M, Eom T, Lim G, Kim J. Secondary trigeminal neuralgia attributed to paranasal sinusitis in a pediatric patient. Child's Nerv Syst. 2017;33:397–8.

113. Graff-Radford S, Gordon R, Ganal J, Tetradis S. Trigeminal neuralgia and facial pain imaging. Curr Pain Headache Rep. 2015;19:19.

114. Chang PC, Fischbein NJ, Holliday RA. Central skull base osteomyelitis in patients without otitis externa: imaging findings. Am J Neuroradiol. 2003;24:1310–6.

115. Chong J, Hinckley LK, Ginsberg LE. Masticator space abnormalities associated with mandibular osteoradionecrosis: MR and CT findings in five patients. Am J Neuroradiol. 2000;21:175–8.

116. Hojaili B, Barland P. Trigeminal neuralgia as the first manifestation of mixed connective tissue disorder. JCR J Clin Rheumatol. 2006;12:145–7.

117. Hagen NA, Stevens JC, Michet CJ. Trigeminal sensory neuropathy associated with connective tissue diseases. Neurology. 1990;40:891–6.

118. Kumar V, Kaur J, Pothuri P, Bandagi S. Atypical trigeminal neuralgia: a rare neurological manifestation of systemic lupus erythematosus. Am J Case Rep. 2017;18:42–5.

119. Kalanie H, Harandi A, Mardani M, Shahverdi Z, Morakabati A, Alidaei S, et al. Trigeminal neuralgia as the first clinical manifestation of Anti-Hu paraneoplastic syndrome induced by a borderline ovarian mucinous tumor. Case Rep Neurol. 2014;6:7–13.

120. Cruccu G, Gronseth G, Alksne J, et al. AAN-EFNS guidelines on trigeminal neuralgia management. Eur J Neurol. 2008;15:1013–28.

121. Gronseth G, Cruccu G, Alksne J, Argoff C, Brainin M, Burchiel K, et al. Practice parameter: the diagnostic evaluation and treatment of trigeminal neuralgia (an evidence-based review): report of the quality standards subcommittee of the American Academy of Neurology and the European Federation of Neurological Societies. Neurology. 2008;71:1183–90.

122. Cruccu G, Truini A. Refractory trigeminal neuralgia. CNS Drugs. 2012;27:91–6.

123. Gu W, Zhao W. Microvascular decompression for recurrent trigeminal neuralgia. J Clin Neurosci. 2014;21:1549–53.

124. Mousavi S, Akpinar B, Niranjan A, Agarwal V, Cohen J, Flickinger J, et al. The clinical significance of persistent trigeminal nerve contrast enhancement in patients who undergo repeat radiosurgery. J Neurosurg. 2017;127:219–25.

Spine Pain: Clinical Features

7

Luigi Murena, Gianluca Canton, Gioia Giraldi, and Stefania Bassini

7.1 Epidemiology of Spine Pain

Spine pain is one of the most common pain conditions worldwide. It affects both men and women in all ethnic groups, increasing dramatically in incidence and prevalence with age. The lifetime prevalence of neck and low back pain in adults is currently estimated to be 66.7% and 91%, respectively. Moreover, spine pain has a great impact on functional capacity and occupational activities, representing a major welfare and economic problem.

Low back pain represents indeed the second leading cause of disability worldwide with 1% of the world population estimated to be involved. One-year recurrence rate of non-specific back pain reaches 20–44% and its lifetime recurrence rate up to 72%. Nonetheless, back pain often evolves in chronic pain, defined as a recurrent or persistent pain lasting at least 3 months, which characterizes the chronic lower back pain (CLBP) syndrome. CLBP has increased more than 100% in the last decade, despite several investments in improving workplace ergonomics and other preventive measures. Low back pain is furthermore the leading chronic health problem forcing older workers to retire prematurely or forcing people out of the workplace (more than

heart disease, diabetes, hypertension, neoplasm, respiratory disease and asthma combined). The economic burden of the disease is then related both to healthcare system spending and decreased productivity. In the USA, among the 116 million people affected by CLBP, 19% lost their job, 13% changed job because of their pain and 60% consulted a doctor for pain relief 2 to 9 times in a 6 months' time lapse [1, 2].

On the other hand, neck pain has an overall prevalence of 27% in female and 17% in male, and the incidence of neck pain reported in various studies ranges from 10% to 21% in the general population, with an increased incidence in office and computer workers [3].

Carroll et al., in their work on the course and prognostic factors of neck pain in general population, have found that 50–85% of people that experience an episode of neck pain will report neck pain 1–5 years later [4].

Although many cases of neck pain resolve with time and require minimal intervention, about one third of people will suffer from chronic neck pain, and 5% will develop significant disability and reduction of quality of life [5].

The factors leading to both low back and neck chronic pain are various, with a significant role of nonanatomical factors such as psychological stress, depression and/or anxiety. This complex scenario determines chronic back pain syndrome to be very challenging for the physician, both for diagnosis and treatment.

L. Murena (✉) · G. Canton · G. Giraldi · S. Bassini
Orthopaedics and Traumatology Unit, Trieste
University Hospital—ASUITS, Trieste, Italy
e-mail: l.murena@units.it

© Springer Nature Switzerland AG 2019
M. A. Cova, F. Stacul (eds.), *Pain Imaging*, https://doi.org/10.1007/978-3-319-99822-0_7

7.2 Pathways and Pathophysiology of Spine Pain

The spine receives its somatic innervation from both somatic fibres (inside spinal nerves) and autonomic fibres (originating from the paravertebral sympathetic ganglia and chains).

Discs and vertebral bodies are innervated all around their circumference by three microscopic plexuses (anterior, lateral and posterior) and inside by their short periosteal and annulus fibres. There are three main sources of pain in consideration of the spine innervation:

- Dorsal branch of the spinal nerves (dorsal rami)

This branch develops from the thick anterior branch at the exit of the foramen. It runs dorsally, between the transverse processes, innervating the posterior structures: facet joints, ligamentum flavum, supra- and interspinous ligaments, spinal muscles and adjacent dorsal skin.

- Sinuvertebral nerve (recurrent nerve of Luschka or recurrent meningeal nerve)

This nerve is a recurrent branch formed by union of the grey ramus communicans (GRC) of the sympathetic system with a little branch coming from the proximal end of anterior primary ramus of the spinal nerve. It penetrates retrogressively through the intervertebral foramen into the spinal canal. It is a polisegmentary mixed nerve containing both somatic and autonomic fibres for the posterolateral annulus, the posterior vertebral body and the periosteum, facet joints, ventral meninges and anterior epidural vessels. Sympathetic trunks and ganglia directly innervate the anterior longitudinal ligament (ALL), the anterior periosteum and vertebral body, the paravertebral muscles and fascia as well as the anterolateral disc. Autonomic nervous afferences may enter the white ramus communicans (WRC) and reach the spinal nerve and the dorsal root ganglion, or they can reach the sinuvertebral nerve through the GRC. Through the sinuvertebral nerves, autonomic fibres reach all the structure they supply and complete the innervation of the anterior spine. Its complex anatomy explains how challenging is to localize the pain derived from Luschka's recurrent nerve.

- Ventral branches of the sympathetic system

These nerves innervate the anterior common vertebral ligament and the anterior and lateral zones of the disc.

Acute transient pain can be efficaciously modulated by supraspinal centres, which determine pain to disappear with the end of the noxious stimulation. Conversely, a persistent pain is able to alter pain pathways. Persistent noxious stimulation, in fact, may decrease neuronal activation threshold, increase response to over-threshold stimuli and even spontaneous neuronal activity. This phenomenon generates allodynia and hyperalgesia (wind-up response).

Chronic pain is biochemically characterized by an imbalance of inhibitory and excitatory neurotransmitters.

In addition, the perpetuation and amplification of pain is promoted by a neuroimmune and neuroinflammatory reaction. This maintaining circle is very difficult to breakdown: while acute pain tends to solve over time, chronic back pain resolution seems to occur in less than 5–10% of cases.

Very similar pathological pathways are observed in chronic affective disorders such as depression, anxiety, pain crises and post-traumatic stress disorders [6, 7].

7.2.1 Nociceptive and Neuropathic Pain

When facing a patient with spine pain, differentiating between nociceptive and neuropathic pain is clinically important because these components require different pain management strategies directed at peripheral and central processes. Nociceptive or mechanical pain results from activation of nociceptors that innervate ligaments, joints, muscles, fascia and tendons as a response to tissue injury or inflammation and biomechanical stress [7–9].

On the other hand, somatic fibres directly reach the spinal cord at every level and mediate a well-localized local pain, known as radicular pain. Nociceptive pain is typically described as aching, dull or throbbing and is adaptive and usually short-lived; it generally resolves once the original physical assault has healed [10]. Noxious stimulation of structures in the spine can also produce referred pain in addition to back pain. This is defined as pain perceived as occurring in a region of the body topographically distinct from the region in which the source of pain is located and arises from central processing of afferent activity in intact nerves.

When somatic tissues of the spine are the source of spinal referred pain, the condition is named somatic referred pain, to differentiate it both from visceral referred pain and radicular pain. Somatic referred pain is produced by noxious stimulation of nerve endings within spinal structures such as discs, zygapophysial joints or sacroiliac joints. Since no involving stimulation of nerve roots is present, there are no neurological signs.

Somatic referred pain is described as dull, aching, gnawing and sometimes an expanding pressure into wide areas that can be difficult to localize, and once established, it tends to be fixed in location. The pattern of pain is not dermatomal, most often it tends to be localized in the gluteal region and less commonly to the foot. However, the distribution of referred pain varies among patients and between studies [11].

Neuropathic back pain is defined as pain arising from an injury or disease that directly affects the nerve roots that innervate the spine and lower limbs or pathological invasive innervation of the damaged lumbar discs [9].

In contrast with nociceptive pain, neuropathic pain is maladaptive and tends to become chronic [10].

Attal et al. in 2011 studied the prevalence of neuropathic pain in CLBP patients. They found a prevalence of 8% in pain restricted to the lumbar area, 15% in pain radiating proximally, 39% in pain radiating below the knee without neurologi-cal signs and 80% in pain radiating towards the foot in a dermatomal distribution with neurological signs corresponding to typical radiculopathy. Other studies reported a prevalence of 16–55% for neuropathic pain in the lumbar area, with one review reporting an aggregate rate of 36.6% [12].

In the cervical region, 43 of 100 patients were found to have non-neuropathic pain, 7% to have predominantly neuropathic pain and 50% to have mixed pain [13].

Characteristics of neuropathic pain are painful signs and symptoms arising from an area of altered sensation. These signs and symptoms can actually vary both between patients and over time in the same individual.

Cardinal features include spontaneous pain, abnormal response to non-painful stimuli and moderate heat or cold (allodynia) or an excessive response to painful stimulation (hyperalgesia).

Spontaneous pain can be paroxysmal (like shooting, stabbing or electric), dysesthetic (unpleasant abnormal sensations of touch) or associated with abnormal thermal sensation. These signs and symptoms can coexist in an area with loss of afferent sensation (numbness) [9].

7.3 Non-Specific Low Back Pain

Traditionally, 80–90% of cases of low back pain are defined as non-specific, a term used to describe a type of low back pain with unknown aetiology.

As mentioned previously, symptoms of low back pain can derive from different sources including aberrant neurological processing causing neuropathic pain and abdominal organs causing referred pain. It is also once more important to consider that low back pain can be influenced by psychological factors such as anxiety, stress and depression. When facing a patient with back pain, the anamnestic investigation should include a detailed health history, information about work (heavy weight lifting, standing or sitting, satisfaction), drugs, habits and psychosocial factors.

In some cases, low back pain could be referred to a specific pain generator, with its own characteristics and with different therapeutic opportunities, but generally the recognition of the specific cause is lacking [1].

As suggested by Hansen, clinicians currently tend to have a purely structural approach that overemphasizes the spine and neuraxis as the primary source of pain with under-recognition of the role of soft tissues as pain generators [14].

The recognition of soft tissues as pain generators in chronic back pain is not a new concept. In 1944 Stimson conducted a study to investigate the aetiology of low back pain, with a structural or an organic aetiology found in 17% of cases. The majority of patient had no underlying disorder but failed in functional test of key posture muscles and responded favourably to a muscle pain treatment protocol including an exercise programme.

Kraus in the 1960s postulated that non-specific back pain is a "disease of civilization" caused by sedentary lifestyle, stress and suppression of the fight and flight response. The author theorized that lack of exercise and emotional stress lead to muscle weakness, stiffness, pain and injury.

Recently Mense et al. found in a rat model that back muscle inflammation and psychological stress sensitize dorsal horn neurons, thus magnifying the input of pain signals from the soft tissues of the low back. The authors hypothesize that inappropriate use or an overuse of low back muscles leads to neuronal sensitization. The latter could be the responsible mechanism for the clinical presentation of chronic low back pain [15].

As CLBP could have simultaneous multiple pain generators, a multidisciplinary diagnosis and multimodal treatment is necessary [1].

7.3.1 Red Flags

Non-specific low back pain is generally considered a benign condition that can be managed in a primary care setting. Some patients, however, present with back pain as the initial manifestation of a more serious pathology, such as malignancy, spinal fracture, infection or cauda

Table 7.1 Reliable red flags according to Downie et al. and Verhnagen et al.

Red flags
Fractures
Older age
Prolonged corticosteroid use
Severe trauma
Contusion or abrasion
Malignancy
History of malignancy
Strong clinical suspicion

equina syndrome. Spinal fracture and malignancy are the most common serious pathologies affecting the spine, but the absolute magnitude of their occurrence may be regarded as rare [16–18]. Patients with low back pain presenting to primary care are estimated to have spinal fracture between 1% and 4% and malignancy (primary tumour or metastasis) in less than 1% [18].

Conventionally clinicians are encouraged by several guidelines to suspect serious underlying pathology in patients with back pain by checking for "red flags" (Table 7.1). This term is used to describe signs or symptoms that may be related to a serious underlying pathology and may therefore indicate more diagnostic testing to be performed before appropriate care offering. Currently the appropriateness and the utility of checking for red flags when approaching a patient with back pain is controversial [16–19]. Current guidelines indeed present a list of red flags that is variable, often without consideration given to the diagnostic accuracy of each sign and with heterogeneity in their precise definition. Several studies have been conducted to establish the actual utility of such practice, with rather disappointing results. Some authors assert that without rigorous evidence on the diagnostic accuracy of red flags, this advice may be associated with unwanted side effects through unnecessary imaging (increase radiation exposure and healthcare costs), alarming of patients (reduction of quality of life) and treatment (including unnecessary surgery) [16].

Henschke et al. [20], in a primary care cohort of 1172 LBP patients, have found that most patients (80.4%) had at least 1 red flag. Leerar et al., in a study focusing on physiotherapist adherence to guidelines, found that 7 of the 11 red flags endorsed in guidelines were documented in 98% of the patients [21].

Cook et al., in their work published in 2017, concluded that red flag symptoms might have a stronger relationship with prognosis than diagnosis [19].

In conclusion, at present for the majority of red flags endorsed by guidelines, there is a strikingly little or no evidence available regarding their diagnostic accuracy, limiting their clinical value.

7.4 Intervertebral Disc Degeneration

The intervertebral disc is the core structure of the main joint between two consecutive vertebrae in the vertebral column. Each disc consists of three different structures: an inner gelatinous nucleus pulposus surrounded by an outer annulus fibrosus and two cartilage endplates that cover the upper and lower surfaces of vertebral bodies. Disc degeneration is a physiological phenomenon beginning in the second decade of men's life and third decade of women's life, as ageing implies cell apoptosis or programmed cellular death. Degeneration is also determined by environmental factors (such as heavy works or sports) and genetic factors.

While disc degeneration is a sort of physiologic age-related event, disc disruption is pathologic and recognized as the most common cause of discogenic pain. Nonetheless, intervertebral discs are responsible of 39% of all CLBP, even though not all degenerated or herniated discs are painful. According to literature, 26–42% of patients with intervertebral disc degeneration are affected by chronic back pain [6].

According to Kirkaldy-Willis classification, disc degeneration can be divided into three stages: dysfunction (*disc disruption syndrome* and, eventually, *disc herniation*), instability and stabilization [6].

The first phase occurs between 20 and 45 years: the disc gradually decreases in height and capacity to bear axial weight. Intervertebral joints synovitis might be associated with disc degeneration and determine an intermittent low back pain. Degeneration of facet joints is usually expected as a consequence. Between 45 and 60–70 years, weight distribution over different spinal areas is usually seen. Even 70% of axial weight might indeed be distributed onto the facet joints, instead of a normal 20%. This is called the instability stage because of the inevitable vertical subluxation of the facet joints. The overloading of the facet joints is inversely proportional to the disc height with a consequent disc collapse, arthritic changes, loss of tension and thickening of ligamentum flavum and posterior longitudinal ligament. These anatomical changings lead to a medullary canal stenosis, initially dynamic with extension and standing, then permanent. Patients often complain chronic or recurrent pain in the low back or irradiated to the lower extremities, relieved by supine position. Degenerative spondylolisthesis secondary to facet joint hypertrophic degenerative changes can generate mechanical pain, radicular pain or neurogenic claudication. The third stage is characterized by bone spurs and osteophytes sprouting that add to the "soft stenosis" of the instability phase to determine a "rigid stenosis". This is the so-called stabilization stage because the increased bony contact stabilizes the spine. Disc collapse and remodelling of vertebral bodies may block the progression of vertebral slippage. Sometimes the degenerative process leads to kyphotic angulation of the spine in the stenotic area. In these cases clinical symptoms may be reduced because of the increase of dural sac volume and foramen area and decrease of ligamentum flavum thickness and disc protrusion. Different manifestations of spine degenerative disease can be clinically recognized. These pathologic scenarios may represent the clinical presentation of different phases of intervertebral disc degeneration, although a strict correlation with Kirkaldy-Willis classification is not demonstrated (Table 7.2).

Table 7.2 Possible clinical presentations of disc degeneration stages according to Kirkaldy-Willis

Disc degeneration (paraphysiologic)	Clinical presentation (pathologic)
Dysfunction	Crock's internal disc disruption Disc herniation Facet joint syndrome
Instability	Dynamic instabilities
Stabilization	Spondylosis and stenosis

7.4.1 Crock's Internal Disc Disruption Syndrome

This syndromic pain pattern seems to be caused by a rupture in the internal structure of the disc without compression of the nervous root. The pathoanatomical feature of the syndrome is disc fissuring, which can be limited to the inner part or spread to the outer part of the annulus. Literature reports that 70% of fissures reaching the outer part of the annulus (Grade III according to Dallas discogram scale) are painful and 70% of all painful discs present with a Grade III or IV fissuration [6].

While a healthy disc in adulthood is avascular and aneural, degenerated discs fissures might be colonized by pathologic neoangiogenesis. The disc neovascularisation can be explained as an attempt to heal from outside to inside. However, in the hostile microenvironment of the intervertebral disc, this process promotes catabolic process and pain rather than repair. Normally nerve endings and their capillaries cannot withstand the high inner hydrostatic pressures of normal discs. Conversely, new blood vessels penetrate into the degenerated disc because of an internal depressurization. These vessels bring inflammatory cytokines (IL6, IL1β, TNF α) and cells (macrophages) leading to inflammatory granulation tissue and neo-innervation. Among all the inflammation molecules, some interesting studies detected higher levels of neurotrophins (NGF, BDNF, NT3, NT4/5) in the degenerated discs, which could be responsible of nerve fibres attraction.

The neo-innervation creates a close association between sympathetic postganglionic efferent and autonomic afferent endings, with the first exerting a neuroregulatory function [22, 23]. This pain pattern is very similar to the enteric one, suggesting that discogenic pain is the only example of visceral-like pain in the muscular skeletal system. Discogenic pain might then present as a combination of chemical and mechanical pain. Inflammation creates a dull constant pain, which is worsened by the mechanical stimulation of the annulus during movements and weight bearing. In addition, the inflammatory process amplifies the response of nerve endings to mechanical stress.

Clinical features of Crock's internal disc disruption syndrome are not specific. Patients more often present with a pseudo-radicular pain: unilateral or bilateral axial pain with frequent referral to lower limbs and non-specific clinical findings (negative Lasegue test, normal osteo-tendinous reflexes, irradiation of pain to the knees). Pain is elicited by posture and activity that raise intradiscal pressure and stress the annulus and relieved during recumbence. Discogenic pain is often referred distant from the anatomic origin, causing diagnosis to be difficult.

7.4.2 Disc Herniation

Disc herniation is defined as the migration of the nucleus pulposus outside its normal location through a torn annulus fibrosus, towards the periphery or cranio-caudal (Schmorl's herniation). Annulus fibres can elongate by up to the 9% during torsional loading (where the failure elongation point is 25% from the baseline) and can bear a stress 4–5 times greater than the nucleus. The nucleus is, on the contrary, a relatively incompressible structure, which bulges approximately 1 mm per physiological load. With disc degeneration elasticity is gradually lost compromising its ability to compress. Shock absorption is no longer spread or absorbed by the surrounding annulus, leading to greater shearing, rotation and traction stress on the disc and adjacent vertebrae [5]. The most frequently involved discs in the lumbar spine are L4-L5 and L5-S1.

Table 7.3 Disc herniation classification and related symptoms

Type of herniation	Description	Symptoms
Bulging	Symmetrical disc enlargement >50% of its perimeter Not pathological	No
Disc protrusion	Displacement outside its boundaries Sessile aspect	No
Disc extrusion	Displacement outside its boundaries Pedicled aspect	Yes
Disc sequestration	Free disc material displacement Frequent resorption	Yes

Table 7.4 RAPIDH score

Item	Points
Monoradicular leg pain	6
Straight leg raise <60° or positive femoral stretch test	4
Unilateral ankle reflex decrease	4
Unilateral muscle weakness	3
Unilateral patient reported pain in legs	3

Disc herniation can be classified as shown in Table 7.3 [6]:

Despite the clinical relevance of disc herniation, it causes only a limited percentage of cases (lower than 30%) of low back pain [7]. Disc herniation is in fact a typical cause of radicular pain: it radiates from the back and buttock onto the limb in a dermatomal distribution, without neurological impairment. When disc herniation involves the cervical spine, it typically presents with acute onset of severe neck and arm pain unrelieved by any position and often results in encroachment on a cervical nerve root. Symptoms are due primarily to nerve root inflammation rather than a real compression.

The International Association for the Spine Pain defines radicular pain as arising in a limb or the trunk wall, caused by either ectopic activation or nociceptive afferent fibres in a spinal nerve and its roots or by other neuropathic mechanism. It may be episodic, recurrent or sudden [5].

Radicular pain, though, is different from radiculopathy even if they often coexist. Radiculopathy is in fact due to an impairment of sensory and motor fibres with the appearance of dermatomic distribution of numbness and myotomal weakness. It may be accompanied by reduced reflexes and is usually painless [7].

Considering the heterogeneous clinical presentation of lumbar herniation syndrome, Genevay and collaborators recently proposed clinical criteria to identify patients with radicular

pain caused by disc herniation and developed the "RAPIDH" (radicular pain caused by disc herniation) score (Table 7.4) [8].

The patient is classified as having RAPIDH if the total score is 11 (range 0–20) or more. RAPIDH score figured out to have a 90.4% specificity and 70.6% sensitivity. This test is an attempt to differentiate patients with radicular symptoms caused by lumbar disc herniation from those with lumbar spinal stenosis or non-specific low back pain with referred leg pain.

7.5 Facet Joint Pain

Zygapophyseal or facet joints are diarthrodial joints with their own articular surfaces, capsula and synovial membrane. These joints are located in pairs on the posterolateral aspect of each motion segment, spanning from the cervical to the lumbar spine. Each facet joint is innervated by the dorsal branch of the corresponding spinal nerve and by the sinuvertebral nerve of the same level and of the level above. Facet pain is defined as pain arising from any structure of facet joints. Being arthritis a prominent cause of facet joint pain, its prevalence increases with age [24].

The most common initial event causing facet pain is a synovial reaction caused by trauma or mechanical stress associated with a fluid distension of the capsule or a capsular damage. These mechanisms provoke the stimulation of joint nociceptors and type-C pain fibres of the densely innervated capsule [24–26].

As previously described, axial weight on the facet joints may increase from 20% to 70% due to intervertebral disc degeneration. This mechanical overload causes different changes in the joints. Hyperpressure of the subchondral bone, trabecular microfractures, capsular distension or impingement of the synovial villi are possible changes that finally cause pain [5].

Degeneration of facet joints is a frequent cause of radicular pain by compression of nerve roots in lateral recesses and in the foramina secondary to hypertrophic and osteophytic remodelling of the facets, sublussation, joint effusion with capsular tension and synovial cysts formation [7]. Manchikanti et al. in their study about chronic spinal pain estimated that facet joints in the cervical region contribute to 55% of spinal pain and in localized thoracic pain the prevalence of facet joint pain amounts to 42% [27]. Depending on diagnostic criteria, zygapophyseal joints account for 5% to 15% of cases of chronic, axial low back pain [24–26].

Cervical facet joint pain can be described as an axial neck pain, without neurological deficit, referred to the occipital, suboccipital, shoulder or mid-back regions. The pain is induced with pressure on the dorsal side of the cervical spine at the level of the facet joints and limits extension and rotation. Specifically, pain emanating from the C2–3 or C3–4 facet joints can extend into the occipital and suboccipital regions, C4–5 or C5–6 facet joint disease can cause pain radiating into the shoulder, and the C6–7 and C7-T1 joints typically refer pain to the mid-back and scapular regions [12, 25].

In the thoracic spine a paravertebral pain without signs of neurological impairment that worsens with prolonged standing, hyperextension or rotation of the spine is suggestive of facet pain. The pain is often bilateral and generally affects several segments [26].

In the lumbar area, facet joint pain is usually characterized by low back pain with or without somatic referral to the legs terminating above the knee, often radiating to the thigh or to the groin without a radicular pattern. Back pain tends to be off-centre and increases with hyperextension, rotation and lateral bending.

It is exacerbated when waking up from bed or trying to stand after prolonged sitting. Patients often complain of back stiffness, which is more evident in the morning [1, 24].

7.6 Dynamic Instabilities

The smallest functional unit in the spine is represented by the Jughanns mobile segment, which is formed by two adjacent vertebrae and the soft tissues between them. Dynamic instabilities affect this functional unit during spine mobilization [6]. Dynamic instability can be minor (soft tissue injuries, with pain and musculoskeletal symptoms), moderate (autonomic nervous system symptoms, positional radiculopathy) or severe (severe neurological complications and persisting somatic nerves symptoms) (Table 7.5).

Cervical spine is the most mobile segment of the entire column and must support high degree of movement. Consequently, a great amount of stability is required to the ligamentous tissues in the cervical spine. This is the reason why this spine segment is highly susceptible to ligamentous injuries and dynamic instabilities. Ligament injuries can be caused by severe neck trauma with rotational stress, with 25% presenting as C0–C2 injuries, and by excessive or abnormal forces during mechanically mediated manipulation. Capsular ligament laxity can either occur instantaneously as a single trauma, such as in whiplash injury (up to 10 times more force is absorbed in the capsular ligaments versus the intervertebral disc), or develop slowly as cumulative microtrauma. Dynamic instabilities are then characterized by an abnormal motion on the spine with sub-failure loads to the facet joints and

Table 7.5 Progression of dynamic spine instability with related symptoms

Normal spine joint motion	Hypermobility	Minor instability	Moderate instability	Severe instability
Asymptomatic	Asymptomatic	Musculoskeletal pain	Positional radiculopathy and autonomic nervous system symptoms	Persistent symptoms and severe neurological complications

the capsular ligaments. Capsular ligament tension is increased during abnormal postures up to 70% of normal elongation. Clinically patients always suffer of a chronic post-trauma neck pain, rarely accompanied by neurological impairment. Instability is accompanied by muscle spasms that cause intense pain because of the ligamentomuscular reflex, which originates from ligamentous mechanoreceptors. This is an attempt to preserve the joint stability using muscular strength instead of ligamentous structures. Unfortunately the joint instability and abnormal loading stimulate integrin-cytoskeleton and ion-stretch mechanoreceptors that induce catabolic pathways. The metalloproteinases cause the breakdown of cartilage and consequent articular cartilage degradation. Thus, instability can be clearly differentiated from hypermobility, which is a loss of normal motion stiffness in a particular spine segment. This determines a greater displacement under mechanical stimulation but is typically asymptomatic.

Among cervical axial rotation instabilities, 30% present intermittent radicular symptoms, worsening with rotation, flexion or extension of the neck. These movements, in fact, reduce the room for cervical nerve roots, which usually occupy at least the 72% of the total neural foramina volume.

Radicular symptoms are related to the facet joint hypertrophy and disc degeneration, which follows the capsular ligament injury.

7.7 Spondylosis and Stenosis

Spondylosis is a disease generally associated with ageing, characterized by degeneration of the intervertebral disc, osteophytosis of the vertebral bodies and hypertrophy of the facet joints and laminar arches. Spondylosis corresponds to the third stage of intervertebral disc degeneration according to Kirkaldy-Willis (stabilization): the spine tries to heal the instability with the formation of marginal osteophytes that can lead to a natural fusion of affected vertebrae. The degenerative cascade is usually slow and initially silent. The first symptoms are non-specific and include spinal pain and stiffness. Clinical findings are non-specific too: a limited range of spine tract motion and poorly localized tenderness can occur. Radicular symptoms are more likely to occur in patients with underlying capsular ligament laxity because the neural foramen is already reduced by the narrowed facet joint hypertrophy and disc degeneration. Spondylosis usually involves several spine tracts; thus the eventual radiculopathy symptoms are more diffuse than those of typical single soft disc herniation.

Only rarely neurologic symptoms (radiculopathy or myelopathy) appear, usually in patients with congenital narrow spinal canal. The bridging bony spurs can in fact induce or worsen a spinal stenosis, which is a narrowing of the central spinal canal, lateral recess and/or neural foramen (Table 7.6). The trefoil shape of lumbar canal at the fifth lumbar level makes L4–L5 the narrowest and more affected level [28].

Central canal stenosis occurs at intervertebral disc level with midline sagittal narrowing and is mainly caused by hypertrophy of ligamentum flavum, facet joint osteophytes and degenerative spondylolisthesis. The symptoms are bilateral leg heaviness, soreness or weakness. The most characteristic is though neurogenic claudication: numbness, weakness or discomfort in the legs with prolonged standing and relieved by sitting or rest.

Table 7.6 Spinal stenosis: topographical classification, causes and symptoms

	Central canal stenosis	Lateral recess stenosis	Foraminal stenosis
Causes	Ligamentum flavum Facet joint osteophytes Degenerative spondylolisthesis	Hypertrophy of superior articular facet and posterior aspect of vertebra and disc	Isthmic spondylolisthesis Far lateral disc herniation
Symptoms	Bilateral radicular	Unilateral radicular	Unilateral/bilateral radicular

Table 7.7 Wiltse-Newmann classification

Wiltse-Newmann classification					
I Dysplastic	II Isthmic	III Degenerative	IV Traumatic	V Pathologic	VI Iatrogenic
	A. Pars' disruption (stress fracture) B. Pars' elongation (multiple microfractures) C. Acute fracture through pars				

Lateral recess stenosis occurs when the nerve root is compressed beneath the medial aspect of a hypertrophic superior articular facet and posterior aspect of vertebral body and disc. In this case unilateral radicular symptoms occur: leg pain along with numbness, paraesthesia or burning in a dermatomal distribution. Foraminal stenosis is the most rare among the three types of canal stenosis. The foramen is the exit zone of the spinal roots of the bony vertebral structure (medial and lateral pedicle border), and its calibre depends on the posture of the spine.

Foraminal stenosis most frequently occurs in case of isthmic spondylolisthesis, where the exiting nerve root is compressed in the distorted foramen. In rare cases nerve root can be compressed in far lateral disc herniation.

In every type of lumbar stenosis, clinical findings are poor: there may be a limitation of spine extension, sensory deficit, muscle weakness, limited straight leg raise and absent peripheral osteo-tendinous reflexes. In 5% of the cases, the most common lumbar spinal canal stenosis is associated with cervical canal narrowing (tandem stenosis), so signs of myelopathy might be found [28].

7.8 Spondylolisthesis

Spondylolisthesis is a spinal disorder characterized by forward slippage of a vertebra over one beneath (especially the fifth lumbar vertebra over the first sacral one). The "listhesis" is actually a rotatory deformity and not just a simple forward or backward displacement.

Various classification systems have been proposed [29].

Marchetti and Bartolozzi classified the pathology in developmental (high or low grade

dysplastic) or acquired [30]. Mac Thiong and Labelle proposed a different classification in eight types of spondylolisthesis, combining the slip grade, degree of dysplasia and sagittal sacro-pelvic balance [31]. Wiltse and collaborators, though, developed the first and most widely used classification, describing 5 types of spondylolisthesis [32] (Table 7.7). At radiographic exam, severity of the pathology is classified in ranging from 1 to 5 in dependence of the percentage of slippage with respect to the beneath vertebral body.

Type I is very rare. It is secondary to congenital lumbosacral articulation abnormalities (such as hypoplastic facet joints or sacral deficiency), representing 14–21% of congenital spondylolisthesis cases. Children and adolescents with this pathology are more likely to develop neurologic complications (cauda equina) and to progress towards severe spine deformity and clinical consequences than Type II (32% versus 4%) [29].

Types IV, V and VI are particular and rare types of spondylolisthesis.

Type IV is a post-traumatic spondylolisthesis with a fracture occurring in a region other than the pars interarticularis but evenly leading to slippage. Type V is a pathological spondylolisthesis which occurs in diffuse or local disease compromising the stability of the vertebra (e.g. in case of metastatic disease, primary bone neoplasia, etc.). Type VI is iatrogenic.

Isthmic and degenerative spondylolisthesis are the most common types.

Isthmic spondylolisthesis has an incidence of 4–8% among the general population, with a high prevalence among athletes. According to Adult Isthmic Spondylolisthesis Work Group of the North American Spine Society (NASS) Evidence-Based Clinical Guideline Development Committee, it is an anterior translation of one lumbar vertebra relative to the next caudal segment as a result of an abnormality in the pars interarticularis [33]. The cause is recognized to be a spondylolysis: a fracture of the pars interarticularis of the vertebra, which can have hormonal, genetic and/or mechanical cause (sports involving hyperlordosis) [34]. At least two thirds of individuals with spondylolysis develop the pathology during childhood and are usually asymptomatic. The remaining one third develops a pars defect in adolescence or early adulthood and are more likely to present symptoms [35]. Spondylolisthesis is unlikely to occur in patients with unilateral spondylolysis but occurs in 40–66% of patients with bilateral spondylolysis [33].

Type IIA, which is the most common subtype, is a complete defect of the pars interarticularis caused by repetitive microtraumas and loading. Type IIB is caused by repeated microfractures that try to heal resulting in an elongated pars. Type IIC is a complete fracture caused by an acute trauma.

Type II spondylolisthesis is associated with a higher pelvic incidence, which is related to an increased sacral slope and an increased lumbar lordosis to maintain sagittal balance.

Isthmic spondylolisthesis has a benign clinical course in the majority of patients considering that osteosclerosis, spur formation and ligaments ossification slowly stop the slippage progression.

When symptomatic, isthmic spondylolisthesis causes a variable clinical syndrome of back and/ or lower extremity pain, and about half of symptomatic patients have radicular lower extremity pain with evidence of neurologic deficits below the injury level [33].

A recent review analysed the diagnostic utility of patient history and physical examination data to detect spondylolysis and spondylolisthesis in athletes with low back pain. It reported that some symptoms such as difficulty falling asleep, waking up because of pain and pain worsening with sitting and walking have a moderate/high to high sensitivity. By the way these patients' history data are not specific: pain worsening with sitting and prolonged weight bearing are also typical of lumbar disc pathology. The commonly cited signs of hamstring tightness and paravertebral muscle symptoms are also not sensitive and specific enough [36].

Approximately 50% of symptomatic spondylolisthesis have a positive straight leg test on examination [30]. The patients experience sciatic pain when laying down on the back when the examinator straightens the leg at 30°–70°. According to Alqarni and collaborators, though, the only accurate clinical test helpful in the spondylolisthesis diagnosis is the palpation of the lumbar spinous processes. The examiner slides his fingertips on the lumbosacral spinous processes, maintaining a lateral view of the patient's spine. The sign is positive when the examiner can feel a lumbar spinous process "step". The lumbar spinous process palpation test has a high specificity (87–100%) and moderate-high sensitivity (60–88%) compared to one-legged hyperextension test (sensitivity 50–73%, specificity 17–32%) [37].

The suggested diagnostic exams include standing plain radiographs (with or without oblique views dynamic views), CT (the most reliable to diagnose a defect in the pars interarticularis) or MRI (in patients with radiculopathy; even though there are insufficient evidence of its utility in differential diagnosis between isthmic and degenerative spondylolisthesis) [33].

Type III is a degenerative spondylolisthesis.

The Degenerative Lumbar Spondylolisthesis Work Group of the North American Spine Society (NASS) Evidence-Based Clinical Guideline Development Committee defined the degenerative spondylolisthesis as an acquired anterior displacement of one vertebra over the subjacent vertebra, associated with degenerative changes, without an associated disruption or defect in the vertebral ring [38]. It is four to five times more common in women and has a higher incidence in African Americans and diabetic patients.

The major local causes of degenerative slippage are the loss of bone support in arthritis of facet joints (that normally bear 30–45% of the torsional forces of the spine), the segmental instability that cause tension on the facet joints capsule, ligaments and muscles and the spinal stenosis and intravertebral foramen stenosis [39].

Degenerative spondylolisthesis can be seen as an accidental finding in asymptomatic patients.

At presentation, in fact, the mean slip is less than 15% and just one third of patients present slip progression. When symptomatic, it usually occurs in patients aged over 40 and has traditionally been considered as one of the major causes of low back pain and spinal canal stenosis. The clinical presentation can be various; thus degenerative spondylolisthesis can be included in classification of spondylolisthesis, spinal stenosis and segmental instability [40].

The symptoms are mainly back pain and radicular pain together. When they present singularly, back pain is more frequent than radicular pain alone, exacerbated with extension due to posterior elements compression. When the rotational slippage component is mild, nerve root involvement is typically bilateral and pluriradicular. The dural sac in the central spinal canal is compressed and a bilateral lateral recess stenosis occurs. On the other hand, in presence of marked rotation, nerve root involvement is usually unilateral and ipsilateral to the maximal facet joint subluxation [29].

One of the most characteristic symptoms of degenerative spondylolisthesis in presence of stenosis is a neurogenic pain that shifts from side to side [39]. A common clinical finding is the hamstrings spasm, the result of an attempt to protect the lumbar spine by limiting lumbar lordosis.

Rarely the progressive degeneration of the disc, thickening of ligamentum flavum and slippage of the vertebra can induce bowel or bladder symptoms. In these cases, symptoms are not acute and devastating as in cauda equina syndrome in lumbar disc herniation, but they have an insidious and subtle presentation.

According to a recent guideline summary review, the most appropriate way to approach a patient with degenerative spondylolisthesis is obtaining an accurate history (through appropriate clinical questions) and physical examination. Lateral radiograph is then suggested as the most appropriate, noninvasive diagnostic test, even though MRI is indicated when spondylolisthesis is accompanied by canal stenosis (or CT if MRI is contraindicated) [38].

7.9   Osteoporotic Compression Fractures

Osteoporosis, defined as loss of bone mineral density, is a major public health problem. This pathology predisposes to fragility fractures, whose incidence increases with age. In Italy, the prevalence of osteoporosis according to the ESOPO study in 2003 by Adami et al. was 23% among all women, ranging from 9% (40–49 years of age) to 45% (70 years of age) and almost 15% in men aged over 60 [40].

Common sites of fragility fracture are the wrist, proximal femur and proximal humerus, but the most common site is the vertebral body. Compression fractures of the vertebral body caused by osteoporosis can be a consequence of a usually low-energy trauma or spontaneous. In the United States, the incidence of recognized vertebral osteoporotic fracture is approximately 700.000 cases/year, which account for half of all fragility fractures. However, many of these fractures are asymptomatic; thus their real impact is probably underestimated [41–43]. Piscitelli et al. in 2011 estimated the number of fragility vertebral fractures in Italy as 61.009 [44].

Fragility vertebral fractures negatively affect the quality of life, limiting the activity of normal daily living. They are associated with reduction of spine mobility, pulmonary dysfunction and with chronic back pain. Several studies reported that one previous vertebral fracture increases the risk for subsequent vertebral fracture approximately fivefold and the risk of hip fracture approximately threefold [41]. The most common sites for osteoporotic vertebral fracture are the midthoracic region and the thoracolumbar junction (respectively T7-T8 and T12-L1) [32]. Many fractures may develop insidiously and chronic compression fractures are commonly detected incidentally on chest X-rays. Conversely, some fractures present with sudden-onset severe, focal back pain that may radiate anteriorly. The reduction of height resulting from a compression vertebral fracture, especially if multiple fractures are present, may result in sagittal imbalance which may lead to chronic back pain and accelerate the degeneration of adjacent segments [43].

7.10 Spinal Infections

Spinal infections account for 2–7% of all infections of the musculoskeletal system with an incidence that varies between 1:100,000 and 1:250,000 in Western countries. Various studies reported a bimodal distribution of incidence with a peak below 20 years and another between 50 and 70 years of age [43, 45].

Some predisposing factors for spinal infections can be recognized, both generally associated with musculoskeletal infections (Table 7.8) and specifically associated with the spine such as a history of previous spine surgery, lumbar puncture or epidural procedures.

The possible routes of pathogens spread in the spine are the haematogenous, direct external inoculation and spread from contiguous tissues. The most common is the haematogenous seeding of the axial skeleton from distant infected foci and more often via the arterial network than the venous [45]. The most common site of infectious disease of the spine in the adult is the corpus vertebrae.

The adult intervertebral disc is an avascular structure. Septic emboli in the adult spine, from distant infected foci, lead to the formation of vascular bone infarcts that often first affects the subchondral region of the vertebral body endplates and spreads in an anterior to posterior direction (spondylitis). The infectious process that spreads to the contiguous spaces, with the involvement of the disc and two adjacent vertebral bodies, is defined as spondylodiscitis. Conversely, in children anastomosis between intraosseous arteries and vessels penetrating the disc is present. Thus a septic embolus from haematogenous spread does not result in bone infarction but reaches the disc where infection finally develops. This scenario is defined as discitis and represents the most common spine infection in paediatric patients [45, 46].

Pyogenic spondylodiscitis caused by haematogenous spread affects mainly the lumbar spine (58%), followed by thoracic (30%) and cervical spine (11%), reflecting the vascular supply of these structures. Tuberculosis lesions preferentially affect the thoracic spine, often involving two or more levels, which differentiates it from pyogenic spondylodiscitis [45]. Currently the majority of spinal infections are bacterial monomicrobial, with a reported incidence of infection caused by *Staphylococcus aureus* between 30 and 80%. Other bacterial agents are causative in selected patient populations (Table 7.9).

The spread of infection into adjacent soft tissues accounts for the development of epidural abscesses, paravertebral muscle abscesses, iliacus and psoas muscle abscesses and prevertebral collections.

The symptoms and signs of spondylodiscitis are non-specific and the average delay in diagnosis reported in studies is 2 months. A new onset of back or neck pain is common; fever is an inconstant finding present in less than half of patients with pyogenic infections and even more rare in case of fungal or mycobacterial aetiology.

Table 7.8 Risk factors for spinal infection

Diabetes mellitus
Advanced age
Immunosuppression and HIV infection
Intravenous drug use
Cancer history
Renal failure
Chronic vascular access
Rheumatologic disease
Liver cirrhosis

Table 7.9 Bacterial agents in spine infections

Enterobacteriaceae (concurrent urinary tract infections)
Pseudomonas aeruginosa (intravenous drug abuse or hospitalized patients)
Streptococcus pneumoniae (diabetes mellitus)
Salmonella species (sickle cell disease or asplenia)
Mycobacterium tuberculosis (immunosuppression, HIV)

Back pain is usually localized at the level of the vertebral body affected by the infection with a localized percussion tenderness, is exacerbated by physical activity and is present at night [43, 45]. Dysphagia and torticollis are symptoms that may be caused by cervical location. Symptoms such as leg weakness, numbness and incontinence that are associated with neurological deficits are present in about one third of patients [45, 46].

In paediatric patients the clinical presentation is largely non-specific with symptoms that may include irritability; refusal to crawl, sit or walk; abdominal pain; or incontinence. Fever and neurological deficits are rare in children, and the most frequent sign found on physical examination is the loss of lumbar lordosis [45].

Sometimes the site of haematogenous localization of the infection can be a degenerated facet joint [43]. The clinical feature of a septic facet joint is characterized by the acuity of its presentation, with a sudden onset of back pain, sometimes in a patient with chronic back pain. The pain is exacerbated with flexion and extension and is not relieved by rest. Patients can usually localize the laterality of back pain, tenderness of the ipsilateral paravertebral muscles at palpation are often present, fever is a more common feature and marked neurologic deficits can be present [43].

References

1. Allegri M, Montella S, Salici F, et al. Mechanisms of low back pain: a guide for diagnosis and therapy. F1000Res. 2016;5:1530.
2. Maher C, Underwood M, Buchbinder R. Non-specific low back pain. Lancet. 2017;389(10070):736–47.
3. Hoy DG, Protani M, De R, et al. The epidemiology of neck pain. Best Pract Res Clin Rheumatol. 2010;24(6):783–92.
4. Carroll LJ, Hogg-Johnson S, van der Velde G, et al. The burden and determinants of neck pain in the general population: results of the bone and joint decade 2000–2010 task force on neck pain and its associated disorders. Spine. 2008;33(4 Suppl):S39–51.
5. Steilen D, Hauser R, Woldin B, et al. Chronic neck pain: making the connection between capsular ligament laxity and cervical instability. Open Orthop J. 2014;8:326–45.
6. Cano-Gómez C, Rodríguez de la Rúa J, García-Guerrero G, et al. Physiopathology of lumbar spine degeneration and pain. Rev Esp Cir Ortop Traumatol. 2008;52:37–46.
7. Izzo R, Popolizio T, D'Aprile P, et al. Spinal pain. Eur J Radiol. 2015;84(5):746–56.
8. Cohen S. Epidemiology, diagnosis, and treatment of neck pain. Mayo Clin Proc. 2015;90(2):284–99.
9. Baron R, Binder A, Attal N, et al. Neuropathic low back pain in clinical practice. Eur J Pain. 2016;20(6):861–73.
10. Muller-Schwefe G, Morlion B, Ahlbeck K, et al. Treatment for chronic low back pain: the focus should change to multimodal management that reflects the underlying pain mechanisms. Curr Med Res Opin. 2017;33(7):1199–210.
11. Bogduk N. On the definitions and physiology of back pain, referred pain, and radicular pain. Pain. 2009;147(1–3):17–9.
12. Cohen S, Hooten M. Advances in the diagnosis and management of neck pain. BMJ. 2017;358:j3221.
13. Attal N, Perrot S, Fermanian J, et al. The neuropathic components of chronic low back pain: a prospective multicenter study using the DN4 questionnaire. J Pain. 2011;12(10):1080–7.
14. Hansen AE, Marcus NJ. Is it time to consider soft tissue as a pain generator in nonspecific low back pain? Pain Med. 2016;17(11):1969–70.
15. Mense S, Hoheisel U, Vogt MA, et al. Immobilization stress sensitizes rat dorsal horn neurons having input from the low back. Eur J Pain. 2015;19(6):861–70.
16. Verhagen AP, Downie A, Chiro M, et al. Most red flags for malignancy in low back pain guidelines lack empirical support; a systematic review. Pain. 2017;158(10):1860–8.
17. Verhagen AP, Downie A, Popal N, et al. Red flags presented in current low back pain guidelines: a review. Eur Spine J. 2016;25(9):2788–802.
18. Downie A, Williams CM, Henschke N, et al. Red flags to screen for malignancy and fracture in patients with low back pain: systematic review. BMJ. 2013;347:f7095.
19. Cook CE, George SZ, Reiman MP. Red flag screening for low back pain: nothing to see here, move along: a narrative review. Br J Sports Med. 2018;52(8):493–6.
20. Henschke N, Maher CG, Refshauge KM, et al. Prevalence of and screening for serious spinal pathology in patients presenting to primary care settings with acute low back pain. Arthritis Rheum. 2009;60(10):3072–80.
21. Leerar PJ, Boissonnault W, Domholdt E, et al. Documentation of red flags by physical therapists for patients with low back pain. J Man Manip Ther. 2007;15:42–9.
22. Wiet MG, Piscioneri A, Khan SN, et al. Mast cell-intervertebral disc cell interactions regulate inflammation, catabolism and angiogenesis in discogenic back pain. Sci Rep. 2017;7(1):12492.
23. Garcia-Cosamalòn J, del Valle ME, Calavia MG, et al. Intervertebral disc, sensory nerves and neu-

rotrophins: who is who in discogenic pain? J Anat. 2010;217(1):1–15.

24. Van Eerd M, Patijn J, Lataster A, et al. Cervical facet pain. Pain Pract. 2010;10(2):113–23.

25. Van Kleef M, Stolker RJ, Lataster A, et al. Thoracic pain. Pain Pract. 2010;10(4):327–38.

26. Van Kleef M, Vanelderen P, Cohen SP, et al. Pain originating from the lumbar facet joints. Pain Pract. 2010;10(5):459–69.

27. Manchikanti L, Boswell MV, Singh V, et al. Prevalence of facet joint pain in chronic spinal pain of cervical, thoracic, and lumbar regions. BMC Musculoskelet Disord. 2004;28:5–15.

28. Rajagopal TS, Marshall RW. Understanding and treating spinal stenosis. J Bone Joint Surg. 2010;1-7.

29. Wang YX, Kaplar Z, Deng M, et al. Lumbar degenerative spondylolisthesis epidemiology: a systematic review with a focus on gender-specific and age-specific prevalence. J Orthop Translat. 2017;11:39–52.

30. Marchetti PG, Bartolozzi P. Classification of spondylolisthesis as a guideline for treatment. Textbook of spinal surgery. Philadelphia: Lippincott-Raven; 1997. p. 1211–54.

31. Labelle H, Roussouly P, Berthounnaud E, et al. Spondylolisthesis; pelvic incidence and sagittal spino-pelvic balance: a correlation study. Spine. 2004;29(18):2049–54.

32. Wiltse LL, Newman PH, Macnab I. Classification of spondylolisis and spondylolisthesis. Clin Orthop Relat Res. 1976;117:23–9.

33. Kreiner DS, Braisden J, Mazanec DJ, et al. Guideline summary review: an evidence-based clinical guideline for the diagnosis and treatment of adult isthmic spondylolisthesis. Spine J. 2016;16(12):1478–85.

34. Niggemann P, Kuchta M, Grosskurth D, et al. Spondylolysis and isthmic spondylolisthesis: impact of vertebral hypoplasia on the use of the Meyerding classification. Br J Radiol. 2012;85(1012):358–62.

35. Haun DW, Kettner NW. Spondylolysis and spondylolisthesis: a narrative review of etiology, diagnosis, and conservative management. J Chiropr Med. 2005;4(4):206–17.

36. Grodahl LH, Fawcett L, Nazareth M, et al. Diagnostic utility of patient history and physical examination data to detect spondylolysis and spondylolisthesis in athletes with low back pain: a systematic review. Man Ther. 2016;24:7–17.

37. Alqarni AM, Schneiders AG, Cook CE, et al. Clinical tests to diagnose lumbar spondylolysis and spondylolisthesis: a systematic review. Phys Ther Sport. 2015;16(3):268–75.

38. Matz PG, Maegher RJ, Lamer T, et al. Guideline summary review: an evidence based clinical guideline for the diagnosis and treatment of degenerative lumbar spondylolisthesis. Spine J. 2016;16(3):439–48.

39. Kalichman L, Hunter DJ. Diagnosis and conservative management of degenerative lumbar spondylolisthesis. Euro Spine J. 2008;17:327–35.

40. Adami S, Giannini S, Giorgino R, et al. The effect of age, weight, and lifestyle factors on calcaneal quantitative ultrasound: the ESOPO study. Osteoporos Int. 2003;14(3):198–207.

41. Lenchik L, Lee FR, Delmas PD, et al. Diagnosis of osteoporotic vertebral fractures: Importance of recognition and description by radiologists. AJR Am J Roentgenol. 2004;183(4):949–58.

42. Babic M, Simpfendorfer CS. Infections of the spine. Infect Dis Clin N Am. 2017;3(2):279–97.

43. Duarte RM, Vaccaro A. Spinal infection: state of the art and management algorithm. Eur Spine J. 2013;22(12):2787–99.

44. Piscitelli P, Tarantino U, Chitano G, et al. Updated incidence rates of fragility fractures in Italy: extension study 2002–2008. Clin Cases Miner Bone Metab. 2011;8(3):54–61.

45. Sundaram VK, Doshi A. Infections of the spine: a review of clinical and imaging findings. Appl Radiol. 2016;45:10–20.

46. Petkova A, Zhelyazkov CB, Kitov BD. Spontaneous spondylodiscitis—epidemiology, clinical features, diagnosis and treatment. Folia Med (Plovdiv). 2017;59(3):254–60.

Imaging of Spine Pain

8

Rosario Francesco Balzano
and Giuseppe Guglielmi

8.1 Introduction

Spinal pain is a common cause of disability, frequently self-limiting, with a high socioeconomic impact on health systems worldwide. The age of onset ranges between 30 and 50 years, and in particular it is estimated that more than 80% of general population will suffer from low back pain (LBP) at least once in their lifetime [1]. The impact on health systems (in the USA it is estimated over $100 billion) is significant for both its wide prevalence and the increasing recourse to novel imaging techniques, such as magnetic resonance, to investigate a possible underlying condition [2, 3]. Even if it is usually a self-limiting condition, symptoms of spinal pain may last for more than 1 year, becoming chronic and impeding both daily activities and working capacity, and consequently being an important cause of work absence [4, 5]. Main causes of spine pain

often include benign diseases, less commonly malignant; clinically several manifestations have been described in the scientific literature which may be eventually divided into three main patterns: cervical, thoracic, and lumbosacral or low back pain [6].

8.2 Etiology

There is no univocal classification of spinal pain causes, even if several ones have been proposed; nevertheless on a practical point of view, they may be schematically distinguished three main categories of etiology: structural, neurogenic, and extraspinal.

8.2.1 Structural Etiology

The spine has two major functions: the protection of the spinal cord and nerve roots and the support head and trunk, conveying forces to the lower limbs [7]; these functions play together with the muscles' actions, under the CNS control, in the maintaining of spinal stability [7]. Any alteration involving one of the vertebral column structures (intervertebral discs, ligaments, synovial intervertebral joints, paravertebral muscles and fasciae) may be source of pain [8]. In this sight, mechanic and inflammatory components play a major role in the onset and maintenance of spinal pain.

Electronic Supplementary Material The online version of this chapter (https://doi.org/10.1007/978-3-319-99822-0_8) contains supplementary material, which is available to authorized users.

R. F. Balzano (✉)
Department of Radiology, University of Foggia, Foggia, Italy

G. Guglielmi
Department of Radiology, University of Foggia, Foggia, Italy

Department of Radiology, Scientific Institute "Casa Sollievo della Sofferenza" Hospital, Foggia, Italy
e-mail: giuseppe.guglielmi@unifg.it

8.2.1.1 Degenerative Disc

Intervertebral disc modifications play a very important role in the genesis of spinal pain. Degenerative disc changes comprehend annular fissures and disc herniation, besides several other manifestations (such as disc dehydration, intradiscal mucinous degradation, gas formation, and somatomarginal osteophytes) which are related to normal aging disc [9] and not always are a source of spinal pain in healthy population [2]. Annular fissures consist in delamination of annular fibers or detachment from vertebral bone; according to the orientation, annular fissures may be concentric, if parallel to the disc contour, radial, if they run through the fiber network from nucleus to periphery, or transverse, which in a narrow sense indicates fissures in the peripheral annulus and separation of annular fibers from the apophyseal bone [9]. The term "tear" instead of "fissure" should be avoided because it may be misleading [9].

Annular fissures are associated to discogenic LBP, which is the most common type of LBP: this is may be secondary to the development of inflammatory response to the annular fissure, probably elicited by disc matrix degradation products, which causes neoangiogenesis and sprouting of nerve endings by the disc lesion. As a consequence, several inflammatory metabolites may stimulate nociceptive receptors on these nerve terminations and determine a painful sensation [10]. Annular fissures should be considered different from degenerative disc changes because this latter may be a simple consequence of normal disc aging and may not be associated to spinal pain; but it is also true that several times, annular fissures and disc degeneration coexist [9].

Disc herniation is defined as displacement of disc material—nucleus, annular tissue, bone fragments—outside the intervertebral disc space outline; it may be distinguished in focal or broad-based if it involves less than 25% or up to 50% of disc circumference [9]. According to the shape, herniation can be further distinguished in protrusion and extrusion [9]. Protrusion is defined when the height of displaced disc material is lower than its base (measured at the outer margins of disc space); extrusion is instead present when the high of herniated disc is greater than its base. If there is no more visible continuity between the displaced disc material and the native disc, the extrusion is further defined as sequestration [9]. If the displacement is away from its first extrusion site, the condition is defined as migration [9]. Furthermore, herniation may be either contained within the external annular fibers or the posterior longitudinal ligament or uncontained if there is no such coverage [9]. Pain may then derive from the conflict between disc herniation and the nerve roots. According to the location and with respect to some anatomic landmarks, disc herniation may occupy the central canal zone, the subarticular zone, and the foraminal or extraforaminal zone [9].

Disc herniation may also take place within the subchondral bone of end plates; it in this occasion is referred as intravertebral herniation or Schmorl's nodes [9].

Bulging disc is considered a generalized disc displacement beyond the disc space, and, by definition, it is not an herniation. It may be both paraphysiological and secondary to disc degeneration [9].

Disc degeneration is often associated with pathological changes in the bone marrow composition that may be in turn connected in the generation of LBP [11]. These alterations are visualized on MRI as Modic changes (see the text below); also, they are not bone marrow lesions related to malignancy, infection, or seropositive rheumatic diseases [11].

Abnormalities of facet joints are another cause implied in the development of spinal pain [12]. These include osteoarthrosis, joint effusions, ligamentous laxity, inflammatory facet synovitis, and synovial cysts [12].

Spondylolysis is a bone defect of the vertebral body at the pars interarticularis which is usually secondary to traumatic events or repetitive high loading [13]; as a consequence, the vertebral body may then slip on the below vertebra, condition known as spondylolisthesis [13]. But spondylolisthesis may also be secondary to degenerative changes in the posterior elements, which in turn determine impairment of ligament stability and consequent slippage of the vertebra on the below one [13]. Spondylolisthesis is classified in four grades [13]: grade 1, 0–25%; grade 2, 26–50%; grade 3, 51–75%; and grade 4, 76–99%; a displacement of 100% is referred as spondyloptosis.

8.2.1.2 Rheumatic Diseases

The spine is frequently involved in course of rheumatic diseases. Among these conditions, rheumatoid arthritis (RA) and axial spondyloarthropathies (axSpA) play an important role. The hallmark pathological of these conditions is enthesopathy.

RA primarily affects the cervical spine and, less frequently, the thoracic and lumbosacral. At the cervical level, the inflammatory process involves ligamentous structures around the occipito-atlantoaxial joints causing bone and ligament erosions with subsequent cervical instability [14]; the intervertebral disc may also be involved in this process. The instability is secondary to the inflammatory involvement of transverse ligament and the nearby synovial bursa [15] and may manifest as atlantoaxial subluxation: this may be anteroposterior, with increase of distance between the atlas and the odontoid process and may also determine canal stenosis; vertical (also known as cranial settling), in which laxity of ligamentous structures results in descent C1 lateral masses and dens entrapping within the foramen magnum (there are several index proposed for the evaluation—see imaging section below) [16]; and lateral, in which the lateral masses of C1 are displaced sideways [14]. In some patients subluxation may also involve cervical levels below C2, for this reason called "subaxial," and produce a characteristic appearance on imaging [16]. Less frequently, inflammatory changes may be evident also in the thoracolumbar spine and at the sacroiliac joints (SIJs) [16].

Spondyloarthropathies are a group of rheumatic diseases which, more frequently than RA, affect the spine and the SIJs. This group includes ankylosing spondylitis (AS), psoriatic arthritis (PsA), reactive spondyloarthropathies (former Reiter syndrome), and spondylitis associated with inflammatory bowel disease (IBD) [16].

AS, the prototype of aSpA, is an inflammatory condition which affects axial synovial joints leading to progressive articular ossification and, in the end, to ankylosis. Usually, at first SIJs are selectively involved, and then the inflammation spreads to the thoracolumbar spine (interapophyseal, costovertebral, atlantoaxial joints, and other entheses such as the spinal processes are implicated): it characteristically involves the tendons and ligaments at their insertion on bone structure with consequent erosions and, in response, new bone production; this process will lead to ankylosing of articulation. These manifestations are distinctive at the level of intervertebral disc, with signs of calcification involving the outsider annular fibers all along the disc contour, but also other synovial joints such as the interapophyseal ones. An important consequence of the diffuse spine ossification is increased risk of vertebral column fractures, especially at the cervicothoracic and thoracolumbar curvatures, following traumas even of minor intensity [17].

PsA is a chronic inflammatory disease which usually involves peripheral joints but may sometimes affects the spine as well [18]; reactive arthritis is an autoimmune disorder secondary to infection developing elsewhere in the body which typically is associated with conjunctival and ureteral inflammation [16]; both entities present common manifestations: spinal enthesopathy is characterized by coarse and asymmetrical soft-tissue calcifications arising from the vertebral body, some millimeters away from the end plate margin, in continuity with the spongious bone, the so-called parasyndesmophytes; similarly to RA there may be also a cervical involvement with subsequent instability [14].

Enteropathic arthritis, which is associated to IBD, may also involve both spine entheses and SIJs [16].

8.2.1.3 Infectious Diseases

Spine infections are another rare but very important cause of spinal pain which involve the vertebral column and/or the endocanal content with possible secondary neurologic manifestations; this condition may be life-threatening at times [19, 20].

Most cases of spondylitis are secondary to pyogenic bacteria (*Staphylococcus aureus* is the most common etiologic agent); other microbial agents implied in the pathogenesis are *Mycobacterium tuberculosis* and fungi (*Candida*, *Aspergillus*), which are more common in immunosuppressive patients [19–21]. Brucellosis is common cause of spinal infection in endemic areas, such as the Mediterranean Basin and the Middle East [22], and should be taken in account into the differential diagnosis.

It is commonly believed that pathogenic agents reach the spine through the hematogenous pathway [19]; rarely the contamination is secondary to contiguous spread from paravertebral soft-tissue infection, as it may happen after spinal surgery—this is mostly valid for pyogenic infection [21]. The urinary tract is the most frequent original site for pyogenic infection, and some risk factors, such as diabetes and history of intravenous drug administration, are often present [19]. The lumbar spine is the most frequent involved site, followed by dorsal (especially for tuberculosis) and then cervical tracts [19]. On a pathogenic point of view, spondylitis begins at the anterior margin of the vertebral body; this may be explained for the richer vascular network at the end plate surfaces; then the infection may extend to the disc and the whole vertebral body, till the opposite end plate, even causing extensive bone infarcts [21]. Disc involvement is more pronounced during pyogenic than mycobacterial infections [21], while it is primary affected in children, probably for its high vascularization in the early lifetime [19].

Infections may also involve the paravertebral muscles, the epidural, and the subdural spaces, and these localizations may then be another cause of back pain [19]. Most of the times, these involvements are secondary to spinal osteomyelitis, but it is also possible they arise as the primary site of infection [19, 21].

8.2.1.4 Vertebral Fractures

Vertebral fractures may represent an extremely disabling condition with significant repercussions on patient's health, social life, and self-sufficiency. On an etiologic point of view, vertebral fractures may be a consequence of moderate-severe entity traumas, above all in young population, as it happens in motor vehicle accidents; while in adults they are frequently secondary to underlying diseases, which often are underestimated, and the fracture with its related symptoms may be the first clinical manifestation.

Traumatic vertebral fracture may be classified according to Magerl on the basis of the traumatic mechanism (extension, flexion, twisting) and the tendinous and muscle-ligamentous structures involved by the fracture line itself [23].

Nevertheless a reduction of bone strength, primarily due to reduced quality of spongious bone trabeculae (either for metabolic causes linked to bone matrix production or for replacement of bone tissue with neoplastic one), may determine an increased risk of fractures even for a minor trauma (also including those vertebral fractures which are secondary to the trunk weight, even without an evident traumatic event) [24]. Clinically the main symptom is spinal pain whose onset maybe either acute, above all following severe vertebral trauma and may be also associated to serious neurological signs and symptoms (following spinal cord compression), or even insidious and slightly worsening [25].

In this latter case, the differential diagnosis may be difficult for several pathologies, both benign and malignant, and may present this type of manifestations; thus clinical findings alone are not specific [26]. It must be taken in account that these pathologies affect patients with similar age, generally senile population, who present several comorbidities (such as diabetes, history of tumor) and likely spinal degenerative changes, which the spinal pain may be wrongly attributed to, and then make the diagnosis even more difficult. Therefore, as we will see, imaging is crucial for the diagnosis [27].

Among bone metabolic diseases, osteoporosis is surely the main cause of vertebral fractures, above all in postmenopausal female population [28]. The vertebral fracture is a secondary to the reduction of bone strength two loading forces due to a relative increasing of osteoclastic activity over the osteoblastic and the consequent loss of trabecular meshwork [25]. Vertebral fractures and manifesting as a reduction in height of vertebral body (in comparison with the adjacent above and below vertebral body) and its severity depend on both which portion of the vertebral body is reduced (anterior, central, or posterior) and the quantitatively height loss [29].

8.2.1.5 Spine Tumors

Another important cause of spinal pain is spinal tumors. The most common spinal tumors arise from the vertebral bone column, from the spinal cord and dorsal roots, or from the paravertebral tissues; more than half of them are extradural; nevertheless a discrete percentage (almost 40%) is intradural [30].

Classically, primitive tumors are quite rare, while secondary tumors represent the very large amount of them (including metastases, multiple myeloma, and lymphoma) [31]. Clinical symptoms, if present, mainly consist in thoracic and lumbar pain with gradual onset which may be worsened by some, neurological symptoms, are usually belated and are often wrongly credited to degenerative changes [27].

In general patients with malignant tumors experience more frequent and intense pain for the secondary compression of the spinal cord and dorsal roots [32].

Concerning bone tumors, primary malignant bone tumors and bone metastases are predominantly affecting adult patients, while benign lesions are more common in young population; primitive bone lesions, both benign

and malignant, have the tendency to arise from the posterior elements: among these, benign lesions become clinically manifest when they reach significant dimensions. It must be also stated that some benign tumors, such as osteoid osteoma, present a typical clinical pattern characterized by recrudescent night pain which is rapidly relieved using salicylates [30]. Metastatic lesions instead tend to involve predominantly the thoracic vertebral body and specifically the posterior third: this location may be favored by the presence of an extensive venous vascular system, the so-called Batson plexus, which largely makes anastomoses with the systemic circulation [32].

An important complication of vertebral tumor is the collapse of the vertebral body and the consequent pathological vertebral fracture [33]. Clinically, as previously stated, the differential diagnosis between benign and malignant vertebral fractures may be difficult for the presence of comorbidities within the same patient, making therefore imaging essential.

A relatively rare cause of spinal pain is represented by intradural neoplasms: they represent a quite rare cause of spine tumor that usually becomes clinically manifest in late stage of disease; most of them are located in the extramedullary space [34]; among these, nerve sheath tumors are the most common and consist in neurofibromas and schwannomas, while meningiomas are secondary for frequency [35].

Leptomeningeal metastases account for a small percentage of intradural extramedullary tumors [35]; the primary site of tumor may be the CNS (in which the implied tumors are in order of frequency medulloblastoma, high-grade astrocytoma, ependymoma, oligodendroglioma, retinoblastoma, pineal tumors, and choroid plexus papilloma) and systemic tumors (breast, lung, melanoma, lymphoma, gastrointestinal, genitourinary, and head and neck tumors) [35].

8.2.2   Neurogenic Etiology

To distinguish between structural (musculo-skeletal) and neurogenic generators in the evaluation of back pain may be challenging because there can be some overlaps of these two entities: in fact, the most common cause of neurogenic back pain, especially in the lumbar spine, is spinal stenosis (SS), which is a frequent complication of several musculoskeletal pathologies and may determine compression of the spinal cord and nerve roots [8]. Structural causes of neurogenic back pain are usually a consequence of other diseases, especially spine degeneration and spinal stenosis, as discussed above and better illustrated below [8, 36, 37]. Prevalence of SS seems to be correlated with age and its severity as well. Clinical manifestations of SS include neurogenic claudication, which may manifest as LBP, sensation of heaviness, pain irradiating to one or both thighs, or even lower limb weakness, and it may be secondary to neurogenic or vascular compression [37–39]. When SS is clinically suspected, further imaging investigations should be advised to confirm the diagnosis.

8.2.3   Extraspinal Etiology

Spinal pain may also be consequent to several visceral diseases which irradiate their painful sensation on the back. Pathological conditions which are associated to back pain include genitourinary, gastrointestinal, cardiovascular, and some other else [1, 3, 8, 40]. Concerning the topic of the book, all these causes will not be discussed in the chapter: for a specific handling, we advise to read the related literature.

8.3   Imaging

Several studies have demonstrated that most patients with acute back pain do not need to seek any radiological investigation, because most of the times, symptoms usually improve spontaneously within few weeks from the onset and imaging does not improve the outcome; on the contrary, the early employment of imaging investigations, especially CT and MRI, is an expensive cost for the health system [3]; for all these reasons, the American College of Physicians does not advice further radiological investigations during the first weeks from the onset of pain, unless symptoms persist for more than 6 weeks or "red flag" symptoms are reported [41]; these latter include onset of neurological symptoms (progressive motor and sensitive changes, sudden anesthesia, impairment in sphincter control), systemic symptoms (fever, night sweats, weight loss), history of trauma (even of minor entity for patients aged more than 50 years), malignancy, or immunosuppression (even iatrogenic) [1–3, 40].

Plain radiography of the lumbar spine, performed with anteroposterior (AP) and latero-lateral (LL) projections, is usually the first imaging modality which, even if it does not provide any specific diagnosis, may exclude vertebral fractures as a consequence of minor spinal traumas (particularly in osteoporotic patients); nevertheless further evaluations with magnetic resonance imaging (MRI) are needed [3]. MRI, whose use in the investigation of back pain has exponentially increased in the last few years [8], should be considered in order to rule out suspicion of vertebral fracture, infection, or tumor [3]. Computerized tomography (CT) should be reserved to patients whom MRI is not indicated for or if anatomical bone details are needed [40]. Nuclear medicine imaging such as SPECT (single photon emission CT) and PET (positron-emission tomography) is useful mostly in the differentiation of benign vertebral fractures from neoplastic ones [40].

8.3.1   Degenerative Disc

Degenerative changes in the spine, even if very common, are usually detected at late stages on conventional radiology. They consist in disc alterations (reduction of disc height, disc generation with gas formation—vacuum phenomenon, intra-discal calcifications), subchondral sclerosis, and marginal osteophytes (Fig. 8.1) [9].

Disc degeneration may be easily assessed using MRI and relating with the T2 signal intensity (Fig. 8.2). One of the most used classifications is Pfirrmann's which evaluate degeneration accord-

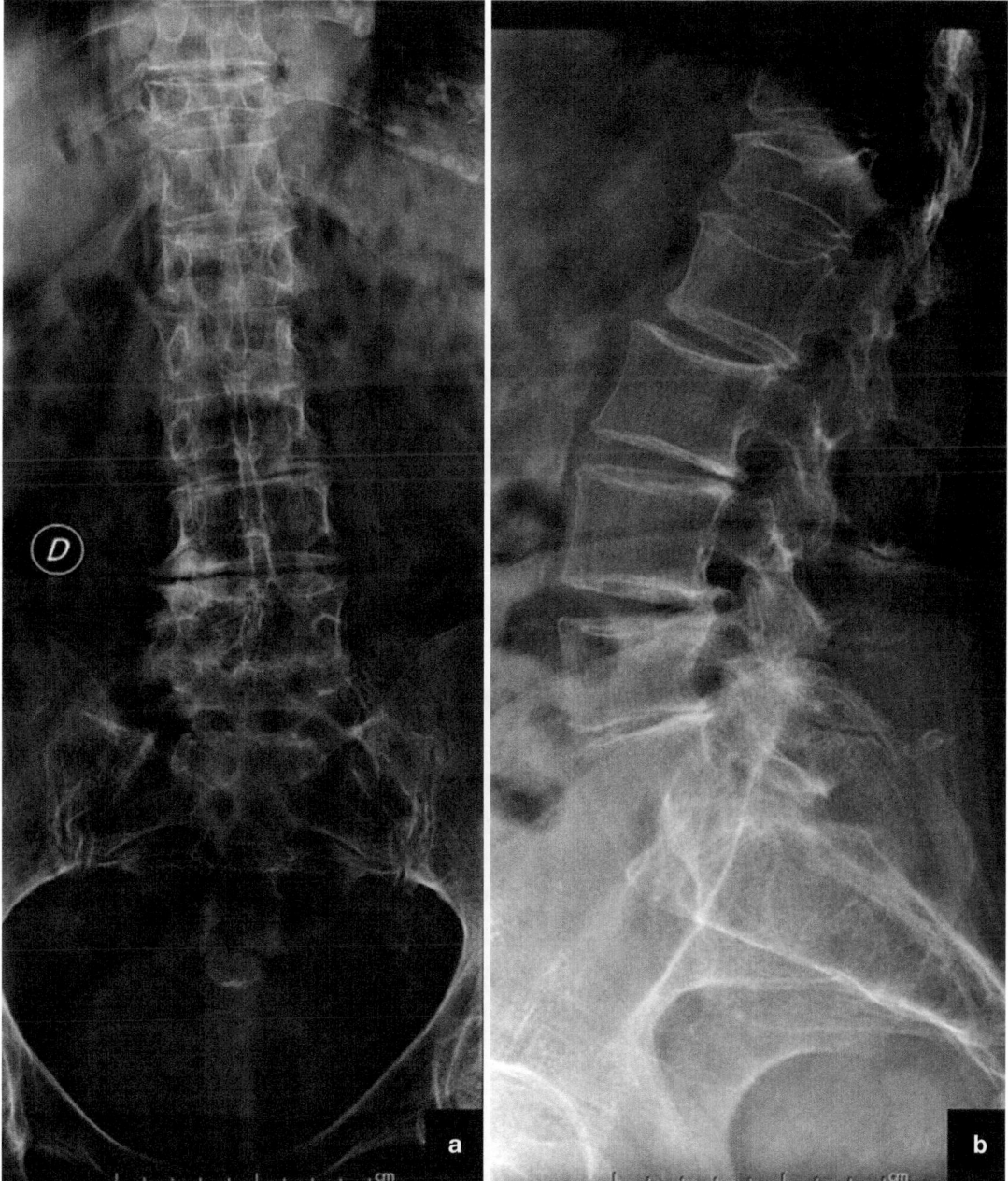

Fig. 8.1 A 65-year-old woman with long history of low back pain. Anteroposterior (**a**) and latero-lateral (**b**) radiograms show lumbar spine instability with multilevel reduction of intersomatic spaces at L3–L4, L4–L5, and L5–S1, subchondral sclerosis, and marginal osteophytes. Compression fracture of T12 is also present

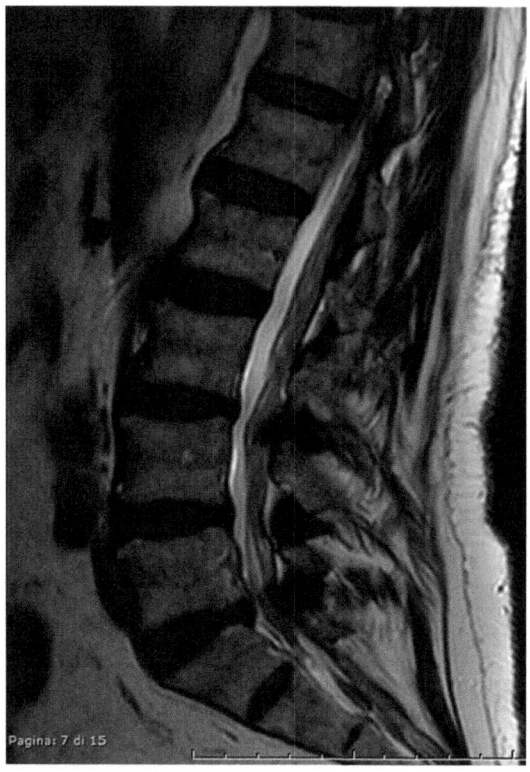

Fig. 8.2 Multilevel disc degeneration with low T2 signal intensity due to loss of proteoglycan and water content

ing to the structure homogeneity, signal intensity, and disc height [42].

For what concerns annular fissure, they can be appreciated as localized hyperintensity zones (HIZ), on T2-wi, in the context of annular fibers and are better visualized if the disc still has a certain degree of normality; they may also undergo enhancement after contrast medium administration [42].

MRI is useful in the assessment of disc herniation concerning its definition, location, and containment within the posterior longitudinal ligament (Figs. 8.3 and 8.4) [9].

Degenerative changes involving the vertebral end plates are classified according to the variation of signal intensity on MRI at these sites, using Modic classification (Fig. 8.5). Three types are recognized: at the beginning the inflammatory changes appear as low signal on T1-wi and high signal on T2-wi, and these changes are referred as type I; with the replacement of bone tissue with the adipose, changes present high intensity signal in both T1 and T2-wi; finally bone sclerosis in late stages appears as decreased signal on both T1 and T2-wi [11].

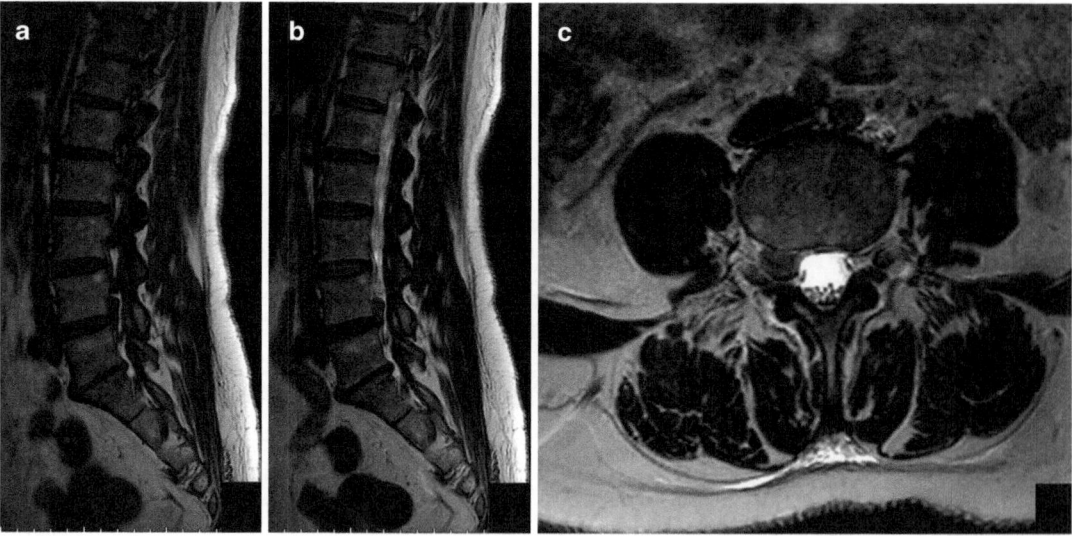

Fig. 8.3 Example of disc herniation migrated cranially, as visible on T1-wi (**a**) and T2-wi (**b**), and located in the right subarticular zone (**c**, axial T2-wi)

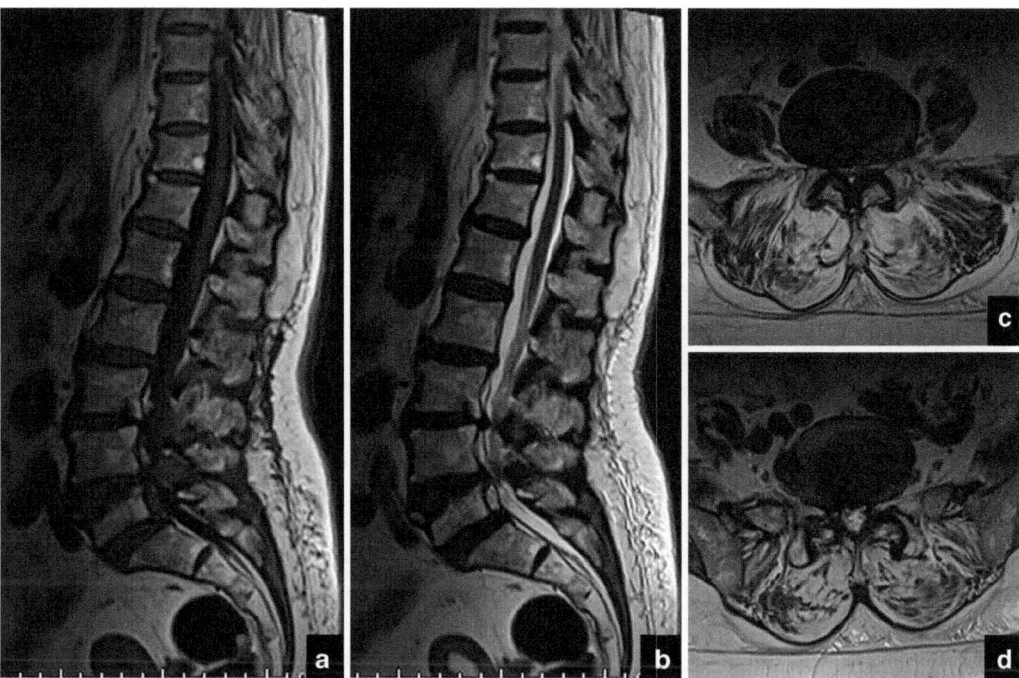

Fig. 8.4 A 75-year-old man suffering of a longtime history of low back pain with bilateral lower limb irradiation. MRI shows diffuse degenerative spine changes [sagittal T1-wi (**a**) and T2-wi (**b**)], multilevel disc herniation, spinal stenosis at the L3–L4 intervertebral space [axial T2-wi (**c**)] which is sustained broad-based herniation, and ligamentum flavum hypertrophy, grade I spondylolisthesis of L5 on S1 possibly secondary to degenerative changes in the zygoapophyseal joints [axial T2-wi (**d**)]

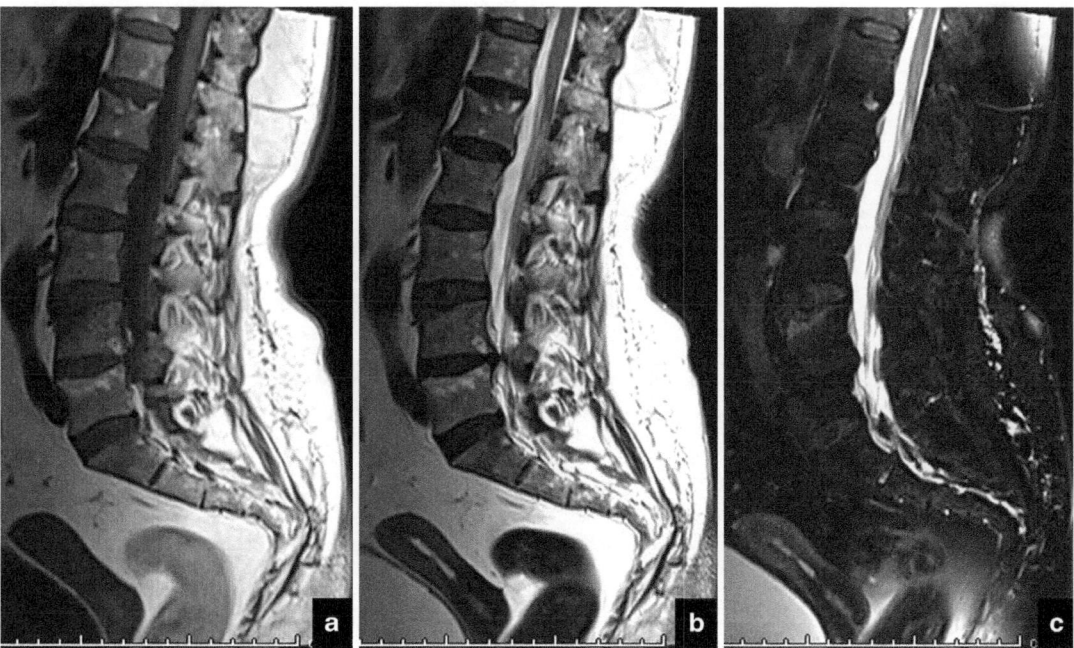

Fig. 8.5 MRI features of Modic changes: type I modification involving L4 superior end plate, appearing hypointense on FSE T1-wi (**a**) and hyperintense on FSE T2-wi (**b**) better evaluated with fat-suppression sequences (**c**); type II modification involving L5 superior end plate, which appears hyperintense on both FSE T1-wi and T2-wi (**a**, **b**) and shows low signal on fat-suppression images (**c**), features compatible with fat infiltration

8.3.2 Degenerative Bone and Ligaments

Spine degeneration may also affect synovial joint, in particular the uncovertebral joints, in the cervical level, and facet joints, in the lumbosacral. Joint osteoarthrosis may be appreciated as reduction of the articular space, subchondral bone sclerosis, and marginal osteophytes on plain radiograms (Figs. 8.6 and 8.7) and better visualized on CT scans [12]. Synovial cyst presents hypointense signal on T1-wi and hyperintense signal on T2-wi; if an acute hemorrhage occurs, the cyst rapidly increases in volume with a signal iso-/hyperintense on T1-wi and hypointense on T2-wi [12]. Facet synovitis appears as T2 hyperintensity, due to inflammatory edema, which is best appreciated using fat-suppressed sequences; it also presents intense CE after contrast medium administration [12].

Laxity of ligamentum flavum may manifest on imaging as edema, inflammation, calcification, and/or bone proliferation at insertion points, and it is in general secondary to disc degeneration

and/or facet subluxation [12]: as these conditions progress, the ligamentum flavum becomes redundant and protrudes into the spinal canal eventually causing it stenosis (Fig. 8.4).

On MRI, signal of bone marrow edema in a pedicle or pars interarticularis may be also indicative of spondylolysis [12], and the presence of spondylolisthesis may strengthen the evidence (Fig. 8.8).

8.3.3 Rheumatic Diseases

The role of imaging in the diagnosis of inflammatory diseases has become crucial, and MRI acts as the leader in this context. Besides the spine, also SIJs are usually involved in these conditions, especially in case of aSpA.

Characteristic of RA is the cervical inflammatory involvement that manifests as occipito-atlantoaxial subluxation, secondary to laxity of ligaments, which may be either anteroposterior, vertical, or lateral. Conventional radiography, which is usually the first investigation in a patient

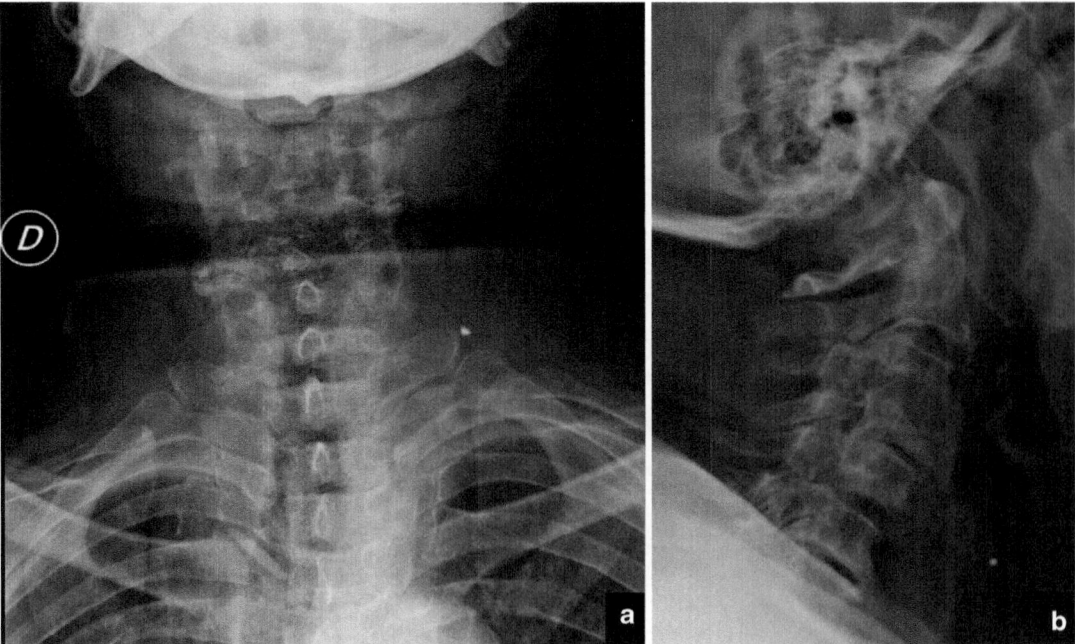

Fig. 8.6 AP (**a**) and LL (**b**) radiographs of cervical spine show spine instability with uncoarthrosis and interapophyseal arthrosis

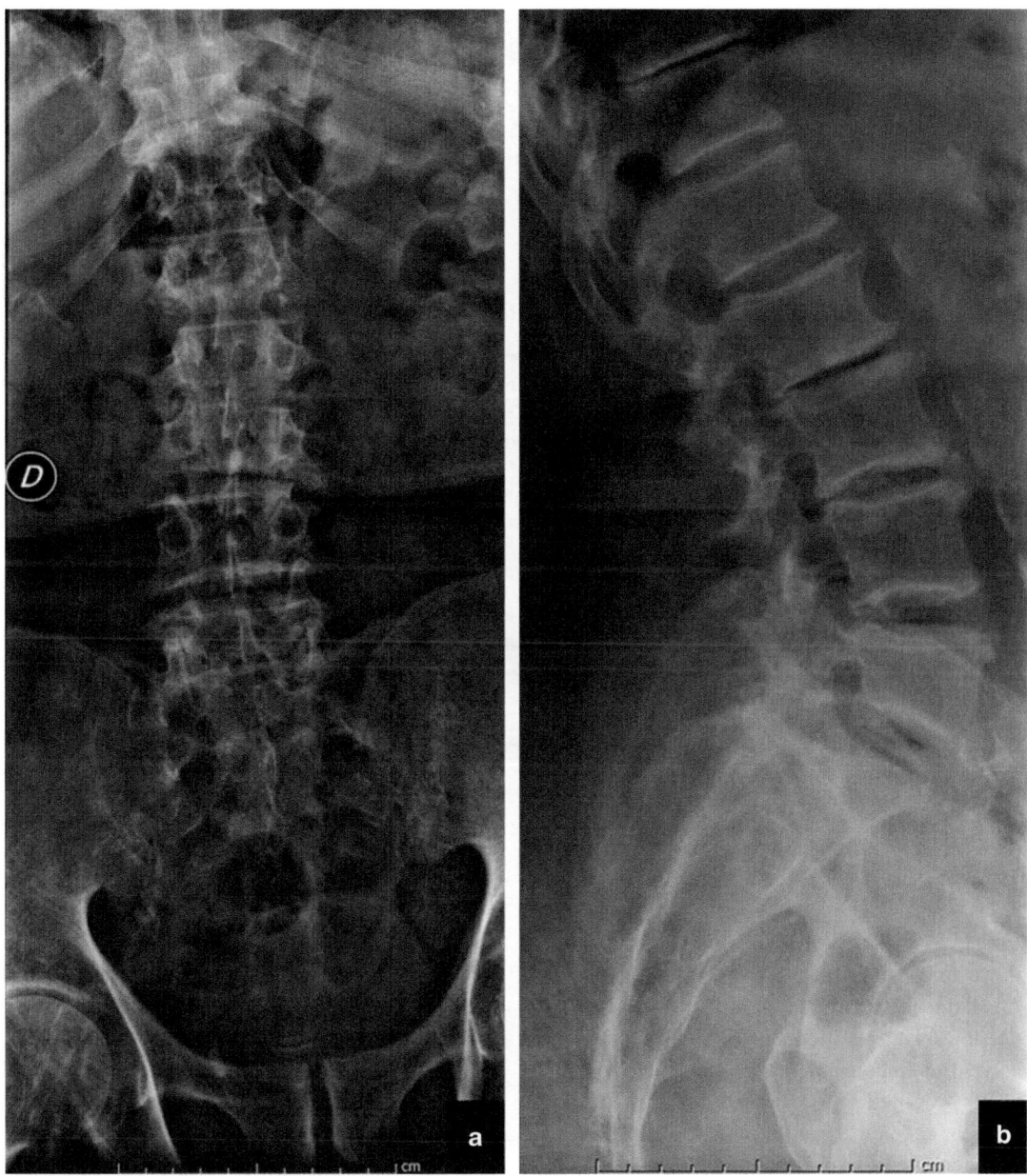

Fig. 8.7 AP (**a**) and LL (**b**) radiographs of the lumbar spine show spine instability with facet joint arthrosis and vertebral anterolisthesis of L5 on S1; multilevel disc degeneration with intradiscal vacuum can be appreciated

with neck pain [14], using dynamics projections may indicate anteroposterior subluxation as an increase of distance between the posterior aspect of the anterior arc of C1 and the odontoid process more than 3 mm on flexion, and if the posterior atlanto-dental interval is shorter than 14 mm, canal stenosis may be suspected [16]; also the

lateral subluxation, using the anteroposterior open-mouth view, may be easily documented as displacement of lateral masses of C1 more than 2 mm on the coronal plane [14, 43]. Vertical subluxation may be suspected on lateral radiographs if the dens apex is more than 4.5 mm above the McGregor's line (which runs from the hard palate

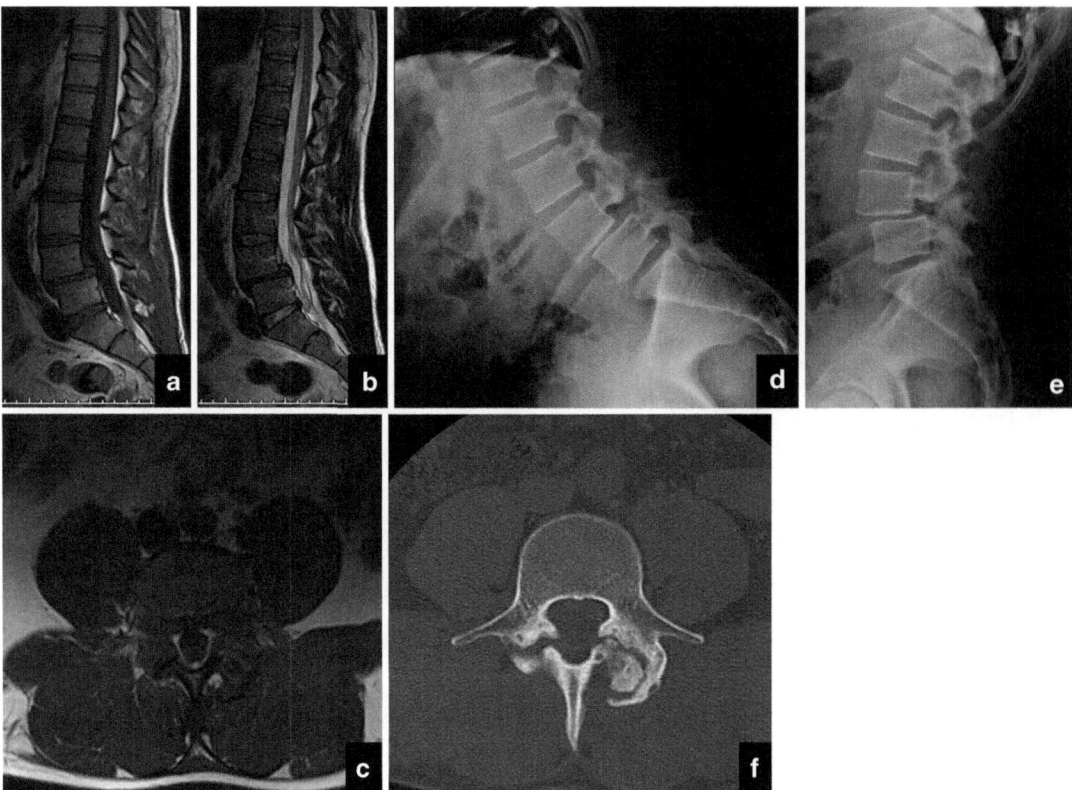

Fig. 8.8 A 32-year-old man with a long history of low back pain; MRI examination [sagittal T1-wi (**a**) and T2-wi (**b**), axial T1-wi (**c**)] shows anterolisthesis of L4 on L5 and widening of the spinal canal. Dynamic evaluation with flexion (**d**) and extension (**e**) radiograms confirms the grade I anterolisthesis. CT scan (**f**) shows bilateral pars interarticularis lysis with new bone production and sclerosis

to the most inferior point of the occipital bone); however the presence of bone erosions and the overlap of bone structures at this level may hinder the exact position of the dens. In order to solve this inconvenience, other methods have been proposed. The Redlund-Johnell method takes in account the minimum distance between McGregor's line and the inferior aspect of C2 body at the midpoint, on a lateral radiograph in a neutral position; if the distance is less than 34 mm in men or less than 29 mm in women, vertical subluxation should be suspected [14]. Clark et al. [44] divided axis into three equal parts on lateral radiograph; if the anterior arc of the atlas descends at the middle or inferior third of C2 body, vertical subluxation may be also suspected [45]. Finally, Ranawat et al. [46] measured the distance between the transverse axis of C1 and the center of the second pedicle; if the distance is

less than 15 mm in men or less than 13 mm in women, vertical subluxation should be suspected [14]. If one of these methods is suspicious for subluxation, MRI investigation is mandatory to evaluate the spinal cord [14]. Combination of these methods greatly increases the chances to individuate vertical subluxation [14].

Subaxial instability is a consequence of inflammation of uncovertebral and/or interapophyseal joints [14]; radiographies, including a dynamic exam, may show anterior slinging of a vertebral on the inferior one, and inflammatory changes may appear as small articular erosions [14].

Besides spinal instability, MRI also provides an excellent evaluation of the inflammatory changes involving the soft tissues nearby the atlantoaxial joint [43]; in particular the inflammatory pannus presents high signal on T2-wi, better appreciated in fat-suppressed or

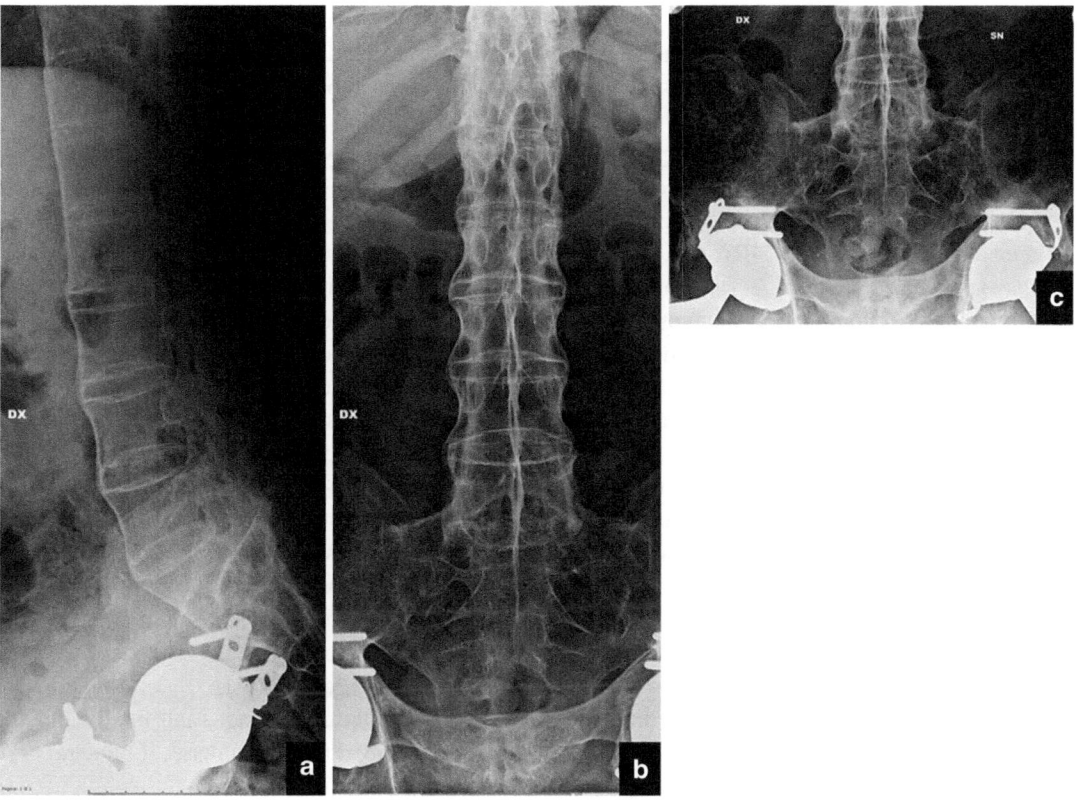

Fig. 8.9 Standard radiograms for the evaluation of the lumbar spine (**a**, **b**) and SIJs (**c**) in a patient affected by AS. The presence of diffuse syndesmophytes provides the classical "bamboo spine" appearance (**a**, **b**). Note SIJs ankylosis (**c**)

short-tau inversion recovery (STIR) sequences, and undergoes an intense contrast enhancement after gadolinium administration [14]. CT allows a direct evaluation of inflammatory erosions mostly involving the dens [43].

On contrast to RA, axSpA are more likely to affect the spine at the thoracolumbar junction and the lumbosacral level: inflammatory changes lead to alterations of vertebral shape and production of bony reactions [16]. SIJs are a common site involved in course of AS, and the Assessment of SpondyloArthritis International Society (ASAS) provides the New York criteria for the radiological assessment of sacroiliitis [47]. Standard imaging protocol consists in anteroposterior view (with cranially angulating the X-ray tube 30–35°), completed with oblique views if necessary [16]. The grading system that distinguishes five grades according to minimal erosions,

subchondral sclerosis, or complete ankyloses is present (Fig. 8.9) [47]. MRI may reveal early inflammatory lesions, which may not be evident on conventional radiographs, as areas of bone marrow edema on T2-wi with fat suppression or STIR that present strong enhancement after intravenous contrast administration; also thickening and enhancement of synovial membrane may be present [47].

Typical inflammatory changes of the spine principally involve the disco-vertebral unit; the earliest changes may be difficult to detect on standard radiographs, while they are better recognized on MRI. Three types of disco-vertebral lesions are described [48]:

- Type I lesions, or Andersson type A lesions, consist in focal erosions centrally in the vertebral end plate; most of the time, they are asymptomatic and thus may go unnoticed on conventional radiograms, while they may appear as increased T2-wi signal on MRI.

- Type II lesions, or Romanus lesions, represent bone erosions most involving the supero-anterior aspect of the vertebral body; standard radiographs may evidence the erosion with the subchondral bone sclerosis (shiny corner appearance), while on MRI the alterations may appear as increased T2-wi signal on MRI; the result of inflammatory changes and bone production results in squaring of the vertebral body.
- Type III lesions, or Andersson type B lesions, usually rare and belated changes, consist in vast central and peripheral end plate erosions associated to incorrect ossification of vertebral fractures, which are in turn secondary to some risk factors (such as osteoporosis, trauma, and increased lumbar kyphosis), when is present multiple level ankylosis.

Syndesmophytes, which also subordinated to entheseal inflammation, derived from Sharpey's fiber ossification, in the outer annulus fibrosus, and appear symmetrical and smooth connecting two vertebral bodies; if extensive, their appearance on conventional radiographs is called "bamboo spine" (Fig. 8.9) [16]. Syndesmophytes must be differentiated from other forms of bony spurs which are instead typical of other kinds of arthropathies [16]; these include:

- Marginal osteophytes typically seen in osteoarthrosis (also known as osteophytes), which consist in marginal bone productions at the level of vertebral end plates, in continuity with cortical and spongious vertebral bone, may be horizontal in shape and become large enough to join another osteophyte.
- Tractional or non-marginal osteophytes, which also present continuity with cortical and spongious vertebral bone but arise 2–3 mm away from the end plate, appear vertical in shape and are common in course of PsA and reactive arthritis.
- Paraspinal phytes, which consist in coarse calcification of paraspinal structures outside the intervertebral disc and the vertebral body

(such as the anterior longitudinal ligament), appear separated from them by a small hyperdiaphanous space.

Enthesitis may also implicate the posterior spine joints and ligaments, leading to ossification of them in late stages; ossification of interapophyseal joints appears on AP radiographs as two couple of parallel lines running across the lumbar spine (the tramline sign) [48].

For what concerns PsA, spine involvement resembles AS but with some differences: in particular, syndesmophytes appear to be coarse and unilateral and do not involve two following vertebral bodies [49] (for this reason they are also called parasyndesmophytes); cervical spine alterations, with subsequent atlantoaxial instability similar to RA, are also very common [49]. SIJs may also be involved in the inflammatory process, and radiological features consist in erosions, subchondral sclerosis, widening and later narrowing of articular space, and finally ankylosis; changes tend to be unilateral; if bilateral they usually are asymmetrical [50].

8.3.4 Infectious Diseases

With a clinical suspect of spine infection, conventional radiology is the first step in the imaging evaluation; however it lacks in sensitivity because bone changes are not visible until a certain amount of the bone (almost 30%) is lost, at 3–6 weeks from the onset (Fig. 8.10) [51]: earliest signs of infection are represented by foci of bone rarefaction nearby the vertebral end plate with irregularity; reduction in disc space may be indication of discitis [52]. CT may also be negative in early stages or document focal areas of bone erosions and bone sclerosis at the level of end plates, but they are more evident in late stages [52]. MRI is the most sensitive technique for spine infection which allows a direct visualization of bone marrow edema as increased T2 signal intensity (Fig. 8.10) [52]; in early stages the alterations are visible on the superomarginal aspects of the vertebral body which later may spread to the whole vertebral body [19].

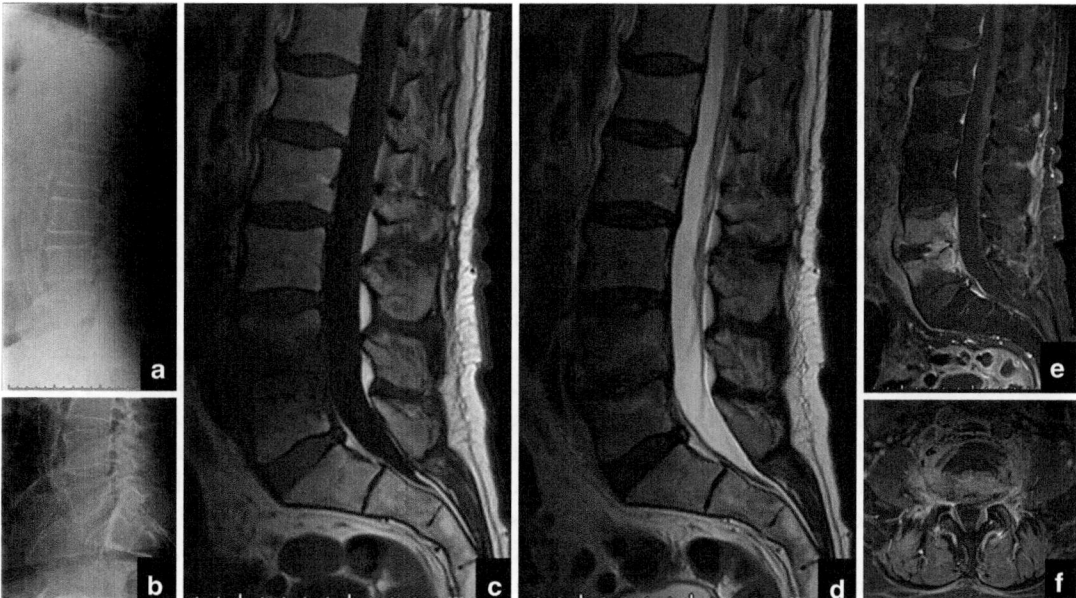

Fig. 8.10 Pyogenic spondylodiscitis. At the time of imaging evaluation, conventional radiograms (**a**, **b**) did not show bone changes yet, while the MRI exam demonstrates coarse area of bone signal changes, hypointense on T1-wi (**c**) and hyperintense on T2-wi (**d**) which underwent homogeneous CE (**e**, **f**), the signs are compatible with an active inflammatory process. A fluid collection in the surrounding anterior and lateral paravertebral space can be also appreciated, with inflammation extending in the epidural space, determining focal dural inflammatory reaction, and involving the ligamentum flavum and the interapophyseal joints (**f**)

MRI also allows an excellent evaluation of endocanal content, which may be involved by the infective spread, and also documents the disc involvement better than conventional radiography and CT [52]. Contrast medium administration, especially for MRI, confirms the findings on the basal exam, provides an adequate delineation of paravertebral abscesses, and permits the differential diagnosis with other pathologies which may mimic spondylodiscitis, especially in early stages (such as Modic and degenerative changes) [52].

There are some imaging findings that can guide in the differential diagnosis of spinal infection etiologies [19, 52]:

- *Pyogenic infection* tends to involve two consecutive vertebral levels, mostly in the lumbar spine, starting at the anterolateral aspects of the vertebral body; the intervertebral disc is usually involved, even if in early stages, it may be spared; posterior vertebral elements are generally not involved; inflammation of paravertebral and epidural spaces with paraspinal abscesses may be present.

- *Tubercular spondylodiscitis* preferentially locates at the thoracic spine, involving multiple vertebral levels with predominant disintegration of anterior margins of the vertebral body; intervertebral disc is generally not involved until late stage of infection and posterior elements are more frequently involved than pyogenic infection; sometimes skip lesions have been described; also large paraspinal abscesses are present, and the infection may spread along the anterior and posterior longitudinal ligaments; meningeal involvement is also common; if the infection is limited to a single vertebral body, it may result in vertebral collapse (vertebra plana), and subsequent ossification may appear as "ivory vertebra" on conventional radiography.

- *Brucellar infection*, on the contrary to the previous ones, is characterized by isolated location of the lower lumbar spine with relative sparing of vertebral body and predominant disc involvement; usually posterior element is not involved, and paraspinal abscesses are not present, but infection may spread posteriorly to the leptomeninges and radicular nerve roots and anteriorly involving the peritoneum nearby the affected vertebral level.

- *Fungal infections*, which are common in immunosuppressed patients, usually involve the lumbar spine at multiple levels and frequently with skip lesions; generally the vertebral body is variably involved without severe bone destruction, and the intervertebral disc is preserved; paravertebral abscesses if present are small and do not undergo intense contrast enhancement for the low inflammatory response in this kind of patients; like tuberculosis, spread of infection beneath the ligaments is common.

As a consequence of the reduction in bone matrix, vertebral fractures may also occur.

8.3.5 Vertebral Fractures

According to the morphology, vertebral fractures are distinguished in wedge, end plates, or crush fractures depending on the reduction of anterior, middle, or posterior vertebral height, respectively, and these features can be already appreciated on conventional radiographs (Fig. 8.11) [29]. Genant and colleagues have developed a grading system for the evaluation of fracture severity [53]: with respect to vertebral height loss and vertebral body shape, fractures are considered mild, moderate, and severe if it is loss up to 25%, from 25 to 40%, or more than 40% of disc height, respectively.

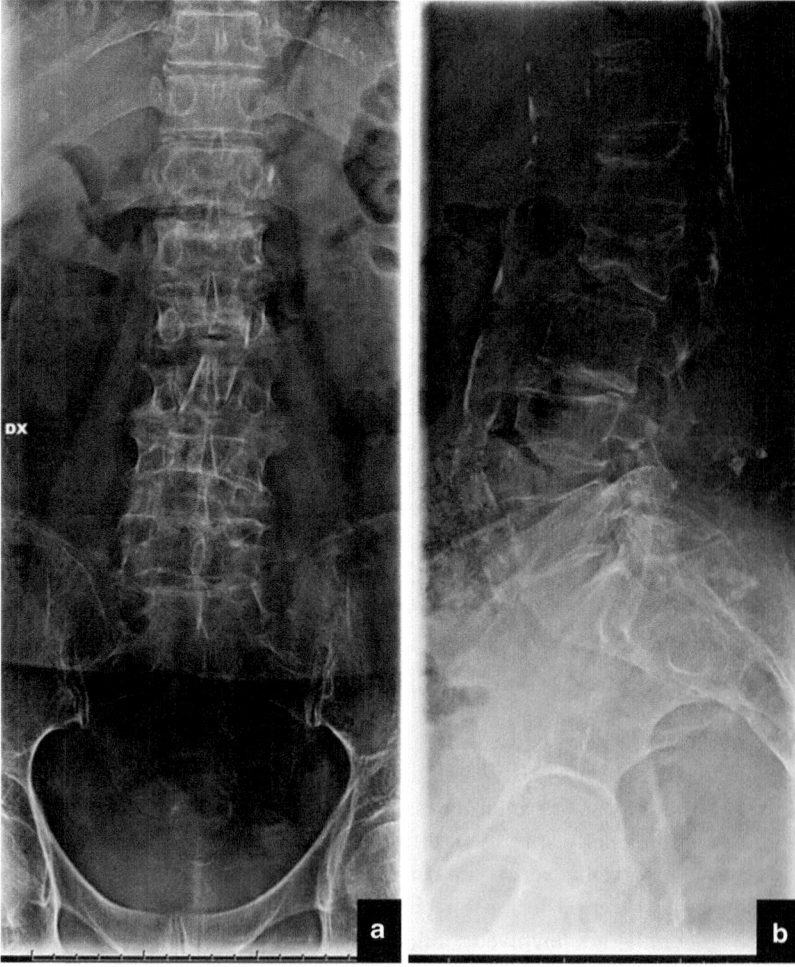

Fig. 8.11 A 70-year-old woman with osteoporosis. Conventional radiography, with AP (**a**) and LL (**b**) radiograms, shows fractures of L1, L2, and L4 vertebral bodies

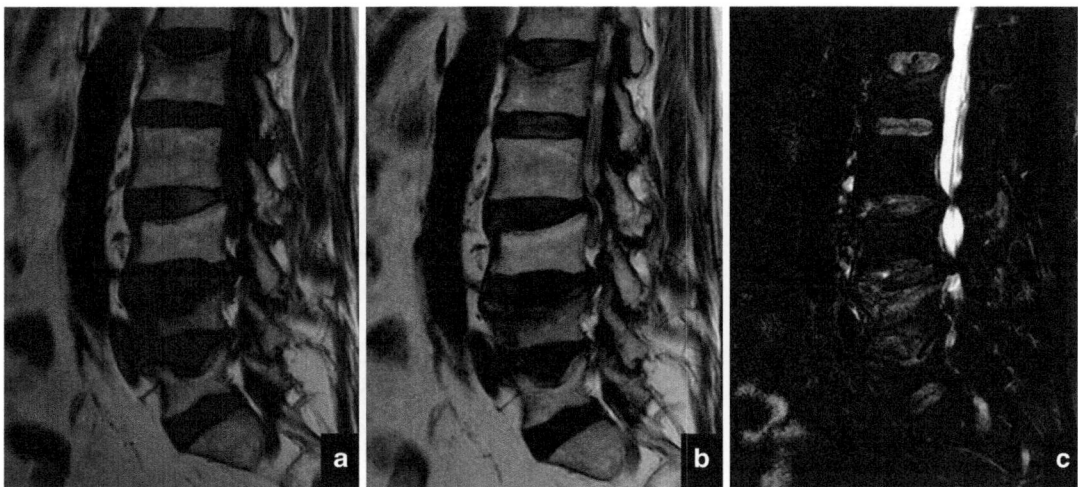

Fig. 8.12 Vertebral fractures. Recent collapse of L4 vertebral body; the bone edema appears hypointense on FSE T1-wi (**a**), has an inhomogeneous signal on T2-wi (**b**), and appears hyperintense on T2 fat-sat images (**c**). Also L1 and L5 vertebral bodies are collapsed, but these fractures are relatively older. Mild anterior height reduction of L3 can be also appreciated

Conventional radiography demonstrates a symmetrical vertebral fracture with both pedicles usually clearly evident; other signs of benignity include the so-called Kümmel or vacuum phenomenon, which consist in vertebral osteonecrosis, usually beneath the end plate, the posterior retropulsion of a bony fragment, and no evidence of osteolysis [25, 54]; these signs are better evaluated using CT, which also may point out the integrity of posterior vertebral wall.

MRI evaluation of vertebral fractures is useful to date the fracture itself: in fact, acute fracture will usually present edematous signal within the spongious bone, appearing as low signal on T1-wi and high T2-wi signal; this latter is better evaluated using fat-suppression or STIR sequences [26] (Fig. 8.12), which sometimes may undergo mild/moderate contrast enhancement [55].

8.3.6   Spine Tumors

Main characteristics of primary bone spine tumors, both benign and malignant, associated to spinal pain are described in Tables 8.1 and 8.2.

For a more extensive discussion on the topic, we suggest to read the related references [30–32].

Bone spinal metastases, which involve the spine more frequently than primary tumors, are another common cause of spinal pain; they generally induce a reaction in the vertebral spongious bone which may be either osteoblastic (that elicits new bone production) or osteoclastic (that is secondary to bone destruction): these changes may be detected on conventional radiographs and CT scans as areas of bone sclerosis or bone lysis, respectively.

According to the spread pathway, posterior vertebral body and elements are more often involved: this aspect may be associated to either loss of integrity or convex appearance of posterior vertebral wall, asymmetrical vertebral fracture, and paravertebral soft-tissue masses that may also invade the spinal canal (these features are better evaluated on CT scans).

MRI investigation is usually advised to further evaluate the bone involvement, the tumor spread into the spinal canal, and paravertebral spaces, and it also helps in the distinction of vertebral fractures secondary to tumoral disease and (so-called malignant fractures) and those

Table 8.1 Primary benign tumors of the spine

	Epidemiology	Spine location	Morphology	Conventional radiography	CT	MRI
Osteoid osteoma	Young patients Slight male predominance	Posterior elements Lumbar > cervical > thoracic > sacrum	< 2 cm Well-represented trabecular bone and fibrous connective tissue often surrounded by bone sclerosis	Difficult to see; generally a radiolucent area within the posterior elements	Radiolucent nidus +/− central calcification surrounded by bone sclerosis	Nidus: low to intermediate signal on T1-wi, intermediate to high signal on T2-wi with surrounding edema which may be extensive
Osteoblastoma	Young adults (second–third decades) M:F = 2:1	Posterior elements	Histologically similar to osteoid osteoma but larger than 2 cm May be associated to ABC	Similar to osteoid osteoma	Multiple small calcifications and peripheral sclerotic rim	Allows a better evaluation of surrounding soft tissues
Aneurismal bone cyst (ABC)	Young patients, predominant in female population	1/3 of all ABC are located in the spine Thoracic > lumbar and cervical Usually extends within the spinal canal	Hemorrhagic lesion which can be primary or secondary to preexisting lesion	Eccentric lytic lesion with bone remodeling and blown out contour	Evaluation of lesion margins, which appear thin but continuous Fluid levels may be observed	Peripheral contour of hypointensity on both T1- and T2-wi Multiloculated lesion with fluid levels which present high signal on both T1- and T2-wi (methemoglobin) Perilesional edema presents high signal on T2-wi with fat suppression
Giant-cell tumor (GCT)	Young patients (second–fourth decades) M:F = 1:2.5	Sacrum (upper segments) > thoracic > cervical > lumbar Generally affects the vertebral body and may extend to the posterior elements; may be associated to secondary ABC	It is rare after skeletal maturity It consists of osteoclastic-like giant cells In some cases may give metastases (lungs)	Well-delimited lytic lesion, in the sacrum may cross the midline and the SIJs	Better evaluation of the lesion margins and matrix, which does not show calcifications	The tumor presents an inhomogeneous signal intensity in all sequences and CE; a central low T2 signal may be related to collagen fibers
Eosinophilic granuloma (EG)	Young patients (3–12 years old) and male predominance	Thoracic > cervical and lumbar Primary involvement of posterior elements is rare	Localized and benign form of Langerhans cell histiocytosis with a variable amount of lymphocytes, polymorphonuclear cells and eosinophils	Lytic lesion is not always visible, but the principal characteristic is the anterior vertebral collapse	Lytic lesion is well visualized, and extracompartimental invasion is also well documented	Tumor presents low T1 signal and high T2 signal with intense enhancement following contrast medium administration

Table 8.2 Primary malignant tumors of the spine

	Epidemiology	Spine location	Morphology	Conventional radiography	CT	MRI
Plasmacytoma/multiple myeloma	Following metastases is the second most common spine tumor	Usually the spine is diffusely involved; rarely the manifestation is focal Vertebral fractures may be present, prevalently at T6–L4	Destructive neoplastic masses of plasma cells	Diffuse osteopenia with multiple lytic lesions (in 20% radiograms are negative)	Allows a better definition of lytic lesions and cortical destruction	Tumoral tissue appears as diffuse/focal T1 hypointensity and T2 hyperintensity (this latter better evaluated with fat suppression sequences) and presents CE
Chordoma	Peak incidence around fifth decade	Sacrum (lower segments) > clivus > other cervical and other segments	Arises from the notochord remnants which extend from Rathke pouch to coccyx, for this reason is almost always detected in the midline Histologically it is composed of physaliphorous cells	Spine: bone destruction predominates with peripheral sclerosis in the mobile segments Sacrum: in more than half of cases, tumor presents calcifications and extends into the paraspinal tissues; it also crosses the SIJs in almost ¼ of cases	Findings are similar to those of standard radiographs, but CT allows a better evaluation of cortical destruction and intratumoral calcifications	Tumor has signal intensity similar to nucleus pulposus (intervertebral disc) with low/ intermediate T1-w signal and high T2-wi signal; intracranial chordoma may present also high T1-w signal for the elevated protein content (mucin). CE may appear thick and peripheral
Chondrosarcoma	It is the third most frequent malignant tumor, after metastases and plasmacytoma M:F = 2–4:1	Thoracic > lumbar > cervical It usually arises from the posterior elements and then involves the vertebral body; location in the vertebral body alone is not common	It may be primary or secondary (deriving from a preexisting osteochondroma) Histologically tumor consists of malignant cartilage (usually low grade)	Lytic lesion, with "arc-and-ring" pattern (chondroid matrix)	Identifies bone destruction and matrix calcification	Tumor presents low/ intermediate signal on T1-wi and high signal on T2-wi, due to the high water content of matrix; calcifications appear as low signal in all sequences Extra-osseous invasion is also well depicted

(continued)

Table 8.2 (continued)

	Epidemiology	Spine location	Morphology	Conventional radiography	CT	MRI
Ewing's sarcoma and PNET (primitive neuroectodermal tumor)	The most common nonlymphoproliferative primary malignant tumors of the spine in children	Primary tumors of the spine are rare, instead metastases at this site are more common Sacrum >lumbar > thoracic; cervical spine is rarely involved Most lesions arise from posterior elements and secondarily involve the vertebral body	Tumor consists of small rounded blue cells and abundant collagen	Lytic lesions, with moth eaten or permeative pattern Ewing's sarcoma is frequently associated with diffuse sclerosis, corresponding to osteonecrosis	Findings are similar to those found in radiographs but better evaluated	Tumor presents intermediate signal on T1-wi and intermediate/high signal on T2-wi; CE is homogeneous Extra-osseous invasion is also well depicted
Osteosarcoma	Peak incidence of spine osteosarcoma is around the fourth decade Relative male predilection	Mostly arise from the posterior elements Predilection for thoracic segments Generally is a singular lesion, sometimes may be multiple	Osteoid matrix with calcification is the most frequent pattern Spinal canal invasion is frequent	Hyperdense lesion which may result in ivory vertebra Vertebral collapse is common	Allows a better delineation of lesion matrix and paravertebral involvement	If the mineralization is intense, the lesion has low signal in all sequences; otherwise, the signal is intermediate Contrast enhancement is slightly inhomogeneous

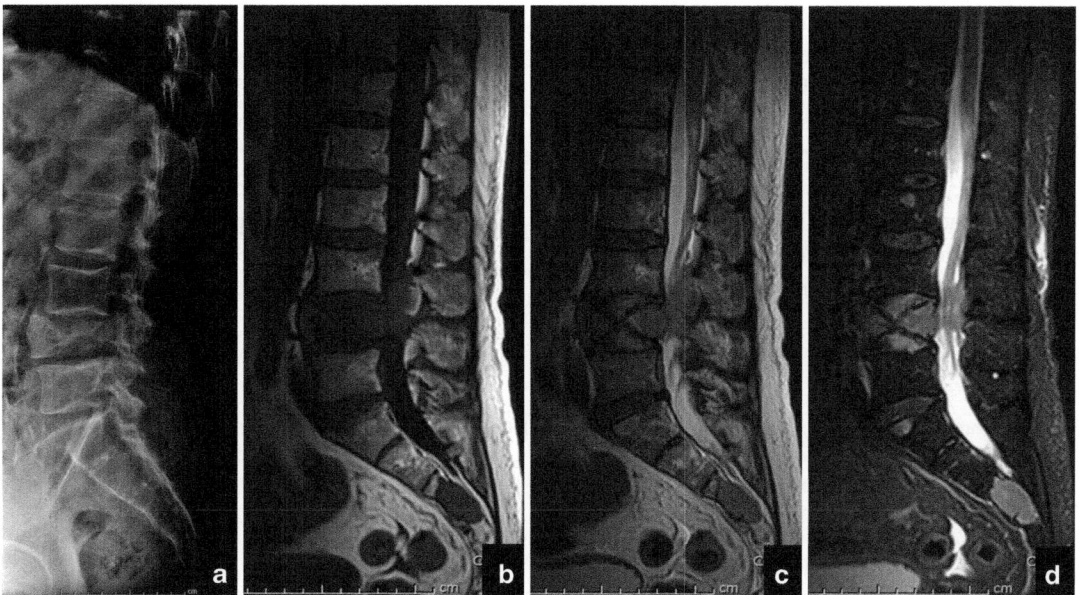

Fig. 8.13 A 65-year-old patient with history of lung tumor. Lateral radiogram (**a**) documents fracture of L4 involving the posterior vertebral body and interruption of posterior vertebral wall. MRI examination [T1-wi (**b**), T2-wi (**c**), T2 fat sat (**d**)] documents replacement of normal bone tissue with neoplastic one which expands within the spinal canal. L2, L3, and S3 vertebral bodies are also involved

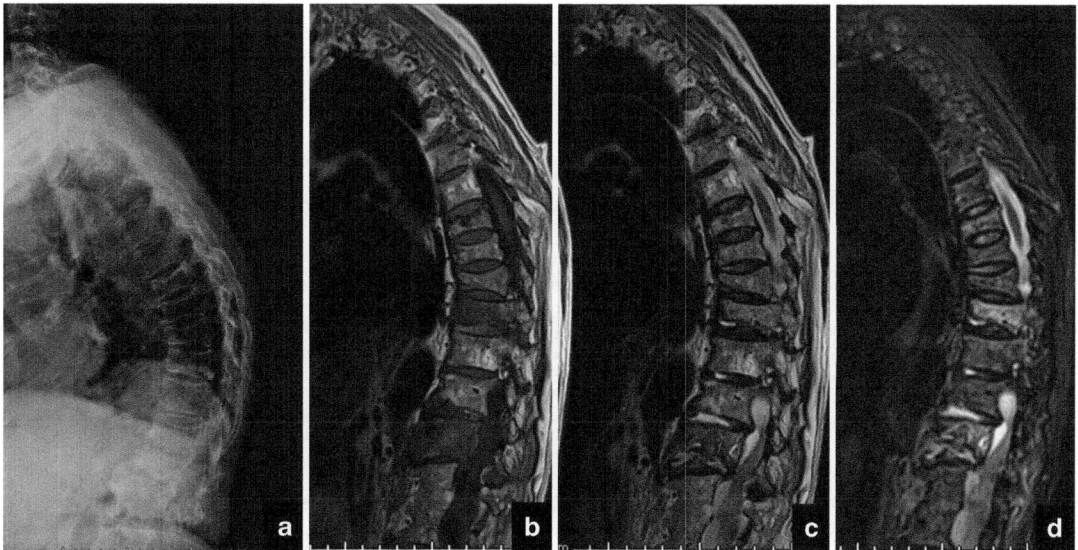

Fig. 8.14 Dorsal spine imaging of a patient affected by multiple myeloma; multilevel spinal fractures are evident secondary to reduction of bone mineralized mass due to lymphomatous tissue infiltration. (**a**) Lateral radiogram, (**b**) sagittal T1-wi, (**c**) sagittal T2-wi, (**d**) sagittal T2 fat-sat image

secondary to osteoporosis or other benign diseases (mostly metabolic) (Figs. 8.13 and 8.14).

The intravenous administration of contrast medium generally determines a variable tumoral uptake, both in the vertebral bone and in the paravertebral tissues, which is also in correlation to necrotic areas within the tumor, and this may result in an inhomogeneous CE pattern.

Recently, several studies have stated the adding value of other MRI sequences, such as diffusion-weighted imaging (DWI) and in-phase and opposed-phase sequences, for the distinction of benign and malignant vertebral fractures.

The role of MRI is also essential in the detection of intradural tumors. The most common neoplasms, which are also extramedullary, are represented by schwannomas, neurofibromas, and meningiomas, whose principal are listed on Table 8.3 [32, 34, 35]. Other lesions include paraganglioma, melanocytoma, melanoma, hemangiopericytoma, and leptomeningeal metastases [34]. On MRI, schwannomas hypo-/isointense on T1-wi and iso-/hyperintense on T2-wi and also present intense and homogeneous CE (Fig. 8.15) [34]; neurofibromas appear with a rounded or fusiform shape, isointense on T1-wi and highly

Table 8.3 Spinal cord tumor

	General characteristics	Site
Schwannoma	Most common benign tumor (55%) (WHO I) Typically found in adult patients Generally are single, well-defined masses provided with capsule	70% intradural, 30% extradural; 15% dumbbell-shaped (intra/extradural) Eccentric to nerve fibers
Meningioma	The second most intradural tumor, benign in 95% of cases (WHO I) Most common in women (45–74 years)	90% are intradural Dorsal spine in women, cervical spine in men
Neurofibroma	Benign slow-growing tumor (WHO I) In 90% of cases is sporadic; it may be associated to genetic syndrome such as NF-1	Dorsal nerve roots, peripheral nerves; in almost 40% of cases are located within the spinal canal
Paraganglioma	Rare benign tumor (WHO I) arising from neural crest cells Slightly predominant in men, with a mean age of 46 years	Typically found in the cauda equina with secondary compression of neural structures
Metastases	Small percentage Secondary to either CNS or, less frequently, systemic neoplasms	Leptomeninges

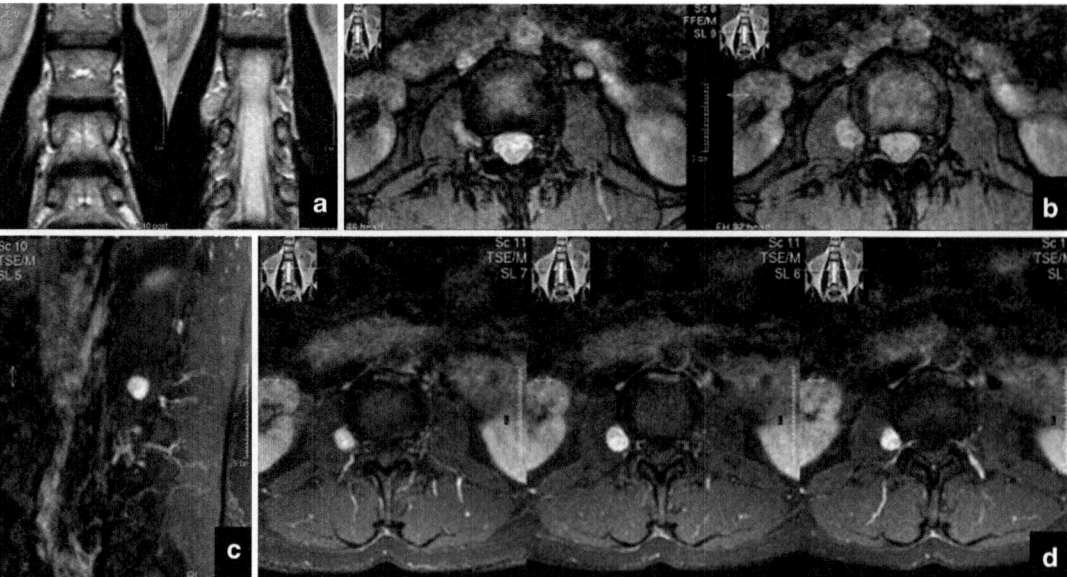

Fig. 8.15 Right L2 schwannoma which enlarges the homonymous canal and presents high T2 signal (**a, b**). The lesions enhance homogeneously (**c, d**) on T1 fat-sat images

hyperintense on T2-wi which undergo homogeneous CE [34]; meningiomas arise from the dura mater, which is connected with a tail, as rounded broad-based mass with isointense T1 and T2 signal intensity and shows intense CE [34]; calcifications may be found in 5% of cases [35]. Paraganglioma usually involves the filum terminale and is then associated to canal stenosis and low back pain [32]; on MRI it appears as a well-defined mass, iso-/hypointense on T1-wi and hyperintense on T2-wi with an hemosiderin cup; it undergoes intense CE [34]. Leptomeningeal metastases present a variable appearance on morphologic sequences, presenting as nodular masses or with an infiltrative pattern, but usually they present a diffuse and marked CE [35].

References

1. Manusov EG. Evaluation and diagnosis of low back pain. Prim Care Clin Office Pract. 2012;39:471–9.
2. Maus T. Imaging the Back Pain Patient. Phys Med Rehabil Clin N Am. 2010;21:725–66.
3. Patrick N, Emanski E, Knaub MA. Acute and chronic low back pain. Med Clin N Am. 2016;100:169–81.
4. Kleinman N, Patel AA, Benson C, Macario A, Kim M, Biondi DM. Economic burden of back and neck pain: effect of a neuropathic component. Popul Health Manag. 2014;17(4):224–32.
5. Costa-Black KM, Loisel P, Anema JR, Pransky G. Back pain and work. Best Pract Res Clin Rheumatol. 2014;24(2):227–40.
6. Parkin-Smith GF, Amorin-Woods LG, Davies SJ, Losco BE, Adams J. Spinal pain: current understanding, trends, and the future of care. J Pain Res. 2015;8:741–52.
7. Muto M, Giurazza F, Guarnieri G, Izzo R, Diano A. Neuroimaging of spinal instability. Magn Reson Imaging Clin N Am. 2016;24(3):485–94.
8. Amirdelfan K, McRoberts P, Deer TR. The differential diagnosis of low back pain: a primer on the evolving paradigm. Neuromodulation. 2014;17:11–7.
9. Fardon DF, Williams AL, Dohring EJ, Murtagh FR, Gabriel Rothman SL, Sze GK. Lumbar disc nomenclature: version 2.0. Recommendations of the combined task forces of the North American Spine Society, the American Society of Spine Radiology and the American Society of Neuroradiology. Spine J. 2014;14:2525–45.
10. Izzo R, Popolizio T, D'Aprile P, Muto M. Spinal pain. Eur J Radiol. 2015;84(5):746–56.
11. Dudli S, Fields AJ, Samartzis D, Karppinen J, Lotz JC. Pathobiology of Modic changes. Eur Spine J. 2016;25(11):3723–34.
12. Kotsenas AL. Imaging of posterior element axial pain generators: facet joints, pedicles, spinous processes, sacroiliac joints, and transitional segments. Radiol Clin N Am. 2012;50(4):705–30.
13. Donnally CJ III, Dulebohn SC. Lumbar spondylolysis and spondylolisthesis. In: StatPearls. Treasure Island: StatPearls Publishing; 2017.
14. Jurik AG. Imaging the spine in arthritis—a pictorial review. Insights Imaging. 2011;2:177–91.
15. Garlaschi G, Satragno L, Silvestri E, La Paglia E. Rachide infiammatorio non infettivo. In: Martino F, Leone A, editors. Imaging del rachide - il vecchio e il nuovo. Milano: Springer-Verlag; 2008.
16. Mattar M, Salonen D, Inman RD. Imaging of spondyloarthropathies. Rheum Dis Clin N Am. 2013;39:645–67.
17. Leone A, Marino M, Dell'Atti C, Zecchi V, Magarelli N, Colosimo C. Spinal fractures in patients with ankylosing spondylitis. Rheumatol Int. 2016;36(10):1335–46.
18. Anandarajah A. Imaging in psoriatic arthritis. Clinic Rev Allerg Immunol. 2013;44:157–65.
19. Diehn FE. Imaging of spine infection. Radiol Clin N Am. 2012;50:777–98.
20. Duarte RM, Vaccaro AR. Spinal infection: state of the art and management algorithm. Eur Spine J. 2013;22:2787–99.
21. DeSanto J, Ross JS. Spine infection/inflammation. Radiol Clin N Am. 2011;49:105–27.
22. Kaya S, Ercan S, Kaya S, Aktas U, Kamasak K, Ozalp H, Cinar K, Duymus R, Boyaci MG, Akkoyun N, Eskazan AE, Temiz H. Spondylodiscitis: evaluation of patients in a tertiary hospital. J Infect Dev Ctries. 2014;8(10):1272–6.
23. Magerl F, Aebi M, Gertzbein SD, Harms J, Nazarian S. A comprehensive classification of thoracic and lumbar injuries. Eur Spine J. 1994;3:184–201.
24. Ruiz Santiago F, Tomás Muñoz P, Moya Sánchez E, Revelles Paniza M, Martínez Martínez A, Pérez Abela AL. Classifying thoracolumbar fractures: role of quantitative imaging. Quant Imaging Med Surg. 2016;6(6):772–84.
25. Guglielmi G, Muscarella S, Bazzocchi A. Integrated imaging approach to osteoporosis: state-of-the-art review and update. Radiographics. 2011;31:1343–64.
26. Cicala D, Briganti F, Casale L, Rossi C, Cagini L, Cesarano E, Brunese L, Giganti M. Atraumatic vertebral compression fractures: differential diagnosis between benign osteoporotic and malignant fractures by MRI. Musculoskelet Surg. 2013;97(Suppl 2):S169–79.
27. Jung HS, Jee WH, McCauley TR, et al. Discrimination of metastatic from acute osteoporotic compression spinal fractures with MR imaging. Radiographics. 2003;23:179–87.
28. Sözen T, Özışık L, Başaran NC. An overview and management of osteoporosis. Eur J Rheumatol. 2017;4:46–56.
29. Griffith JF. Identifying osteoporotic vertebral fracture. Quant Imaging Med Surg. 2015;5(4):592–602.

30. Erlemann R. Imaging and differential diagnosis of primary bone tumors and tumor-like lesions of the spine. Eur J Radiol. 2006;58:48–67.

31. Orguc S, Arkun R. Primary tumors of the spine. Semin Musculoskelet Radiol. 2014;18:280–99.

32. Wald JT. Imaging of spine neoplasm. Radiol Clin N Am. 2012;50:749–76.

33. Sung JK, Jee WH, Jung JY, Choi M, Lee SY, Kim YH, Ha KY, Park CK. Differentiation of acute osteoporotic and malignant compression fractures of the spine: use of additive qualitative and quantitative axial diffusion-weighted MR imaging to conventional MR imaging at 3.0 T. Radiology. 2014;271(2):488–98.

34. Merhemic Z, Stosic-Opincal T, Thurnher MM. Neuroimaging of spinal tumors. Magn Reson Imaging Clin N Am. 2016;24(3):563–79.

35. Beall DP, Googe DJ, Emery RL, Thompson DB, Campbell SE, Ly JQ, DeLone D, Smirniotopoulos J, Lisanti C, Currie TJ. Extramedullary intradural spinal tumors: a pictorial review. Curr Probl Diagn Radiol. 2007;36(5):185–98.

36. Kalichman L, Cole R, Kim DH, Li L, Suri P, Guermazi A, Hunter DJ. Spinal stenosis prevalence and association with symptoms: the Framingham Study. Spine J. 2009;9(7):545–50.

37. Middleton K, Fish DE. Lumbar spondylosis: clinical presentation and treatment approaches. Curr Rev Musculoskelet Med. 2009;2(2):94–104.

38. Melancia JL, Francisco AF, Antunes JL. Spinal stenosis. Handb Clin Neurol. 2014;119:541–9.

39. Deasy J. Acquired lumbar spinal stenosis. JAAPA. 2015;28(4):19–23.

40. Becker JA, Stumbo JR, et al. Prim Care Clin Office Pract. 2013;40:271–88.

41. Qaseem A, Wilt TJ, McLean RM, Forciea MA, Clinical Guidelines Committee of the American College of Physicians. Noninvasive treatments for acute, subacute, and chronic low back pain: a clinical practice guideline from the American College of Physician. Ann Intern Med. 2017;166(7):514–30.

42. Pfirrmann CW, Metzdorf A, Zanetti M, Hodler J, Boos N. Magnetic resonance classification of lumbar intervertebral disc degeneration. Spine (Phila Pa 1976). 2001;26(17):1873–8.

43. Joaquim AF, Appenzeller S. Cervical spine involvement in rheumatoid arthritis--a systematic review. Autoimmun Rev. 2014;13(12):1195–202.

44. Clark CR, Goetz DD, Menezes AH. Arthrodesis of the cervical spine in rheumatoid patients. J Bone Joint Surg Am. 1989;71:381–92.

45. Riew KD, Hilibrand AS, Palumbo MA, Sethi N, Bohlman HH. Diagnosing basilar invagination in the rheumatoid patient. J Bone Joint Surg Am. 2001;83(2):194–200.

46. Ranawat CS, O'Leary P, Pellicci P, Tsairis P, Marchisello P, Dorr L. Cervical spine fusion in rheumatoid arthritis. J Bone Joint Surg Am. 1979;61(7):1003–10.

47. Sudoł-Szopinska I, Urbanik A. Diagnostic imaging of sacroiliac joints and the spine in the course of spondyloarthropathies. Pol J Radiol. 2013;78(2):43–9.

48. Bazzocchi A, Aparisi Gómez MP, Guglielmi G. Conventional radiology in spondyloarthritis. Radiol Clin N Am. 2017;55(5):943–66.

49. Baraliakos X, Coates LC, Braun J. The involvement of the spine in psoriatic arthritis. Clin Exp Rheumatol. 2015;33(93):S31–5.

50. Porter GG. Psoriatic arthritis. Plain radiology and other imaging techniques. Baillieres Clin Rheumatol. 1994;8(2):465–82.

51. Márquez Sánchez P. Espondilodiscitis. Radiologia. 2016;58(S1):50–9.

52. Prodi E, Grassi R, Iacobellis F, Cianfoni A. Imaging in spondylodiskitis. Magn Reson Imaging Clin N Am. 2016;24(3):581–600.

53. Genant HK, Wu CY, van Kuijk C, Nevitt MC. Vertebral fracture assessment using a semiquantitative technique. J Bone Miner Res. 1993;8(9):1137–48.

54. Freedman BA, Heller JG. Kummel disease: a not-so-rare complication of osteoporotic vertebral compression fractures. J Am Board Fam Med. 2009;22(1):75–8.

55. Biffar A, Sourbron S, Dietrich O, Duerr HR, Reiser MF, Baur-Melnyk A. Combined diffusion-weighted and dynamic contrast-enhanced imaging of patients with acute osteoporotic vertebral fractures. Eur J Radiol. 2010;76:298–303.

Thoracic Pain: Clinical Features

9

Antonio Cannata', Jessica Artico, Valerio De Paris,
Jacopo Cristallini, Piero Gentile, Paola Naso,
Benedetta Ortis, Enrico Fabris,
and Gianfranco Sinagra

9.1 Definition and Epidemiology of Chest Pain

Thoracic pain, or chest pain, represents one of the most challenging and life-threatening situations in everyday clinical practice. Often referred as a syndrome, chest pain may be the epiphenomenon of a large series of almost any medical condition of the thorax and the abdomen ranging from medical emergencies, such as acute aortic syndromes and myocardial infarction, to non-specific discomforts of benign origin [1, 2].

Though the first description of chest pain has been made by Erasistratus of Chios (around 300 BC), it is William Heberden who medically described chest pain, in 1768: "There is a disorder of the breast marked with strong and peculiar symptoms, considerable for the kind of danger belonging to it, and not extremely rare, which deserves to be mentioned more at length. The seat of it, and sense of strangling, and anxiety with which it is attended, may make it not improperly be called angina pectoris" [3]. However, the first correlation between chest pain and heart appeared in 1809 by Allen Burns, who linked the chest pain with an "insufficient blood supply" [4]. With

time, the dogma chest pain-myocardial ischemia has been broken by several observations of patients with chest pain of non-cardiac origin. Yet in 1950, Rhodes Allison highlighted that "mistakes are frequent and 16% of patients referred to hospitals with a diagnosis of angina are found in fact to be suffering from pain arising in the chest wall only, with no evidence whatsoever of underlying heart disease" [5].

Generally, chest pain is defined as any kind of thoracic pain, from the jaw to the epigastria and/or from the neck to the 12th thoracic vertebra, and may be classified as visceral or somatic. Somatic pain refers to neuromuscular structures, skeletal pain, and dermatological issues, whereas visceral pain includes pain from internal organs such as the heart, stomach, or lungs [1, 6]. Furthermore, chest pain may be referred as cardiac, when caused by cardiovascular-related diseases either of ischemic or nonischemic origin, or non-cardiac, when cardiovascular causes have been ruled out in the emergency department.

Typical presentation of chest pain ranges from a sharp stab in the chest to a dull, oppressive discomfort (Table 9.1). Sometimes it may be described as burning or crushing and in specific cases may radiate to the neck, into the jaws, to the back or throughout the arms. Often, epigastric pain may be also referred as chest pain due to the close proximity of the regions.

The prevalence of chest pain is extremely variable, and it is estimated that in the USA more than five million of people every year present to

A. Cannata' · J. Artico · V. De Paris · J. Cristallini
P. Gentile · P. Naso · B. Ortis · E. Fabris · G. Sinagra (✉)
Cardiovascular and Thoracic Department, Azienda
Sanitaria Universitaria Integrata di Trieste and
University of Trieste, Trieste, Italy
e-mail: Gianfranco.sinagra@asuits.sanita.fvg.it

© Springer Nature Switzerland AG 2019
M. A. Cova, F. Stacul (eds.), *Pain Imaging*, https://doi.org/10.1007/978-3-319-99822-0_9

Table 9.1 Typical and atypical presentation of chest pain

	Typical	Atypical
Site	Left sided	Right sided
Appearance	Exercise induced/at rest	Inducible by pressure/dependent of position, cough respiration/no relation with exercise
Character	Dull/crushing/oppressive/squeezing	Stabbing/sharp/superficial/burning
Radiation	Arms/neck/jaw/back	No radiation
Vegetative signs	Dyspnea/diaphoresis/nausea	No vegetative signs
Relief	Nitrates/rest	Unresponsive

Table 9.2 Etiology of chest pain

	General practitioner	Ambulance	Emergency department
Cardiovascular	20	69	45
Musculoskeletal	43	5	14
Pulmonary	4	4	5
Gastrointestinal	5	3	6
Psychiatric	11	5	8
Other	16	14	22

Modified from Erhardt L, Herlitz J, Bossaert L, et al. Task force on the management of chest pain. Eur Heart J 2002; 23 (15):1153–1176

the emergency department for chest pain. Approximately 25–40% of the entire population experienced once in their lifetime a chest pain [7–9], and it represent 2% of the primary care visits and around 40% of emergency admissions [10]. Life-threatening situations, including acute coronary syndromes, aortic dissection, pulmonary embolism (PE), ruptured aortic aneurysm, and tension pneumothorax, account for approximately 20% of all cases of chest pain, and more than 1,500,000 people undergo annual workup of acute coronary syndrome [11]. Mortality of patients with chest pain remains still high, and more than 2% of people admitted in the emergency department died at 1 year [11]. In children, on the contrary, chest pain represents a rare cause of medical examination, accounting for less than 0.6% of the pediatric emergency visits [12].

Similarly to the wide clinical presentation, the etiology of chest pain varies from benign conditions such as musculoskeletal conditions to life-threatening disease. According to the place where the patient is seen, the probability of those conditions varies as well. Indeed, general practitioner more often visit patients with chest pain of non-cardiac origin, whereas chest pain requiring emergency transportation to the hospital are more frequently caused by cardiovascular disease

rather than other non-emergent conditions. Interestingly, approximately 50% of patients admitted in the emergency department are discharged with non-cardiac chest pain (Table 9.2) [1, 2, 7, 11].

9.2 Initial Evaluation of Patients with Chest Pain

Correct chest pain assessment represents a major achievement in early evaluation of patients. Proper and prompt identification of life-threatening situations is fundamental in patients presenting with chest pain. Either patients' and physicians' factors may delay the prompt recognition of chest pain, such as language, culture, socioeconomic status, complexities of the cases, biases, and queues in the service.

The first approach to patients complaining chest paint should rule out patients with cardiovascular conditions, which require emergent evaluation. A detailed clinical history, documenting the age and sex of the patient, the characteristics of the pain, any associated symptoms, any history of cardiovascular disease, and risk factors, is important to differentiate those patients to that with stable or benign conditions.

Fig. 9.1 Typical
locations of chest pain

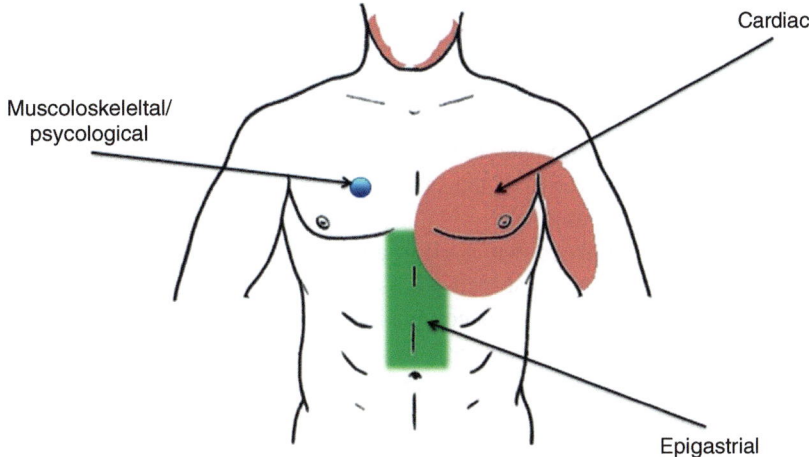

Non-cardiac chest pain usually is sharp, long lasting, not related to effort or exercise, and frequently not associated with other cardiac symptoms or cardiac risk factors, such as hypertension, smoking, and diabetes. Specific location of the discomfort may aid the identification of cardiac or non-cardiac chest pain. Serious intrathoracic or subdiaphragmatic diseases are usually associated with chest pain beginning in the anterior chest, left shoulder or arm, interscapular region, or epigastrium (Fig. 9.1).

9.3 Cardiac Chest Pain

Main symptom of coronary artery disease is typical chest pain or angina. The term angina originates from the Latin verb *angere*, which means to strangle. Commonly, angina refers to chest pain; however, in pediatrics it may refer also to throat pain. Angina pectoris is a dull chest pain, or a discomfort, caused by myocardial ischemia [13, 14]. The causes underlying the oxygen imbalance are extremely wide ranging from coronary atherosclerosis to afterload mismatch, arrhythmias, anemia, and microvascular dysfunction. Typical "stable" angina is the presence of chest pain or discomfort provoked by exertion or emotional stress and relieved by rest or nitroglycerin [13, 14]. Furthermore, cardiac chest pain is radiated to the chest, jaw, neck, shoulders, and usually left arm. Classical Levine's sign, a pounding hand or fist held over the chest, and dull and diffuse pain,

radiated to the left arm or to the jaw and neck, are frequently of cardiac origin [15]. Furthermore, the palm sign, palm of the hand to the chest, and the arm sign, touching the left arm, are classically associated with cardiac chest pain. Often underestimated, patient's gestures may guide the correct diagnosis. Though sometimes unspecific, patient's gestures may underlie the size of chest discomfort. Larger areas, highlighted by the Levine's sign, the palm sign, and the arm sign, are suggestive of ischemic origin of the pain, whereas the pointing sign, pointing the chest with one finger, is suggestive of nonischemic chest pain [16].

Thanks to the effort of the Canadian Cardiovascular Society (CCS), severity of pain may be divided into four different grades, according to its intensity [17]:

Grade I: Ordinary physical activity does not cause angina, such as walking and climbing stairs. Angina with strenuous or rapid or prolonged exertion at work or recreation.

Grade II: Slight limitation of ordinary activity. Walking or climbing stairs rapidly; walking uphill; walking or stair-climbing after meals, in cold, in wind, or under emotional stress; or only during the few hours after awakening. Walking more than two blocks on the level and climbing more than one flight of ordinary stairs at a normal pace and in normal conditions.

Grade III: Marked limitation of ordinary physical activity. Walking one or two blocks on the level and climbing one flight of stairs in normal conditions and at normal pace.

Grade IV: Inability to carry on any physical activity without discomfort, anginal syndrome may be present at rest.

Angina pectoris may also be clinically classified in stable and unstable according to the time of onset, the severity of the symptoms, and the frequency of the angina.

Stable angina, also known as effort angina, is the classical type of chest pain. It is a chest discomfort, frequently accompanied by associated symptoms such as dyspnea or diaphoresis. Usually, stable angina is precipitated by effort, such as running or walking, with fast relief, within 3–5 min, at rest or after the administration of sublingual nitrates [18]. Chest pain recurs often at the same level of effort in the same conditions. Furthermore, precipitant factors, such as heavy meals, anemia, tachycardia, cold weather, and emotional stress, may exacerbate the frequency and the severity of symptoms. However, once removed the precipitant factor, pain characteristics often return to the previous level. Stable angina is caused by stable coronary artery disease and usually requires medical management or percutaneous revascularization according to patient's status and the patient's risk profile [19]. Usually, this form of chest pain is seen and treated by primary care physicians; however, a non-negligible number of admissions in the emergency department are due to stable chest pain [20].

Whenever the onset of the chest pain is recent, ingravescent, or at rest, clinicians are facing unstable angina. *Unstable angina* (UA) is the typical chest pain due to myocardial ischemia at rest or after minimal exertion. While unstable angina requires no myocyte necrosis, whenever a significant release of troponin occurs, this situation is called non-ST elevation myocardial infarction (NSTEMI) [21]. Therefore it appears pivotal to discriminate between UA and NSTEMI, since patients with UA, who do not experience myocyte necrosis and troponin release, are at lower risk of death and require less intensified treatments [22]. Historically, UA has three specific clinical presentations: (1) angina at rest, (2) new onset of severe exertional angina (CCS grade III or more), and (3) intensification of previously stable angina [23]. However, in 2008, the World Health Organization (WHO) revised the clinical spectrum of UA, proposing a new definition. According to the WHO, UA is diagnosed when "there are new or worsening symptoms of ischemia (or changing symptom pattern) and ischemic ECG changes...with normal biomarkers. The distinction between new angina, worsening angina and UA is notoriously difficult and based on a clinical assessment and a careful and full clinical history" [24]. Since the clinical spectrum of UA is tangled together with the one of NSTEMI, a clear distinction is somehow lacking. The only distinctive feature is the absence of biomarker elevation, such as troponin. However, with the advent of more sensitive biomarker essays for myocardial necrosis, the number of patients with UA has been reduced compared to those admitted for NSTEMI [24].

9.4 Causes of Cardiac Chest Pain

Cardiac chest pain may be the epiphenomenon of different conditions involving the heart, the mediastinum, and the great vessels. Ideally, causes of cardiac chest pain may be divided into two distinct categories: ischemic and non-ischemic. While collecting patient's history, the presence of cardiovascular risk factors, the type of pain, and its association may guide the correct identification of the underlying condition [13, 14].

9.4.1 Ischemic Chest Pain

Although several causes may ultimately lead to imbalance between myocardial oxygen demand and supply, the most common cause is the reduced myocardial perfusion due to atherosclerotic coronary artery disease (CAD) [25]. Coronary artery disease appears the most common cause of cardiac chest pain. In this scenario, chest pain is often associated with dyspnea, nausea/vomiting, and diaphoresis. In case of overt myocardial infarction, 78% of patients had diaphoresis besides chest pain, 52% had also nausea, and 47% complained shortness of breath [26]. Classically, patients with CAD have stable or unstable angina according to the severity of the disease; usually they may complain ischemic chest pain in the days/months before hospital admission. Clinical characteristics of chest pain and associated symptoms may increase or lower the likelihood of myocardial infarction. The presence of cardiovascular risk factors, such as smoke, diabetes, dyslipidemia, and hypertension of familial history of CAD, may also help the differential diagnosis of those patients, reducing the time from the first medical contact to the effective treatment. The five main hallmarks of ischemic chest pain (Fig. 9.2) explaining the clinical scenario are (1) thrombotic occlusion of the epicardial coronary artery leading to ST elevation myocardial infarction, (2) nonocclusive thrombosis of a preexistent atherosclerotic plaque, (3) dynamic obstruction, (4) microvascular dysfunction, and (5) nonstenotic imbalance between oxygen demand and supply. All those causes are not mutually exclusive, and sometimes oxygen imbalance due to severe anemia may concur for the worsening of an otherwise stable atherosclerotic plaque.

Besides the stable, abrupt, or progressive atherosclerotic occlusion of a coronary artery, coronary spasm may also concur in the genesis of the cardiac pain. Variant angina can be divided into two distinct subgroups of coronary vasospasm: (1) the Prinzmetal's variant angina, caused by focal spasm of an epicardial coronary artery without underlying coronary atherosclerotic plaque, and (2) the so-called Prinzmetal's angina, when the spasm occurs in the proximity of a nonobstructive atherosclerotic lesion worsening the functional status of the plaque resulting in myocardial oxygen imbalance [23, 27].

Furthermore microvascular dysfunction may play a critical role in the genesis of chest pain. Small coronary vasoconstriction and increased intramural coronary artery resistance, caused by adrenergic stimuli, cold, drugs, and release of vasoactive substances such as thrombin, serotonin, thromboxane A2, and endothelin together with the reduction of relaxing factors on top of a dysfunctional coronary endothelium, are responsible for the myocardial ischemia, regardless of myocyte necrosis, at the basis of ischemic chest pain [28].

Lastly, concurrent afterload mismatch, due to aortic stenosis or hypertrophic cardiomyopathy, or severe anemia may suddenly worsen the frail balance between oxygen demand and supply even in the absence of atherosclerotic lesions.

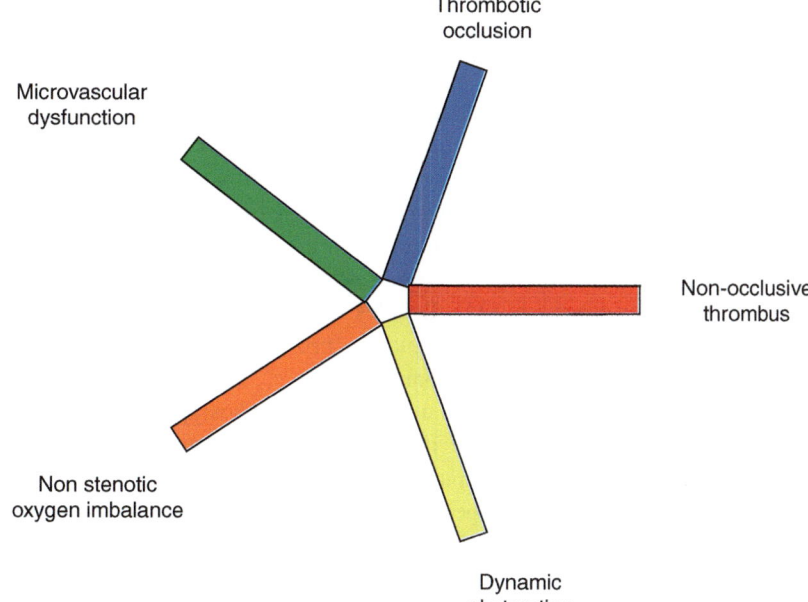

Fig. 9.2 Hallmarks of cardiac chest pain

Those scenarios may cause either unstable or stable angina, depending by the level of effort, the severity of the underlying disease, and the patient's functional status. Typically, the chest pain due to aortic stenosis is exertional and sometimes may be accompanied by signs and symptoms of heart failure and/or exertional syncope due to the afterload mismatch [29]. Hypertrophic cardiomyopathy, on the other side, causes chest pain due to both causes outflow obstruction of the left ventricle and increased diastolic pressures resulting in reduced coronary filling and myocardial oxygen supply [30]. Whenever on top of these conditions occur other causes of augmented myocardial oxygen demand, such as hyperkinetic states or thyrotoxicosis, or reduced myocardial oxygen supply, such as anemia or coronary artery disease, chest pain becomes overt.

9.4.2 Nonischemic Chest Pain

Although ischemic chest pain may be the most common, nonischemic chest pain may require particular attention since several life-threatening situations may be often misdiagnosed.

One of the most common causes of nonischemic chest pain may be myocarditis. Inflammatory myocardial damage, at the basis of myocarditis, may produce typical cardiac chest pain. It is reported that approximately 30–40% of patients with myocarditis are seen in the emergency department because of cardiac chest pain [31]. However, despite sometimes the abrupt presentation of those patients, patients presenting with chest pain and/or supraventricular arrhythmias with preserved left ventricular function typically have an excellent prognosis [32]. Besides myocarditis, pericardial involvement typically produces a chest pain with peculiar characteristics. Inflammation of the pericardium may produce visceral pain similarly to pleural inflammation. Indeed, it may be either a sharp pain or a diffuse chest discomfort. However, in pericarditis, chest pain usually resembles pleuritic pain in most of the cases and sometimes may be disguised for. Usually, it may be episodic, may last for hours,

may worsen with deep breathing, and relieves with antalgic positions, such as lying forward or on the left side. In some cases radiation to the left arm or to the jaw may be common, and a sharp sensation toward the cardiac apex may be complained. However clinical characteristics, biomarker elevation, ECG features, and imaging techniques aid the clinician to safely rule out life-threatening situations.

Disease of the aorta may sometimes require medical attention. Stable conditions such as small aortic aneurysm or arteriovenous may present with atypical chest pain.

Sudden onset of relentless sharp pain, usually tearing in the middle of the sternum/thorax, like a knife on the anterior chest, often radiating to the back between the shoulders and associated with hypertension, connective tissue disorders, aortic insufficiency, and asymmetric peripheral pulse represent the clinical hallmark of aortic dissection, an extremely life-threatening situation with sky-high mortality rate, on average more than 60%, requiring immediate surgical treatment [33]. However, involvement of the coronary artery ostia in small dissections may complicate the scenario. In those cases, ischemic chest pain may be the referring symptom and signs of myocardial ischemia, ultimately with ST-segment elevation, and hinder the correct diagnosis leading to dangerous delays harmful for the patient [34]. Those situations are the most challenging because ischemic chest pain diverges the attention to the real underlying condition, the dissection, and a sharp pain often is hidden by the more severe oppressive chest pain secondary to myocardial ischemia. In this scenario, a correct clinical examination, a good patient's history, and imaging techniques may help the clinicians to rule out the atherosclerotic origin of the chest pain shedding the light to the vascular problem.

Lastly, mitral valve disease may also cause chest pain. Indeed, patients with mitral valve prolapse and severe mitral stenosis may refer to physicians often with atypical chest pain. Mitral valve prolapse represent one of the most challenging situation in cardiac pathophysiology. Apparently benign, several reports highlighted the role of mitral valve abnormalities as the basis for arrhythmias and sudden death [35]. In this light, patients with mitral valve prolapse may also present at the emergency department with atypical chest pain, often of psychological origin, accompanied by anxiety. On the other side, severe mitral stenosis with large left atrium, which invades the mediastinum, may press on vascular structures, bronchi, and nerves leading to atypical chest pain. However, associated symptoms, such as coarse, and the very low incidence nowadays of rheumatic disease bound this condition among the rare situations [13, 14].

9.5 Rule-Out Scores for Cardiac Chest Pain

Clinical decisions may often be extremely challenging. Since the spectrum of causes leading to thoracic pain is wide, ranging from absolutely benign condition to rapidly evolving life-threatening scenarios, rapid rule-in and rule-out protocols should be adopted to reduce the risk of misdiagnosed life-threatening situations and to aid prompt discharge for patients with chest pain from benign conditions [13].

For this purpose, several algorithms have been proposed, and most of the hospitals adopt its own strategy for the best treatment.

In the last years two distinct scores have been widely used to identify patients at higher risk for coronary syndromes requiring urgent hospitalization from those with non-cardiac chest pain. This kind of diagnosis may be relatively easy in the case of overt ST elevation whereas extremely challenging in overlap situations or in non-ST elevation acute coronary syndromes [13, 14].

The first score proposed has been the HEART score [36]. It categorizes patients using five different items composing the acronym of HEART: history, ECG, age, risk factors, and troponin, scored with 0, 1, or 2 points with a maximum score of 10 points (Tables 9.3 and 9.4). This risk score has been retrospectively validated in more than 2400 patients in different centers underlining how the HEART score may be extremely useful because it provides a quick and reliable predictor of outcome in patients admitted

for thoracic pain. Low HEART scores (0–3) are associated with less than 2% of short-term major adverse cardiac events (MACE), whereas in patients with intermediate HEART scores (values 4–6) and in patients with high HEART scores (values 7–10), MACE was diagnosed in 16.6% and in 50.1%, respectively, suggesting that patients with high HEART scores should undergo more aggressive strategies [37].

The second, less utilized risk score has been proposed in 2012. The North American Chest Pain Rule has been designed to identify patients with symptoms suggestive of acute coronary syndromes from those with non-cardiac chest pain to speed up the discharge process without other cardiac testing [38].

Table 9.3 Chest pain scores

HEART score		
History	Highly suspicious	2
	Moderately suspicious	1
	Slightly suspicious	0
ECG	Significant ST depression	2
	Non-specific abnormality	1
	Normal	0
Age	>65 years	2
	Between 45 and 65 years	1
	<45 years	0
Risk factors	>3 risk factors	2
	1–2 risk factors	1
	None	0
Troponin	>3 times upper limit	2
	1–3 times upper limit	1
	Normal	0
	Total	
	Low risk	0–3
	Intermediate risk	4–6
	High risk	7–10

Table 9.4 North American chest pain rule

High-risk criteria	Yes/no
Typical symptoms of ischemia	
Acute ischemic changes (ECG)	
Age > 50 years	
Known coronary artery disease	
Troponin >99th percentile	
Low risk	All no
Intermediate/high risk	Any yes

However, while the HEART score has nearly 100% sensitivity and approximately 25% specificity, the North American Chest Pain Rule has less than 6% specificity, severely limiting its feasibility in everyday clinical practice [39]. Furthermore, the HEART score outperformed the previously validated and widely diffused GRACE and TIMI scores in discriminating between high-risk and lower-risk patients and those with and without MACE in patients admitted for thoracic pain. Therefore the HEART score appears to safely identify the largest group of low-risk patients, ameliorating the rule-in/rule-out process [40].

More recently, a prospective observational study validated a novel predefined 2-h accelerated protocol in patients admitted to the emergency department with thoracic pain to the ED, the ASPECT study [41].

9.6   Non-cardiac Chest Pain

Whether the most severe and life-threatening situation is cardiac chest pain, non-cardiac chest pain is the most common referral symptom to the emergency department. Frequently, non-cardiac chest pains are seen by different specialists, such as cardiologist, pneumologist, rheumatologist, and gastroenterologists, drowning time and resources.

Potential risk factors for non-cardiac chest pain include younger age, family history for noncardiac chest pain, gastrointestinal conditions, heartburn, dysphagia, acid regurgitation, anxiety or depression, alcohol consumption, pregnancy, specific food, or beverages (i.e., coffee, lemon juice, chocolate, mint, carbonated beverages). Patients complaining chest pain should be investigated for those risk factors in order to tailor treatment and to avoid excessive management.

In the last years, several approaches have been proposed to evaluate the chest pain. So far, one of the most useful tools appears to be the BLADE approach [42]. To evaluate and validate this approach, 160 patients with thoracic pain have been followed for 2 years after the first presentation by a team of physicians, nurse, and medical students. The BLADE approach joins together six examination steps (E) with four initial assessment of the patient (background, location, association, duration).

9.6.1   Background

Initial assessment requires investigation of common risk factors for cardiac disease. Patients with visceral disease, such as reflux disease, pleuritic pain, fibromyalgia, chronic pain, or osteochondral pain, are more likely to have recurrences of their original pain rather than cardiac chest pain.

9.6.2   Location

The chest is divided in four quadrants using the midsternal lines. The likelihood of cardiac chest pain is reduced in the right quadrants whereas elevated in the inferior left quadrant.

9.6.3   Association

Chest pain secondary to direct trauma, infections, anxiety/depression, unusual physical activity, and association with particular sleeping positions or movements or activity are more likely to be of non-cardiac origin. Reproducibility by palpation safely excludes chest pain of cardiac origin.

9.6.4   Duration

Very short duration of pain or extremely longlasting pain without any other sign of cardiac ischemia or aortic syndromes is very likely to be non-cardiac.

The BLADE approach is useful to identify patients with non-cardiac chest pain.

Indeed, when applied in a hospital setting, correct use of the BLADE approach help to identify more than 80% of patients with noncardiac chest pain. In the remaining 20%, however, further examinations are required for safe discharge. In those patients, reassurance is the most useful management once the source of pain can be easily identified. Moreover, further investigations are often unnecessary in those with a benign specific diagnosis.

9.6.5 Non-cardiac Chest Pain May Have Different Origin

9.6.5.1 Respiratory

Respiratory chest pain is quite common. It is estimated that approximately 10% of all admissions to emergency departments were secondary to respiratory chest pain [43]. Respiratory chest pain is mainly due to noxae affecting pleura (mainly parietal), the chest wall, and the other mediastinal structures, since the lung parenchyma and the visceral pleura are often nonsensitive to painful stimuli. Pleuritic pain or chest wall pain is frequently worsened by deep inspiration, coughing, and movement of the trunk, and their intensity widely varies ranging from nearly asymptomatic to severely painful scenarios. Though dramatic, sometimes the intensity of the pain does not correlate with the underlying disease and its severity. Sudden onset of the pain, usually after cough or isometric effort, may suggest a pneumothorax or a rib fracture, whereas pleuritic pain, either benign or malign, might be subtle.

Causes of respiratory chest pain are the following.

Pleural Disease

Pleuritis or malignant involvement of the pleura may onset with thoracic chest pain. Dyspnea and chest pain are frequently the presenting symptoms of cancers of the pleura or the chest wall [44]. Malignant chest pain is usually an asymmetric dull ache, and it is caused by malignant pleural or chest wall infiltration. The Pancoast tumor of the lung apex may present with localized shoulder and chest pain; however patient with thoracic cancer and chest pain often have other presenting symptoms (dyspnea, cough, hemoptysis, and weight loss) suggesting the diagnosis. On the other hand, pleuritic pain associated with signs and symptoms of infection (fever and inflammatory markers) and a pleural effusion are highly suggestive of inflammation pleuritic/pleural infection [45].

Pneumothorax

A pneumothorax may be spontaneous, after trauma or surgery, or iatrogenic. Spontaneous pneumothorax may occur either in otherwise well subjects (primary) or in those with underlying lung disease (secondary) such as chronic obstructive pulmonary disease (COPD). A sudden, localized pleuritic chest pain, highly susceptible to breathing variation and often originating from intense coughing, is highly suggestive of spontaneous pneumothorax [46]. In some cases, free air is found within the mediastinum, a rare condition called pneumomediastinum. Usually it is not preceded by trauma or surgical procedures and is sometimes a benign condition, in which conservative management is particularly useful [47].

Pulmonary Embolism

Sudden onset of chest pain, dyspnea, and syncope may be suggestive of pulmonary embolism (PE). Patients with PE may experience either a pleuritic chest pain, secondary to irritation of the parietal pleura after the infarction of the underlying lung segment affected by the embolus and the following inflammation of the visceral pleura, or a central dull pain secondary to the distension of the mechanoreceptors in the pulmonary artery in case of massive PE [48].

Pneumonia

Localized and often sharp thoracic pain associated with fever, productive cough, and signs of infection such as leukocytosis is suggestive of pneumonia. Approximately 50% of the patients with pneumonia are admitted with chest pain arising from the irritation of the parietal pleura secondary to the infection of the lung [49]. Chest pain is, however, uncommon in bronchiectasis and cystic fibrosis due to the lack of pleural involvement and in patients with viral pneumonia, such as H1N1 infection [50].

Other Causes of Respiratory Chest Pain

Other rare causes of thoracic chest pain secondary to respiratory tract involvement are due to connective tissue disease, pulmonary arterial hypertension, epidemic myalgia (Bornholm disease), asbestosis, sarcoidosis, tracheobronchitis, and iatrogenic causes, such as thoracentesis, pericardiocentesis, or other procedures involving the pleura [45].

9.6.5.2 Gastrointestinal

Thoracic pain, usually a burning epigastrial pain, may sometimes originate from the esophagus. Potentially, gastroesophageal reflux disease (GERD), hiatal hernia, esophageal motility disorders, and esophageal hypersensitivity may cause chest pain [51].

GERS is the most common cause of gastrointestinal (GI) cause of chest pain, and approximately 40–60% of patients with non-cardiac chest pain have GERD disease [52]. However still unknown is the mechanism why GERD may cause either heartburn or chest pain. Erosive esophagitis is present in approximately 50–70% of patients with GERD and thoracic pain, and more than 50% of patients have abnormal acid exposure to the esophagus [53].

Non-GERD causes of thoracic pain secondary to esophageal disease vary from diffuse esophageal spasm, nutcracker esophagus, achalasia, and hypertensive lower esophageal sphincter [51]. Central and peripheral hypersensitivity, esophageal abnormalities, and sustained contractions of the esophageal longitudinal muscle may be the cause of motion abnormalities causative of esophageal functional chest pain [54].

Symptom relief following antiacids or proton pump inhibitors is suggestive of GI chest pain.

9.6.5.3 Other Causes of Chest Pain

Chest pain may be secondary to several other conditions ranging from neuromuscular disease to psychological status and anxiety.

Neuromuscular disorders, such as neuritis/nevritis, radiculitis, chest pain wall syndrome, and herpes zoster, are commonly associated with chest pain. Neuromuscular chest pain is usually exacerbated by trunk movement, breathing, and pressure on specific points. Usually, neuromuscular disorders cause long-lasting pain (hours or days), rarely relieved by nitrates and unrelated to the effort, whereas anti-inflammatory drugs may relieve symptoms [42]. Tietze syndrome, a rare inflammatory disorder, may also cause chest pain, which usually is gradual and may affect one or both arms and shoulders. Tietze syndrome is easily recognized by the association of chest pain and swelling of the cartilage of the chondrosternal joints [55].

Chest pain is common in patients with or without cardiac disease who are admitted in the emergency department with psychological pain. Previous experience of cardiac disease may exacerbate the awareness of chest pain even of non-cardiac origin. Psychological assessment and treatment are fundamental in those patients and may improve quality of life reducing inappropriate admissions to the hospital for benign conditions [56].

9.7   Physical Examination

The physical examination of patients admitted for thoracic pain is fundamental to guide the following therapeutic choices. Physical examination is pivotal in assessing patients with chest pain since correct observation of associated signs may provide direct or indirect evidence for cardiac involvement and life-threatening situations. Identifying all the contributing factors for increased myocardial oxygen demand or reduced oxygen supply, such as hypertension, anemia, thyrotoxicosis, cardiomyopathies, and heart failure, is crucial to drive the proper diagnosis. Furthermore, correct physical examination helps to rule out cardiac causes of chest pain; to identify the other non-cardiac emergencies, such as aortic dissection or open pneumothorax; and to provide a general assessment of the patient's status [14].

Patients admitted with cardiac chest pain or with life-threatening situation usually may appear anxious, uncomfortable, or diaphoretic. Sometimes cyanosis or pallor may be also present. Besides the cardiogenic shock, which requires emergent treatment, hypotension and tachycardia may also be present. Fever may aid the diagnosis of inflammatory causes rather than ischemic causes; however the presence of low-grade fever does not exclude the presence of myocardial infarction [13].

In patients with chest pain, jugular venous pressure is usually normal, except for those with underlying heart failure. Third or fourth heart sound may also be present together with systolic murmurs (mitral regurgitation or aortic stenosis) and, sometimes, harsh murmurs of ventricular septal defects, and complication of acute myocardial infarction. In patients with pleuritic or pericardial pain and fever, pericardial rubs may be present as well.

Acute limb ischemia, asymmetric pulses, pallor of the limbs, should immediately warn for possible aortic dissection.

Lastly, abdominal and musculoskeletal examination may reveal other causes of chest pain. Localized swelling, redness, or tenderness of the joints may be suggestive of costochondritis. Pain on palpation of the chest may reveal trauma or other mucoloskeletal causes of thoracic pain rather than myocardial ischemia [13, 14].

However, since clinical examination may be normal in most of the patients with thoracic pain, negative physical examination do not per se exclude life-threatening situations.

References

1. Knockaert DC, Buntinx F, Stoens N, Bruyninckx R, Delooz H. Chest pain in the emergency department: the broad spectrum of causes. Eur J Emerg Med. 2002;9(1):25–30.
2. Erhardt L, Herlitz J, Bossaert L, et al. Task force on the management of chest pain. Eur Heart J. 2002;23(15):1153–76.
3. Heberden W. Some account of a disorder of the breast. Med Trans Coll Physician London. 1772;2:59–67.
4. Burns A. Observations on some of the most frequent and important diseases of the heart: aneurism of the thoracic aorta; on preternatural pulsation in the epigastric region; and on the unusual origin and distribution of some of the large arteries of the human body. Edinburgh: T. Bryce; 1809.
5. Allison DR. Pain in the chest wall simulating heart disease. Br Med J. 1950;1(4649):332–6.
6. Stochkendahl MJ, Christensen HW. Chest pain in focal musculoskeletal disorders. Med Clin North Am. 2010;94(2):259–73.
7. Eslick GD, Fass R. Noncardiac chest pain: evaluation and treatment. Gastroenterol Clin N Am. 2003;32(2):531–52.
8. Geyser M, Smith S. Chest pain prevalence, causes, and disposition in the emergency department of a regional hospital in Pretoria. Afr J Prim Health Care Fam Med. 2016;8(1):e1–5.
9. Wong WM, Lam KF, Cheng C, et al. Population based study of noncardiac chest pain in southern Chinese: prevalence, psychosocial factors and health care utilization. World J Gastroenterol. 2004;10(5):707–12.
10. Goodacre S, Cross E, Arnold J, Angelini K, Capewell S, Nicholl J. The health care burden of acute chest pain. Heart. 2005;91(2):229–30.
11. Ruigomez A, Rodriguez LA, Wallander MA, Johansson S, Jones R. Chest pain in general practice: incidence, comorbidity and mortality. Fam Pract. 2006;23(2):167–74.
12. Thull-Freedman J. Evaluation of chest pain in the pediatric patient. Med Clin North Am. 2010;94(2):327–47.
13. Mann DL, Zipes DP, Libby P, Bonow R. Braunwald's heart disease: a textbook of cardiovascular medicine. Philadelphia: Elsevier/Saunders; 2015.
14. Kasper D, Fauci A, Hauser S, Longo D, Jameson J. Harrison's principles of internal medicine. 19th ed. New York: McGraw-Hill Education; 2015.
15. Edmondstone WM. Cardiac chest pain: does body language help the diagnosis? BMJ. 1995;311 (7021):1660–1.
16. Marcus GM, Cohen J, Varosy PD, et al. The utility of gestures in patients with chest discomfort. Am J Med. 2007;120(1):83–9.
17. Campeau L. Letter: grading of angina pectoris. Circulation. 1976;54(3):522–3.
18. Ohman EM. Clinical practice. Chronic stable angina. N Engl J Med. 2016;374(12):1167–76.
19. Task Force M, Montalescot G, Sechtem U, et al. 2013 ESC guidelines on the management of stable coronary artery disease: the Task Force on the management of stable coronary artery disease of the European Society of Cardiology. Eur Heart J. 2013;34(38):2949–3003.
20. Beltrame JF, Weekes AJ, Morgan C, Tavella R, Spertus JA. The prevalence of weekly angina among patients with chronic stable angina in primary care practices: The Coronary Artery Disease in General Practice (CADENCE) Study. Arch Intern Med. 2009;169(16):1491–9.
21. Thygesen K, Alpert JS, Jaffe AS, et al. Third universal definition of myocardial infarction. Circulation. 2012;126(16):2020–35.
22. Mueller C. Biomarkers and acute coronary syndromes: an update. Eur Heart J. 2014;35(9):552–6.
23. Braunwald E, Morrow DA. Unstable angina: is it time for a requiem? Circulation. 2013;127(24):2452–7.
24. Mendis S, Thygesen K, Kuulasmaa K, et al. World Health Organization definition of myocardial infarction: 2008-09 revision. Int J Epidemiol. 2011;40(1):139–46.
25. Theroux P, Fuster V. Acute coronary syndromes: unstable angina and non-Q-wave myocardial infarction. Circulation. 1998;97(12):1195–206.
26. Horne R, James D, Petrie K, Weinman J, Vincent R. Patients' interpretation of symptoms as a cause of delay in reaching hospital during acute myocardial infarction. Heart. 2000;83(4):388–93.
27. Braunwald E. Unstable angina: an etiologic approach to management. Circulation. 1998;98(21):2219–22.

28. Diver DJ, Bier JD, Ferreira PE, et al. Clinical and arteriographic characterization of patients with unstable angina without critical coronary arterial narrowing (from the TIMI-IIIA Trial). Am J Cardiol. 1994;74(6):531–7.

29. Vandeplas A, Willems JL, Piessens J, De Geest H. Frequency of angina pectoris and coronary artery disease in severe isolated valvular aortic stenosis. Am J Cardiol. 1988;62(1):117–20.

30. Marian AJ, Braunwald E. Hypertrophic cardiomyopathy: genetics, pathogenesis, clinical manifestations, diagnosis, and therapy. Circ Res. 2017;121(7):749–70.

31. Anzini M, Merlo M, Sabbadini G, et al. Long-term evolution and prognostic stratification of biopsy-proven active myocarditis. Circulation. 2013;128(22): 2384–94.

32. Sinagra G, Anzini M, Pereira NL, et al. Myocarditis in clinical practice. Mayo Clin Proc. 2016;91(9): 1256–66.

33. Criado FJ. Aortic dissection: a 250-year perspective. Tex Heart Inst J. 2011;38(6):694–700.

34. Fruergaard P, Launbjerg J, Hesse B, et al. The diagnoses of patients admitted with acute chest pain but without myocardial infarction. Eur Heart J. 1996;17(7):1028–34.

35. Lancellotti P, Garbi M. Malignant mitral valve prolapse: substrates to ventricular remodeling and arrhythmias. Circ Cardiovasc Imaging. 2016;9(8):e005248.

36. Six AJ, Backus BE, Kelder JC. Chest pain in the emergency room: value of the HEART score. Neth Heart J. 2008;16(6):191–6.

37. Backus BE, Six AJ, Kelder JC, et al. A prospective validation of the HEART score for chest pain patients at the emergency department. Int J Cardiol. 2013;168(3):2153–8.

38. Hess EP, Brison RJ, Perry JJ, et al. Development of a clinical prediction rule for 30-day cardiac events in emergency department patients with chest pain and possible acute coronary syndrome. Ann Emerg Med. 2012;59(2):115–125 e111.

39. Mahler SA, Miller CD, Hollander JE, et al. Identifying patients for early discharge: performance of decision rules among patients with acute chest pain. Int J Cardiol. 2013;168(2):795–802.

40. Poldervaart JM, Langedijk M, Backus BE, et al. Comparison of the GRACE, HEART and TIMI score to predict major adverse cardiac events in chest pain patients at the emergency department. Int J Cardiol. 2017;227:656–61.

41. Than M, Cullen L, Reid CM, et al. A 2-h diagnostic protocol to assess patients with chest pain symptoms in the Asia-Pacific region (ASPECT): a prospective observational validation study. Lancet. 2011;377(9771):1077–84.

42. Lanham DA, Taylor AN, Chessell SJ, Lanham JG. Non-cardiac chest pain: a clinical assessment tool. Br J Hosp Med (Lond). 2015;76(5):296–300.

43. Pitts SR, Niska RW, Xu J, Burt CW. National Hospital Ambulatory Medical Care Survey: 2006 emergency department summary. Natl Health Stat Report. 2008;7:1–38.

44. Opitz I. Management of malignant pleural mesothelioma-The European experience. J Thorac Dis. 2014;6(Suppl 2):S238–52.

45. Brims FJ, Davies HE, Lee YC. Respiratory chest pain: diagnosis and treatment. Med Clin North Am. 2010;94(2):217–32.

46. Kalomenidis I, Moschos C, Kollintza A, et al. Pneumothorax-associated pleural eosinophilia is tumour necrosis factor-alpha-dependent and attenuated by steroids. Respirology. 2008;13(1):73–8.

47. Iyer VN, Joshi AY, Ryu JH. Spontaneous pneumomediastinum: analysis of 62 consecutive adult patients. Mayo Clin Proc. 2009;84(5):417–21.

48. Rubin LJ. Pathology and pathophysiology of primary pulmonary hypertension. Am J Cardiol. 1995;75(3):51A–4A.

49. Fine MJ, Stone RA, Singer DE, et al. Processes and outcomes of care for patients with community-acquired pneumonia: results from the Pneumonia Patient Outcomes Research Team (PORT) cohort study. Arch Intern Med. 1999;159(9):970–80.

50. Perez-Padilla R, de la Rosa-Zamboni D, Ponce de Leon S, et al. Pneumonia and respiratory failure from swine-origin influenza A (H1N1) in Mexico. N Engl J Med. 2009;361(7):680–9.

51. Schey R, Villarreal A, Fass R. Noncardiac chest pain: current treatment. Gastroenterol Hepatol (N Y). 2007;3(4):255–62.

52. Liuzzo JP, Ambrose JA. Chest pain from gastroesophageal reflux disease in patients with coronary artery disease. Cardiol Rev. 2005;13(4):167–73.

53. Fass R, Naliboff B, Higa L, et al. Differential effect of long-term esophageal acid exposure on mechanosensitivity and chemosensitivity in humans. Gastroenterology. 1998;115(6):1363–73.

54. Hobson AR, Furlong PL, Sarkar S, et al. Neurophysiologic assessment of esophageal sensory processing in noncardiac chest pain. Gastroenterology. 2006;130(1):80–8.

55. Ayloo A, Cvengros T, Marella S. Evaluation and treatment of musculoskeletal chest pain. Prim Care. 2013;40(4):863–887, viii.

56. White KS. Assessment and treatment of psychological causes of chest pain. Med Clin North Am. 2010;94(2):291–318.

Imaging of Vascular Thoracic Pain

10

Manuel Belgrano and Matilda Muça

10.1 Introduction

Chest pain is the most common cause of first aid access in the emergency room and causes high mortality if not treated properly (2–4%) [1, 2]. About 15% to 25% of patients presenting for the evaluation of acute chest pain in emergency departments (EDs) have acute myocardial infarction (MI) or unstable angina [3]. Therefore, in a typical population of patients, a systematic and well-coded approach is necessary. In this chapter we will primarily consider cardiogenic causes of chest pain and partly non-cardiogenic causes.

A high accuracy and efficiency of the evaluation of patients with acute chest pain are necessary, including better blood markers for myocardial injury [4], early exercise testing [5], radionuclide scanning for lower-risk patients [6] and multi-slice computed tomography (MSCT), essential tools for the anatomic evaluation of coronary artery disease, exclusion of pulmonary

embolism, and aortic dissection. Conti et al. demonstrated that chest pain was secondary to acute coronary syndrome (ACS) in almost 45% of cases, pulmonary embolism in 4%, and spontaneous pneumothorax in 3%, and only in 1% of cases, it depends on aortic dissection or acute pericarditis. Among the life-threatening pathologies, ACS is the most common cause of chest pain [3, 7, 8].

10.2 Acute Coronary Syndrome

Acute coronary syndromes (ACS) have different presentations, including unstable angina pectoris, non-ST-elevation myocardial infarction (NSTEMI), and ST-elevation myocardial infarction (STEMI) [9, 10].

Any pain located anteriorly between the root of the nose and navel and posteriorly between the neck and the XII backbone vertebrae which has no traumatic origin is considered of cardiac origin. In patients with ACS chest pain and sometimes dyspnea and fatigue may be the only presenting symptoms [7, 11]. Age >75 years, female gender, nonwhite patients, a previous stroke or congestive heart failure, and diabetes mellitus are conditions more frequently associated with the presentation without chest pain [7, 12, 13].

The known cardiovascular risk factors are familiarity for an ischemic event (father <55 years, mother <50 years), diabetes mellitus, arterial

Electronic Supplementary Material The online version of this chapter (https://doi.org/10.1007/978-3-319-99822-0_10) contains supplementary material, which is available to authorized users.

M. Belgrano (✉) · M. Muça
SC (UCO) Radiologia Diagnostica e Interventistica, Dipartimento di Scienze Mediche, Chirurgiche e della Salute - Università degli Studi di Trieste, Azienda Sanitaria Universitaria Integrata di Trieste (ASUITS), Trieste, Italy
e-mail: mbelgrano@units.it

© Springer Nature Switzerland AG 2019
M. A. Cova, F. Stacul (eds.), *Pain Imaging*, https://doi.org/10.1007/978-3-319-99822-0_10

hypertension, smoke, and hypercholesterolemia. However, it is not clear how much these factors increase the probability of a cardiac event. Among the cardiac causes of chest pain, ischemic heart disease remains the most frequent cause and often that with fatal or debilitating consequences [14].

Of course in case of a suspected ACS with ST-elevation myocardial infarction (STEMI) or in non-ST-elevation myocardial infarction (NSTEMI) with an intermediate-high Global Registry of Acute Coronary Events (GRACE) score, an early angiography is highly recommended [15].

A 12-lead ECG must be performed in triage and evaluated within 10 min from the patient arrival in ED. The persistent ST-segment elevation is the most sensitive (>90%) and specific (>90%) marker of transmural myocardial ischemia therefore of ACS with acute myocardial infarction (STEMI) even if this aspect is present only in 30–40% of cases of myocardial infarction [1, 7]. With a sensitivity lower than 50%, the ST-segment depression (NSTEMI) indicates non-transmural myocardial ischemia [14, 16].

10.2.1 Imaging Techniques

There are several different imaging techniques to approach a patient with ACS, many of which are mainly of pertinence of cardiologist and will be briefly described in this chapter that is mainly focused on CT and MR.

10.2.1.1 Echocardiography
Despite the echocardiogram sensitivity for identification of myocardial infarction is high (93%), the specificity is limited to patients with a history of previous myocardial infarction [7, 17]. Echocardiography can highlight/exclude segmental kinetic abnormalities of the left ventricle in patients with chest pain, and its execution is indicated during and/or immediately after the chest pain episode, since alterations in segmental kinetics may persist sufficiently long after the symptom resolution due to the myocardial stunning [7, 18]. This method potentially allows dif-

ferential diagnosis with other potentially lethal cardiovascular pathologies (aortic dissection, pulmonary embolism, aortic stenosis, pericardial infarction) and is indicated in patients with persisting pain at the time of observation and with nondiagnostic 12-lead ECG and those with hemodynamic or arrhythmic instability [7].

10.2.1.2 Stress Ultrasound
The stress ultrasound (stress-US) is a useful tool for recognizing coronary artery disease in patients with a recent episode of acute chest pain. The most physiological stress-US is the physical effort followed by the use of pharmacologic agents such as dobutamine (the most used), dipyridamole, or adenosine. In cases where the patient is unable to perform adequate physical exercise, a pharmacological eco-stress is used. When both cycloergometer and the treadmill are used for the eco-stress, the echocardiographic survey is performed at baseline and immediately after reaching the stress peak. The average sensitivity is about 88% for the recognition of angiographic documented coronary artery disease (stenosis >50% in at least one of the major coronary branches) with a specificity of 83% when performed by experienced personnel, which is similar to that of myocardial scintigraphy [7, 19].

The execution of stress-US is crucial in patients with acute chest pain where the pretest probability of coronary artery disease is intermediate with normal/nondiagnostic 12-lead ECG and negative biomarkers or when 12-lead ECG is not interpretable (e.g., bundle branch block) or when it is impossible to perform an ergometric test [7, 20].

10.2.1.3 Myocardial Scintigraphy
Thallium-201 and technetium-99m sestamibi or tetrofosmin are excellent tracers of myocardial perfusion, whose uptake is proportional to the regional blood flow and depends on the vitality of myocardial tissue. Considering its easier availability and the lack of redistribution, technetium-99m sestamibi is the more favorable to obtain the best image quality, particularly in emergency situations, so the images always document the myocardial flow at the time of the radiotracer

infusion, even if they are reviewed minutes/hours from the injection. Scintigraphy is an excellent diagnostic method for recognizing the presence of coronary artery disease in patients with an intermediate stage of pretest probability of disease [7, 21, 22]. Underwood et al. documented an average sensitivity of scintigraphy equal to 87% and a specificity of 73% for the recognition of angiographically documented coronary artery disease [23]. Considering the clinical utility of scintigraphy in terms of diagnosis, prognosis, and cost-effectiveness, we understand why it has recently received a Class I indication for the evaluation of acute chest pain [22].

Despite this it is poorly usable and therefore of little practical application [7].

10.2.1.4 Chest Radiography

Chest radiograph is performed in about one quarter of patients accessing in the ED, and often significant findings may be present, including cardiomegaly, pneumonitis, and pulmonary edema. Nevertheless, the chest X-ray utility has never been evaluated in patients previously defined with low probability of cardiac origin chest pain due to anamnesis and objective examination [7].

10.2.1.5 Calcium Score

Calcium score (Ca-Score) is a CT scan performed with cardiac synchronization without administration of contrast medium, to identify calcific coronary plaques; a specific software calculates a score based on the volume of calcium measured in the different vessels.

If we look to the atherosclerotic plaque evolution, the presence of calcium is the final stage of the evolution of the coronary plaque, which implies a relative stability with low opportunity of plaque rupture and sudden coronary occlusion and ACS [24]. Therefore Ca-Score appears to be a bad predictor of further cardiovascular events, because it is missing the more unstable soft plaques, but it is a good indicator of the global plaque burden and is a powerful tool to stratify the patient based on his other cardiovascular risk factors. A negative coronary calcium scan alone is generally not sufficient to rule out ACS in patients with chest pain, but the absence of calcium in low-risk acute chest pain indicates a low probability of ACS and good overall prognosis [25, 26].

10.2.1.6 CT Coronary Angiography

Computed tomography (CT) is the most accurate noninvasive test for the diagnosis of coronary artery disease [27]. The greatest clinical value of cardiac CT (CCT) may be its ability to reliably rule out obstructive coronary artery disease in patients with atypical presentation and thus with a low-to-intermediate pretest probability of disease [28, 29]. Coronary CTA is more sensitive (98–100%) than any other noninvasive technique for the coronary pathology identification [30, 31] and is recommended in patients with a low-to-intermediate probability of CAD, or after an inconclusive functional test, because of its high-negative predictive value (99–100%) [32].

In those patients, the use of coronary CTA in the early phase is safe and demonstrated a high effectiveness with shortened total length of stay in hospital with consequent cost reduction and more cost-effective care in the triage [33].

In case of absence of any coronary plaque, other cardiac reasons for the acute chest pain can be excluded and, if the patient does not have any other relevant comorbidities (e.g., pneumothorax), can be safely discharged from the ED [33] and will remain virtually event-free [25, 34].

CCT also presents a high accuracy (96% sensitivity and 99% specificity) in the evaluation of coronary bypass, avoiding invasive procedures like coronary angiography [35, 36] with a consequent reduction of the volume of contrast medium and radiation dose [37].

The main technical limit of CT is related to the low temporal resolution of the method, with poor image quality in patients with high heart rate or cardiac arrhythmias (e.g., atrial fibrillation) [38]. The last generation of multi-slice CT (MSCT) allows minimizing or eliminating the impact of such limits.

A meta-analysis that included 18 studies that compared 64-slice coronary computed tomography angiography (CTA) with invasive angiography showed that CTA has obtained a good diagnostic

Table 10.1 SCCT guidelines on the use of coronary computed tomographic angiography for patients presenting with acute chest pain to the emergency department

Risk category	Level 1	Level 2	Level 3	Level 4	Level 5
Suspected diagnosis	Low risk (TIMI score 0)	Intermediate risk (TIMI score 2–4)	High risk (TIMI >4)	NSTEMI UAP	STEMI
Appropriate diagnostic strategy	Coronary CTA or functional assessment	Coronary CTA or functional assessment	Functional assessment and/or admission	ICA	ICA

CTA CT angiography, *ICA* invasive coronary angiography, *NSTEMI* non-ST segment elevation myocardial infarction, *STEMI* ST-elevation myocardial infarction, *TIMI* thrombolysis in myocardial infarction risk score, *UAP* unstable angina pectoris

accuracy for detecting significant stenosis with a mean sensitivity of 99% and specificity of 89% [39]. The presence of calcifications can overestimate stenosis severity, and this explains the lower reported specificity (≈85%) which anyway is not inferior to other noninvasive techniques.

Coronary CTA potentially allows to visualize and characterize coronary atherosclerotic plaque, both in obstructive and nonobstructive lesions, and to classify plaque composition as calcified or noncalcified. Furthermore CT can detect characteristics associated with plaque instability, such as low attenuation (<30 HU), high total plaque burden, spotty calcifications, and outward vessel remodeling, and can assess the functional relevance of coronary artery disease (CAD) on CT [40].

However, the MSCT provides only anatomical data on the presence of coronary artery disease, but does not provide information about the functional relevance of stenosis [41]. Goldstein et al. [42] compared the diagnostic strategy based on MSCT with the classic clinical practice. MSCT demonstrated not only to be safe in diagnosing SCA without "missing" any patient, with a consequent reduction of the need to perform coronary angiography (2 vs 7%), but also that it is faster in the diagnosis (3.4 h vs 15 h to establish the definitive diagnosis). However, MSCT has limitations in determining the physiological significance of intermediate grade coronary pathology and in cases of inadequate image quality has brought in a wide use (~25% of MSCT cases) of perfusional scintigraphy.

CT-STAT [42], ACRIN [43], and ROMICAT II [44] trials, in which more than 3000 patients were included, have established CCT as a viable alternative to functional testing for triage of low-risk patients with acute chest pain. In fact, follow-up analysis from these three trials demonstrated that no patient was discharged with a missed diagnosis of ACS, based on the CT results, and this supports the conclusion that coronary CTA-guided management at the ED is safe.

Considering guidelines, the 2014 SCCT guidelines are substantially in line with what has been described in Table 10.1, indicating the execution of the coronary CTA in patients considered at low-intermediate risk for coronary origin of the chest pain, whereas the CTA is not indicated in high-risk patients [45].

Although doses have decreased substantially over the past decade, risks due to radiation exposure are still associated with CTA [30].

In clinical practice patient-specific scan protocols should be used, especially in patients susceptible of harm from X-ray exposure to the chest such as women and younger patients. Considering and selecting carefully the setting parameters, a significant amount of radiation could be spared for many patients without compromising image quality [46].

Nowadays doses <5 mSv are common practice using state-of-the-art technology. However, increasingly personalized exams for each individual patient and very recent innovations permit doses <1 mSv in selected patients [30, 47].

The patient's cardiac frequency may limit the image quality especially on slow scanners [38] and must be lowered as much as possible with beta-blockers, and if arrhythmia is present it should be pharmacologically controlled (by cardiologist or trained radiologist).

In absence of contraindications, sublingual administration of nitroglycerine, increasing the coronary diameter, improves significantly the exam and is strongly recommended.

To reduce the radiation dose and to increase the vascular attenuation, low-tube voltage (80–100 kV) may be used but only in low body mass index patients.

According to literature [48] a high iodine concentration contrast medium should be used and administered with a high flow (5–6 ml/s); low concentration contrast medium may be used especially in low kV acquisitions.

Cardiac CTA may be a valuable tool to rule out CAD in patients with minor high-sensitive-troponin elevations, and early triage by coronary CTA can be a viable and potentially more accurate alternative to functional testing in low-risk patients with acute chest pain. Of course, coronary CTA requires advanced equipment, expertise in data acquisition and image interpretation, and most importantly an appropriate patient selection. If we put together the CT capabilities to determine the morphological plaque characteristics and the assessment of the functional severity of CAD, we can confirm that CCT could add diagnostic value to examinations in the ED [30].

10.2.1.7   Magnetic Resonance

7–10% of patients presenting with STEMI and 10–15% of patients presenting with NSTEMI have unobstructed coronary artery disease (CAD) on urgent angiography. Cardiac magnetic resonance (CMR) has a potentially important diagnostic role, in these cases, especially in distinguishing ischemic from nonischemic causes of ACS with unobstructed coronary arteries. Different studies have shown that the mortality rate or reinfarction is not negligible following ACS with unobstructed CAD. The clinical presentation in up to 95% of cases of acute chest pain, elevated troponin, and unobstructed coronary arteries can be explained by an underlying acute myocarditis, acute myocardial infarction (MI), and cardiomyopathy, in particular Takotsubo cardiomyopathy (TCM), and all these conditions can be accurately diagnosed with an appropriate CMR study. The added diagnostic value of CMR is in its high temporal and con-trast resolution, noninvasive myocardial tissue characterization, and the 3D image acquisition [15]. There are some fundamental sequences including long- and short-axis cine, T2-weighted, and late gadolinium enhancement (LGE) imaging that can, respectively, assess some important elements, such as the presence of regional wall motion abnormalities and ventricular volume calculation, presence, and extent of myocardial edema/inflammation and myocardial scar/fibrosis. The most commonly used sequence to image edema in clinical practice is T2-weighted short-tau inversion recovery (T2-STIR).

A large part of patients presenting with suspected ACS and unobstructed coronary arteries have an underlying etiology of myocarditis. The prevalence of myocarditis is variable and ranges from 15 to 75% [15, 49–55].

In patients with a suspicion of underlying **myocarditis,** three CMR sequences have diagnostic role:

(1) LGE sequences for detection of myocardial necrosis and/or fibrosis
(2) T2-weighted images for assessment of myocardial edema
(3) T1-weighted sequences before and after contrast injection for detection of myocardial hyperemia

If two of three sequences of CMR demonstrate myocardial edema, hyperemia, and fibrosis—late enhancement—the CMR findings are consistent with the diagnosis of myocarditis. The gold standard for the diagnosis of myocarditis continues to be the endomyocardial biopsy (EMB). Nevertheless, CMR allows to obtain fundamental elements for the diagnosis of myocarditis, and moreover it is a noninvasive technique. It is known that CMR is superior to echocardiography for the identification of ventricular thrombi, especially in conditions where small and apical thrombi are present. As demonstrated in autopsy studies of young adults, myocarditis is responsible for 5–20% of sudden deaths [15, 56].

CMR can also provide further valuable prognostic information during follow-up, including myocardial wall motion, global function, perfusion, and viability which can be decisional to start or not secondary atherosclerotic prevention treatment. The noninvasive myocardial tissue characterization of CMR is important not only for its diagnostic role but even for the risk stratification [15]. CMR has an important role to detect other complications of MI including ventricular aneurysm, pseudoaneurysm, papillary muscle infarction associated with mitral regurgitation [15].

Cardiomyopathy is the third common cause of suspected ACS with unobstructed coronary arteries. If a characteristic mid-apical myocardial edema with corresponding regional wall motion abnormalities and apical ballooning, but with no or only subtle LGE, is identified at CMR, a **TCM** can be diagnosed. According to literature, TCM is the most frequent and occurs in 10–15% of this patient group [15, 49–55]. Typically TCM is characterized by mid-cavity to apical regional wall motion abnormalities (apical ballooning) with sparing of the left ventricular basal segments. Although TCM is usually considered to be a benign reversible condition, its arrhythmic risk is to be feared, and for that it requires a correct and prompt identification [15].

10.2.2 Imaging Findings

The Ca-Score exam, generally performed just before the CT coronary angiography, gives information on the presence of calcific plaques and, in case of values over 400 AU, may be considered as a contraindication to the execution of subsequent angiographic scan (Fig. 10.1).

As a result of CT coronary angiography, we may have several levels of pathology:

- The most common finding is a negative exam without evidence of coronary artery plaques with all the coronary free of disease and with good visibility of either distal branches (Fig. 10.2) or presence of atherosclerotic plaques without significant stenosis (Fig. 10.3); in those cases, it is possible to exclude the cardiac origin of chest pain.
- CT may show a severe atherosclerosis associated with significant coronary stenosis

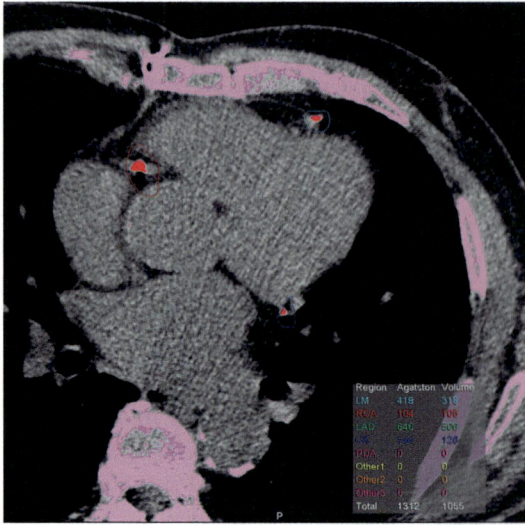

Fig. 10.1 Elderly male patient with chest pain and elevated Ca-Score. A score higher than 400 AU reduces significantly the accuracy of CT coronary angiography with an overestimation of the pathology due to the high calcium burden

(Fig. 10.4) that usually directs the patient to cardiology department for further investigation and monitoring.
- In some cases an intermediate lesion is possible (Fig. 10.5), with a borderline stenosis that does not permit to rule out the presence of pathology; in this case additional functional tests are needed.

In rare cases the coronary stenosis may originate from an aortic dissection extended to the coronary arteries (Fig. 10.6); this condition is extremely dangerous, especially if involving the left main trunk, because an acute fatal coronary occlusion may occur.

The CT may also highlight a bypass stenosis or occlusion, causing chest pain and heart failure (Figs. 10.7, 10.8, 10.9); this information is important for the interventional cardiologist in the cath lab that can focus the procedure only on the occluded graft.

A subendocardial hypodensity (Fig. 10.10) is indicative of past ischemic events and is generally associated to CAD [57, 58]. Both chronic myocardial scar and acute hypoperfusion show lower contrast enhancement on CTA, while chronic

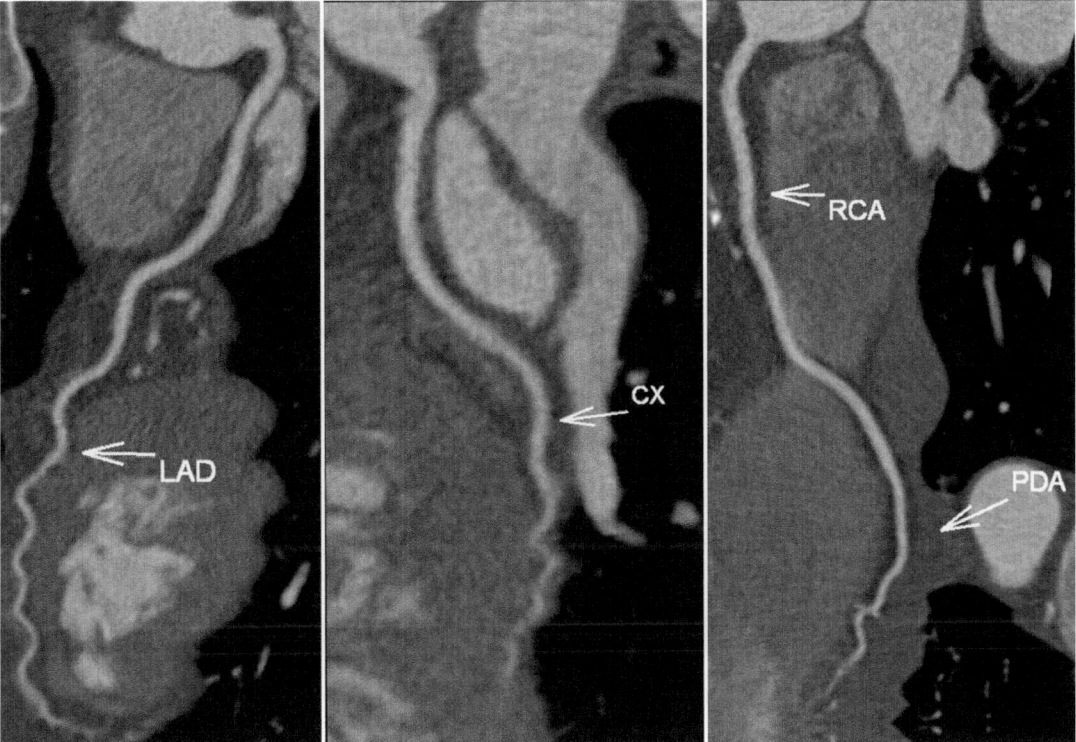

Fig. 10.2 Young female with suspected Takotsubo syndrome; the low-dose coronary CT angiography (80 kV; 0.8 mSv) shows fully patent and disease-free coronaries

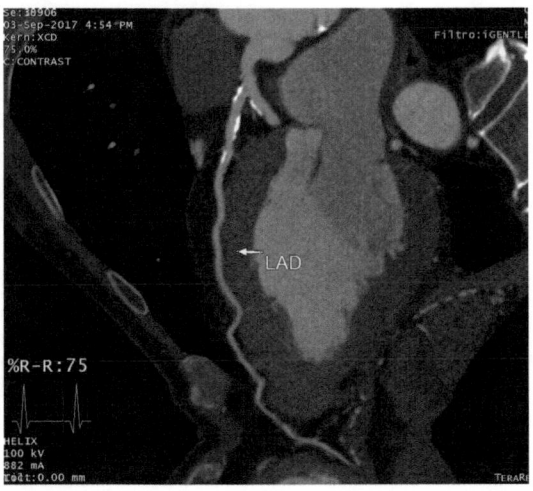

Fig. 10.3 Mid-age patient with chest pain; CT coronary angiography shows noncritical stenosis due to calcific plaques

infarction can often be associated with wall thinning or lower attenuation values (<0 HU) as a result of fat tissue within the scar [59].

In cardiac MR, the identification of a subendocardial or transmural LGE pattern (Fig. 10.11) can be diagnostic for **myocardial infarction (MI)**. Acute MI with unobstructed coronary artery is a common clinical presentation and is the second most common etiology in patients presenting with chest pain (5–29%) [15, 49–55]. The rupture or erosion of a vulnerable plaque (causing transitory occlusion that resolves spontaneously) and distal vessels or small-caliber side branches disease could be the pathological mechanisms to explain this phenomenon. Other mechanisms including coronary dissections, coronary vasospasm, distal embolization, or inflammation can rarely cause a MI with unobstructed coronary artery.

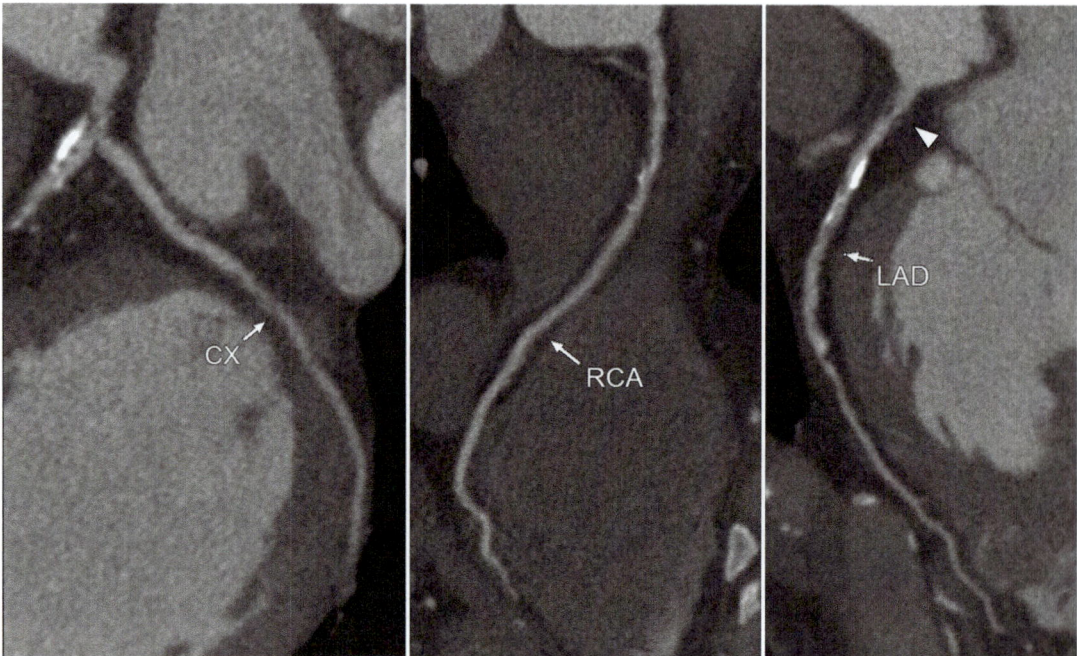

Fig. 10.4 Young male with mild chest pain and nonconclusive stress echocardiography; CT coronary angiography showed critical three vessel disease (arrowhead), confirmed by coronary angiography; the patient underwent coronary bypass

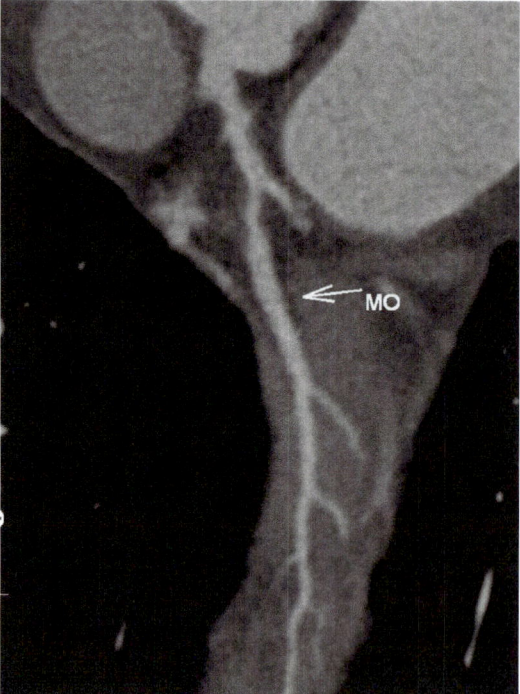

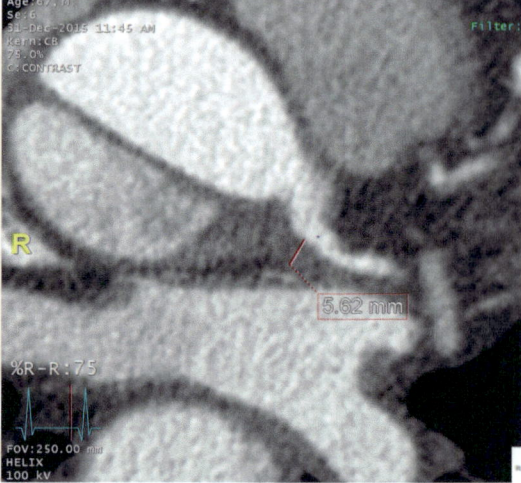

Fig. 10.6 ECG-triggered scan of the aortic root shows a dissection that involves the origin of the left main coronary artery that presents a significant stenosis

Fig. 10.5 This CT coronary angiography shows a borderline stenosis that does not allow excluding the cardiac origin of the chest pain; further functional tests are needed

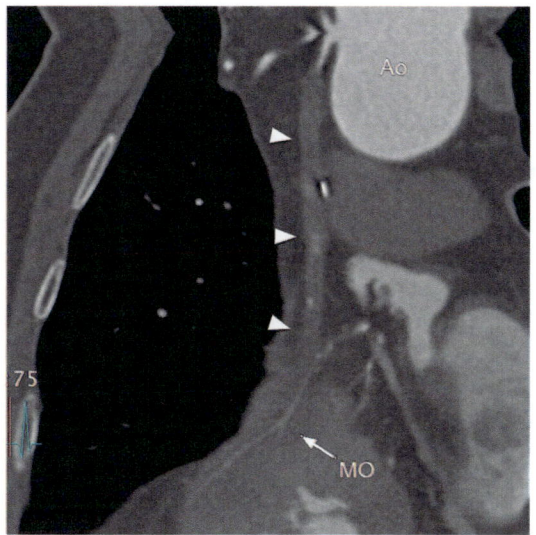

Fig. 10.7 Occluded saphena venous graft coronary bypass (arrowheads) in patient with chest pain and heart failure

10.3   Acute Aortic Syndrome (AAS)

Acute aortic syndrome assembles a set of aortic diseases which have in common the acute, irreversible change of aortic wall such as dissection, intramural hematoma, penetrating ulcer, non-dissecting aneurysm, and traumatic or non-traumatic rupture. Acute aortic syndrome is characterized by high mortality and morbidity, and early recognition of these conditions is crucial to ensure prompt treatment [60, 61].

10.3.1 Imaging Techniques

10.3.1.1   Chest Radiography
The study of Yskert et al. describes the diagnostic accuracy of chest radiography (CXR) among patients with suspected acute aortic syndrome. In

Fig. 10.8 MPR reconstruction of a diseased saphena venous graft coronary bypass with two stents that present a kinking (arrowhead) due to their rigidity that limits the blood flow in the graft

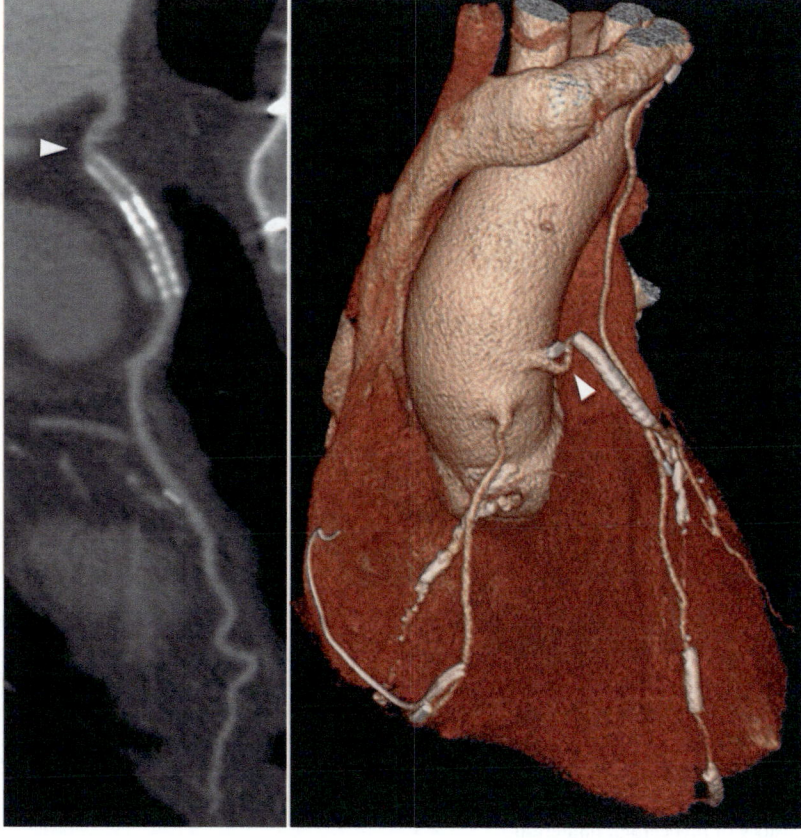

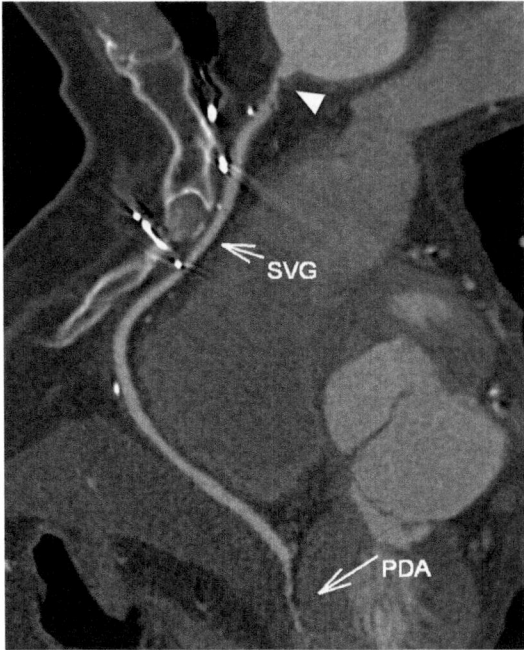

Fig. 10.9 Proximal significant stenosis of saphena venous graft (arrowhead) coronary bypass in patient with chest pain

this study CXR had a sensitivity of 64% and a specificity of 86% for the identification of aortic disease, with a lower sensitivity for aortic disease confined to the proximal aorta compared to the distal aortic segments. The description of kinking or tortuosity of the thoracic aorta, displacement of intimal calcifications, and a widened aortic contour were associated with a high-positive likelihood ratio for the detection of aortic disease. Both single (anteroposterior or posteroanterior) and double (with lateral) views of the initial chest radiograph had similar sensitivity (58% for single views vs 67% for double views) and specificity (89% for single views vs 85% for double views) for the diagnosis of aortic disease. There were no differences in the diagnostic accuracy between aortic dissection, non-dissecting aneurysm, intramural hemorrhage, and penetrating ulcer. Of course, due to the intrinsical proprieties of the investigation, chest radiography cannot distinguish different causes of the acute aortic syndrome, and furthermore a negative result does not rule out acute aortic disease. For this reason,

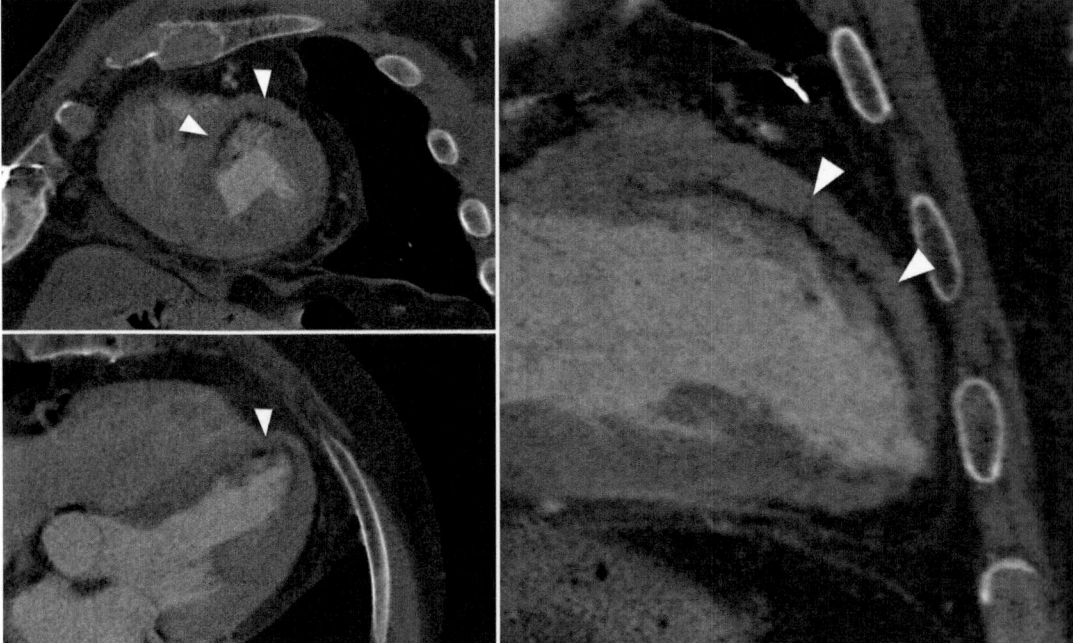

Fig. 10.10 Subendocardial hypodensity (arrowheads) of left ventricle due to perfusion defect in patient with previous history of myocardial infarction

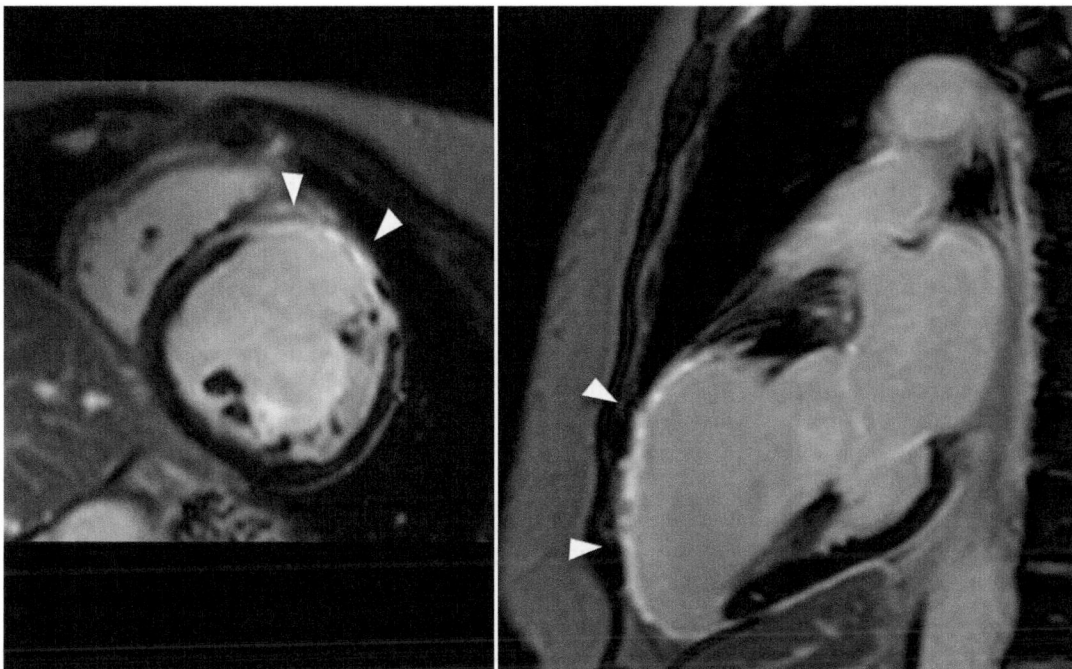

Fig. 10.11 Transmural and subendocardial late enhancement (arrowheads) in patient with acute myocardial infarction

it requires diagnostic confirmation in all patients with suspected acute aortic syndrome and should be replaced by first-line CT aortic imaging. Since a definitive diagnosis is required in any patient with clinically suspected acute aortic syndrome, routine chest radiography should be replaced by CT aortic imaging [62].

10.3.1.2 CT

In the last decade, the speed, isotropic spatial resolution, accessibility, and constant availability of multi-slice CT have made this technique the gold standard in the evaluation of the acute aorta.

The opportunity to perform cardiac synchronized acquisitions considerably improved the image quality of the ascending aorta, eliminating motion artifacts due to the normal cardiac pulsatility and allowing a precise visualization of the aortic root [63].

Clinical presentation of AAS is typically dramatic, with patients often presenting sweat, hypo- or hypertension, dyspnea, and loss of pulses.

All those symptoms are related to injuries of the aortic wall: site, extension of the intimal tear,

and wall hematoma that strictly correlate with the site and the characteristics of pain that typically modify with the evolution of the lesions.

The aortic evaluation should include the origin of the aortic arch and proximal great vessels and continue to the common femoral arteries. The exam should start with a non-contrast-enhanced scan that allows detection of an acute aortic wall hematoma and is then followed by a contrast-enhanced CT (CTA) for the evaluation of abnormal filling defects of the aorta. In young patients who need repeated CT evaluations, the radiation dose could be a problem [61], but using low-tube voltage techniques, a dramatic reduction in cardiac CT doses has been observed during the years [61, 64]. Almost all exams should be acquired with retrospective electrocardiogram-gated CT that acquires diastolic images of the aorta reducing cardiac motion artifacts. Despite this for most cases, beta-blockers may be necessary to obtain slow and regular heart rates which allow good-quality imaging.

The thoracic aorta is well evaluated with CTA, and the dataset obtained can be easily manipulated in multiple planes for a more accurate assessment of the anatomy and relationship of adjacent structures. Curved multiplanar reconstructions (MPRs) can be performed with almost all recent workstations allowing true perpendicular measurements of the lumen.

10.3.1.3 MRI

MRI is an exam that may complete the information regarding the aorta and generally has a role in examinations performed electively and not in an acute setting. MRI has some limitations like the exclusion of patients who have metallic devices, such as stents or valve prosthesis that cause artifacts that preclude adequate evaluation of the aorta. Sequences can be combined with respiratory and ECG gating to reduce motion artifacts of the aorta. In case of slow flow or static blood within the lumen due to a dissection, "black blood" double inversion recovery spin echo are very useful sequences, and they can also assess the vessel wall, for example, in Takayasu's disease, where a thickened vessel wall can be evaluated, while the so-called "white blood" cine sequences, balanced steady-state free precession, allow appreciation of flow turbulence within the lumen in case of stenosis and planning of phase contrast sequences to determine peak velocity and degrees of regurgitation. Indeed phase contrast sequences can better assess the peak velocity at the stretch of stenosis in the aorta, which can estimate a gradient and calculate the direction of flow and velocity using the changes in phase in flowing blood [61]. Non-contrast MR angiography sequences balanced steady-state free precession (bSSFP), which ensure a three-dimensional (3D) dataset to be produced including motion-free images of the aorta when combined with ECG gating and respiratory navigation [61, 65], is susceptible to flow disturbance and high velocity resulting in artifacts. Contrast-enhanced MR angiography, which provides the use of gadolinium, reduces the artifact from inhomogeneous flow and produces consistently good-quality 3D datasets. Ultrafast gradient echo cine sequences have been surpassed by bSSFP but can be still useful when there are areas of disturbed high-velocity flow of the aorta because they tend to

be less susceptible to flow-related artifacts than bSSFP [61]. MRI has no role in the acute aneurysmal rupture.

10.3.2 Imaging Findings

Aneurysmal disease is the principal thoracic aortic disease and is a challenge in both elective and emergency cases. The decision when and if to operate, established on the surgical risk and hazard of rupture, may be problematic in borderline cases, but in case of thoracic aortic rupture, the mortality is remarkably high (94–100%) [66]. When rupture is imminent, as in acute proximal aortic dissection, the operative mortality and morbidity is about 25% [67].

When acute rupture of an aortic aneurysm occurs, it can be seen as extensive ill-defined heterogeneous periaortic hematoma (Fig. 10.12), a focal new saccular pseudoaneurysm (Fig. 10.13) or active contrast extravasation at the site of rupture can also be present, and if the rupture is involving the aortic root, hemopericardium may be visible (Fig. 10.14).

Aortic dissection is the most common acute aortic pathology, and it provides the presence of an intimal tear which allows blood to interrupt the media and penetrate the aortic wall forming a false lumen with reentry at a variable distance along the

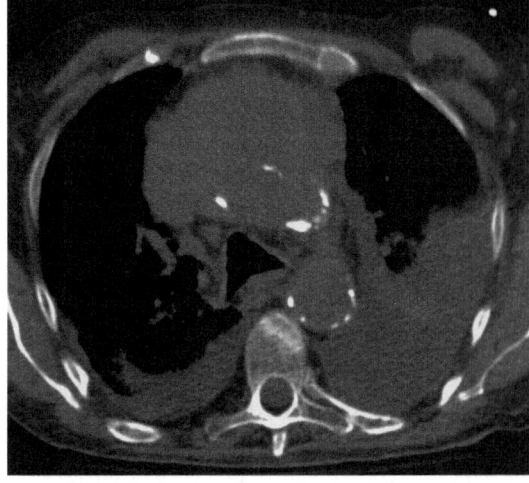

Fig. 10.12 Large mediastinum hematoma in patient with ruptured thoracic aortic aneurysm

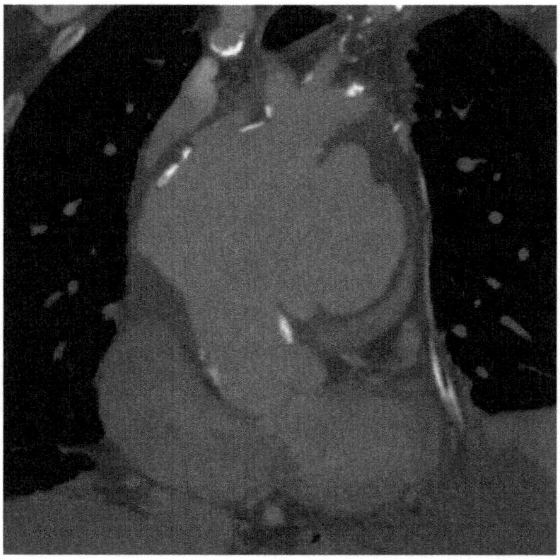

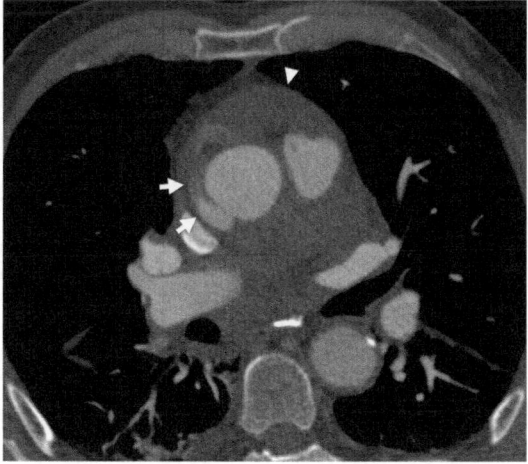

Fig. 10.13 Large pseudoaneurysm in patient with ruptured thoracic aortic aneurysm

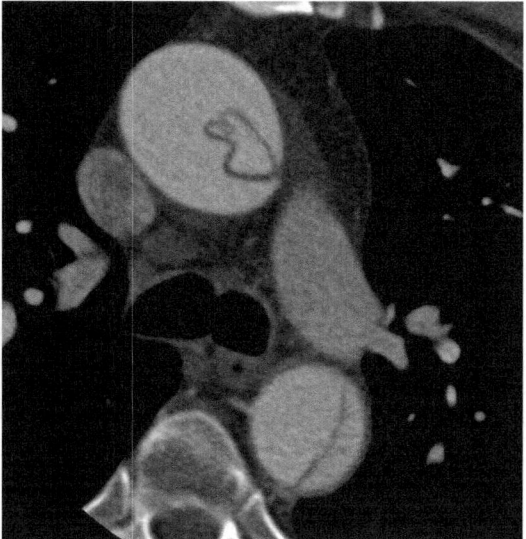

Fig. 10.15 Aortic dissection; ECG-triggered CT angiography shows the typical linear filling defect within the lumen representing the intimal flap

Fig. 10.14 Patient with ruptured ascending aorta aneurysm; active bleeding (arrows) and hemopericardium (arrowhead) are visible

vessel course [61]. For its identification, the CT is the method of choice. The typical appearance on CT is a linear filling defect within the lumen representing the intimal flap (Fig. 10.15; Video 10.1); despite the false lumen is generally identified by the acute angulation between the flap and the wall [61, 68], during the cardiac cycle, the intimal flap is waving, and the angulation may appear as opposite (Fig. 10.16; Video 10.2). The presence of calcifications that are attached to the intimal flap

(Fig. 10.17) and the vasa vasorum attached to the intimal layer (cobweb sign), visible as hypodense stripes (Fig. 10.18), are both useful to identify the false lumen.

The involvement of branches with their occlusion is often responsible for stroke (Fig. 10.19) or chest pain radiating to the neck and jaw which is common in patients with type-A aortic dissection, while abdominal pain is more frequent in type-B aortic dissection [69–71]. Syncope often indicates the development of dangerous complications such as cardiac tamponade, obstruction of cerebral vessels, or activation of cerebral baroreceptors. It is reported in 13% of patients, and it is a negative prognostic factor because 34% of patients with syncope die versus 23% without syncope. Pulmonary edema, neurologic findings due to carotid artery obstruction (hemiplegia, hemianesthesia) or spinal cord ischemia (paraplegia), bowel or myocardial ischemia, hematuria, and compression of adjacent structures (superior vena cava syndrome, hoarseness, dysphagia, and dyspnea due to airways obstruction) represent the most serious manifestations of AAS [11–14]. However, in some cases patients are asymptomatic.

There are two main classification of aortic dissection (Stanford and DeBakey classifications)

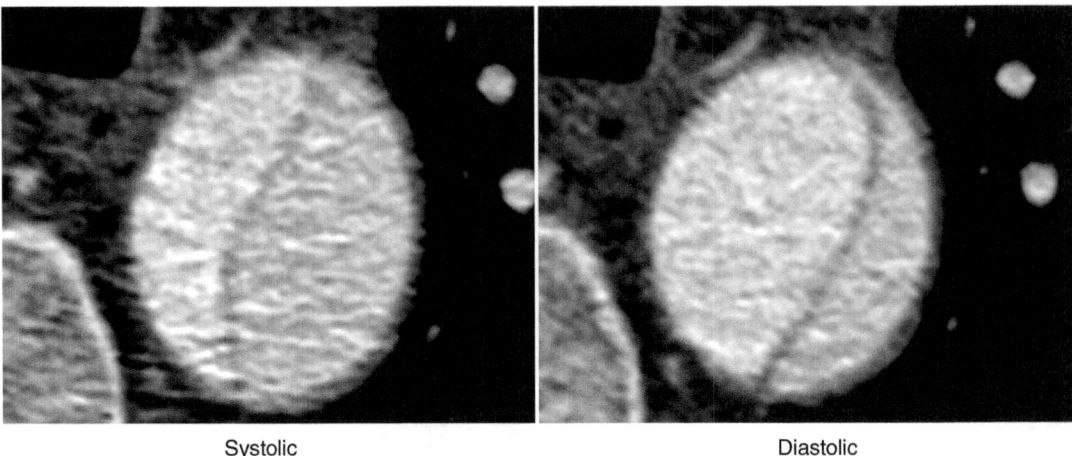

Systolic   Diastolic

Fig. 10.16 ECG-triggered CT angiography of dissected aorta reconstructed in both systolic and diastolic phases shows the intimal flap waving during the cardiac cycle changing its orientation

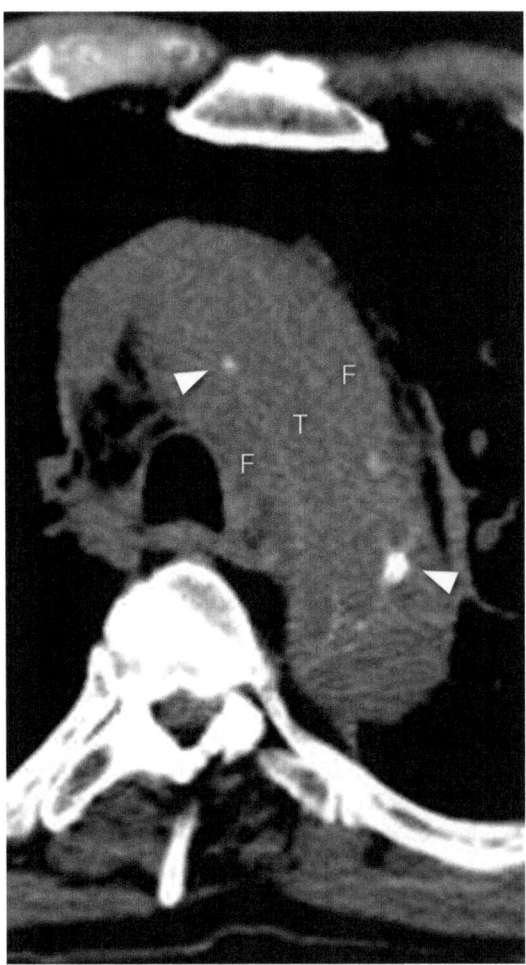

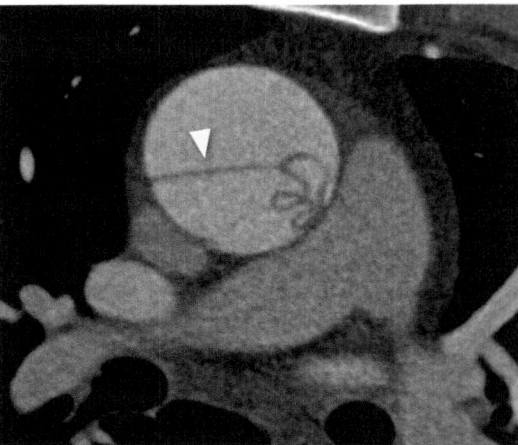

Fig. 10.18 ECG-triggered CT angiography of dissected aorta: the vasa vasorum attached to the intimal layer (cobweb sign) are visible as hypodense stripes (arrowhead)

that are based on the involvement of the ascending and/or descending aorta (Fig. 10.20).

In the dissection of the ascending aorta, it is crucial to exclude the involvement of the coronary artery (Fig. 10.21) and of the aortic valve (Fig. 10.22) that represent a clinical emergency, in this suspect, an ECG-triggered scan in mandatory.

Penetrating atherosclerotic ulcers can potentially evolve in aortic dissection, intramural hematoma, or rupture and are characterized by interruption of an atherosclerotic lesion of the intimal and elastic lamina which leads to a hematoma within the media (Fig. 10.23). Penetrating

Fig. 10.17 Direct CT scan in dissection of thoracic aorta shows calcifications attached to the intimal layer delineating the true lumen (arrowheads)

atherosclerotic ulcers appear on CT as focal protrusions of contrast through atherosclerotic plate into the aortic wall (Fig. 10.24) [61] and most commonly occur in the descending aorta [72].

Intramural hematoma can be spontaneous or underlying imaging features of intimal flap, or penetrating atherosclerotic ulcer can be seen (Fig. 10.25). Rupture of the vasa vasorum [73] or underlying microscopic intimal tears is other potential mechanisms of genesis [61]. On noncontrast CT it appears as a half-moon hyperdense rim in the aortic wall (Fig. 10.26), while no

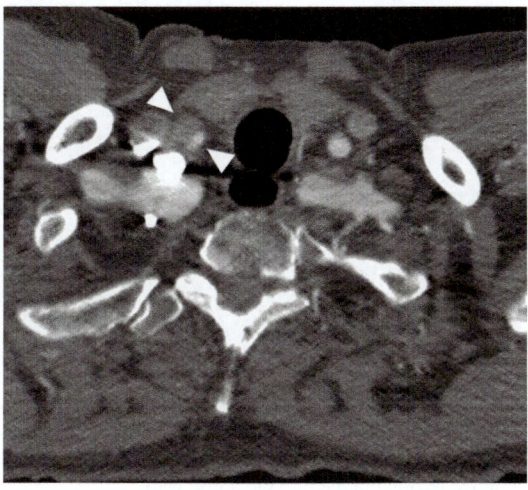

Fig. 10.19 CT angiography of dissected aortic arch shows a dissected common carotid artery (arrowheads) in patient with stroke

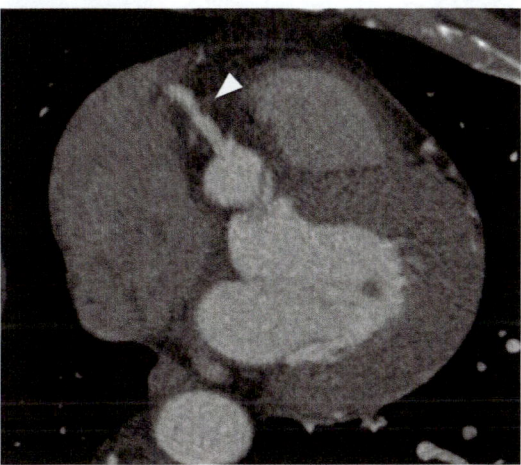

Fig. 10.21 ECG-triggered CT angiography shows right coronary artery irregularities (arrowhead) suggestive for coronary dissection

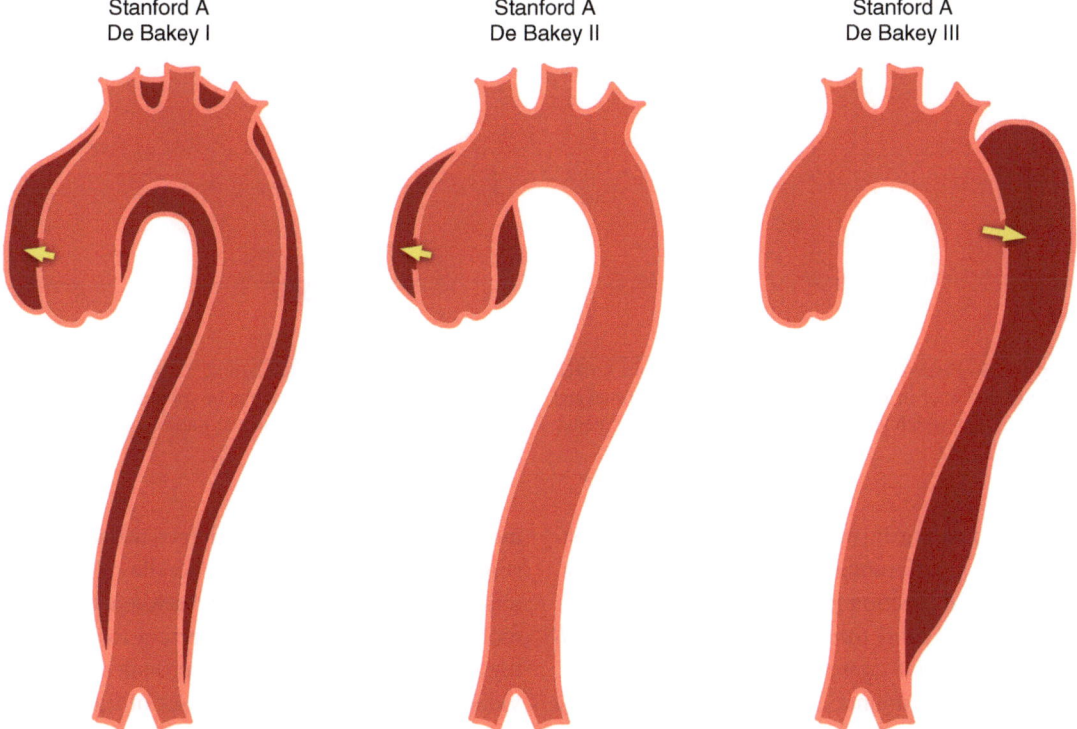

Stanford A
De Bakey I

Stanford A
De Bakey II

Stanford A
De Bakey III

Fig. 10.20 Classification of aortic dissection

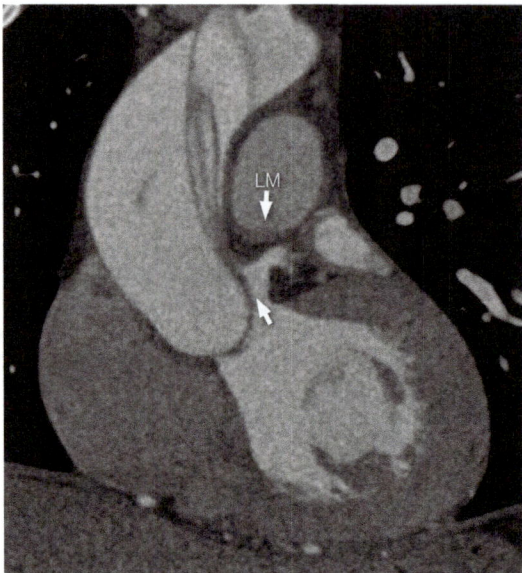

Fig. 10.22 ECG-triggered CT angiography of dissection of aortic arch with involvement of aortic valve (arrow) that is missing below the left main (LM) coronary artery (due to a lesion of left coronary sinus)

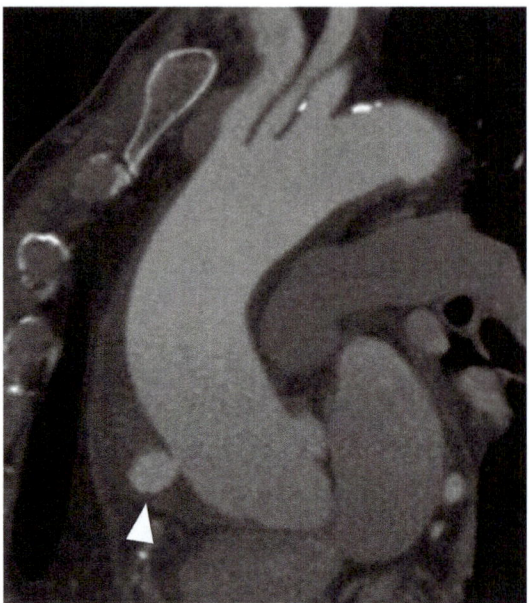

Fig. 10.24 ECG-triggered CT angiography of penetrating atherosclerotic ulcers that appear on CT as focal protrusions of contrast medium (arrowhead) through atherosclerotic plaque into the aortic wall

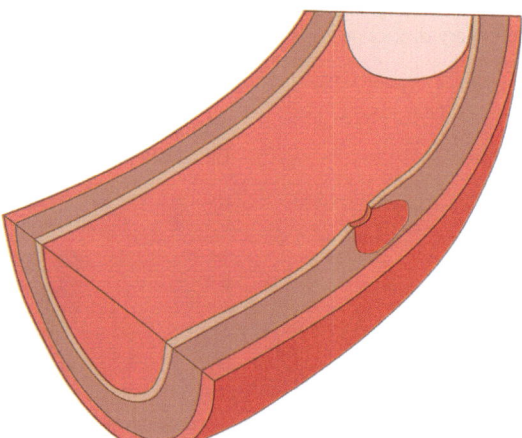

Fig. 10.23 Penetrating atherosclerotic ulcer characterized by interruption of an atherosclerotic lesion of the intimal and elastic lamina which leads to a hematoma within the media

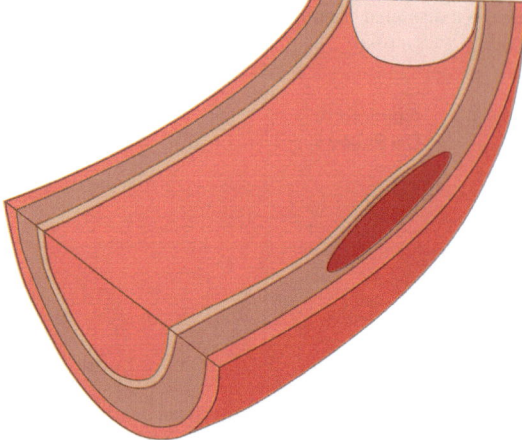

Fig. 10.25 Intramural hematoma is a bleeding in the context of the media layer. It can be spontaneous or underlying imaging features of intimal flap or penetrating atherosclerotic ulcer

contrast flowing in the false lumen on contrast-CT allows differentiation of intramural hematoma from dissection [61].

Partial or total transection of the aortic wall can be a mortal consequence of thoracic aortic injury in blunt trauma. The aortic isthmus is the most frequent site of transection of the aortic wall (Fig. 10.27) [74]. Blanking, bending forces, or torsion stress at the junction between fixed and mobile points of the aorta represent the underlying damage mechanism. CTA provides excellent views of the thoracic aorta in cases of trauma, and

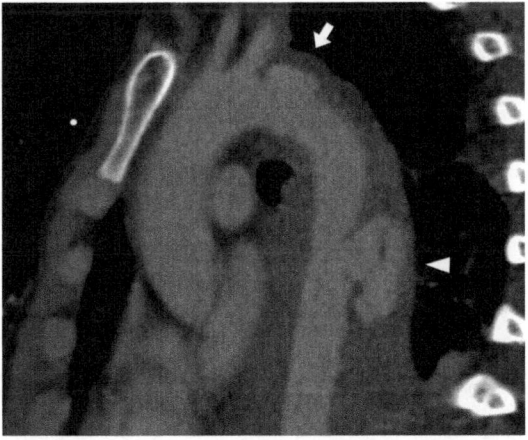

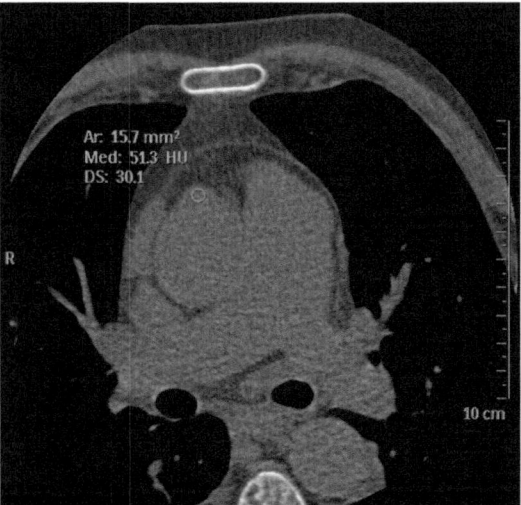

Fig. 10.26 ECG-triggered direct CT scan of an intramural hematoma that appears as a half-moon hyperdense rim in the aortic wall (arrowheads)

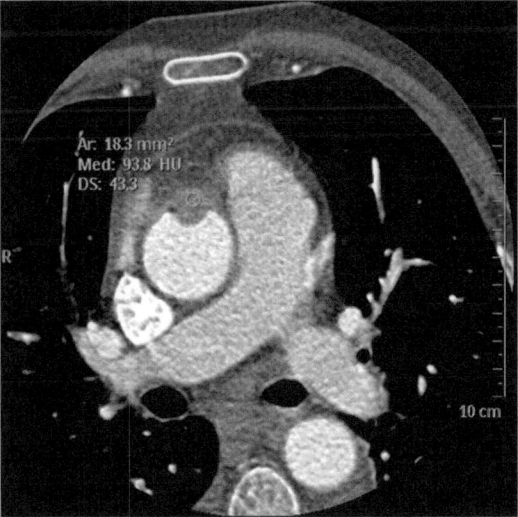

Fig. 10.27 CT angiography of a traumatic partial transection of aortic wall in a young male shows active extravasation at the isthmus (arrow) and at the descending aorta (arrowhead)

Fig. 10.28 ECG-triggered CT image of ascending aorta shows a wall thickening with contrast enhancement and intraluminal thrombus in a septic patient presented with stroke due to a mycotic aortitis

the presence of dissection, intimal flaps, intramural hematoma, pseudoaneurysm or contour irregularities represent direct signs of aortic injury [61].

Vasculitis of the aortic wall may occur in case of multisystem disorder like Takayasu's disease or after systemic infections caused by staphylococcus and streptococcus aureus that lead to a mycotic flogosis of the aorta. They are characterized by wall thickening with contrast enhancement (Fig. 10.28) with possible association of intraluminal thrombo-

sis and may evolve in aneurysm or pseudoaneurysm formation with eventually rupture of the wall [75]. Generally, they are more frequently seen in descending and abdominal aorta [76].

10.4   Acute Pericarditis

Pericarditis is due to a primary inflammation of the pericardium or as a manifestation of a systemic disorder. Chest pain is the most frequent manifestation of acute pericarditis, typically sudden onset, retrosternal, and exacerbated by inspiration pain [77]. Typical electrocardiography alteration is seen in up to 60% [78] of patients and includes widespread upward concave ST-segment elevation and PR-segment depression [77].

10.4.1 Technique and Imaging Findings

10.4.1.1 Chest Radiography
Chest radiography is usually normal in patients with pericarditis. The presence of cardiomegaly may indicate the presence of pericardial effusion, although it is a rare finding [77].

10.4.1.2 Echocardiography
In patients with a suspect of acute pericarditis with hemodynamic instability, a transthoracic echocardiography is recommended [79]. Beyond the presence of pericardial effusion in some cases, there can be a cardiac tamponade which needs an emergent pericardiocentesis [77].

10.4.1.3 CT
CT is very sensitive in the detection of generalized or loculated effusions, and an increased pericardial thickness may be present in a patient with acute pericarditis, nevertheless this last finding is not diagnostic for pericarditis (Fig. 10.29; Video 10.1) [77].

10.4.1.4 MRI
Also MRI is a very sensitive technique in the detection of generalized or loculated effusions, and the delayed enhancement of the pericardium (Fig. 10.30; Video 10.3) is even more sensitive for the detection of pericarditis. Furthermore, MRI allows the evaluation of the myocardium which can be involved in cases of pericarditis becoming a myopericarditis. If after the evaluation of the clinical history, of the objective examination and the serologic test, the diagnosis remains uncertain, an MRI should always be performed [77].

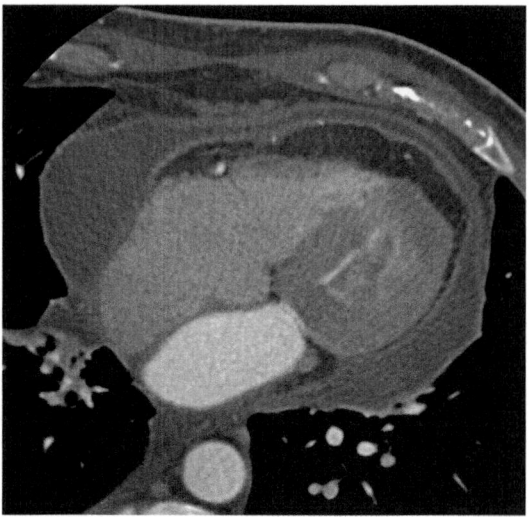

Fig. 10.29 ECG-triggered CT angiography in a patient with acute pericarditis shows pericardial effusions and pericardial thickening

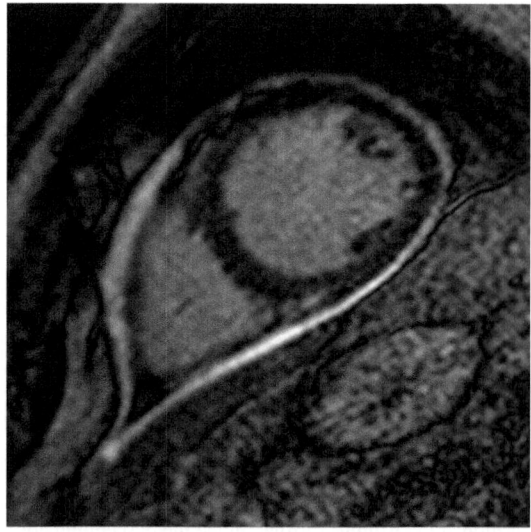

Fig. 10.30 Cardiac MR shows pericardial thickening associated with late enhancement in a patient with pericarditis

10.5 Pulmonary Thromboembolism

Pulmonary thromboembolism (PTE) is a potentially fatal condition caused principally by thrombosis of the lower limbs with a high morbidity and mortality. For these reasons imaging plays a crucial role in the diagnosis of PTE.

10.5.1 Technique and Imaging Findings

10.5.1.1 Chest Radiography
There are different radiographic signs with a relatively high specificity but low sensitivity which may indicate the presence of a pulmonary thromboembolism condition. Westermark sign is an expression of decreased vascularity in the peripheral lung. Fleischner sign consists in an enlargement of the central pulmonary artery, and Hampton sign represents pleura-based areas of increased opacity. Other findings that may be seen in PTE are hemidiaphragm elevation, focal areas of increased density, linear atelectasis, and pleural effusion, but even these findings are non-specific. Radiography has also the role to exclude other diseases that may mimic PTE such as pneumonia and pneumothorax [80].

10.5.1.2 Scintigraphy
Progressively CT has replaced scintigraphy in pulmonary embolism diagnosis, but scintigraphy still has a role in the diagnosis of peripheral embolism. For perfusion scintigraphy technetium-99m-labeled human albumin microsphere or macroaggregated albumin is the radiopharmaceuticals of choice, while xenon-133 is used for ventilation scintigraphy. Ventilation and perfusion scintigraphy may have a high percentage of nondiagnostic intermediate probability scans, and this is the main limitation of this technique, and scan results remain uncertain in up to 73% of cases. Some scintigraphic abnormalities suggestive for diagnosis of PTE, including non-segmental perfusion abnormalities, are perfusion defects smaller than the corresponding regions of increased opacity at radiography, triple-matched defects in the upper or middle lung zone, matched V-P abnormalities in two or three zones of one lung, and one to three small segmental perfusion defects. Anyway these signs have a positive predictive value (PPV) of less than 10% [80].

10.5.1.3 CT Angiography
CT is actually a fast and reliable diagnostic technique for pulmonary embolism showing an intraluminal filling defect (Fig. 10.31). CT allows an

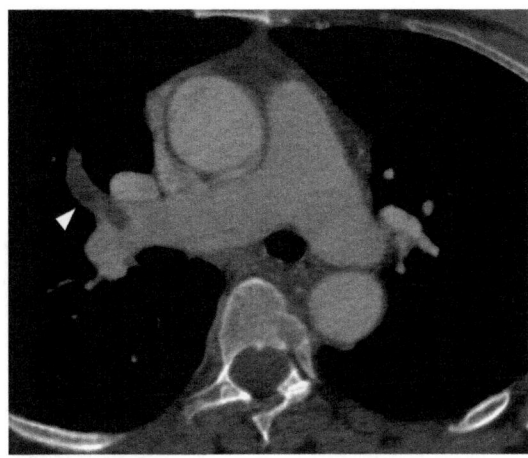

Fig. 10.31 CT angiography in patient with suspect of pulmonary embolism showing an intraluminal filling defect (arrowhead)

evaluation also of subsegmental pulmonary arteries identifying even small dimension pulmonary embolisms. Actually, after positioning region of interest (ROI) at the origin of pulmonary artery, automatic acquisition is performed. If this is not possible and manual acquisition is necessary, a 15–17 second scan delay during contrast medium administration is adequate in most cases. In addition to the filling defect, other signs that can coexist with PTE are pleural effusion, parenchymal opacity, lobar or segmental volume loss, and dilatation of the pulmonary artery. Cardiac abnormalities (right ventricular or atrial enlargement, thrombi in the right atrium or ventricle), vascular abnormalities like abrupt narrowing of the vessel diameter or abrupt cutoff of distal lobar or segmental artery (Fig. 10.32), and parenchymal abnormalities are usually seen in chronic PTE [80]. CT can also exclude other causes of chest pain that may mimic PTE like pulmonary, cardiac, or mediastinal pathologies.

10.5.1.4 Magnetic Resonance Angiography
Although MRI can potentially allow visualization of intravascular filling defects and provide physiologic information including the regional distribution of ventilation and perfusion, its limited availability and long acquisition time have made MRI seldom performed in PTE diagnosis [80].

10.5.1.5 Pulmonary Angiography

Angiography was considered the standard of reference in PTE diagnosis, but considering that angiography is an invasive technique and complications include bleeding, recurrent ventricular arrhythmias, and respiratory complications, it is actually little used. It demonstrates filling defects and secondary signs like abrupt occlusion of a pulmonary artery and areas of oligemia with pruning of branching vessels [80].

10.5.2 Triple Rule Out

In few problematic cases, the differential diagnosis of chest pain may be a challenge for the clinician that could have difficulties to formulate a diagnostic hypothesis.

In this case the radiologist can make a particular CT angiography that consists in a triggered scan performed injecting an increased amount of contrast medium, to opacify simultaneously the pulmonary artery, the coronaries, and the thoracic aorta (Fig. 10.33), to exclude pulmonary embolism, coronary stenosis, and aortic dissection that represent the most common and dangerous causes of thoracic pain.

This protocol however, represents a compromise due to the suboptimal vessel opacification that is obtained and to the high dose of radiation related to the triggered scan.

For these reasons, the use of this particular protocol should be limited as much as possible.

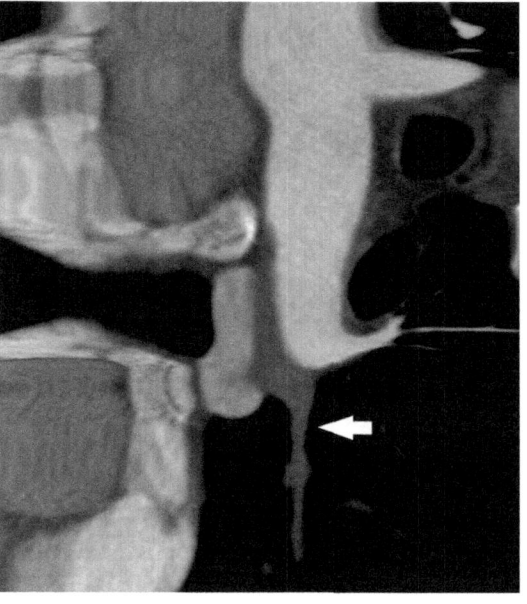

Fig. 10.32 CT angiography in patient with chronic pulmonary embolism shows abrupt cutoff of distal lobar or segmental artery (arrow)

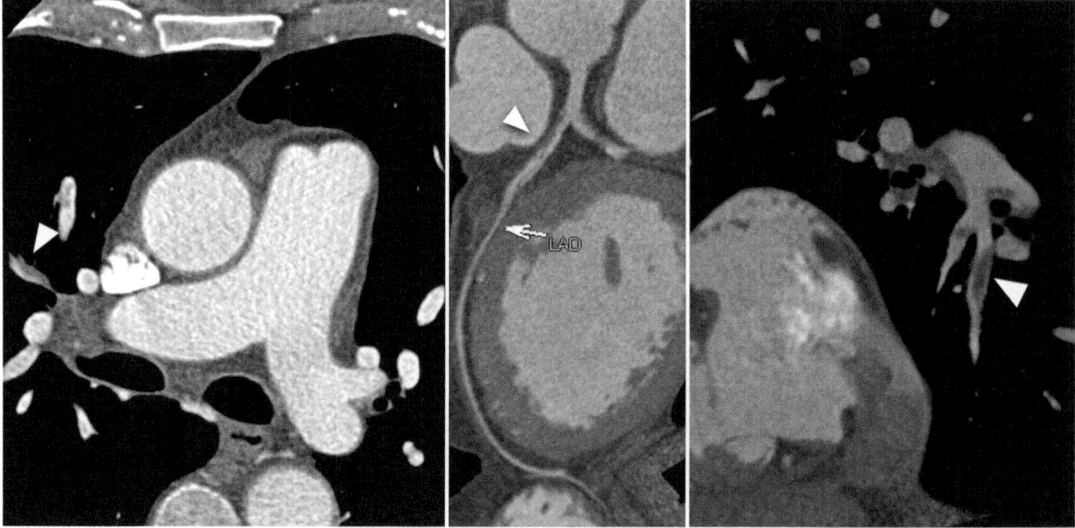

Fig. 10.33 Triple rule out protocol with simultaneous opacification of pulmonary arteries, aorta, and coronary arteries, showing filling defects in pulmonary arteries and dissection of proximal left anterior descending coronary artery

References

1. Lee TH, Goldman L. Evaluation of the patient with acute chest pain. N Engl J Med. 2000;342(16):1187–95.
2. Pope JH, Aufderheide TP, Ruthazer R, Woolard RH, Feldman JA, Beshansky JR, et al. Missed diagnoses of acute cardiac ischemia in the emergency department. N Engl J Med. 2000;342(16):1163–70.
3. Sabatine MS, Cannon CP. Approach to the patient with chest pain. Philadelphia: Elsevier; 2012. p. 1076–86.
4. Morrow DA. Clinical application of sensitive troponin assays. N Engl J Med. 2009;361(9):913–5.
5. Amsterdam EA, Kirk JD, Diercks DB, Lewis WR, Turnipseed SD. Exercise testing in chest pain units: rationale, implementation, and results. Cardiol Clin. 2005;23(4):503–16. vii.
6. Ekelund U, Forberg JL. New methods for improved evaluation of patients with suspected acute coronary syndrome in the emergency department. Emerg Med J. 2007;24(12):811–4.
7. Ottani F, Binetti N, Casagranda I, Cassin M, Cavazza M, Grifoni S, Lenzi T, Lorenzoni R, Sbrojavacca R, Tanzi P, Vergara G. Percorso di valutazione del dolore toracico. Valutazione dei requisiti di base per l'implementazione negli ospedali italiani ANMCO.
8. Conti A, Paladini B, Toccafondi S, Magazzini S, Olivotto I, Galassi F, et al. Effectiveness of a multidisciplinary chest pain unit for the assessment of coronary syndromes and risk stratification in the Florence area. Am Heart J. 2002;144(4):630–5.
9. Taylor AJ, Cerqueira M, Hodgson JM, Mark D, Min J, O'Gara P, et al. ACCF/SCCT/ACR/AHA/ASE/ASNC/NASCI/SCAI/SCMR 2010 appropriate use criteria for cardiac computed tomography. A report of the American College of Cardiology Foundation Appropriate Use Criteria Task Force, the Society of Cardiovascular Computed Tomography, the American College of Radiology, the American Heart Association, the American Society of Echocardiography, the American Society of Nuclear Cardiology, the North American Society for Cardiovascular Imaging, the Society for Cardiovascular Angiography and Interventions, and the Society for Cardiovascular Magnetic Resonance. J Am Coll Cardiol. 2010;56(22):1864–94.
10. Antman EM, Anbe DT, Armstrong PW, Bates ER, Green LA, Hand M, et al. ACC/AHA guidelines for the management of patients with ST-elevation myocardial infarction--executive summary: a report of the American College of Cardiology/American Heart Association Task Force on Practice Guidelines (Writing Committee to Revise the 1999 Guidelines for the Management of Patients With Acute Myocardial Infarction). Circulation. 2004;110(5):588–636.
11. Stern S. Symptoms other than chest pain may be important in the diagnosis of "silent ischemia," or "the sounds of silence". Circulation. 2005;111(24):e435–7.
12. Canto JG, Shlipak MG, Rogers WJ, Malmgren JA, Frederick PD, Lambrew CT, et al. Prevalence, clinical characteristics, and mortality among patients with myocardial infarction presenting without chest pain. JAMA. 2000;283(24):3223–9.
13. Culic V, Eterovic D, Miric D, Silic N. Symptom presentation of acute myocardial infarction: influence of sex, age, and risk factors. Am Heart J. 2002;144(6):1012–7.
14. Binetti N, Lenzi T, Strada A. Medicina di Emergenza-Urgenza. Approccio al paziente con dolore toracico. Amsterdam: Elsevier; 2011. p. 345–9.
15. Dastidar AG, Rodrigues JC, Ahmed N, Baritussio A, Bucciarelli-Ducci C. The role of cardiac MRI in patients with troponin-positive chest pain and unobstructed coronary arteries. Curr Cardiovasc Imaging Rep. 2015;8(8):28.
16. Karlson BW, Herlitz J, Wiklund O, Richter A, Hjalmarson A. Early prediction of acute myocardial infarction from clinical history, examination and electrocardiogram in the emergency room. Am J Cardiol. 1991;68(2):171–5.
17. Sabia P, Afrookteh A, Touchstone DA, Keller MW, Esquivel L, Kaul S. Value of regional wall motion abnormality in the emergency room diagnosis of acute myocardial infarction. A prospective study using two-dimensional echocardiography. Circulation. 1991;84(3 Suppl):I85–92.
18. Jeroudi MO, Cheirif J, Habib G, Bolli R. Prolonged wall motion abnormalities after chest pain at rest in patients with unstable angina: a possible manifestation of myocardial stunning. Am Heart J. 1994;127:1241–50.
19. Schinkel AF, Bax JJ, Geleijnse ML, Boersma E, Elhendy A, Roelandt JR, et al. Noninvasive evaluation of ischaemic heart disease: myocardial perfusion imaging or stress echocardiography? Eur Heart J. 2003;24(9):789–800.
20. Douglas PS, Khandheria B, Stainback RF, Weissman NJ, Peterson ED, Hendel RC, et al. ACCF/ASE/ACEP/AHA/ASNC/SCAI/SCCT/SCMR 2008 Appropriateness Criteria for Stress Echocardiography. A report of the American College of Cardiology Foundation Appropriateness Criteria Task Force, American Society of Echocardiography, American College of Emergency Physicians, American Heart Association, American Society of Nuclear Cardiology, Society for Cardiovascular Angiography and Interventions, Society of Cardiovascular Computed Tomography, and Society for Cardiovascular Magnetic Resonance endorsed by the Heart Rhythm Society and the Society of Critical Care Medicine. Catheter Cardiovasc Interv. 2008;71(5):E1–19.
21. Fox K, Garcia MA, Ardissino D, Buszman P, Camici PG, Crea F, et al. Guidelines on the management of stable angina pectoris: executive summary: the task force on the management of stable Angina Pectoris of the European society of cardiology. Eur Heart J. 2006;27(11):1341–81.
22. Marcassa C, Bax JJ, Bengel F, Hesse B, Petersen CL, Reyes E, et al. Clinical value, cost-effectiveness, and

safety of myocardial perfusion scintigraphy: a position statement. Eur Heart J. 2008;29(4):557–63.

23. Underwood SR, Anagnostopoulos C, Cerqueira M, Ell PJ, Flint EJ, Harbinson M, et al. Myocardial perfusion scintigraphy: the evidence. Eur J Nucl Med Mol Imaging. 2004;31(2):261–91.

24. Naghavi M, Libby P, Falk E, Casscells SW, Litovsky S, Rumberger J, et al. From vulnerable plaque to vulnerable patient: a call for new definitions and risk assessment strategies: Part I. Circulation. 2003;108(14):1664–72.

25. Hoffmann U, Bamberg F, Chae CU, Nichols JH, Rogers IS, Seneviratne SK, et al. Coronary computed tomography angiography for early triage of patients with acute chest pain: the ROMICAT (rule out myocardial infarction using computer assisted tomography) trial. J Am Coll Cardiol. 2009;53(18): 1642–50.

26. Dedic A, Ten Kate GJ, Neefjes LA, Rossi A, Dharampal A, Rood PP, et al. Coronary CT angiography outperforms calcium imaging in the triage of acute coronary syndrome. Int J Cardiol. 2013;167(4):1597–602.

27. Dewey M, Rief M, Martus P, Kendziora B, Feger S, Dreger H, et al. Evaluation of computed tomography in patients with atypical angina or chest pain clinically referred for invasive coronary angiography: randomised controlled trial. BMJ. 2016;355:i5441.

28. Genders TS, Petersen SE, Pugliese F, Dastidar AG, Fleischmann KE, Nieman K, et al. The optimal imaging strategy for patients with stable chest pain: a cost-effectiveness analysis. Ann Int Med. 2015;162(7):474–84.

29. Schlattmann P, Schuetz GM, Dewey M. Influence of coronary artery disease prevalence on predictive values of coronary CT angiography: a meta-regression analysis. Eur Radiol. 2011;21(9):1904–13.

30. Nieman K, Hoffmann U. Cardiac computed tomography in patients with acute chest pain. Eur Heart J. 2015;36(15):906–14.

31. Yang L, Zhou T, Zhang R, Xu L, Peng Z, Ding J, et al. Meta-analysis: diagnostic accuracy of coronary CT angiography with prospective ECG gating based on step-and-shoot, Flash and volume modes for detection of coronary artery disease. Eur Radiol. 2014;24(10):2345–52.

32. Task Force M, Montalescot G, Sechtem U, Achenbach S, Andreotti F, Arden C, et al. 2013 ESC guidelines on the management of stable coronary artery disease: the task force on the management of stable coronary artery disease of the European society of cardiology. Eur Heart J. 2013;34(38):2949–3003.

33. Schlett CL, Hoffmann U, Geisler T, Nikolaou K, Bamberg F. Cardiac computed tomography for the evaluation of the acute chest pain syndrome: state of the art. Radiol Clin North Am. 2015;53(2):297–305.

34. Schlett CL, Banerji D, Siegel E, Bamberg F, Lehman SJ, Ferencik M, et al. Prognostic value of CT angiography for major adverse cardiac events in patients with acute chest pain from the emergency department: 2-year outcomes of the ROMICAT trial. JACC Cardiovasc Imaging. 2011;4(5):481–91.

35. Di Lazzaro D, Crusco F. CT angio for the evaluation of graft patency. J Thorac Dis. 2017;9(Suppl 4):S283–S8.

36. Chan M, Ridley L, Dunn DJ, Tian DH, Liou K, Ozdirik J, et al. A systematic review and meta-analysis of multidetector computed tomography in the assessment of coronary artery bypass grafts. Int J Cardiol. 2016;221:898–905.

37. Pesenti-Rossi D, Baron N, Georges JL, Augusto S, Gibault-Genty G, Livarek B. Assessment of coronary bypass graft patency by first-line multi-detector computed tomography. Ann Cardiol Angeiol (Paris). 2014;63(5):284–92.

38. Schroeder S, Achenbach S, Bengel F, Burgstahler C, Cademartiri F, de Feyter P, et al. Cardiac computed tomography: indications, applications, limitations, and training requirements: report of a Writing Group deployed by the Working Group Nuclear Cardiology and Cardiac CT of the European Society of Cardiology and the European Council of Nuclear Cardiology. Eur Heart J. 2008;29(4):531–56.

39. Mowatt G, Cook JA, Hillis GS, Walker S, Fraser C, Jia X, et al. 64-Slice computed tomography angiography in the diagnosis and assessment of coronary artery disease: systematic review and meta-analysis. Heart. 2008;94(11):1386–93.

40. Achenbach S, Ropers D, Hoffmann U, MacNeill B, Baum U, Pohle K, et al. Assessment of coronary remodeling in stenotic and nonstenotic coronary atherosclerotic lesions by multidetector spiral computed tomography. J Am Coll Cardiol. 2004;43(5): 842–7.

41. Goldstein JA, Gallagher MJ, O'Neill WW, Ross MA, O'Neil BJ, Raff GL. A randomized controlled trial of multi-slice coronary computed tomography for evaluation of acute chest pain. J Am Coll Cardiol. 2007;49(8):863–71.

42. Goldstein JA, Chinnaiyan KM, Abidov A, Achenbach S, Berman DS, Hayes SW, et al. The CT-STAT (coronary computed tomographic angiography for systematic triage of acute chest pain patients to treatment) trial. J Am Coll Cardiol. 2011;58(14):1414–22.

43. Hoffmann U, Truong QA, Schoenfeld DA, Chou ET, Woodard PK, Nagurney JT, et al. Coronary CT angiography versus standard evaluation in acute chest pain. N Engl J Med. 2012;367(4):299–308.

44. Litt HI, Gatsonis C, Snyder B, Singh H, Miller CD, Entrikin DW, et al. CT angiography for safe discharge of patients with possible acute coronary syndromes. N Engl J Med. 2012;366(15):1393–403.

45. Raff GL, Chinnaiyan KM, Cury RC, Garcia MT, Hecht HS, Hollander JE, et al. SCCT guidelines on the use of coronary computed tomographic angiography for patients presenting with acute chest pain to the emergency department: a report of the Society of Cardiovascular Computed Tomography Guidelines Committee. J Cardiovasc Comput Tomogr. 2014;8(4):254–71.

46. Halliburton SS, Abbara S, Chen MY, Gentry R, Mahesh M, Raff GL, et al. SCCT guidelines on radiation dose and dose-optimization strategies in cardiovascular CT. J Cardiovasc Comput Tomogr. 2011;5(4):198–224.

47. Fuchs TA, Stehli J, Bull S, Dougoud S, Clerc OF, Herzog BA, et al. Coronary computed tomography angiography with model-based iterative reconstruction using a radiation exposure similar to chest X-ray examination. Eur Heart J. 2014;35(17):1131–6.

48. Cademartiri F, de Monye C, Pugliese F, Mollet NR, Runza G, van der Lugt A, et al. High iodine concentration contrast material for noninvasive multislice computed tomography coronary angiography: iopromide 370 versus iomeprol 400. Invest Radiol. 2006;41(3):349–53.

49. Leurent G, Langella B, Fougerou C, Lentz PA, Larralde A, Bedossa M, et al. Diagnostic contributions of cardiac magnetic resonance imaging in patients presenting with elevated troponin, acute chest pain syndrome and unobstructed coronary arteries. Arch Cardiovasc Dis. 2011;104(3):161–70.

50. Monney PA, Sekhri N, Burchell T, Knight C, Davies C, Deaner A, et al. Acute myocarditis presenting as acute coronary syndrome: role of early cardiac magnetic resonance in its diagnosis. Heart. 2011;97(16):1312–8.

51. Chopard R, Jehl J, Dutheil J, Genon VD, Seronde MF, Kastler B, et al. Evolution of acute coronary syndrome with normal coronary arteries and normal cardiac magnetic resonance imaging. Arch Cardiovasc Dis. 2011;104(10):509–17.

52. Gerbaud E, Harcaut E, Coste P, Erickson M, Lederlin M, Labeque JN, et al. Cardiac magnetic resonance imaging for the diagnosis of patients presenting with chest pain, raised troponin, and unobstructed coronary arteries. Int J Cardiovasc Imaging. 2012;28(4):783–94.

53. Mahmoudi M, Harden S, Abid N, Peebles C, Nicholas Z, Jones T, et al. Troponin-positive chest pain with unobstructed coronary arteries: definitive differential diagnosis using cardiac MRI. Br J Radiol. 2012;85(1016):e461–6.

54. Collste O, Sorensson P, Frick M, Agewall S, Daniel M, Henareh L, et al. Myocardial infarction with normal coronary arteries is common and associated with normal findings on cardiovascular magnetic resonance imaging: results from the Stockholm Myocardial Infarction with Normal Coronaries study. J Intern Med. 2013;273(2):189–96.

55. Kawecki D, Morawiec B, Monney P, Pellaton C, Wojciechowska C, Jojko J, et al. Diagnostic contribution of cardiac magnetic resonance in patients with acute coronary syndrome and culprit-free angiograms. Med Sci Monit. 2015;21:171–80.

56. Doolan A, Langlois N, Semsarian C. Causes of sudden cardiac death in young Australians, 2004. Available from: http://www.ncbi.nlm.nih.gov/pubmed/14748671.

57. Schepis T, Achenbach S, Marwan M, Muschiol G, Ropers D, Daniel WG, et al. Prevalence of first-pass myocardial perfusion defects detected by contrast-enhanced dual-source CT in patients with non-ST segment elevation acute coronary syndromes. Eur Radiol. 2010;20(7):1607–14.

58. Feuchtner GM, Plank F, Pena C, Battle J, Min J, Leipsic J, et al. Evaluation of myocardial CT perfusion in patients presenting with acute chest pain to the emergency department: comparison with SPECT-myocardial perfusion imaging. Heart. 2012;98(20):1510–7.

59. Nieman K, Cury RC, Ferencik M, Nomura CH, Abbara S, Hoffmann U, et al. Differentiation of recent and chronic myocardial infarction by cardiac computed tomography. Am J Cardiol. 2006;98(3):303–8.

60. Hagan PG, Nienaber CA, Isselbacher EM, Bruckman D, Karavite DJ, Russman PL, et al. The international registry of acute aortic dissection (IRAD): new insights into an old disease. JAMA. 2000;283(7):897–903.

61. Holloway BJ, Rosewarne D, Jones RG. Imaging of thoracic aortic disease. Br J Radiol. 2011;84(3):S338–54.

62. von Kodolitsch Y, Nienaber CA, Dieckmann C, Schwartz AG, Hofmann T, Brekenfeld C, et al. Chest radiography for the diagnosis of acute aortic syndrome. Am J Med. 2004;116:73–7.

63. Salvolini L, Renda P, Fiore D, Scaglione M, Piccoli G, Giovagnoni A. Acute aortic syndromes: role of multidetector row CT. Eur J Radiol. 2008;65(3):350–8.

64. Feuchtner GM, Jodocy D, Klauser A, Haberfellner B, Aglan I, Spoeck A, et al. Radiation dose reduction by using 100-kV tube voltage in cardiac 64-slice computed tomography: a comparative study. Eur J Radiol. 2010;75(1):e51–6.

65. Miyazaki M, Lee VS. Nonenhanced MR angiography. Radiology. 2008;248(1):20–43.

66. Johansson G, Markstrom U, Swedenborg J. Ruptured thoracic aortic aneurysms: a study of incidence and mortality rates. J Vasc Surg. 1995;21(6):985–8.

67. Trimarchi S, Nienaber CA, Rampoldi V, Myrmel T, Suzuki T, Mehta RH, et al. Contemporary results of surgery in acute type A aortic dissection: the international registry of acute aortic dissection experience. J Thorac Cardiovasc Surg. 2005;129(1):112–22.

68. LePage MA, Quint LE, Sonnad SS, Deeb GM, Williams DM. Aortic dissection: CT features that distinguish true lumen from false lumen. AJR Am J Roentgenol. 2001;177(1):207–11.

69. Suzuki T, Mehta RH, Ince H, Nagai R, Sakomura Y, Weber F, et al. Clinical profiles and outcomes of acute type B aortic dissection in the current era: lessons from the International Registry of Aortic Dissection (IRAD). Circulation. 2003;108(Suppl 1):II312–7.

70. Mehta RH, Suzuki T, Hagan PG, Bossone E, Gilon D, Llovet A, et al. Predicting death in patients with acute type a aortic dissection. Circulation. 2002;105(2):200–6.

71. Mehta RH, O'Gara PT, Bossone E, Nienaber CA, Myrmel T, Cooper JV, et al. Acute type A aortic dissection in the elderly: clinical characteristics, man-

agement, and outcomes in the current era. J Am Coll Cardiol. 2002;40(4):685–92.

72. Kazerooni EA, Bree RL, Williams DM. Penetrating atherosclerotic ulcers of the descending thoracic aorta: evaluation with CT and distinction from aortic dissection. Radiology. 1992;183(3):759–65.

73. Nienaber CA, Sievers HH. Intramural hematoma in acute aortic syndrome: more than one variant of dissection? Circulation. 2002;106(3):284–5.

74. Richens D, Kotidis K, Neale M, Oakley C, Fails A. Rupture of the aorta following road traffic accidents in the United Kingdom 1992–1999. The results of the co-operative crash injury study. Eur J Cardiothorac Surg. 2003;23(2):143–8.

75. Gotway MB, Araoz PA, Macedo TA, Stanson AW, Higgins CB, Ring EJ, et al. Imaging findings in Takayasu's arteritis. AJR Am J Roentgenol. 2005;184(6):1945–50.

76. Lin MP, Chang SC, Wu RH, Chou CK, Tzeng WS. A comparison of computed tomography, magnetic resonance imaging, and digital subtraction angiography findings in the diagnosis of infected aortic aneurysm. J Comput Assist Tomogr. 2008;32(4):616–20.

77. Khandaker MH, Espinosa RE, Nishimura RA, Sinak LJ, Hayes SN, Melduni RM, et al. Pericardial disease: diagnosis and management. Mayo Clin Proc. 2010;85(6):572–93.

78. Imazio M, Demichelis B, Parrini I, Giuggia M, Cecchi E, Gaschino G, et al. Day-hospital treatment of acute pericarditis: a management program for outpatient therapy. J Am Coll Cardiol. 2004;43(6):1042–6.

79. Cheitlin MD, Armstrong WF, Aurigemma GP, Beller GA, Bierman FZ, Davis JL, et al. ACC/AHA/ASE 2003 guideline update for the clinical application of echocardiography: summary article: a report of the American College of Cardiology/American Heart Association Task Force on Practice Guidelines (ACC/AHA/ASE Committee to Update the 1997 Guidelines for the Clinical Application of Echocardiography). Circulation. 2003;108(9):1146–62.

80. Han D, Lee KS, Franquet T, Muller NL, Kim TS, Kim H, et al. Thrombotic and nonthrombotic pulmonary arterial embolism: spectrum of imaging findings. Radiographics. 2003;23(6):1521–39.

Imaging of Non-vascular Thoracic Pain

11

Gianluca Milanese, Aldo Carnevale, João Cruz, and Nicola Sverzellati

In patients with chest pain [1], ruling out parenchymal, pleural, musculoskeletal, oesophageal, psychogenic or neurologic diseases is crucial [2, 3]. It is worth bearing in mind that lung tissue itself has no pain fibres. Indeed, pneumonia or pulmonary infarction-related chest pain usually arises from inflammation of the adjacent parietal pleura or from muscle strain from prolonged recurrent coughing [4].

Imaging plays a pivotal role in the diagnosis and characterization of parenchymal and pleural diseases. Chest radiography (CXR) remains the initial investigation for the majority of subjects with acute chest pain. However, radiographic findings are often non-specific and need some integration with other imaging modalities [5]. Over the past decade, lung ultrasonography (US) has gained an important role in the diagnosis of thoracic diseases, especially in acute care setting [6, 7]. US is particularly helpful in children, owing to their suitability for US investigation and radiation exposure avoidance [8, 9]. Computed tomography (CT) remains the gold standard technique for pleuro-parenchymal imaging as it may determine aetiology and extent of the underlying disease. Both thin-section volumetric CT acquisition and multiplanar reconstructions (MPRs) may show subtle abnormalities in the early phase of the disease [5, 10].

11.1 Lung Parenchyma Disorders Causing Chest Pain

11.1.1 Lung Cancer

Pain is one of the most common and debilitating symptoms experienced by patients with advanced lung cancer. Pain most commonly follows the invasion of the parietal pleura and ribs, compression or infiltration of neural structures or metastatic dissemination (e.g. osseous). In addition, both short- and long-term sequelae of surgery or radiotherapy can be painful [11].

CT is currently the gold standard imaging technique in lung cancer staging. However, it is limited in the evaluation of pleural infiltration by peripheral cancer. The presence of pleural tags is a highly sensitive but not very specific predictor of visceral pleural infiltration. The contact of tumour to the adjacent chest wall or mediastinum

Electronic Supplementary Material The online version of this chapter (https://doi.org/10.1007/978-3-319-99822-0_11) contains supplementary material, which is available to authorized users.

G. Milanese · N. Sverzellati (✉)
Division of Radiology, Department of Medicine and Surgery, University of Parma, Parma, Italy
e-mail: nicola.sverzellati@unipr.it

A. Carnevale
Section of Radiology, Department of Morphology, Surgery and Experimental Medicine, University of Ferrara, Ferrara, Italy

J. Cruz
Department of Radiology, Hospital Garcia de Orta, Almada, Portugal

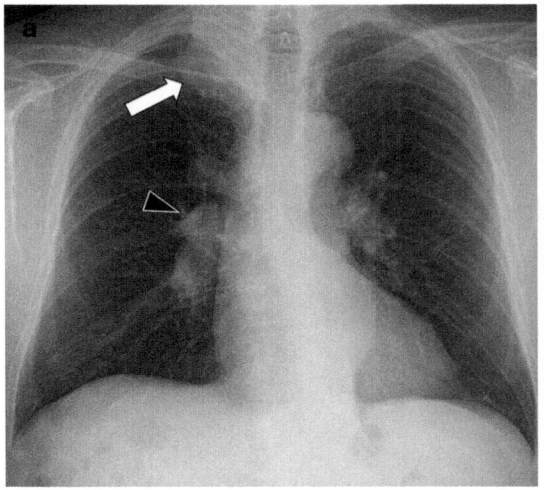 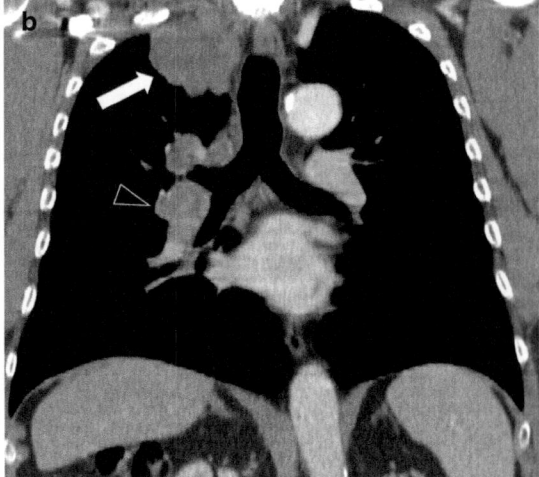

Fig. 11.1 Pancoast tumour. (**a**) Chest radiograph (frontal view) of a patient suffering from upper chest and right shoulder pain shows a mass (*white arrow*) located in the upper portion of the lung, associated with ipsilateral mediastinal widening (*black arrowhead*). (**b**) The CT-MPR reformatted image (coronal view) confirmed the presence of a soft tissue mass infiltrating the mediastinal fat tissue (*white arrow*) and ipsilateral lymphadenopathies (*black arrowhead*)

is not necessarily indicative for invasion. However, the greater the degree of contact, the more probable is their involvement. Bone destruction with or without soft-tissue mass extending into the chest wall is the only CT finding with a 100% positive predictive value for infiltration of both parietal pleura and chest wall [12]. Obliterations of the extrapleural fat, pleural thickening and soft tissue mass are considered signs of highly probable pleural invasion.

Magnetic resonance imaging (MRI) may detect chest wall invasion caused by peripheral lung tumours, similarly to CT. In particular, the depiction on STIR sequence of a small amount of fluid between the visceral and parietal pleural linings may be used to exclude chest wall infiltration [13].

Malignant brachial plexopathy—causing shoulder pain radiating to lateral arm and hand—can derive from the infiltration of the plexus by the tumour. A Pancoast tumour (or superior sulcus tumour) is defined as a non-small-cell tumour arising from the lung apex and invading any of the structures at the apex of the chest, including the most superior ribs or periosteum, the lower nerve roots of the brachial plexus and the sympathetic chain or the

subclavian vessels (Fig. 11.1). This type of lung tumour is currently subcategorized as anterior, middle and posterior, depending on the site of the chest wall infiltration in relation to the insertions of the anterior and middle scalene muscles on the first rib, delineating anterior, middle and posterior compartments, respectively [14]. Superior sulcus tumours may be missed at CXR, particularly when presenting as a small apical cap or mimicking a benign apical pleural thickening [15]. CT is considered the best imaging tool for assessing both bone involvement and patency of subclavian vessels, which may both influence the therapeutic management (Fig. 11.2; Video 11.2). However, CT may be not sufficiently accurate in the evaluation of both tumour extension into vertebral foramina and spinal canal and brachial plexus involvement. In patients candidated to curative-intent surgical resection, MRI of the thoracic inlet and brachial plexus is recommended to exclude infiltration of unresectable vascular structures and to evaluate the extradural space [14]. Owing to its superior contrast resolution, sagittal T1-weighted image (WI) MRI improves reader confidence in the diagnosis of such structures' compromise.

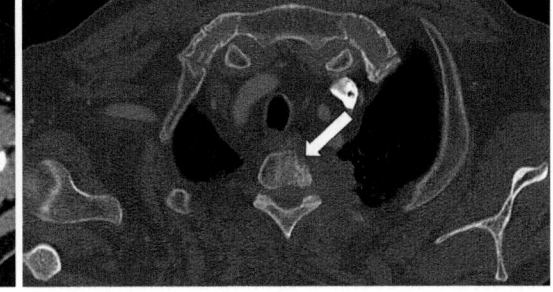

Fig. 11.2 Pancoast tumour. (**a**) CT-MPR image (oblique axial view, soft tissue reconstruction algorithm) shows a soft tissue mass (*white arrow*) in the apicoposterior segment of the left lung, infiltrating into an ipsilateral neural foramen (*black arrowhead*) causing radicular pain. (**b**) The CT-MPR image (oblique axial view, sharp reconstruction algorithm) depicts the erosion of the vertebral body (*white arrow*)

11.1.2 Post-surgery Pain

Chest surgery can cause the development of persistent postoperative pain. The pathogenesis of post-thoracotomy pain is complex, although nerve damage seems to be a major risk factor. Video-assisted thoracoscopic surgery is expected to reduce postoperative pain in comparison with traditional accesses [11]. A postoperative complication is generally defined as "immediate" if it occurs within the first 30 days after surgery, "early" if within the first 6 months and "late" if afterwards. Complications are often further subcategorized into "minor" and "major". The former includes supraventricular arrhythmias, persistent air leak more than 5 postoperative days, accumulation of bronchial secretions with atelectasis and vocal cord paralysis. Major and potentially lethal complications include postoperative bleeding, pleural empyema (with or without fistula formation), pneumonia, respiratory failure requiring mechanical ventilation, acute respiratory distress syndrome (ARDS), pulmonary oedema and embolism, ventricular arrhythmias, acute myocardial infarction and stroke [16]. Both CXR and CT play a crucial role in the surveillance of patients undergoing lung resection for primary tumour.

11.1.3 Pneumonia and Abscess

Chest pain is one of the most useful symptoms for suspecting an underlying pneumonia, and it suggests an associated pleural inflammatory involvement [17]. Community-acquired pneumonia (CAP) is usually diagnosed by both clinical and imaging features, the latter allowing detection, characterization and evaluation of changes during treatment as well as the depiction of complications [18].

CXR is the first-line imaging modality required for the diagnosis of CAP, and it should be performed when pneumonia is clinically suspected [19]. The most frequent imaging appearance of CAP is lobar pneumonia, namely, an airspace consolidation of one segment or lobe, limited by pleural surfaces. Ground-glass opacities (GGO) adjacent to the consolidation may be observed, caused by a partial filling of the alveoli. Small pleural effusions—suggestive for reactive pleural inflammation (i.e. parapneumonic effusions)—are common associated findings [20]. US may represent a promising alternative to CXR and CT in emergency, paediatrics and resource-limited settings, as well as during follow-up, due to the lack of ionizing radiation exposure and ease of longitudinal evaluation [9]. Indeed, recent guidelines for paediatric patients recommended not to use CXR because of poor agreement for the identification of CAP as well as difficulties to differentiate between bacterial and viral diseases [17]. Imaging is generally non-specific, and it may be difficult to determine the causative micro-organism pathogens. Indeed, many pathogens can cause pneumonia with various imaging patterns, and consolidation, peribronchial nodules and GGO may coexist in the same patient [21]. Furthermore, antibiotics can modify the classical appearance of pneumococcal infection, as it may present as patchy confluent areas that may be multilobar or bilateral [20].

Pulmonary abscess following a bacterial pneumonia can cause pleuritic chest pain. It represents a necrotic evolution, with possible bronchopulmonary fistula formation, generally seen in anaerobic bacterial diseases (e.g. aspiration pneumonia).

On CXR, pulmonary abscess appears as a peripheral round opacity with air-fluid level and acute chest wall angles [22] (Fig. 11.3). CT demonstrates single or multiple masses with central hypoattenuation or thick-walled cavities with air-fluid level, representing purulent liquefying necrosis. Peripheral enhancement after intravenous contrast administration is frequent [23] (Fig. 11.4). Bronchi and vessels terminate abruptly at the wall of the abscess,

without being compressed or distorted, and this finding may be useful to distinguish a peripheral lung abscess from an empyema.

11.2 Pleural Causes of Chest Pain

11.2.1 Pneumothorax

Pneumothorax (PTX) is the abnormal presence of air between visceral and parietal pleura [24] and may be classified as spontaneous, post-traumatic or iatrogenic. The incidence of spontaneous PTXs is 16.7/100.000/year (for male patients), whereas the incidence of iatrogenic form is difficult to calculate, although it is probably increasing following the use of mechanical ventilation and interventional procedures [25–27].

On CXR, classical findings are represented by a visceral pleural line parallel to the chest wall and a hyper-transparent area—without lung markings—located between lung surface and

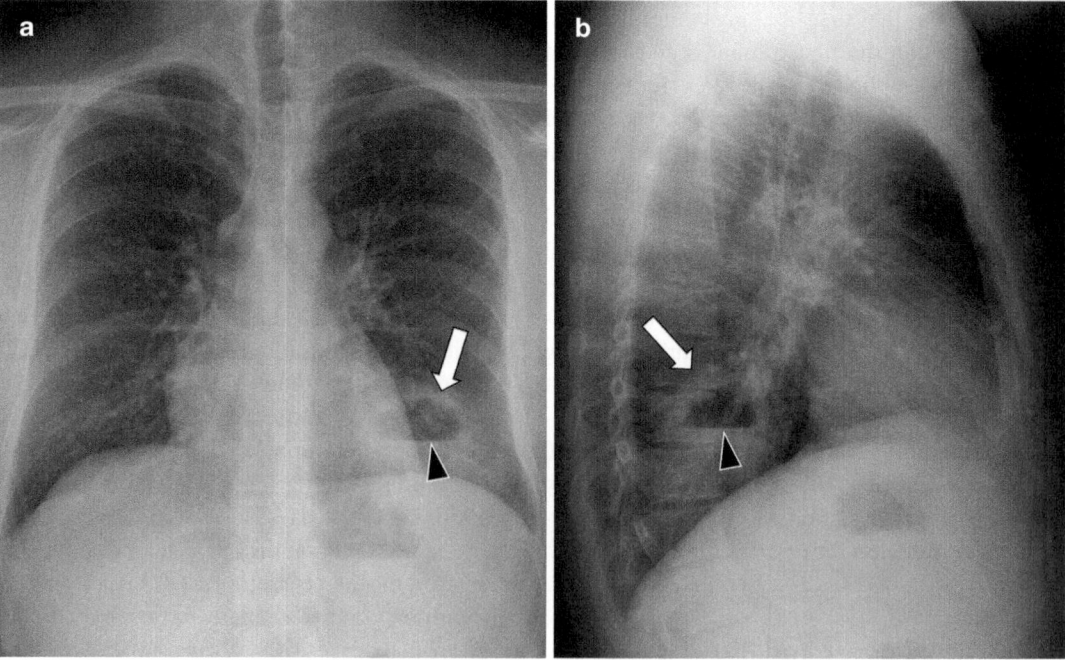

Fig. 11.3 Pulmonary abscess. (**a**, **b**) Chest radiograph of a young patient suffering from chest pain, cough and fever shows a round peripheral opacity (*white arrow*) located in the left lower lobe, associated with an air-fluid level (*black arrowhead*)

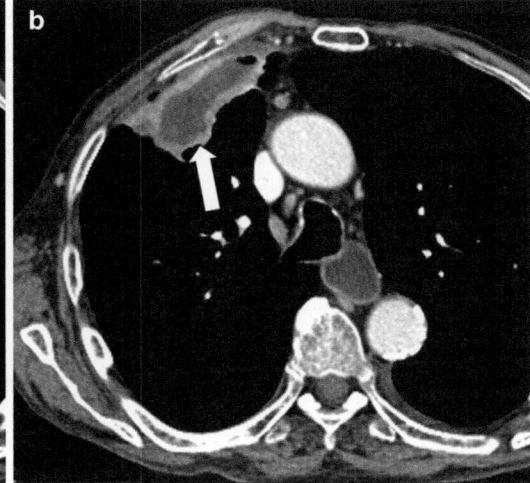

Fig. 11.4 Pulmonary abscess. (**a**) Axial CT image shows a mass in the anterior segment of the right upper lobe with central hypoattenuation, thick walls and gas bubble (*black arrowhead*). (**b**) Axial CT after contrast administration shows intense peripheral enhancement (*white arrow*)

chest wall [24, 26]. Sometimes, an adherence of the inflamed pleura to the chest wall may confine a PTX to a loculated portion of the pleural space around the site of the air leak. However, CXR has suboptimal sensitivity in depicting small PTX, especially in supine patients, in whom the air tends to collect anteriorly and inferiorly, appearing as a hyper-transparent area in the cardio-phrenic and costophrenic sulcus (i.e. "the deep sulcus sign") [24, 26]. Contralateral side decubitus and expiratory views may be helpful in the detection of small PTXs when inspiratory supine CXR appears normal. Indeed, in trauma and intensive care unit settings, as much as 30–50% of PTXs may be missed on supine CXR. Radiologists must be aware of potential pitfalls when imaging patients with suspected PTX, as follows:

- The medial border of the scapula, skin folds, clothing or bed sheets may mimic a visceral pleural line; however, they can be differentiated from a PTX as they continue either with the rest of the bone or beyond the chest wall [26, 28].
- Further shadows—which may be smooth, homogeneous or radiopaque—running parallel along inferior border of lower ribs, upper borders of clavicles and scapula may

correspond to soft tissues and intercostal muscles.

- In patients that underwent pleurectomy because of recurrent PTXs, a radiopaque line representing surgical suture materials or staples can be misdiagnosed as a new air leak [26].

US may be more sensitive in the assessment of traumatic PTX [20, 29–31]. However, its accuracy decreases in the presence of coexisting lung diseases such as consolidation, ARDS, lung fibrosis or atelectasis [6]. Main US signs of PTX are:

- Absence of lung sliding: absence of the typical "up and down" movement (also known as "seashore sign") of the pleural line in M-mode US. The resultant tracing will only display one pattern of parallel horizontal lines above and below the pleural line, exemplifying the lack of movement, often called the "stratosphere or barcode sign". Despite its negative predictive value (99.2–100%), there is a high rate of false positives when other lung pathologies are associated.
- Lung-point sign: the point where alternating "seashore" and "stratosphere" patterns are depicted in M-mode US over time, at the border of a PTX, allowing for the sizing of the PTX (specificity, 100%; sensitivity, 66%) [6].

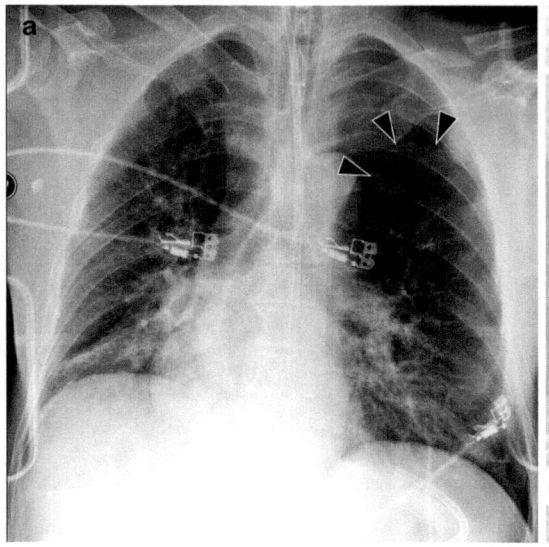 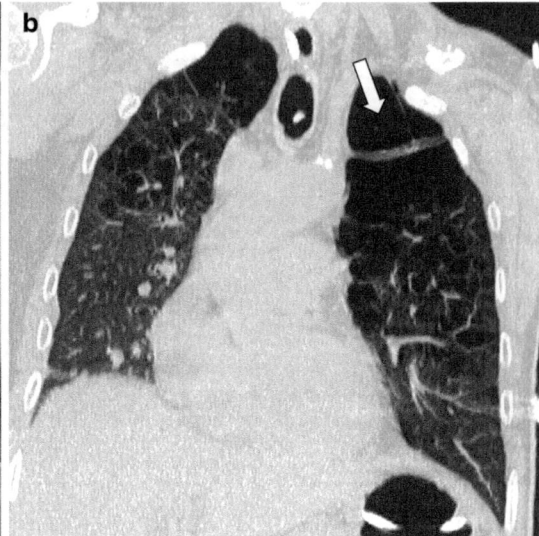

Fig. 11.5 Pitfalls for pneumothorax. (**a**) Supine chest radiograph of a patient admitted to the emergency department after a trauma, depicting a linear opacity (*black arrowheads*) suspicious for the visceral pleural line associated with a hyper-transparent area. The findings were considered consistent with left apical pneumothorax. (**b**) CT-MIP image (MPR coronal view) obtained shortly after shows diffuse bilateral emphysematous alterations, with a large left apical bulla (*white arrow*) mimicking pneumothorax

CT remains the gold standard as it can easily depict an occult PTX. The detection of small PTX is of clinical importance, since mechanic ventilation may worsen this condition [27, 28, 32]. CT is also helpful in identifying any underlying pulmonary predisposing condition, such as emphysema, lung fibrosis or cystic interstitial lung diseases [28, 33]. The main differential diagnosis is with large emphysematous bullae. When both CXR findings and patient symptoms are ambiguous, CT scans should be obtained [28, 34] (Fig. 11.5).

Tension PTX is a medical emergency. It is characterized by the presence of a fistula acting as a check-valve mechanism, letting the air progressively accumulate into the pleural space, with a consequent raise in the intrapleural pressure and possible inadequate diastolic filling of the heart with cardiorespiratory arrest. Large PTX with hyper-expansion of ipsilateral hemithorax, lung collapse, widening of costal arches, depression/inversion of the ipsilateral hemidiaphragm and contralateral mediastinal shift with atelectasis of the contralateral lung are all CXR signs consistent with tension PTX [24, 32].

A bronchopleural fistula—a communication between the pleural space and bronchial tree—may sometimes be depicted on CT. The use of MPR, thin collimation and sharper image reconstruction algorithms are all very helpful tools to identify this subtle complication [24, 27].

11.2.2 Pleural Effusion

Chest pain secondary to pleural effusion results from pleural irritation and usually implies some degree of inflammation, raising the likelihood of an exudative aetiology, such as pleural infection or malignancy [35].

PA and lateral CXR views may depict pleural effusions greater than 200 and 50 ml, respectively [35]. In standing patients, smaller effusions tend to collect in the most dependent part of the pleural space (e.g. the posterior costophrenic recess), blunting the posterior costo-diaphragmatic angles on lateral view. On PA view, CXR depicts the obliteration of the lateral costophrenic angle [24, 28, 35]. As effusions increase in size, they produce the characteristic "meniscus sign", which represents fluid tracking superiorly along the pleural surface after filling of the costophrenic recess. Subpulmonic effusions conform to the shape of the hemidiaphragm, and they are frequently overlooked on PA views. Elevation and lateral displacement of the peak of the hemidiaphragm, paucity of vessels below the hemidiaphragm and a widened distance between gastric bubble and hemidiaphragm should raise the suspicion of a subpulmonic effusion.

Dorsal decubitus may occult large pleural effusion, especially when bilateral, due to the symmetric and posterior layering distribution of the effusion. Expiratory ipsilateral decubitus has been shown to be the most sensitive CXR view for detecting pleural effusion.

Effusion in pulmonary fissures may get a lentiform shape, mimicking a thoracic lesion. Indeed, this kind of pleural effusion has been termed as "pseudotumour" or "vanishing tumour".

US is sensitive in detecting small pleural effusions, with special importance for loculated/septate effusions, which may mimic thoracic lesions on CXR. US is valuable in detecting small amounts of pleural fluid: it can even appreciate physiologic amounts of pleural liquid (i.e. 5 ml), but a minimal volume of 20 ml is more reliably detected, and US is 100% sensitive for effusions >100 ml [36]. US may distinguish solid and fluid pleural abnormalities, thus differentiating peripheral lung lesions from pleural fluid [37].

US can even suggest the nature of an effusion, as it may identify areas of focal pleural thickening or nodules, raising suspicion of malignancy and enabling imaging-guided biopsy. Transudates are typically recognized as anechoic without pleural thickening, whereas exudates—seen in empyema, malignancy, parapneumonic effusions or haemothorax—are more often complex in echogenicity with septations or stranding.

Empyema may not be easy to distinguish from other pathological conditions involving the pleural linings or peripheral lung parenchyma at CXR. US is particularly useful in differentiating transudative from exudative pleural effusions: ultrasonographic findings of empyema comprise heterogeneous appearance, varying according to the stage—US can show internal echoes, septations due to fibrin deposition or a hyperechoic morphology mimicking the normal lung US pattern [38]. Nevertheless, there could be an overlap of findings between transudative and exudative effusions [39]. Although CT is more sensitive than both CXR and US in differentiating pleural fluid from pleural thickening, it cannot differentiate between transudate and exudate [10, 24]. CT may help in differentiating empyema from uncomplicated parapneumonic effusion and peripherally located lung abscess [37]. The "split pleura" CT sign is a reliable finding to differentiate an empyema from a pulmonary abscess, and it shows diffuse pleural thickening and contrast enhancement of the parietal and visceral pleura, separated by an exudative effusion [40]. Pleural thickening and enhancement are seen in 80–100% of empyemas compared with 60% of parapneumonic effusions [24, 28]. Other possible findings are represented by small gas bubble collections or gas-fluid levels [37] (Fig. 11.6; Video 11.6).

Pleural malignancies can be categorized as primary or secondary (by contiguity from a lung or chest wall malignancy or distant spread from other sites of the body).

Mesothelioma is the most common primary pleural tumour. On CXR, mesothelioma may be suspected with moderate or profuse unilateral pleural effusion (30–80% of patients) and contralateral mediastinal shift. However, ipsilateral mediastinal shift can be caused by underlying pleural changes. Findings such as isolated pleural thickening or pleural-based mass—without associated pleural effusions—are less frequent (<25% of patients). Tumour growth leads to circumferential rind-like lobulated pleural thickening encasing the pulmonary parenchyma, causing an impairment in respiratory functions [5]. Imaging findings of volume loss can be detected on CXR, such as elevation of the ipsilateral hemidiaphragm, ipsilateral mediastinal shift, and narrowing of the intercostal spaces [41]. Calcified pleural plaques more prominent on the domes of the diaphragm, on the mediastinal pleura and in the inferior and posterior portions of the hemithoraces are a common radiographic manifestation of asbestos exposure. The partial obscuration of the heart

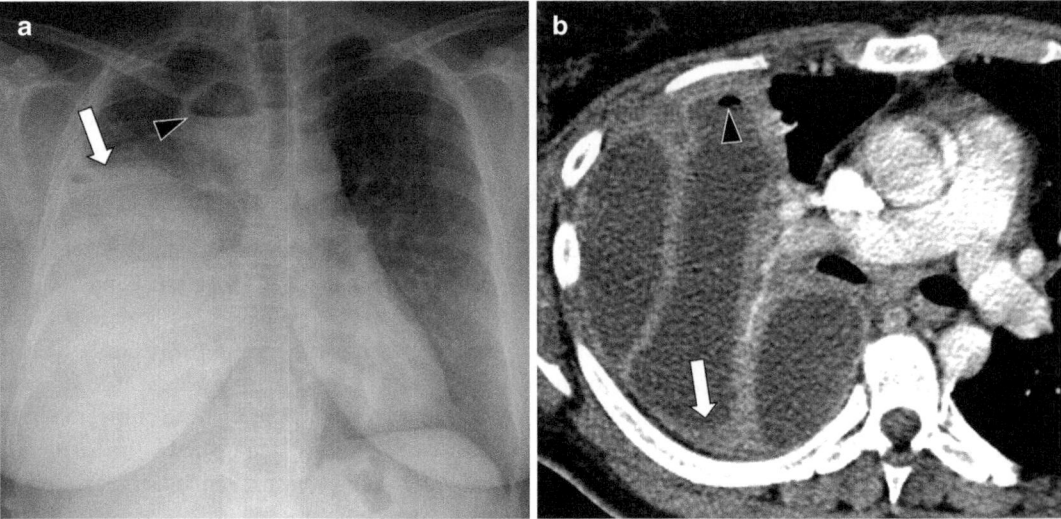

Fig. 11.6 Pleural empyema. (**a**) Chest radiograph (frontal view) of a young female patient shows a large right pleural effusion (*white arrow*), associated with an ipsilateral medially located round peripheral opacity with an air-fluid level (*black arrowhead*). (**b**) The magnification of the axial CT image shows a loculated pleural collection, with thickening and contrast enhancement of the pleural layers (*white arrow*) and small gas bubbles (*black arrowhead*)

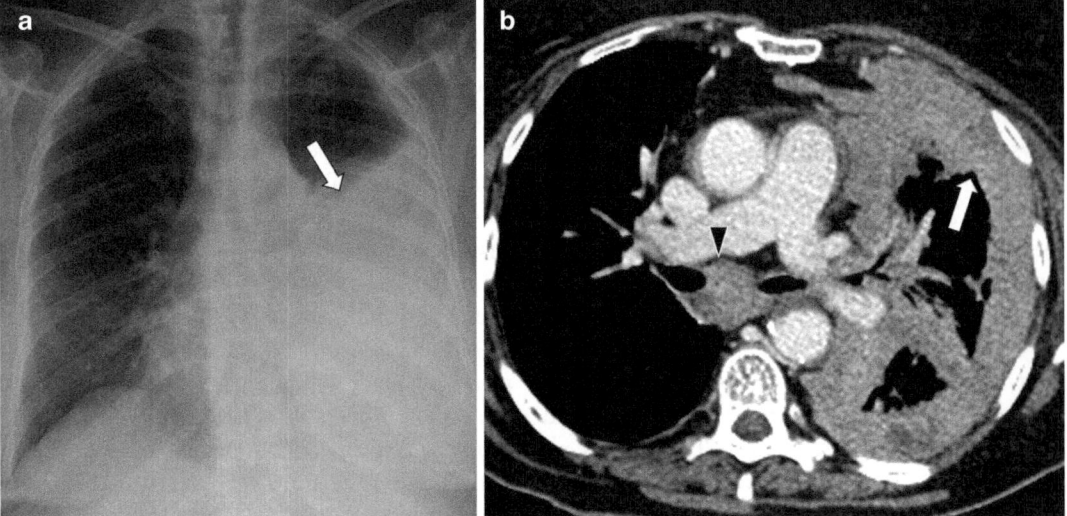

Fig. 11.7 Mesothelioma. (**a**) Chest radiograph (frontal view) of an old female patient shows a large left pleural effusion (*white arrow*). (**b**) The axial CT image shows a circumferential lobulated pleural thickening with intense contrast enhancement (*white arrow*) and mediastinal lymph nodal involvement (*black arrowhead*)

border, known as "shaggy" heart sign, may also be present and follows both pleural and parenchymal changes [42]. On US, mesothelioma may manifest as nodular or irregular pleural thickening. US is characterized by a sensitivity of 79% and a specificity of 100% in distinguishing malignant from benign effusions [43]. On contrast-enhanced CT, suspicious findings for a malignant pleural disease are a circumferential (sensitivity 22–41%), nodular (sensitivity 37–51%) pleural thickening and mediastinal pleural involvement (sensitivity 31–56%) [28, 44] (Fig. 11.7). Features suggestive of chest wall invasion include intercostal muscle invasion, loss of

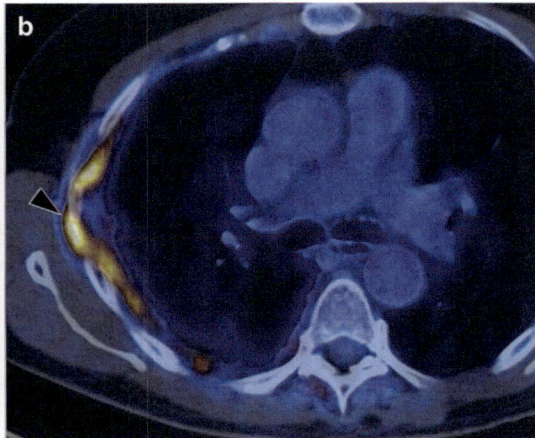

Fig. 11.8 Mesothelioma. (**a**) Axial CT image of a patient suffering from right pleural mesothelioma, depicting loss of the extrapleural fat planes and bone destruction (*white arrow*). (**b**) ^{18}F-FDG PET-CT clearly demonstrating the chest wall invasion by a tumoural nodule with a high tracer uptake (*black arrowhead*)

the extrapleural fat planes and bone destruction (Fig. 11.8; Video 11.8). The differential diagnosis for pleural thickening includes diffuse pleural metastasization (from bronchogenic, breast, ovarian or gastric carcinoma or from lymphoma). It can be impossible to radiologically differentiate pleural metastases from mesothelioma in cases of unilateral malignant pleural thickening. MRI is not routinely performed in patients with mesothelioma because most present with locally advanced and inoperable disease, a condition clearly delineated on CT. However, MRI may be performed when contrast-enhanced CT is contraindicated or in problematic cases, especially in those under consideration for radical surgery, in whom extrapleural infiltration has not been clearly delineated. MRI allows excellent soft tissue contrast, permitting a ready assessment of early chest wall, diaphragmatic and vascular invasion [5, 28, 45]. Mesothelioma is characterized by intermediate or mild high SI on T1-WI, moderate high SI on T2-WI compared to thoracic musculature, with moderate enhancement after contrast administration [45]. DWI may be used to differentiate malignant from benign pleural diseases, and restricted diffusion of water molecules, traduced by low SI on ADC maps, is usually seen [5, 45, 46]. ^{18}F-FDG positron emission tomography (PET) shows sensitivity of 91–100% and specificity of 78–100% in differentiating malignant from benign pleural disease. However, the high rate of false positives (e.g. due to asbestos-related disease or parapneumonic effusion) and false negatives (e.g. due to low-grade malignancies) of this technique remains its drawback. PET may also have a role for monitoring treatment response and detecting recurrent disease [5, 28, 47, 48].

11.3   Painful Chest Wall Conditions

11.3.1   Chest Trauma

US has been reported to be superior to CXR in the diagnosis of rib fractures, haemothoraces and peripheral lung contusions in a blunt trauma setting [49]. However, it is not routinely performed due to its time-consuming and operator-dependency characteristics. Initial CXR may miss about 50% of rib fractures, and CT may be useful in doubtful cases to depict rib fractures and associated thoracic abnormalities [32, 50, 51]. Indeed, CT is more sensitive than CXR in the detection and characterization of thoracic injuries and is considered the gold standard imaging tool for trauma [32, 52, 53].

Rib fractures are common lesions occurring in about 50% of blunt chest trauma [54]. The fourth to the eighth ribs are the most susceptible to external forces causing fractures [55, 56], while fractures of the first three ribs are usually caused by high-energy trauma, given the protection exerted by the shoulder girdle, and injuries to the brachial plexus or subclavian vessels must be ruled out [32, 56]. Lower ribs are relatively mobile and less susceptible to fracture. However, their injury can be associated with upper abdominal organ lesions (e.g. liver, spleen, kidney) [54, 56–58]. Flail chest is a traumatic condition in which three or more consecutive ribs are fractured in two or more places, creating a flail segment that moves paradoxically relative to the other ribs during respiration. Its recognition is of utmost importance and surgical treatment may be required [54, 58]. Sternal fractures usually involve body and manubrium and are caused by high-energy trauma. Sternal fractures are frequently associated with mediastinal hematoma and pulmonary, cardiac or spinal injuries. Importantly, respiratory artefacts and sternal constitutional abnormalities may mimic fractures and should be differentiated [32, 53, 59]. Clavicle and scapular fractures are also relatively common and easily depicted with CT, which is particularly useful in the assessment of sternoclavicular dislocations. Both these conditions are associated with high-energy trauma and may be a cause of serious morbidity, due to the impingement of the underlying vascular and nervous structures. If vascular injury is suspected, intravenous contrast should be administered [32, 58, 60].

Chest wall hematoma is a relatively uncommon condition associated with chest trauma, secondary to rib fractures injuring intercostal, internal mammary or subclavian arteries. The vascular lesion causes the accumulation of spontaneously hyperdense blood between the parietal pleura and the endothoracic fascia that may lead to large, biconvex hematomas [57, 61–63].

Diaphragmatic injury is seen in less than 8% of blunt trauma cases [55, 64]. The left side is more frequently involved than the right one (3:1 ratio) [32, 53]. Specific CXR findings for diaphragmatic injury are the presence of intrathoracic gastrointestinal air and an abnormal positioning of the nasogastric tube tip projecting above the left hemidiaphragm [65].

Diagnosis based on CXR is challenging, as suggestive findings for diaphragmatic injury, such as abnormal contours or elevation of the hemidiaphragm, and contralateral mediastinal shift can be detected in synchronous pulmonary abnormalities. Hence, the 12–66% of diaphragmatic rupture can be initially missed on CXR [64]. Sensitivity and specificity of CT are above 71 and 98%, respectively [65]. MPR images may show even small diaphragmatic tears, the latter allowing the herniation of peritoneal fat or abdominal viscera. The "collar sign" represents a waist-like constriction of the herniated viscera by the surrounding diaphragm (possibly detectable on CXR as well) [55]. Other findings consistent with diaphragmatic rupture are the lack of visualization of the hemidiaphragm or the focal loss of its continuity, although the latter can be congenital or acquired diaphragmatic defects also detectable in an asymptomatic individual [32, 33, 64, 65]. The "dependent viscera sign" is depicted as a herniated viscera (e.g. the stomach on the left side or the liver on the right side) in direct contact with the posterior thoracic wall and ribs, without the support of the intervening diaphragm [55, 65]. Like CT-MPR images, MRI could provide coronal and sagittal views useful to detect hemidiaphragmatic ruptures. Nevertheless, in the emergency setting, MRI applicability is limited by respiratory artefacts, long acquisition times and the need for patient cooperation [66]; thus, MRI should be proposed in cases of uncertain CT diagnosis [64].

11.3.2 Costochondritis

Tietze's syndrome, also known as costochondritis, is an idiopathic non-suppurative inflammatory process involving one or more costochondral cartilages. Tietze's syndrome more often affects females and typically manifests as a benign, painful swelling localised at costosternal, costochondral or sternoclavicular joints (Tietze's area) [67]. The diagnosis is primarily clinical, and radiology plays a role in doubtful cases to rule out other underlying

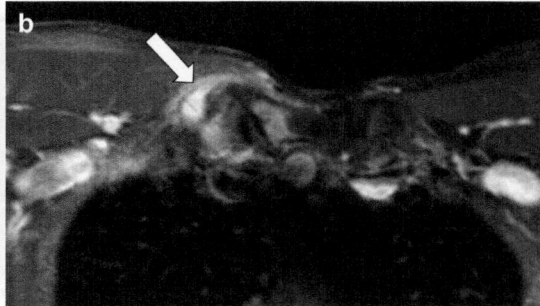

Fig. 11.9 Tietze's syndrome. (**a**) Coronal T1-WI TSE sequence of the right sternoclavicular joint depicting subchondral bone oedema on both articular surfaces (*black arrowhead*). (**b**) Axial T1-WI SPIR TSE sequence after contrast administration shows contrast enhancement of articular and periarticular structures (*white arrow*)

processes, firstly malignancy. CXR helps to exclude bone lesions, whereas US examination displays a heterogeneous increase of echogenicity and thickness in pathological cartilage. CT findings include cartilage enlargement and ventral angulation. MRI is an excellent technique for delineating cartilage and bone abnormalities, demonstrating cartilage enlargement and cartilage and subchondral bone oedema, in association with contrast enhancement of periarticular structures [67] (Fig. 11.9; Video 11.9). Scintigraphy with ^{99m}Tc or ^{67}Ga may show abnormal accumulation in the costochondritic area; however, the tracer accumulation is unspecific [67, 68]. Scintigraphy can be helpful in the management as it can estimate the inflammatory disease [69]; nevertheless, chest wall tumours may mimic Tietze's syndrome, and in such clinical setting, neither CT nor scintigraphy was found to be specific enough to rule out malignant diseases [70].

11.3.3 SAPHO Syndrome

The SAPHO syndrome is a rare condition characterized by a combination of skin and osteo-articular abnormalities (synovitis, acne, pustulosis, hyperostosis and osteitis) [71], affecting all age groups, with a slightly higher incidence reported in the female population [72]. The most common clinical feature is represented by anterior chest wall pain; indeed pain, swelling and limitation of movements are present at any site of articular active inflammation. Skin and skeletal abnormalities may be separated by many years.

In adults, the anterior chest wall is the most commonly involved site, in particular, the sternoclavicular (48%), costochondral (52%), manubriosternal (34%) and costosternal (7%) junctions [73]. In children and adolescents, it involves predominantly the metaphysis of long bones, especially distal femur, proximal and distal tibia and clavicles. The spine, particularly the thoracic segment, is the second most common localisation in children and adults.

On CXR, concomitant osteolysis and osteosclerosis are usually encountered: indeed, early lesions are mainly osteolytic, whereas later abnormalities tend to be osteoproliferative [74]. Bone expansion and medullary canal stenosis are evident, resulting from diffuse thickening of the periosteum, cortex and endosteum. Ossifications of the costoclavicular ligament with sclerosis and hyperostosis at the medial end of the clavicles, sternum and the first ribs are important findings, gradually progressing to ankylosis. MRI is useful in revealing subclinical foci and to identify active lesions by the presence of bone oedema on T2-WI and STIR sequences. Inflamed periarticular soft tissues are also well depicted on MRI. Due to the polyostotic nature of the disease, whole-body MRI has proved to be useful to detect subclinical and radiographically occult sites, depicted as areas of ill-defined oedema-like SI. Whole-body ^{99m}Tc scintigraphy can identify subclinical foci and symmetric high tracer uptake in the

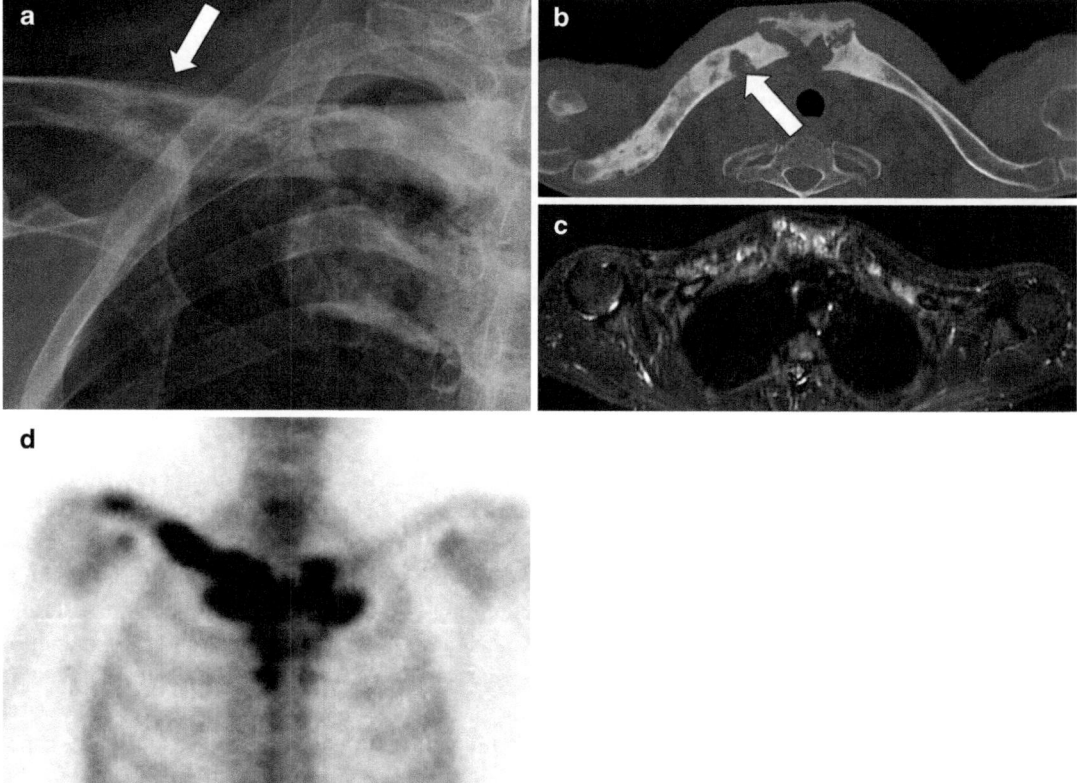

Fig. 11.10 SAPHO syndrome. (**a**) Magnification of the right clavicle radiograph of a patient suffering from anterior chest wall pain showing osteolytic and osteosclerotic osseous alterations with lamellar periosteal reaction (*white arrow*). (**b**) CT-MPR image depicts diffuse sclerosis and hyperostosis of both clavicles and sternal manubrium with concomitant osteolytic lesion of the right clavicle (*white arrow*). (**c**) Axial STIR sequence shows diffuse bone oedema. (**d**) Magnification of a whole-body ^{99m}Tc scintigraphy showing "bull's head" sign demonstrated by high tracer uptake in the sterno-costo-clavicular joints

sterno-costo-clavicular joints can produce a typical "bull's head" sign [71] (Fig. 11.10; Video 11.10). Since repeated follow-up imaging is likely to be necessary, the use of whole-body MRI is preferable to reduce the radiation burden.

11.3.4 Chest Wall Neoplasms

Rarely, chest pain can be caused by neoplasms and tumour-like lesions originating from any tissue of the chest wall, more frequently reported in malignant neoplasms [75]. In particular, cancer-induced bone pain can be considered a type of mixed pain, involving both inflammatory (nociceptive) and neuropathic mechanisms, as tumour expansion induces tissue damage and release of various inflammatory mediators [76].

Chest wall tumours, arising from both osseous and soft tissues, may display non-specific findings. However, a systematic approach based on patient age, clinical history, location, extent, mineralization pattern and intrinsic MRI features of the lesion can narrow the differential diagnosis [77].

While metastases are the most commonly encountered skeletal tumours, particularly in elderly patients, primary malignancies are rare; among them, the most frequent are represented by chondrosarcomas (originating from costo-

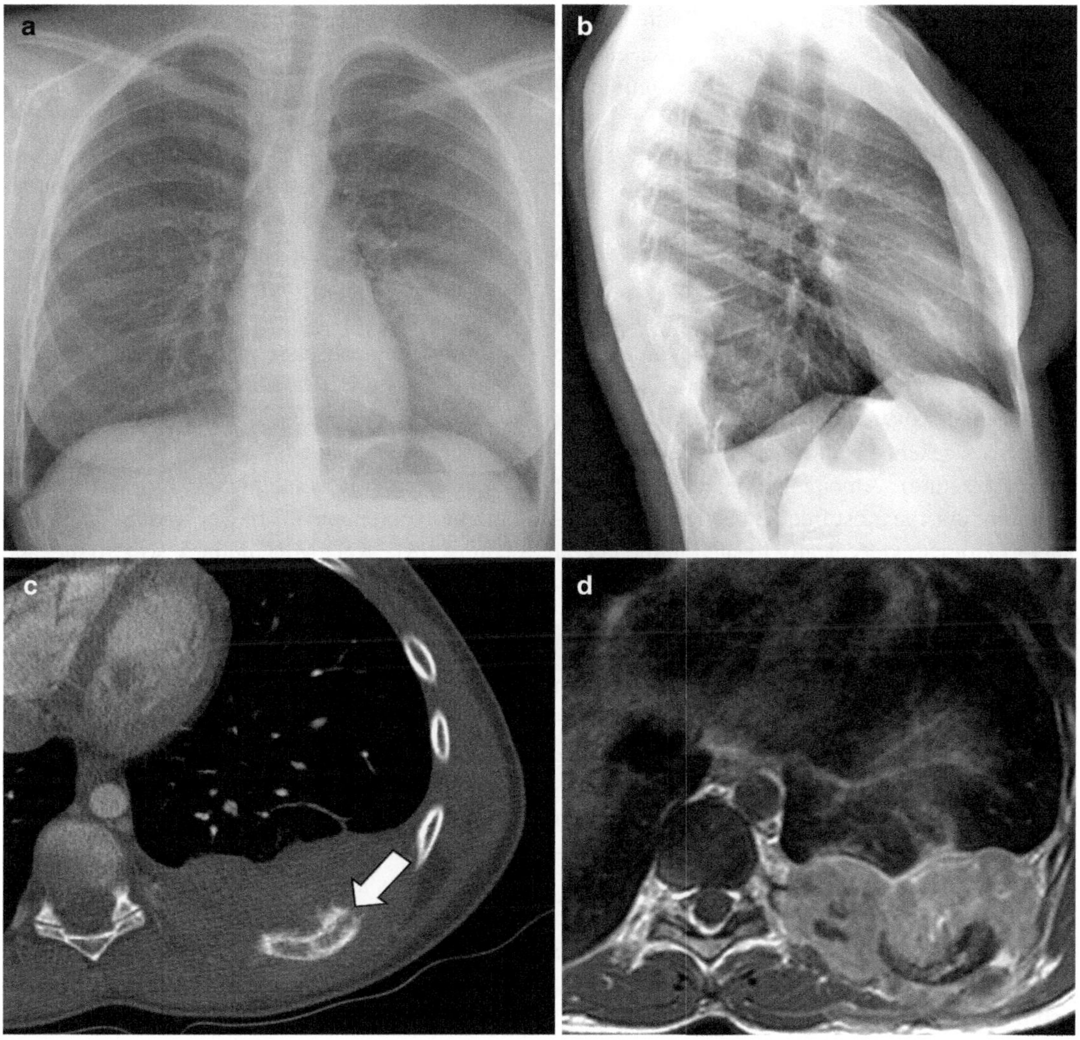

Fig. 11.11 Ewing sarcoma. (**a, b**) Chest radiograph (frontal and lateral views) of a young female patient with chest pain showing a large lobulated opacity in the left hemithorax. (**c**) Magnification of an axial CT image after contrast administration shows a soft tissue mass causing destruction of the posterior arch of the ninth left rib with spiculated periosteal reaction (*white arrow*). (**d**) Magnification of a MRI T1-WI TSE sequence after contrast administration shows a heterogeneous soft tissue mass with intense and diffuse contrast enhancement

chondral arches or sternum) and myelomas [77]. In paediatric individuals, the most frequent chest wall primary bone tumour is Ewing sarcoma [75] (Fig. 11.11; Video 11.11). Signs of malignancy are the extensive cortical destruction (evaluable on CT) and the extraosseous soft tissue mass formation (better characterized on MRI).

Furthermore, CT is valuable in narrowing the differential diagnosis by differentiating between mineralization patterns of the tumorous matrix (i.e. chondroid from osteoid). On CT, chondrosarcoma usually presents as a well-circumscribed lobulated soft tissue mass with "arc-and-ring" appearance, flocculent or stippled or dense calcifications and cortical destruction [77, 78]; on MRI, SI is similar to muscular tissues on T1-WI and hyperintense on T2-WI, associated with areas of signal void on both T1- and T2-WI, reflecting areas of mineralization [78, 79].

Chest wall osteosarcoma is a rare entity, usually arising in ribs, scapula and clavicle and displaying as a soft tissue mass with typical osteoid matrix CT features, i.e. dense, cloudy or ivory-like calcifications predominantly located in the central portion, with a lesser extent of mineralization in the periphery [77–79]. On MRI, it shows a SI higher to muscular tissues on T1-WI and high SI on T2-WI [79]. Matrix mineralization areas show low SI on both T1- and T2-WI MRI [78].

Benign osseous lesions usually manifest as slow-growing palpable masses in asymptomatic patients. Sometimes, chest wall bone neoplasms are indeed discovered only after a fracture occurs in a bone weakened by tumour growth (i.e. pathological fracture). Among benign osseous chest wall tumours, the most frequent is fibrous dysplasia (30% of cases), typically located in the lateral or posterior arc of a rib and in the clavicle; osteochondroma and enchondroma are less frequent, and chondroblastoma, aneurysmal bone cyst and giant cell tumours are rare. Fibrous dysplasia can be evaluated as an osteolytic lesion, with amorphous calcification or cartilaginous mineralization, without osseous erosion [77, 78]. CT findings consistent with osteochondroma are the detection of a cartilage cap, associated with a cortex in continuity with the medullary bone; on MRI, the cartilage cap is hyperintense in T2-WI [75].

Globally, many soft tissue neoplasms share similar characteristics at imaging examination, and the differential diagnosis can be challenging; therefore, biopsies are frequently required.

The most common soft tissue malignant tumour is the undifferentiated pleomorphic sarcoma (or malignant fibrous histiocytoma), detectable as a non-specific heterogeneously enhancing mass, located in the muscle and fascia planes. In the paediatric population, rhabdomyosarcoma and peripheral primitive neuroectodermal tumour ("Askin tumour") are more frequently encountered. On CT, Askin tumour may be depicted as large heterogeneous soft tissue mass with or without pleural effusion and rib destruction, demonstrating inhomogeneous contrast enhancement. On MRI, the mass shows high SI on T1-WI and on T2-WI [80].

11.3.5 Chest Wall Infections

Primary chest wall infections are rare life-threatening conditions and may rise spontaneously or in association with various predisposing factors, such as diabetes mellitus, intravenous drug addiction, immunosuppression, history of trauma or chest wall surgery. Secondary forms are more frequent, following pulmonary or pleural infections [81, 82].

Common causative micro-organisms are *Staphylococcus*, *Pseudomonas* and *Klebsiella* species. CT can show osseous destruction with periosteal reaction, adjacent soft tissue mass and loss of deep soft tissue planes; furthermore, CT can guide percutaneous biopsy and drainage procedures [81, 82]. MRI defines soft tissue and bone involvement, also allowing demonstration of bone oedema on fluid-sensitive sequences.

Tubercular chest wall involvement is unusual (1–5% of all cases of musculoskeletal tuberculosis). It may be due to contiguous spread from pulmonary or pleural diseases or, more frequently, to hematogenous dissemination. Affected sites are sternum, costochondral and costo-vertebral junctions, ribs and vertebral bodies [83]. CXR and CT show osseous and cartilaginous destruction associated with a soft tissue mass with calcification and rim enhancement after intravenous contrast administration [81]. PET-CT and PET-MRI evaluating ^{18}F-FDG uptake can be used to detect active granulomatous inflammatory foci [83].

11.4 Oesophageal Causes of Chest Pain

Chronic and acute oesophageal diseases frequently cause noncardiac chest pain [2, 3, 84]. Barium contrast-enhanced oesophagography (barium swallow, BS) evaluates swallowing function, oesophageal motility and morphology [85]. Multiphasic BS includes upright double-contrast views—obtained after ingestion of effervescent agents and a high-density barium suspension—for the visualization of the mucosal

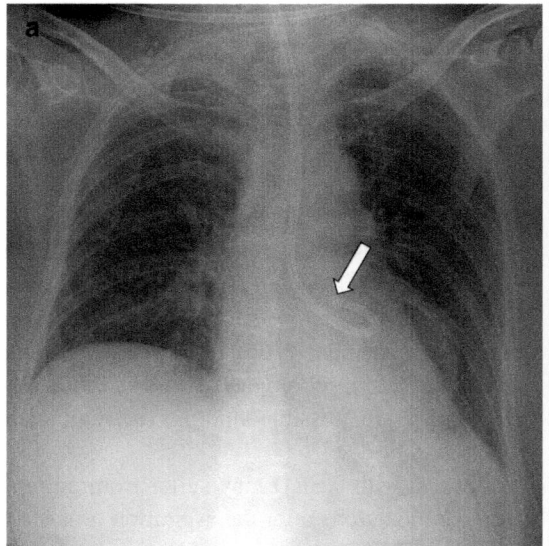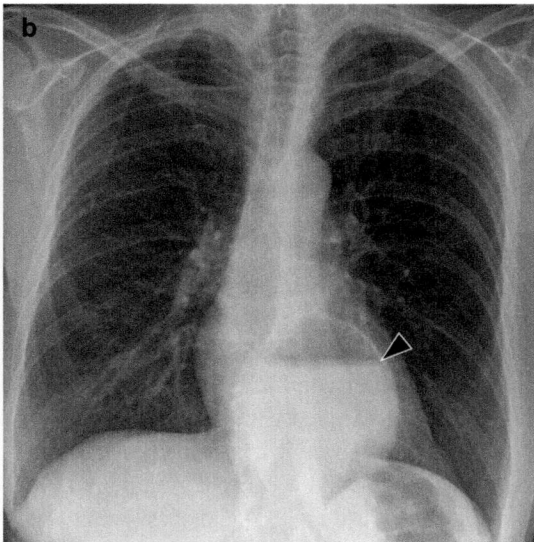

Fig. 11.12 Hiatal hernia. (**a**) Chest radiograph (supine position) of a patient demonstrating a loop of the nasogastric tube with the tip (*white arrow*) in a supradiaphragmatic position. (**b**) A previous chest radiograph shows a large medial opacity with air-fluid level (*black arrowhead*), reflecting a hiatal hernia thus justifying the abnormal tube position

layer, associated with prone single-contrast views acquired with a low-density barium suspension [85, 86].

11.4.1 Hiatal Hernia

Acquired alterations of the phreno-oesophageal membrane with reduced stability of the gastroesophageal junction (GEJ) allow the gastric herniation through the oesophageal hiatus. Different types of hiatal hernia are possible, namely, type I, sliding-hernia; type II, paraesophageal-hernia [87]; type III, in which features of sliding- and paraesophageal-hernias are associated; and type IV, in which abdominal organs (e.g. spleen, colon and small intestine) herniate into the thoracic cavity through a large phreno-oesophageal membrane defect [88, 89]. Hiatal hernias can cause retrosternal and epigastric pain [90]. On CXR, they are suspected when the gastric air bubble—possibly with air-fluid level—is detected in a supradiaphragmatic position, either in the frontal (air bubble in the midline) or in the lateral (air bubble behind

heart) view [87] (Fig. 11.12). Type IV intestinal hernias show intestinal gas, eventually with air-fluid levels, in the thoracic cavity [90]. BS has a high sensitivity to detect hiatal hernias [91]. To diagnose a type I hernia, the GEJ (traduced by the "B" ring) and the diaphragmatic hiatus should be more than 2 cm apart (i.e. gastric cardia at least 2 cm above the hiatus) [89]. Radiological pitfalls (i.e. dynamic location of GEJ, anatomical variability) can be overcome through provocative manoeuvres depicting even small hernias [88]. For type II hernia, BS shows the GEJ located below the diaphragm and the gastric fundus in a supradiaphragmatic para-oesophageal location [87]. When a complicated hernia is suspected, the patient should be administered a hydro-soluble contrast media, given the risk of aspiration pneumonia [92]; type IV hernias complicated by intestinal obstruction depict proximally dilated intestinal portions [90]. At CT, herniated gastric folds and abdominal organs are frequently clearly depicted [87, 90]. Similarly, coronal and sagittal MRI images allow the evaluation of the diaphragm and the hernial orifice [90].

11.4.2 Gastroesophageal Reflux Disease

About 60% of patients with noncardiac chest pain [93] suffer from gastroesophageal reflux disease (GERD), a common disease (prevalence, 10–20%) caused by a combination of frequent transient lower oesophageal sphincter (LES) relaxations, reduced LES tone and ineffective oesophageal motility [94, 95]. Regurgitation (i.e. the perception of refluxed gastric secretions) and heartburn (i.e. substernal discomfort/burning) are common and may be associated with laryngeal manifestations (chronic laryngitis, laryngospasm, vocal cord dysfunction and vocal fold granuloma) [96], chronic cough, asthma [95] and chest pain [97].

GERD is diagnosed according to clinical findings, oesophageal pH monitoring (either with trans-nasal catheter or wireless capsule), upper endoscopy and oesophageal manometry [94]. BS has been excluded from the diagnostic workup because it was thought to have a limited role in detecting GER [3, 94]. Nevertheless, provocative manoeuvres (e.g. water-siphon test) increase the sensitivity of BS for GERD from 26 to 70% [95], and a recent consensus stated that BS—being inexpensive, non-invasive and widely available—detects morphologic and functional alterations, such as hiatal hernia, short oesophagus or achalasia, that may modify the surgical approach [97, 98]. In particular, a short oesophagus may appear as a not reducing hiatal hernia with the patient in the upright position [88]. Fluoroscopy may directly highlight the oesophageal reflux, and its level and the clearance time are useful information for the surgeon to evaluate the extent and severity [88]. Single-contrast views show advanced findings of reflux oesophagitis, while the double-contrast views had greater sensitivity for superficial reflux ulcers and early findings, such as an extensive granularity oedema of the distal mucosa and thickened submucosal folds [88]. Reflux ulcers appear as polymorphous barium collections (punctate, linear or serpiginous), mainly located in the proximal area of the GEJ [85]. CT scans after intravenous contrast media administration may demonstrate thickened or highly enhanced oesophageal mucosa [84].

The persistent mucosal damage caused by refluxed gastric secretions leads to collagen deposition and to the development of peptic strictures (PS) [7]. On BS, PS appear as not-distensible distal narrowing or ring-like structures, with proximal oesophageal dilation [85]. Most PS are 1–4 cm long and 0.2–2 cm wide and they may be associated with pseudodiverticula [99]. Differential diagnoses are Schatzki rings, scleroderma, Barrett's oesophagus and nasogastric tube placement [100]. Luminal narrowing with irregular morphologies, ulcers and mucosal granularity are possible findings of malignant strictures [99].

Patients with GERD may suffer from pulmonary complications after the aspiration of gastric secretions; CXR and CT may show segmental/lobar consolidations, tree-in-bud opacities, eventually with lower lobes' predominance and pleural effusion [101, 102].

11.4.3 Infectious Oesophagitis

Individuals with oesophageal infections (e.g. candidiasis and herpesvirus) may suffer from odynophagia, dysphagia and retrosternal pain [103]. While candidiasis is the most common opportunistic oesophageal infection and may be secondary to achalasia, herpesvirus is the most common among viral oesophagitis [85, 86, 104]. In candidiasis, double-contrast oesophagogram shows linear, longitudinally oriented, plaque-like defects with discrete borders interposed to normal mucosa [85, 104]. This pattern has a sensitivity of about 90% and patients can be directly administered with antifungal therapy [85]. In patients with AIDS and candidiasis, oesophagus may have a "shaggy" appearance, with innumerable coalescent plaques and pseudomembranes trapping the barium [86, 104]. Double-contrast oesophagogram depicting small (<1 cm), multiple and superficial ulcers with discrete borders in the upper and mid-oesophagus, located in a background of normal mucosa (without plaques), is suggestive of herpesvirus oesophagitis [86, 104]. Giant ulcers (>1 cm) are found in cytomegalovirus oesophagitis [85].

11.4.4 Achalasia

Achalasia is a primary oesophageal motility disorder of unknown aetiology, characterized by absent oesophageal peristalsis and impaired LES relaxations [105]. Achalasia has a prevalence of 10/100.000; individuals report dysphagia (98% of patients), regurgitation (72%), chest pain (42%), and—eventually—weight loss [106]. A secondary form of achalasia is caused by tumours or benign conditions (e.g. Chagas disease) [107]. CXR may show the oesophageal dilation as a greater right-sided convexity of the azygo-oesophageal recess associated with an opacity behind the right heart border. In long-standing achalasia, the dilated oesophagus, eventually full of fluid and food debris, can be observed in the midline or above the azygos arch appearing as consolidation, or it can anteriorly displace the trachea. The gastric air bubble is frequently absent [108]. Furthermore, CXR allows the detection of complications like aspiration pneumonitis.

Oesophagography may show oesophageal dilation associated with a narrow GEJ with "bird beak" appearance, lack of oesophageal peristalsis, reduced barium clearance with retained food and saliva producing an air-fluid level [109, 110] (Fig. 11.13). BS in patients with long-standing achalasia may show morphologic changes (i.e. sigmoid oesophagus or megaoesophagus) [106, 109]. In older individuals (>60 years) with a recent onset of symptoms, a narrowed distal oesophageal segment longer than 3.5 cm—with little or absent proximal dilation—is consistent with pseudo-achalasia, secondary to malignant neoplasm, even without other suspicious findings, such as eccentricity, nodularity, shouldering of the oesophageal segment or gastric cardia and fundic lesions [86, 107]. The "timed" BS quantifies oesophageal emptying, either before or after therapy, through the evaluation of changes of the barium column's height. The "timed" oesophagograms are acquired 1 and 5 min after the ingestion of a low-density barium suspension in the upright position [111]. CT findings of primary and secondary achalasia are distal oesophageal narrowing that appears smooth in primary and irregular in secondary forms. Furthermore, secondary

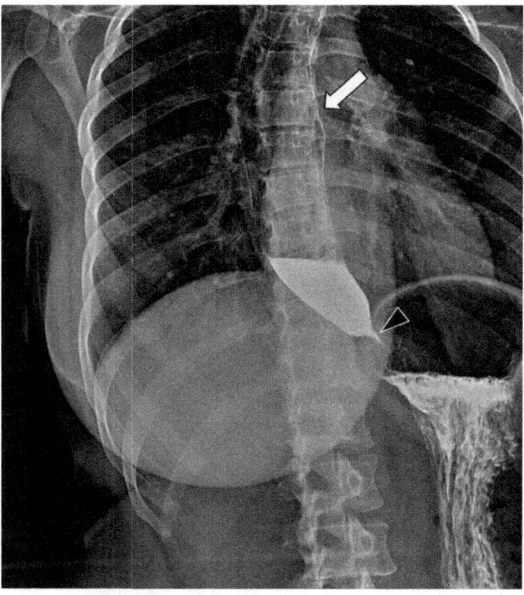

Fig. 11.13 Achalasia. (**a**) Oesophagography of a female patient suffering from long-standing chest pain and dysphagia showing a narrow gastro-oesophageal junction with "bird beak" appearance and oesophageal dilation (*white arrow*) with air-fluid level

achalasia depicts asymmetric nodular or lobulated thickened walls. Adjunctive CT findings consistent with secondary achalasia are soft tissue masses at the GEJ, mediastinal lymphadenopathies and/or distant metastases [112].

11.4.5 Diffuse Oesophageal Spasm

Diffuse oesophageal spasm (DES) is a motility disorder of unknown aetiology, characterized by intermittently abnormal peristalsis with multiple, simultaneous non-peristaltic contractions [86]. The "corkscrew" compartmentalized oesophageal appearance is a classic finding of DES and derives from a combination of intermittently absent primary peristalsis with severe lumen-obliterating non-peristaltic repetitive contractions [86, 113]. However, the "corkscrew" finding may be absent in patients with DES characterized by non-lumen-obliterating non-peristaltic contractions and impaired opening of the LES [114, 115]. BS may define the oesophageal bolus transit and stasis, as well as the presence of epiphrenic diverticula [115].

11.4.6 Oesophageal Emergencies

11.4.6.1 Oesophageal Rupture

Oesophageal rupture can be iatrogenic (most common, caused by non-surgical and surgical procedures), traumatic, spontaneous or neoplastic (rare, malignant neoplasms account for about 1% of cases) [116, 117]. CXR may show indirect findings, such as pneumomediastinum (PNM), PTX, subcutaneous emphysema, pleural effusion, hydrothorax, and lung collapse [118]. In patients with oesophageal perforation and PNM, frontal view may show Naclerio's V sign, a V-shaped air lucency that outlines the left lower mediastinal area and the left medial hemidiaphragm [119]. Hydro-soluble contrast media oesophagography should be preferred over BS; indeed, although barium has a higher diagnostic accuracy for cervical and thoracic perforations, it may cause inflammatory reaction leading to mediastinitis and granuloma formations [117, 120]. Mediastinal or pleural extravasation of contrast material is a key finding [120] (Fig. 11.14; Video 11.14). The procedure should be repeated after 4–6 h in case of

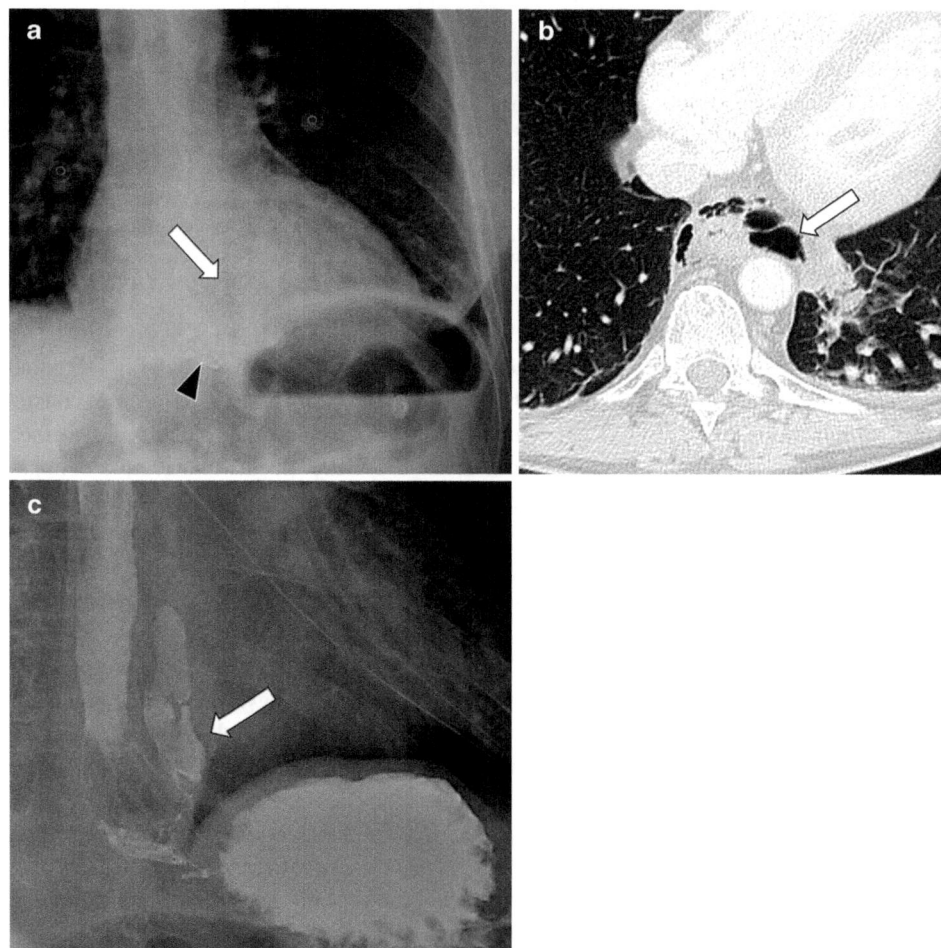

Fig. 11.14 Oesophageal perforation. (**a**) Chest radiograph (frontal view) of a male patient with chest pain and hematemesis after an endoscopic procedure causing an oesophageal perforation; during the procedure endoscopic clips (*black arrowhead*) were positioned. Mediastinal air can be highlighted (*white arrow*). (**b**) Axial CT image confirming pneumomediastinum (*white arrow*). (**c**) Hydro-soluble contrast media oesophagography clearly demonstrates mediastinal extravasation of contrast material (*white arrow*)

negative results with persistent strong clinical suspicion of oesophageal perforation, given that 10–38% of cases can be falsely negative [118, 121]. On CT, presence, location and severity of perforation are depicted by extravasation of oral contrast media. Additional findings are mediastinal gas bubble/fluid, oesophageal wall thickening, pneumopericardium, PTX and pneumoperitoneum [118, 120]. CT is particularly useful to define the underlying cause of the oesophageal perforation, e.g. foreign bodies or tumours, as well as complications such as oesophago-respiratory fistulas [122].

11.4.6.2 Boerhaave Syndrome

Spontaneous oesophageal perforations (Boerhaave syndrome) are rare life-threatening surgical emergencies, usually occurring in middle-aged men presenting with severe chest pain, vomiting and subcutaneous emphysema. The complete transmural laceration—usually in the left posterior wall immediately above the diaphragm—results from an increased intra-oesophageal pressure caused by straining or vomiting associated with an incomplete cricopharyngeal relaxation [100, 116, 121]. CXR may show a widened mediastinum, subcutaneous emphysema, PNM (eventually suggested by Naclerio's V sign), hydro-PTX, large pleural effusions and pulmonary consolidations [116, 120]. Hydro-soluble contrast media, preferred over barium to reduce the risk of mediastinitis, may extravasate at a supradiaphragmatic level. Other findings are submucosal contrast media collections, oesophago-pleural fistulas and gas collections, most frequently in the left distal oesophageal portion [116]. To increase sensitivity for perforations, during follow-up the patients can be administered with barium [116]. Axial and MPR CT images allow to detect supradiaphragmatic perioesophageal gas collections, thickened oesophageal wall, intramural hematoma and mediastinal fluid [123]. The oral administration of 10% diluted iodinated contrast medium ("CT-oesophagography") was demonstrated to be capable of visually documenting the oesophageal perforation through extraluminal contrast leakage [121], which may be associated with air (with possible air-contrast media levels) and debris [124].

11.4.6.3 Mallory-Weiss Syndrome

Mallory-Weiss syndrome is characterized by longitudinal mucosal lacerations located in the distal oesophagus or across the GEJ, usually associated with forceful retching or vomiting. On oesophagography, barium can—rarely—be depicted into linear mucosal tear; indeed, the latter is usually not radiologically detectable. Nevertheless, on CT haemorrhage or extraluminal gas can occasionally be present at the site of the mucosal tear [124].

11.4.6.4 Intramural Hematoma of the Oesophagus

Intramural hematoma of the oesophagus (IHE) is an uncommon condition resulting from haemorrhage within the oesophageal wall, usually in the distal portion. The resulting hematoma may dissect the submucosa and eventually disrupt the mucosa or the muscularis mucosae. IHE can be spontaneous, traumatic, emetogenic or a consequence of abnormal haemostasis or an aortic disease [116, 125]. CXR may show a widened mediastinum (with large intramural hematoma) or an elongated high-density mass in the oesophageal anatomic location, reflecting a distended oesophagus. PNM, PTX and pleural effusion suggest oesophageal perforation [125]. Hydro-soluble contrast media oesophagography depicts a well-defined filling defect and the "double-barrelled" oesophagus, in case of a communication between the hematoma and the oesophageal lumen secondary to mucosal rupture. Contrast media extravasation suggests an oesophageal rupture [116, 125]. CT scans show oesophageal wall thickening, either symmetric or asymmetric, and a well-defined concentric or eccentric intramural posterior mass, not enhancing after intravenous contrast media administration; exceptions are IHE secondary to aorto-oesophageal fistulas, which adjunctively may show irregular aortic outpouching with air in or around the vessel, and passage of contrast media between aorta and oesophagus [126]. Air within the hematoma suggests mucosal tear or infection; air within the mediastinum suggests transmural rupture [116, 125]. CT densitometric measurements reveal blood attenuation values, varying with the age of the hematoma (i.e. high values for fresh blood and subsequent gradual decrease) [127]. MRI precisely delineates the age of the hematoma and—given the lack or radiation exposure—can be proposed during follow-up [127, 128].

11.4.6.5 Oesophageal Fistulas

Fistulas between the oesophagus and its adjacent structures (e.g. trachea, pericardium, aorta) follow inflammatory and/or infective tissue destruction caused by either benign or malignant diseases [100, 124] (Fig. 11.15; Video 11.15). Patients suffering from oesophago-respiratory fistulas usually refer coughing attacks after swallowing, xerostomia and neck and chest pain [116]. For oesophago-respiratory fistulas, CXR can show the presence of aspiration pneumonitis, with unilateral/bilateral pulmonary consolidations [129]. Oesophagography performed after oral administration of non-ionic hydro-soluble contrast media usually allows the diagnosis of oesophago-respiratory fistulas, demonstrating the fistulous tract with contrast media flowing into the tracheobronchial tree and the pulmonary parenchyma [116, 129]. Other types of fistulas are similarly depicted as oesophagography

shows the fistulous tract (e.g. between the oesophagus and stomach) [124]. CT highlights fistulas even not detected at the contrast-enhanced oesophagography and can define presence, number, location and extent of the fistulous tract [116, 130]; furthermore, the detectability can be increased with oral administration of contrast media to expand the fistulous tract. MIP and MPR images allow a multiplanar evaluation of the fistulous tract. Virtual endoscopy can define size and location of the fistula guiding endoscopic biopsy and treatment [131, 132].

11.4.7 Foreign Body Impaction

Sites of physiological oesophageal luminal narrowing (the upper oesophageal sphincter at the thoracic inlet, the mid-oesophagus at the aortic arch and the LES at the GEJ) are the locations where ingested foreign bodies (FB) most commonly impact [100].

In infants and young children, the ingestion of coins or batteries may be associated with chest pain, and—particularly for batteries—the mucosal corrosive damage can lead to critical consequences [133, 134]. Frontal and lateral radiographies of the neck, chest and abdomen depict the presence and number of radiopaque FB

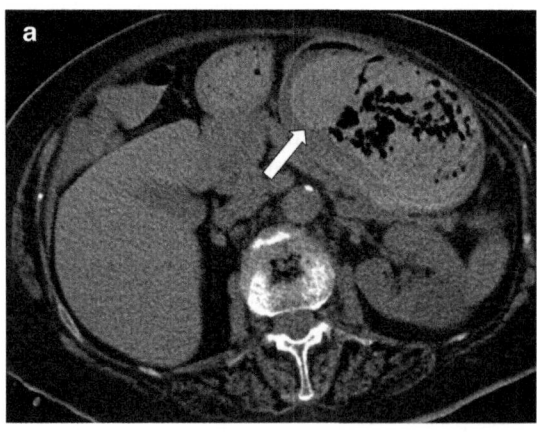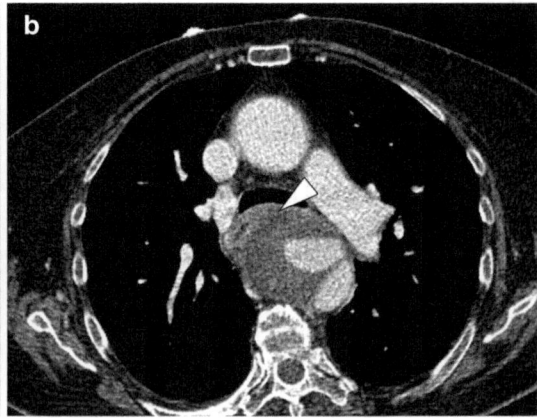

Fig. 11.15 Aorto-oesophageal fistula. (**a**) Native CT image of a female patient with digestive haemorrhage and previous diagnosis of type B aortic dissection showing hyperdense material in the gastric lumen (*white arrow*), consistent with blood clots. (**b**) CT image after contrast administration at a carinal level with a lack of visualization of fatty planes between the oesophagus and thoracic descending aorta (*white arrowhead*). The findings were suggestive of an aorto-oesophageal fistula

and can differentiate between coins, magnets and button batteries [134, 135]. Visibility and detection of low-opacity FB on neck radiographs can be increased through a low peak kilovoltage technique (65–70 kVp), to increase contrast between tissues and FB [136]. In case of non-radiopaque foreign bodies (e.g. plastic toys, aluminium objects, fish bones, plant materials), fluoroscopic studies can be evaluated to detect FB—appearing as a filling defect after administration of hydro-soluble oral contrast media—and its locations, as well as the presence of obstruction [134]. In case of suspected obstruction or oesophageal perforation, the administration of barium should be avoided because of the risk of spillage into the mediastinal or pleural space [133] and because it can obscure the visualization of the FB during the endoscopic removal procedure [122]. CT can be performed if the FB is not detected on radiographies in patients with persistent symptoms, with clinical suspicion of abscess or gastrointestinal obstruction. MPR images may help to evaluate FB greater than 5 cm, with sharp margins [134], and to detect complications (perforations, fistulas, abscesses) [133].

11.4.8 Acute Mediastinitis

Acute mediastinitis (AM) is a life-threatening condition resulting from acute inflammation of the connective and adipose tissues surrounding the mediastinal structures secondary to surgery, oesophageal perforation or spread of infections such as sternal osteomyelitis, sternoclavicular septic arthritis and oropharyngeal, cervical and odontogenic infections (i.e. descending necrotizing mediastinitis) [116]. CXR may depict mediastinal widening associated with gas bubbles or air-fluid levels [137]. CT findings suspicious for AM are mediastinal fat haziness, mediastinal free gas bubbles, fluid collections, enlarged lymph nodes, pleural or pericardial effusions, lung infiltrates and sternal dehiscence. Among these findings, mediastinal fluid collections and free gas bubbles provide the higher diagnostic yield [138]. Furthermore, CT can guide the positioning of drainage tubes [137], if a low-density fluid collection is detected in a febrile patient [130, 139].

AM occurs in 0.5–5% of patients after trans-sternal cardiac procedures, and it is associated with high morbidity and mortality rates (7–80%) [137, 139]. The mediastinal widening on CXR is not a specific finding as it can reflect postsurgical haemorrhage and oedema. Furthermore, fluids and gas bubbles can persist for weeks after the removal of drainage tubes [139]. Sternal dehiscence is associated with AM and can be suspected in case of displacement or disruption of the sternal wires observed in serial CXR [116, 140].

11.4.9 Spontaneous Mediastinal Hematoma

Spontaneous mediastinal hematoma (SMH) is a rare condition occurring in patients with bleeding disorders, clotting abnormalities, mediastinal structures/masses' haemorrhage, mediastinal small-vessel injury following a sudden increase in intrathoracic pressure or a sustained hypertension [116, 141, 142]. CXR may depict mediastinal widening, eventually associated with signs of mediastinal haemorrhage detectable on supine CXR, such as abnormalities of the aortic contours [116, 143]. At CT, mediastinal hematomas may appear as soft tissue masses including areas of haemorrhage (high densitometric values in case of recent bleeding) with possible displacement/compression of mediastinal structures. Aortic dissection or extravasation is excluded after intravenous administration of contrast media. MRI can delineate the age of the hematoma according to changes of the signal intensity [116, 141, 142, 144].

References

1. Verschakelen JA, Bogaert J, De Wever W. Computed tomography in staging for lung cancer. Eur Respir J Suppl. 2002;35:40s–8s.
2. Gruettner J, Henzler T, Sueselbeck T, Fink C, Borggrefe M, Walter T. Clinical assessment of chest pain and guidelines for imaging. Eur J Radiol. 2012;81(12):3663–8.

3. Eslick GD, Fass R. Noncardiac chest pain: evaluation and treatment. Gastroenterol Clin North Am. 2003;32(2):531–52.

4. Lee LY, Yu J. Sensory nerves in lung and airways. Compr Physiol. 2014;4(1):287–324.

5. Cardinale L, Ardissone F, Gned D, Sverzellati N, Piacibello E, Veltri A. Diagnostic imaging and workup of Malignant Pleural Mesothelioma. Acta Biomed. 2017;88(2):134–42.

6. Husain LF, Hagopian L, Wayman D, Baker WE, Carmody KA. Sonographic diagnosis of pneumothorax. J Emerg Trauma Shock. 2012;5(1):76–81.

7. Dietrich CF, Mathis G, Blaivas M, Volpicelli G, Seibel A, Wastl D, et al. Lung B-line artefacts and their use. J Thorac Dis. 2016;8(6):1356–65.

8. Manson DE. Magnetic resonance imaging of the mediastinum, chest wall and pleura in children. Pediatr Radiol. 2016;46(6):902–15.

9. Trovato FM, Catalano D, Trovato GM. Thoracic ultrasound: an adjunctive and valuable imaging tool in emergency, resource-limited settings and for a sustainable monitoring of patients. World J Radiol. 2016;8(9):775–84.

10. McLoud TC, Flower CD. Imaging the pleura: sonography, CT, and MR imaging. Am J Roentgenol. 1991;156(6):1145–53.

11. Mercadante S, Vitrano V. Pain in patients with lung cancer: pathophysiology and treatment. Lung Cancer. 2010;68(1):10–5.

12. Hsu JS, Han IT, Tsai TH, Lin SF, Jaw TS, Liu GC, et al. Pleural tags on CT scans to predict visceral pleural invasion of non-small cell lung cancer that does not abut the pleura. Radiology. 2016;279(2):590–6.

13. Shiotani S, Sugimura K, Sugihara M, Kawamitsu H, Yamauchi M, Yoshida M, et al. Diagnosis of chest wall invasion by lung cancer: useful criteria for exclusion of the possibility of chest wall invasion with MR imaging. Radiat Med. 2000;18(5):283–90.

14. Shen KR, Meyers BF, Larner JM, Jones DR, American College of Chest P. Special treatment issues in lung cancer: ACCP evidence-based clinical practice guidelines (2nd edition). Chest. 2007;132(3 Suppl):290S–305S.

15. Bruzzi JF, Komaki R, Walsh GL, Truong MT, Gladish GW, Munden RF, et al. Imaging of non-small cell lung cancer of the superior sulcus: part 2: initial staging and assessment of resectability and therapeutic response. Radiographics. 2008;28(2):561–72.

16. Cardinale L, Priola AM, Priola SM, Boccuzzi F, Dervishi N, Lisi E, et al. Radiological contribution to the diagnosis of early postoperative complications after lung resection for primary tumor: a revisional study. J Thorac Dis. 2016;8(8):E643–52.

17. Shah SN, Bachur RG, Simel DL, Neuman MI. Does this child have pneumonia?: The rational clinical examination systematic review. JAMA. 2017;318(5):462–71.

18. Vilar J, Domingo ML, Soto C, Cogollos J. Radiology of bacterial pneumonia. Eur J Radiol. 2004;51(2):102–13.

19. Kaysin A, Viera AJ. Community-acquired pneumonia in adults: diagnosis and management. Am Fam Physician. 2016;94(9):698–706.

20. Zhang M, Liu ZH, Yang JX, Gan JX, Xu SW, You XD, et al. Rapid detection of pneumothorax by ultrasonography in patients with multiple trauma. Crit Care. 2006;10(4):R112.

21. Ball L, Vercesi V, Costantino F, Chandrapatham K, Pelosi P. Lung imaging: how to get better look inside the lung. Ann Transl Med. 2017;5(14):294.

22. Stark DD, Federle MP, Goodman PC, Podrasky AE, Webb WR. Differentiating lung abscess and empyema: radiography and computed tomography. AJR Am J Roentgenol. 1983;141(1):163–7.

23. Beigelman-Aubry C, Godet C, Caumes E. Lung infections: the radiologist's perspective. Diagn Interv Imaging. 2012;93(6):431–40.

24. Campos P. 109: Imagiologia das Lesões Pleurais. In: Marques Gomes S-M, editor. Tratado de Pneumologia; Sociedade Portuguesa de Pneumologa: Permanyer; 2003. p. 1429–42.

25. Gupta D, Hansell A, Nichols T, Duong T, Ayres JG, Strachan D. Epidemiology of pneumothorax in England. Thorax. 2000;55(8):666–71.

26. Connor ARO, Morgan WE. Clinical review radiological review of pneumothorax. BMJ. 2005;330:1493–7.

27. Chaturvedi A, Lee S, Klionsky N, Chaturvedi A. Demystifying the persistent pneumothorax: role of imaging. Insights Imaging. 2016;7(3):411–29.

28. Qureshi NR, Gleeson FV. Imaging of pleural disease. Clin Chest Med. 2006;27(2):193–213.

29. Kirkpatrick AW, Sirois M, Laupland KB, Liu D, Rowan K, Ball CG, et al. Hand-held thoracic sonography for detecting post-traumatic pneumothoraces: the extended focused assessment with sonography for trauma (EFAST). J Trauma. 2004;57(2):288–95.

30. Ball CG, Ranson K, Dente CJ, Feliciano DV, Laupland KB, Dyer D, et al. Clinical predictors of occult pneumothoraces in severely injured blunt polytrauma patients: a prospective observational study. Injury. 2009;40(1):44–7.

31. Blaivas M, Lyon M, Duggal S. A prospective comparison of supine chest radiography and bedside ultrasound for the diagnosis of traumatic pneumothorax. Acad Emerg Med. 2005;12(9):844–9.

32. Palas J, Matos AP, Mascarenhas V, Herédia V, Ramalho M. Multidetector computer tomography: evaluation of blunt chest trauma in adults. Radiol Res Pract. 2014;2014:864369.

33. Ho ML, Gutierrez FR. Chest radiography in thoracic polytrauma. AJR Am J Roentgenol. 2009;192(3):599–612.

34. Waseem M, Jones J, Brutus S, Munyak J, Kapoor R, Gernsheimer J. Giant bulla mimicking pneumothorax. J Emerg Med. 2005;29(2):155–8.

35. Froudarakis ME. Diagnostic work-up of pleural effusions. Respiration. 2008;75(1):4–13.

36. Soni NJ, Franco R, Velez MI, Schnobrich D, Dancel R, Restrepo MI, et al. Ultrasound in the diagnosis and management of pleural effusions. J Hosp Med. 2015;10(12):811–6.

37. Hansell DM, Lynch DA, McAdams HP, Bankier AA. Imaging of Diseases of the Chest: Mosby; 2010, 11th December 2009. 1208 p.

38. Nelson M, Stankard B, Greco J, Okumura Y. Point of care ultrasound diagnosis of empyema. J Emerg Med. 2016;51(2):140–3.

39. Heffner JE, Klein JS, Hampson C. Diagnostic utility and clinical application of imaging for pleural space infections. Chest. 2010;137(2):467–79.

40. Raju S, Ghosh S, Mehta AC. Chest CT signs in pulmonary disease: a pictorial review. Chest. 2017;151(6):1356–74.

41. Nickell LT Jr, Lichtenberger JP 3rd, Khorashadi L, Abbott GF, Carter BW. Multimodality imaging for characterization, classification, and staging of malignant pleural mesothelioma. Radiographics. 2014;34(6):1692–706.

42. Miller BH, Rosado-de-Christenson ML, Mason AC, Fleming MV, White CC, Krasna MJ. From the archives of the AFIP. Malignant pleural mesothelioma: radiologic-pathologic correlation. Radiographics. 1996;16(3):613–44.

43. Qureshi NR, Rahman NM, Gleeson FV. Thoracic ultrasound in the diagnosis of malignant pleural effusion. Thorax. 2009;64(2):139–43.

44. Kim JS, Shim SS, Kim Y, Ryu YJ, Lee JH. Chest CT findings of pleural tuberculosis: differential diagnosis of pleural tuberculosis and malignant pleural dissemination. Acta Radiol. 2014;55(9):1063–8.

45. Gill RR, Patz S, Muradyan I, Seethamraju RT. Novel MR imaging applications for pleural evaluation. Magn Reson Imaging Clin N Am. 2015;23(2):179–95.

46. Coolen J, De Keyzer F, Nafteux P, De Wever W, Dooms C, Vansteenkiste J, et al. Malignant pleural disease: diagnosis by using diffusion-weighted and dynamic contrast-enhanced MR imaging--initial experience. Radiology. 2012;263(3):884–92.

47. Yildirim H, Metintas M, Entok E, Ak G, Ak I, Dundar E, et al. Clinical value of fluorodeoxyglucose-positron emission tomography/computed tomography in differentiation of malignant mesothelioma from asbestos-related benign pleural disease: an observational pilot study. J Thorac Oncol. 2009;4(12):1480–4.

48. Orki A, Akin O, Tasci AE, Ciftci H, Urek S, Falay O, et al. The role of positron emission tomography/computed tomography in the diagnosis of pleural diseases. Thorac Cardiovasc Surg. 2009;57(4):217–21.

49. Wustner A, Gehmacher O, Hammerle S, Schenkenbach C, Hafele H, Mathis G. Ultrasound diagnosis in blunt thoracic trauma. Ultraschall Med. 2005;26(4):285–90.

50. Chardoli M, Hasan-Ghaliaee T, Akbari H, Rahimi-Movaghar V. Accuracy of chest radiography versus chest computed tomography in hemodynamically stable patients with blunt chest trauma. Chin J Traumatol. 2013;16(6):351–4.

51. Livingston DH, Shogan B, John P, Lavery RF. CT diagnosis of Rib fractures and the prediction of acute respiratory failure. J Trauma. 2008;64(4):905–11.

52. Traub M, Stevenson M, McEvoy S, Briggs G, Lo SK, Leibman S, et al. The use of chest computed tomography versus chest X-ray in patients with major blunt trauma. Injury. 2007;38(1):43–7.

53. Ozmen A, Press D. Radiologic findings of thoracic trauma. Ther Clin Risk Manag. 2017;13:1085–9.

54. Dunham GM, Perez-Girbes A, Linnau KF. Core curriculum illustration: rib fractures. Emerg Radiol. 2017;24(3):325–7.

55. Oikonomou A, Prassopoulos P. CT imaging of blunt chest trauma. Insights Imaging. 2011;2(3):281–95.

56. Assi A-AN, Nazal Y. Rib fracture: different radiographic projections. Polish J Radiol. 2012;77(4):13–6.

57. Sangster GP, Gonzalez-Beicos A, Carbo AI, Heldmann MG, Ibrahim H, Carrascosa P, et al. Blunt traumatic injuries of the lung parenchyma, pleura, thoracic wall, and intrathoracic airways: multidetector computer tomography imaging findings. Emerg Radiol. 2007;14(5):297–310.

58. Kaewlai R, Avery LL, Asrani AV, Novelline RA. Multidetector CT of blunt thoracic trauma. Radiographics. 2008;28(6):1555–70.

59. Van Hise ML, Primack SL, Israel RS, Müller NL. CT in blunt chest trauma: indications and limitations. Radiographics. 1998;18(5):1071–84.

60. Miller LA. Chest wall, lung, and pleural space trauma. Radiol Clin North Am. 2006;44(2):213–24. viii.

61. Gavilanes EP. Current management of arterial blush and other vascular lesions identified by multidetector-CT in trauma patients. Eur Congress Radiol. 2014:1970. https://doi.org/10.1594/ecr2014/C-0375.

62. Mirka H, Ferda J, Baxa J. Multidetector computed tomography of chest trauma: indications, technique and interpretation. Insights Imaging. 2012;3(5):433–49.

63. Yao DC, Jeffrey RB, Mirvis SE. Using contrast-enhanced helical CT to visualise arterial extravasation after blunt abdominal trauma: incidence and organ distribution. AJR Am J Roentgenol. 2002;178:2000–3.

64. Iochum S, Ludig T, Walter F, Sebbag H, Grosdidier G, Blum AG. Imaging of diaphragmatic injury: a diagnostic challenge? Radiographics. 2002;22:Spec No:S103–16; discussion S16–8.

65. Desir A, Ghaye B. CT of blunt diaphragmatic rupture. Radiographics. 2012;32(2):477–98.

66. Bonatti M, Lombardo F, Vezzali N, Zamboni GA, Bonatti G. Blunt diaphragmatic lesions: Imaging findings and pitfalls. World J Radiol. 2016;8(10):819–28.

67. Volterrani L, Mazzei MA, Giordano N, Nuti R, Galeazzi M, Fioravanti A. Magnetic resonance imaging in Tietze's syndrome. Clin Exp Rheumatol. 2008;26(5):848–53.

68. Mendelson G, Mendelson H, Horowitz SF, Goldfarb CR, Zumoff B. Can (99m)technetium methylene diphosphonate bone scans objectively document costochondritis? Chest. 1997;111(6):1600–2.

69. Koc ZP, Balci TA, Ozyurtkan MO. The role of the three phase bone scintigraphy in the management of the patients with costochondral pain. Mol Imaging Radionucl Ther. 2013;22(3):90–3.

70. Kaplan T, Gunal N, Gulbahar G, Kocer B, Han S, Eryazgan MA, et al. Painful chest wall swellings: tietze syndrome or chest wall tumor? Thorac Cardiovasc Surg. 2016;64(3):239–44.

71. Rukavina I. SAPHO syndrome: a review. J Child Orthop. 2015;9(1):19–27.

72. Khanna L, El-Khoury GY. SAPHO syndrome--a pictorial assay. Iowa Orthop J. 2012;32:189–95.

73. Depasquale R, Kumar N, Lalam RK, Tins BJ, Tyrrell PN, Singh J, et al. SAPHO: what radiologists should know. Clin Radiol. 2012;67(3):195–206.

74. Schaub S, Sirkis HM, Kay J. Imaging for synovitis, acne, pustulosis, hyperostosis, and osteitis (SAPHO) syndrome. Rheum Dis Clin North Am. 2016;42(4):695–710.

75. Zapala MA, Ho-Fung VM, Lee EY. Thoracic neoplasms in children: contemporary perspectives and imaging assessment. Radiol Clin North Am. 2017;55(4):657–76.

76. Falk S, Dickenson AH. Pain and nociception: mechanisms of cancer-induced bone pain. J Clin Oncol. 2014;32(16):1647–54.

77. Nam SJ, Kim S, Lim BJ, Yoon CS, Kim TH, Suh JS, et al. Imaging of primary chest wall tumors with radiologic-pathologic correlation. Radiographics. 2011;31(3):749–70.

78. Carter BW, Benveniste MF, Betancourt SL, de Groot PM, Lichtenberger JP 3rd, Amini B, et al. Imaging evaluation of malignant chest wall neoplasms. Radiographics. 2016;36(5):1285–306.

79. Tateishi U, Gladish GW, Kusumoto M, Hasegawa T, Yokoyama R, Tsuchiya R, et al. Chest wall tumors: radiologic findings and pathologic correlation: part 2. Malignant tumors. Radiographics. 2003;23(6):1491–508.

80. Xu Q, Xu K, Yang C, Zhang X, Meng Y, Quan Q. Askin tumor: four case reports and a review of the literature. Cancer Imaging. 2011;11:184–8.

81. Jeung MY, Gangi A, Gasser B, Vasilescu C, Massard G, Wihlm JM, et al. Imaging of chest wall disorders. Radiographics. 1999;19(3):617–37.

82. Kuhlman JE, Bouchardy L, Fishman EK, Zerhouni EA. CT and MR imaging evaluation of chest wall disorders. Radiographics. 1994;14(3):571–95.

83. Boruah DK, Sanyal S, Sharma BK, Prakash A, Dhingani DD, Bora K. Role of cross sectional imaging in isolated chest wall tuberculosis. J Clin Diagn Res. 2017;11(1):TC01–TC6.

84. Kienzl D, Prosch H, Topker M, Herold C. Imaging of non-cardiac, non-traumatic causes of acute chest pain. Eur J Radiol. 2012;81(12):3669–74.

85. Levine MS, Rubesin SE. History and evolution of the barium swallow for evaluation of the pharynx and esophagus. Dysphagia. 2017;32(1):55–72.

86. Levine MS, Rubesin SE, Laufer I. Barium esophagography: a study for all seasons. Clin Gastroenterol Hepatol. 2008;6(1):11–25.

87. Sandstrom CK, Stern EJ. Diaphragmatic hernias: a spectrum of radiographic appearances. Curr Probl Diagn Radiol. 2011;40(3):95–115.

88. Canon CL, Morgan DE, Einstein DM, Herts BR, Hawn MT, Johnson LF. Surgical approach to gastroesophageal reflux disease: what the radiologist needs to know. Radiographics. 2005;25(6):1485–99.

89. Kahrilas PJ, Kim HC, Pandolfino JE. Approaches to the diagnosis and grading of hiatal hernia. Best Pract Res Clin Gastroenterol. 2008;22(4):601–16.

90. Eren S, Ciris F. Diaphragmatic hernia: diagnostic approaches with review of the literature. Eur J Radiol. 2005;54(3):448–59.

91. Weitzendorfer M, Kohler G, Antoniou SA, Pallwein-Prettner L, Manzenreiter L, Schredl P, et al. Preoperative diagnosis of hiatal hernia: barium swallow X-ray, high-resolution manometry, or endoscopy? Eur Surg. 2017;49(5):210–7.

92. Di Saverio S, Lombardi R, Bianchi E, Tugnoli G, Jovine E. An elderly woman with chest pain and constipation. BMJ. 2015;350:h166.

93. Faybush EM, Fass R. Gastroesophageal reflux disease in noncardiac chest pain. Gastroenterol Clin North Am. 2004;33(1):41–54.

94. Badillo R, Francis D. Diagnosis and treatment of gastroesophageal reflux disease. World J Gastrointest Pharmacol Ther. 2014;5(3):105–12.

95. Lacy BE, Weiser K, Chertoff J, Fass R, Pandolfino JE, Richter JE, et al. The diagnosis of gastroesophageal reflux disease. Am J Med. 2010;123(7):583–92.

96. Hu X, Lee JS, Pianosi PT, Ryu JH. Aspiration-related pulmonary syndromes. Chest. 2015;147(3):815–23.

97. Levine MS, Carucci LR, DiSantis DJ, Einstein DM, Hawn MT, Martin-Harris B, et al. Consensus statement of society of abdominal radiology disease-focused panel on barium esophagography in gastroesophageal reflux disease. AJR Am J Roentgenol. 2016;207(5):1009–15.

98. Moore M, Afaneh C, Benhuri D, Antonacci C, Abelson J, Zarnegar R. Gastroesophageal reflux disease: a review of surgical decision making. World J Gastrointest Surg. 2016;8(1):77–83.

99. Karasick S, Lev-Toaff AS. Esophageal strictures: findings on barium radiographs. AJR Am J Roentgenol. 1995;165(3):561–5.

100. Marini T, Desai A, Kaproth-Joslin K, Wandtke J, Hobbs SK. Imaging of the oesophagus: beyond cancer. Insights Imaging. 2017;8(3):365–76.

101. Prather AD, Smith TR, Poletto DM, Tavora F, Chung JH, Nallamshetty L, et al. Aspiration-related lung diseases. J Thorac Imaging. 2014;29(5):304–9.

102. Cardasis JJ, MacMahon H, Husain AN. The spectrum of lung disease due to chronic occult aspiration. Ann Am Thorac Soc. 2014;11(6):865–73.

103. Grossi L, Ciccaglione AF, Marzio L. Esophagitis and its causes: who is "guilty" when acid is found "not guilty"? World J Gastroenterol. 2017;23(17):3011–6.

104. Carucci LR, Turner MA. Dysphagia revisited: common and unusual causes. Radiographics. 2015;35(1):105–22.

105. Vaezi MF, Pandolfino JE, Vela MF. ACG clinical guideline: diagnosis and management of achalasia. Am J Gastroenterol. 2013;108(8):1238–49. quiz 50.

106. Stavropoulos SN, Friedel D, Modayil R, Parkman HP. Diagnosis and management of esophageal achalasia. BMJ. 2016;354:i2785.

107. Woodfield CA, Levine MS, Rubesin SE, Langlotz CP, Laufer I. Diagnosis of primary versus secondary achalasia: reassessment of clinical and radiographic criteria. AJR Am J Roentgenol. 2000;175(3):727–31.

108. Cole TJ, Turner MA. Manifestations of gastrointestinal disease on chest radiographs. Radiographics. 1993;13(5):1013–34.

109. Ates F, Vaezi MF. The pathogenesis and management of achalasia: current status and future directions. Gut Liver. 2015;9(4):449–63.

110. Patel DA, Kim HP, Zifodya JS, Vaezi MF. Idiopathic (primary) achalasia: a review. Orphanet J Rare Dis. 2015;10:89.

111. de Oliveira JM, Birgisson S, Doinoff C, Einstein D, Herts B, Davros W, et al. Timed barium swallow: a simple technique for evaluating esophageal emptying in patients with achalasia. AJR Am J Roentgenol. 1997;169(2):473–9.

112. Licurse MY, Levine MS, Torigian DA, Barbosa EMJ. Utility of chest CT for differentiating primary and secondary achalasia. Clin Radiol. 2014;69(10):1019–26.

113. Fonseca EK, Yamauchi FI, Tridente CF, Baroni RH. Corkscrew esophagus. Abdom Radiol (NY). 2017;42(3):985–6.

114. Prabhakar A, Levine MS, Rubesin S, Laufer I, Katzka D. Relationship between diffuse esophageal spasm and lower esophageal sphincter dysfunction on barium studies and manometry in 14 patients. AJR Am J Roentgenol. 2004;183(2):409–13.

115. Roman S, Kahrilas PJ. Distal esophageal spasm. Dysphagia. 2012;27(1):115–23.

116. Katabathina VS, Restrepo CS, Martinez-Jimenez S, Riascos RF. Nonvascular, nontraumatic mediastinal emergencies in adults: a comprehensive review of imaging findings. Radiographics. 2011;31(4):1141–60.

117. Madan R, Bair RJ, Chick JF. Complex iatrogenic esophageal injuries: an imaging spectrum. AJR Am J Roentgenol. 2015;204(2):W116–25.

118. Faggian A, Berritto D, Iacobellis F, Reginelli A, Cappabianca S, Grassi R. Imaging patients with alimentary tract perforation: literature review. Semin Ultrasound CT MR. 2016;37(1):66–9.

119. Sinha R. Naclerio's V sign. Radiology. 2007;245(1):296–7.

120. Carter BW, Erasmus JJ. Acute thoracic findings in oncologic patients. J Thorac Imaging. 2015;30(4):233–46.

121. Tonolini M, Bianco R. Spontaneous esophageal perforation (Boerhaave syndrome): diagnosis with CT-esophagography. J Emerg Trauma Shock. 2013;6(1):58–60.

122. Del Gaizo AJ, Lall C, Allen BC, Leyendecker JR. From esophagus to rectum: a comprehensive review of alimentary tract perforations at computed tomography. Abdom Imaging. 2014;39(4):802–23.

123. Ghanem N, Altehoefer C, Springer O, Furtwangler A, Kotter E, Schafer O, et al. Radiological findings in Boerhaave's syndrome. Emerg Radiol. 2003;10(1):8–13.

124. Young CA, Menias CO, Bhalla S, Prasad SR. CT features of esophageal emergencies. Radiographics. 2008;28(6):1541–53.

125. Restrepo CS, Lemos DF, Ocazionez D, Moncada R, Gimenez CR. Intramural hematoma of the esophagus: a pictorial essay. Emerg Radiol. 2008;15(1):13–22.

126. Sipe A, McWilliams SR, Saling L, Raptis C, Mellnick V, Bhalla S. The red connection: a review of aortic and arterial fistulae with an emphasis on CT findings. Emerg Radiol. 2017;24(1):73–80.

127. Yuen EH, Yang WT, Lam WW, Kew J, Metreweli C. Spontaneous intramural haematoma of the oesophagus: CT and MRI appearances. Australas Radiol. 1998;42(2):139–42.

128. Abbey P, Sharma R, Garg PK. Spontaneous intramural haematoma of the oesophagus: complete resolution on follow-up magnetic resonance imaging. Singapore Med J. 2009;50(9):e318–20.

129. Franquet T, Gimenez A, Roson N, Torrubia S, Sabate JM, Perez C. Aspiration diseases: findings, pitfalls, and differential diagnosis. Radiographics. 2000;20(3):673–85.

130. Gimenez A, Franquet T, Erasmus JJ, Martinez S, Estrada P. Thoracic complications of esophageal disorders. Radiographics. 2002;22:S247–58.

131. Hegde RG, Kalekar TM, Gajbhiye MI, Bandgar AS, Pawar SS, Khadse GJ. Esophagobronchial fistulae: diagnosis by MDCT with oral contrast swallow examination of a benign and a malignant cause. Indian J Radiol Imaging. 2013;23(2):168–72.

132. Sonomura T, Kishi K, Ishii S, Kawai N, Masuda M, Terada M, et al. Usefulness of CT virtual endoscopy in imaging a large esophagorespiratory fistula. Eur J Radiol. 2000;34(1):60–2.

133. Pinto A, Lanza C, Pinto F, Grassi R, Romano L, Brunese L, et al. Role of plain radiography in the assessment of ingested foreign bodies in the pediatric patients. Semin Ultrasound CT MR. 2015;36(1):21–7.

134. Pugmire BS, Lim R, Avery LL. Review of ingested and aspirated foreign bodies in children and their clinical significance for radiologists. Radiographics. 2015;35(5):1528–38.

135. Semple T, Calder AD, Ramaswamy M, McHugh K. Button battery ingestion in children-a potentially catastrophic event of which all radiologists must be aware. Br J Radiol. 2018;91(1081):20160781.

136. Guelfguat M, Kaplinskiy V, Reddy SH, DiPoce J. Clinical guidelines for imaging and reporting ingested foreign bodies. AJR Am J Roentgenol. 2014;203(1):37–53.

137. Athanassiadi KA. Infections of the mediastinum. Thorac Surg Clin. 2009;19(1):37–45. vi.

138. Exarhos DN, Malagari K, Tsatalou EG, Benakis SV, Peppas C, Kotanidou A, et al. Acute mediastinitis: spectrum of computed tomography findings. Eur Radiol. 2005;15(8):1569–74.

139. Akman C, Kantarci F, Cetinkaya S. Imaging in mediastinitis: a systematic review based on aetiology. Clin Radiol. 2004;59(7):573–85.

140. Restrepo CS, Martinez S, Lemos DF, Washington L, McAdams HP, Vargas D, et al. Imaging appearances of the sternum and sternoclavicular joints. Radiographics. 2009;29(3):839–59.

141. Mikubo M, Sonoda D, Yamazaki H, Naito M, Matsui Y, Shiomi K, et al. Spontaneous non-traumatic mediastinal hematoma associated with oral anticoagulant therapy: a case report and literature review. Int J Surg Case Rep. 2017;39: 221–4.

142. Chida Y, Inokuchi R, Ishida T, Shinohara K. Spontaneous mediastinal haematoma. BMJ Case Rep. 2016;2016.

143. Woodring JH, Loh FK, Kryscio RJ. Mediastinal hemorrhage: an evaluation of radiographic manifestations. Radiology. 1984;151(1):15–21.

144. Iskander M, Siddique K, Kaul A. Spontaneous atraumatic mediastinal hemorrhage: challenging management of a life-threatening condition and literature review. J Investig Med High Impact Case Rep. 2013;1(2):2324709613484451.

Abdominal Pain: Clinical Features

12

Marina Pace and Fabio Pace

12.1 Introduction

Abdominal pain is a frequent complaint and reason for consultation both in primary care [1] and emergency department [2]. It affects nearly every person once in their lifetime independent from age, gender, and social background [3, 4].

The evaluation of any patient with a complaint of abdominal pain is challenging. Abdominal pain can be caused by a broad spectrum of diseases from primarily trivial and self-limited (e.g., acute gastroenteritis) to life-threatening conditions (e.g., abdominal aortic aneurysm).

The distinction between acute, subacute, and chronic abdominal pain is related to the time frame: abdominal pain is considered acute when it has been occurring for several days (see below for an operative definition), subacute when it has been occurring more than several days but less than 6 months, and chronic when it has been occurring constantly or intermittently over at least 6 months [5].

In this chapter we will mainly focus on acute abdominal pain (AAP), which is frequently a challenging clinical situation, where a correct diagnosis is mandatory in the shortest possible time in order to start the proper medical or surgical therapy. Chronic abdominal pain is generally a clinical picture more frequently encountered in ambulatory patients seen by GPs or specialists outside the setting of an emergency department. Basically, the same organic causes may be present as those found in AAP, but differently from AAP, a functional etiology may be present, such as irritable bowel syndrome (IBS) or functional abdominal pain (FAP), in which all diagnostic laboratory or imaging tests are by definition negative (cfr Rome definition) [6]). For example, in a recent meta-analysis [1], it was found that in 14 studies considered, conducted in primary care, in about one-third of patients, the underlying cause of abdominal pain cannot be specified. The most common etiologies were gastroenteritis (7.2–18.7%), irritable bowel disease (2.6–13.2%), urological cause (5.3%), and gastritis (5.2%). About one in ten abdominal pain patients were suffering from an acute disease like appendicitis (1.9%), diverticulitis (3.0%), biliary/pancreatic (4.0%), or neoplastic (1.0%) diseases needing immediate therapy.

For these reasons, chronic abdominal pain will not be further considered here.

In the present chapter, we will briefly present the definition of AAP, consider the possible etiologies of AAP focusing on the abdominal sources, and describe the clinical features of them, examining the link between specific locations and specific causes of AAP. Finally, we will

M. Pace (✉)
Department of Radiology, Bicocca University, Milan, Italy
e-mail: m.pace10@campus.unimib.it

F. Pace
Gastrointestinal Unit, Bolognini Hospital, Seriate (Bergamo), Italy
e-mail: fabio.pace@unimi.it

© Springer Nature Switzerland AG 2019
M. A. Cova, F. Stacul (eds.), *Pain Imaging*, https://doi.org/10.1007/978-3-319-99822-0_12

consider the relevant diagnostic role of the physical examination, possibly coupled with a core of laboratory tests.

12.2   Epidemiology and Definition

The overall prevalence of AAP is difficult to estimate, since AAP is a heterogeneous and spectrum condition, which is both a frequent reason for presentation at the emergency department, with a reported figure ranging from 5 to 10% of total causes [2], and of consultation in the primary care setting, with a mean consultation prevalence of 2.8% [1]. AAP can be caused by conditions stemming from abdominal and extra-abdominal organs and by a variety of diseases ranging from mild and self-limiting to life-threatening diseases [2]. Clearly, an accurate and timely diagnosis is mandatory to an optimal triage and management of different causes of AAP, since urgent conditions often need a diagnosis within 24 h to prevent complicated or even fatal outcomes. Among common urgent causes, acute appendicitis, acute diverticulitis, and bowel obstruction are the most prevalent ones, whereas most frequent nonurgent causes are nonspecific abdominal pain (NSAP) and gastrointestinal diseases.

Despite several terms and definitions are currently used to describe patients with AAP, with the most common terms used being "acute abdomen" and "acute abdominal pain," we suggest to avoid the former because it misleadingly suggests an urgent condition needing a surgical management; we prefer, among others, the term "acute abdominal pain" which should be defined as abdominal pain of nontraumatic origin with a maximum duration of 5 days [7].

12.3   Clinical Assessment

The first step in the diagnostic pathway is clinical evaluation [7]. In everyday practice, a preliminary diagnosis will be made based on medical history, physical examination, and subsequently some laboratory parameters. Only after this first step, it can be decided whether or not additional diagnostic investigations are needed to increase the likelihood of the diagnosis. Thus, the distinctive features of pain must be carefully assessed, starting with location, intensity, and character of abdominal pain. Additionally, alleviating or aggravating factors could be considered and additional symptoms searched for.

Location Probably the first clue to understand the cause of AAP is to consider the exact location of pain, and therefore it should drive the evaluation [8]. Pain occurring in the right upper quadrant should suggest the possibility of cholelithiasis, cholangitis, colitis, diverticulitis, abscess, hepatitis, masses, pneumonia, and embolus. Pain occurring in the epigastrium can raise the suspicion of cholelithiasis, cholangitis, myocardial infarction, pericarditis, esophagitis, gastritis, peptic ulcer, pancreatitis, masses, aortic dissection, and mesenteric ischemia. In case of pain in the left upper quadrant, angina, myocardial infarction, pericarditis, esophagitis, gastritis, peptic ulcer, pancreatitis, masses, nephrolithiasis, pyelonephritis, aortic dissection, and mesenteric ischemia can be considered. Periumbilical pain location can suggest early appendicitis, esophagitis, gastritis, peptic ulcer, small bowel mass or obstruction, aortic dissection, or mesenteric ischemia, while in case pain occurs in the right lower quadrant, appendicitis, colitis, diverticulitis, IBD, IBS, ectopic pregnancy, fibroids, ovarian mass, torsion, PID, nephrolithiasis, or pyelonephritis should be ruled out. Similar possibilities (appendicitis, colitis, diverticulitis, IBD, IBS, ectopic pregnancy, fibroids, ovarian mass, torsion, PID, cystitis, nephrolithiasis, pyelonephritis) should be considered in case of soprapubic pain, while pain in the left lower quadrant is suggestive of colitis, diverticulitis, IBD, IBS, ectopic pregnancy, fibroids, ovarian mass, torsion, PID, nephrolithiasis, or pyelonephritis. Additionally, some disease can induce abdominal pain without any location preference (herpes zoster, muscle strain, hernia, bowel obstruction, mesenteric ischemia, peritonitis, narcotic withdrawal, sickle cell crisis, porphyria, IBD, heavy metal poisoning).

For some diagnoses, such as appendicitis, the location of pain has a very strong predictive value [9]. Based on this consideration, the American College of Radiology has developed clinical guidelines, called "Appropriateness Criteria," to help physicians choose the most appropriate imaging study based on AAP location. For appendicitis, right lower quadrant pain has the highest positive predictive value, although migration from periumbilical to right lower quadrant and fever also suggest appendicitis. Following the delineation of the pain's location, further characteristics of AAP to be assessed are radiation and movement (as an example, appendicitis-associated pain frequently moves from the periumbilical area to the right lower quadrant of the abdomen). Finally, the physician should obtain general information about onset, intensity, and character of pain.

Onset The onset of biliary pain is more likely to occur during periods of weight reduction and marked physical inactivity such as prolonged bed rest than at other times. In case of acute pancreatitis, the onset of pain is rapid but not as abrupt as that of a perforated viscus, which usually reaches its maximal intensity in 10–20 min.

Intensity and Character Acute abdominal pain usually follows one of four patterns, which are useful but at the same time require caution, both because patient's description may be unclear or vague and because a given descriptor may be attributable to a number of conditions. Basically the pain may be [5] (a) spontaneously remitting, (b) colicky, (c) progressive, and (d) immediately incapacitating. The first type of pain is typical of trivial causes, such as acute gastroenteritis. Patients with obstruction of a hollow viscus, as in intestinal obstruction, renal colic, or biliary pain, present with the gradual onset of cramping pain that follows a sinusoidal pattern of intense pain alternating with a period of relief. Nausea and vomiting are characteristic symptoms associated with this group of disorders. The absence of colic pain is useful for ruling out diseases such as acute cholecystitis; less than 25% of patients with acute cholecystitis present without right upper quadrant or colic pain [10].

The third pattern is of gradually increasing discomfort, usually vague and poorly localized at the start but becoming more localized as the pain intensifies. This picture is usually caused by inflammation, as with acute appendicitis or diverticulitis. Finally, pain that is prostrating, physically incapacitating the sufferer, is usually caused by a severe, life-threatening disease such as a perforated viscus, ruptured aneurysm, or severe pancreatitis. Some disorders, such as acute cholecystitis, may start out as colicky pain but evolve into a constant pain as cystic duct obstruction leads to gallbladder inflammation [5].

Contrary to common belief, analgesia does not mask the signs and symptoms of AAP [11], and therefore pain relief and even the use of opioids in case of severe pain do not actually increase the risk of error in the diagnostic and therapeutic pathway, neither in adults (Level A) [12] nor in children [13] (Level B).

Initial evaluation of patients with acute abdominal pain should rapidly and objectively assess the intensity of the pain in order to guide appropriate pain management. The intensity of pain is a subjective perception, which does not correlate with clinical findings, laboratory parameters, or diagnostic imaging findings [14]. Several studies have demonstrated that the medical staff underestimates patient's pain in comparison with the way patients appraise themselves [15, 16]. Simple and repeatable pain measurements using one-dimensional and multidimensional scales have been developed for objective assessment of individual pain perception. One-dimensional scales such as the visual analogue scale (VAS), verbal rating scale (VRS), and numerical rating scale (NRS), as well as the "smiley analogue scale" (SAS), are used in the acute setting [14] (Fig. 12.1).

Aggravating and Alleviating Factors The relationship of pain with positional changes, meals, bowel movements, and stress may gather important diagnostic informations. Patients with peritonitis, for example, lie motionless, whereas those with renal colic may writhe in an attempt to find a comfortable position [5]. In acute pancreatitis, there is little pain relief with changing

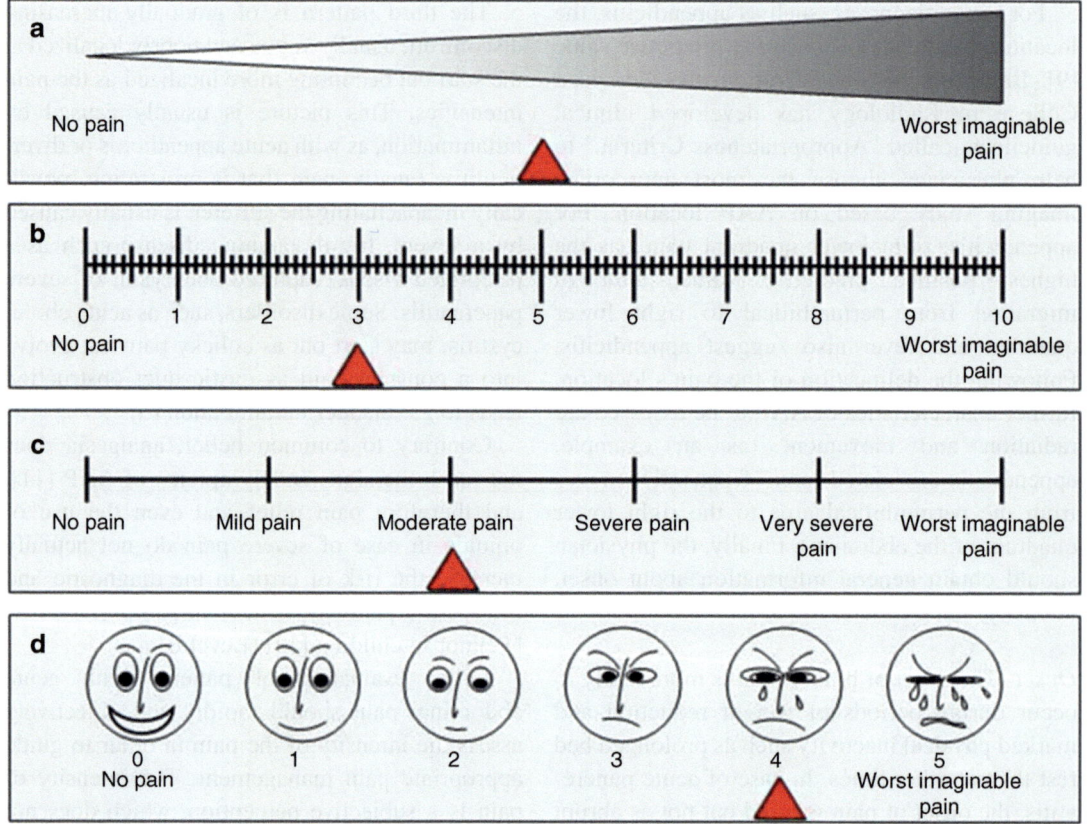

Fig. 12.1 One-dimensional pain scales depicting examples of pain ratings. Pain is assigned to a range between 0 and 100 mm (VAS), a selection of possible answers (VRS), a numerical value between 0 and 10 (NRS), or a facial expression (SAS). (A) Visual analogue scale (VAS). (B) Numerical rating scale (NRS). (C) Verbal rating scale (VRS). (D) The 'Smiley' analogue scale (SAS) (from Falch C, Vicente D, Häberle H, et al. Treatment of acute abdominal pain in the emergency room: A systematic review of the literature. Eur J Pain 2014;14: 902–913)

position. Patients with appendicitis, like other patients with peritonitis, tend to lie still rather than move about.

Sometimes, certain foods exacerbate pain. A classic example is the relationship between the intake of fatty foods and the development of biliary pain. Pain associated with duodenal ulcer often is alleviated by meals [5]. By contrast, patients with gastric ulcer or chronic mesenteric ischemia may report exacerbation of pain while eating. Patients often self-medicate to alleviate symptoms. A history of chronic antacid or of nonsteroidal anti-inflammatory drug use, for example, may suggest the presence of gastroduodenal ulcer disease.

Associated Symptoms Information regarding recent occurrence of systemic symptoms (e.g., fever, chills, night sweats, weight loss, myalgias, arthralgias) or changes in digestive function (e.g., anorexia, nausea, vomiting, flatulence, diarrhea, constipation), jaundice, dysuria, changes in menstruation, and pregnancy should be gathered from the patient. A careful review of these symptoms may reveal important diagnostic information. For example, clear vomitus may be suggestive of gastric outlet obstruction, whereas fecal vomitus suggests more distal small bowel or colonic obstruction. Symptoms in patients with abdominal pain that are suggestive of surgical or emergent conditions include fever, protracted vomiting, syncope or presyncope, and evidence of gastrointestinal blood loss [8]. Combining all the informations together may increase the likelihood of a particular disease entity.

Past Medical History A careful medical history should be obtained from a nonsedated patient, when this proves possible. Previous experience with similar symptoms suggests a recurrent problem. Patients with a history of partial small bowel obstruction, renal calculi, or pelvic inflammatory disease are likely to have recurrences [8]. To further increase the likelihood of a diagnosis, the history of chronic symptoms needs to be evaluated; for example, constipation has a high predictive value for bowel obstruction, whereas a history of chronic abdominal pain resembling the one exhibited by patients with IBS but frequently lasting more than 24 h is to be found in patients with acute diverticulitis [17]. As recalled above, many patients who prove to have peptic ulcer disease (with a positive or negative status for *H. pylori* infection) report recent use of nonsteroidal anti-inflammatory drugs, pain relieved by food, and nighttime awakening with pain. Patients with a systemic illness such as scleroderma, systemic lupus erythematosus, nephrotic syndrome, porphyria, or sickle cell disease often have abdominal pain as a manifestation of the underlying disorder. Abdominal pain also may arise as a side effect of a medication taken for another disease.

12.4   Physical Examination

In the emergency department, the physical examination of the patient with acute abdominal pain begins with an assessment of the patient's appearance and airway, breathing, and circulation (ABC rule) [5]. (A) *Airway*: Is the patient able to maintain an airway? Does an impaired sensorium endanger the patient's airway or pose a risk for aspiration of vomit or oral secretions? (B) *Breathing*: How effectively is the patient breathing? Are breaths rapid and shallow? Is the use of accessory muscles evident? Does the patient appear tachypneic? (C) *Circulation*: Circulation encompasses three areas of assessment – (1) Is the patient in shock, as suggested by pallor, cyanosis,

mottling, prostration, hypotension, tachycardia, or other signs of hypoperfusion? (2) Has intravenous access been established? (3) Is there evidence of active bleeding? If hemodynamic instability is apparent, including clinical evidence of shock, surgical consultation should be sought immediately, and consideration should be given to endotracheal intubation and resuscitation early in the encounter. The adage in acute care surgery that "death begins in radiology" should be a reminder that hemodynamic resuscitation should precede diagnostic imaging. Patients who are in shock demand urgent care and should not be sent for imaging studies without aggressive resuscitation and monitoring.

Following this, the physician should pay attention to the patient's ability to talk, breathing pattern, position in bed, posture, degree of discomfort/pain (see earlier), as well as facial expression. Peritonitis is highly suggested by a picture of a patient lying still in bed, in fetal position and reluctant to move or speak, with a distressed facial expression. On the other hand, a patient who looks restless and changes frequently position likely has an intestinal obstruction. Tachypnea may be a sign of metabolic acidosis caused by shock. All patients should undergo a careful, systematic examination, regardless of the differential diagnosis suggested by the history.

Abdominal Examination Examination of the abdomen is central to the evaluation of a patient with acute abdominal pain, and the four canonical steps of physical examination, i.e., inspection, auscultation, palpation, and (less importantly) finger percussion, should begin with a careful inspection. The entire abdomen, from the nipple line to the thighs, needs to be exposed. Obese patients should be asked whether the degree of protrusion of the abdominal wall is more than usual. Assessment for the presence of bowel sounds and their character should precede any maneuvers that might alter the abdominal contents. Traditionally, it is reported that before concluding that an abdomen is silent, the examiner should listen for at least 2 minutes and in more than one quadrant of the abdomen [5]. Experienced listeners will distinguish the high-pitched churning of a mechanical small intestinal obstruction from the more hollow sounds of toxic megacolon (like dripping in a cavern). Palpation should be very prudent, and possibly the examiner should begin to palpate the abdomen with the head of the stethoscope while carefully watching the patient's facial expression. If tenderness is detected, an assessment for rebound tenderness should be elicited by finger percussion. Hand palpation is performed next. One important trick is to palpate last the area which seems to be the epicenter of pain to prevent involuntary guarding and muscular rigidity. Patients with a rigid abdomen rarely reveal any additional findings (such as a mass) on physical examination. Because these patients usually have a surgical emergency, abdominal examination might be postponed after the completion of general anesthesia, just before laparotomy. Finally, the pelvic organs and external genitalia should be examined in every patient with acute abdominal pain. The rectum and vagina provide additional avenues for gentle palpation of pelvic viscera. Gynecologic pathology should be excluded in all women with acute abdominal pain.

Interestingly, for these three different acute conditions, the highest value of likelihood ratio is achieved by a different feature: for appendicitis it is the location of pain in the right lower abdominal quadrant (8.4); for bowel obstruction it is the clinical finding of a history of constipation (8.8); and for cholecystitis it is an information gathered at bowel examination, namely, a positive Murphy's sign (5.0). Thus, a constellation of different findings may contribute with different diagnostic weight to suggest a particular disease entity.

12.5 Laboratory Data

The history and physical examination findings generally rarely are sufficient per se to establish a firm diagnosis in a patient with AAP. The suggested core of laboratory examinations for AAP patients presenting at an emergency department includes a complete blood count, with a differential count, urinalysis, the determination of serum electrolyte, blood urea nitrogen, creatinine, and glucose levels. These tests allow to assess the patient's fluid and acid-base status, renal function, and metabolic state. A mandatory examination in all women of reproductive age with abdominal pain is a urine pregnancy testing. Liver biochemical tests and serum amylase/lipase levels should be ordered for patients with upper abdominal pain or with jaundice. An increase of serum amylase may follow not only acute pancreatitis but also a perforated ulcer or an acute cholecystitis. The determination of serum lipase, which peaks with a slightly delayed interval compared with amylase in acute pancreatitis, may have greater accuracy. Leukocytosis, particularly when associated with immature band forms, is an important finding. However, it should never be the single deciding factor leading or not to a surgical approach. A white blood cell count >20,000/μL may be encountered in a visceral perforation, but it can also be found in patients with acute pancreatitis, acute cholecystitis, and intestinal infarction, and on the other hand, a normal white blood cell count is not rare in patients with abdominal viscera perforation. The finding of anemia may be more helpful in suggesting a viscus perforation than the white blood cell count, especially when combined with the clinical history. Metabolic acidosis, an elevated serum lactate level, and a depressed bicarbonate level are all associated with tissue hypoperfusion and shock. Patients who manifest these findings are likely to require urgent surgical intervention or intensive care.

At the end of this section, it must be pointed out that, according to some recent studies [2, 18], the diagnosis solely based on medical history and physical examination has a high sensitivity but a low specificity. For example, in the study by Lameris et al. [2], the respective values were 88% and 41%, with 12% of missed diagnoses but 27% of false-positive ones. The consequences for a high sensitivity for urgent conditions are clinically important, as patients with an urgent diagnosis being discharged home and left untreated are undesirable; false-positive urgent diagnoses, on the other hand, could lead to overtreatment, with undue costs and time efforts. Even the addiction of selected laboratory examinations would lead to a low rate of correct diagnoses (46–48% only) of patients with abdominal pain ((evidence level (EL) B) [7]. The diagnostic accuracy increased when the outcome of clinical evaluation was the differentiation between urgent and nonurgent conditions and not so much a specific diagnosis.

Sensitivity of medical history, physical examination, and laboratory values is higher for differentiating urgent from nonurgent conditions than for a specific diagnosis (EL A2) [2, 7]. Therefore, according to a recent evidence-based guideline developed for the diagnostic pathway of patients with abdominal pain of nontraumatic origin, the diagnostic accuracy of medical history and physical examination is insufficient to reach a correct diagnosis with or without laboratory parameters (EL 2). However, the diagnostic accuracy of medical history, physical examination, and/or laboratory parameters is sufficient to discriminate between urgent and nonurgent causes and justify the choice for additional imaging in suspected urgent conditions (EL 2). Patients suspected of a nonurgent condition need no admission and can return to the outpatient clinics for re-evaluation the next day [19].

Which additional imaging test and in which order are beyond the scope of the present chapter, although different conditional strategies have been reported to improve the diagnostic performance of medical history and physical examination combined [2].

Finally, it appears that nonspecific abdominal pain is the main differential diagnostic problem in the emergency department (ED) also for diagnoses requiring surgery [18]. In a study designed to identify the differential diagnostic difficulties in acute abdominal pain at the ED and during hospitalization, conducted on 2851 patients with abdominal pain lasting for up to 7 days seen at ED and re-evaluated 1 year after discharge, it was found that some diagnosis had low sensitivity at entry but markedly increased sensitivity at discharge. They were nonspecific abdominal pain with a sensitivity value at the ED of 0.43, appendicitis 0.80, gallstones 0.68, constipation 0.74, and peptic ulcer 0.26. Corresponding kappa values for concordance between the two observations were 0.48, 0.74, 0.84, 0.88, and 0.93, respectively. Malignancy, gynecological complaints, dyspepsia, urinary tract infection, and diverticulitis displayed fairly good concordance between the preliminary and discharge judgments, but the predictive diagnostic value was still low at discharge. Sensitivity values at discharge were 0.40, 0.75, 0.73, 0.77, and 0.83, respectively. Among 479 surgically treated patients, 104 initially received a diagnosis usually not requiring surgery and had a median delay until operation of 22 h (95% CI 30–50 h), compared with 8 h (12–18 h) for referrals. The conclusion of the authors was that nonspecific abdominal pain is the main differential diagnostic problem in the emergency department also for diagnosis requiring surgery. Constipation is a diagnostic pitfall, and when making this diagnosis a careful re-evaluation is necessary.

References

1. Viniol A, Keunecke C, Biroga T, et al. Studies of the symptom abdominal pain—a systematic review and meta-analysis. Family Pract. 2014;31:517–29.
2. Lameris W, van Randen A, van Es HW, van Heesewijk JP, van Ramshorst B, Bouma WH, et al. Imaging strategies for detection of urgent conditions in patients with acute abdominal pain: diagnostic accuracy study. BMJ. 2009;338:b2431.
3. Hyams JS, Burke G, Davis PM, Rzepski B, Andrulonis PA. Abdominal pain and irritable bowel syndrome in adolescents: a community-based study. J Pediatr. 1996;129:220–6.
4. Kay L. Abdominal symptoms, visits to the doctor, and medicine consumption among the elderly. A population based study. Dan Med Bull. 1994;41:466–9.
5. Yarze JC, Friedman LS. Chronic abdominal pain. In: Feldman M, Friedman LS, Brandt LJ, editors. Sleisenger and Fordtran's gastrointestinal and liver disease. 9th ed. Philadelphia: Saunders Elsevier; 2010. p. 163–71.
6. Lacy BE, Mearin F, Chang L, Chey WD, et al. Bowel disorders. Gastroenterology. 2016;150:1393–407.
7. Gans SL, Pols MA, Stoker J, Boermeester MA. Guideline for the diagnostic pathway in patients with acute abdominal pain. Dig Surg. 2015;32:23–31.
8. Cartwright SL, Knudson MP. Evaluation of acute abdominal pain in adults. Am Fam Phys. 2008;77:972–8.

9. Cartwright SL, Knudson MP. Diagnostic imaging of acute abdominal pain in adults. Am Fam Phys. 2015;91:452–9.

10. Trowbridge RL, Rutkowski NK, Shojania KG. Does this patient have acute cholecystitis? JAMA. 2003;289(1):80–6.

11. Ranji SR, Goldman LE, Simel DL, Shojania KG. Do opiates affect the clinical evaluation of patients with acute abdominal pain? JAMA. 2006;296:1764–74.

12. Manterola C, Vial M, Moraga J, Astudillo P. Analgesia in patients with acute abdominal pain. Cochrane Database Syst Rev. 2011;1:CD005660.

13. Klein-Kremer A, Goldman RD. Opioid administration for acute abdominal pain in the pediatric emergency department. J Opioid Manag. 2007;3:11–4.

14. Falch C, Vicente D, Häberle H, et al. Treatment of acute abdominal pain in the emergency room: A systematic review of the literature. Eur J Pain. 2014;14:902–13.

15. Mäntyselkä P, Kumpusalo E, Ahonen R, Takala J. Patients' versus general practitioners' assessments of pain intensity in primary care patients with non-cancer pain. Br J Gen Pract. 2001;51:995–7.

16. Davoudi N, Afsharzadeh P, Mohammadalizadeh S, Haghhdoost AA. A comparison of patients' and nurses' assessments of pain intensity in patients with coronary artery disease. Int J Nurs Pract. 2008;14:347–56.

17. Annibale B, Lahner E, Maconi G, et al. Clinical features of symptomatic uncomplicated diverticular disease: a multicentre Italian survey. Int J Colorectal Dis. 2012;27:1151–9.

18. Laurell H, Hansson LE, Gunnarrson U. Diagnostic pitfalls and accuracy of diagnosis in acute abdominal pain. Scand J Gastroenterol. 2006;41:1126–31.

19. Toorenvliet BR, Bakker RF, Flu HC, Merkus JW, Hamming JF, Breslau PJ. Standard outpatient re-evaluation for patients not admitted to the hospital after emergency department evaluation for acute abdominal pain. World J Surg. 2010;34:480–6.

Imaging of Biliary Colic and Cholecystitis

13

Bordonaro Veronica, Carchesio Francesca,
Larosa Luigi, Anna Maria De Gaetano,
and Manfredi Riccardo

13.1 Introduction

Gallbladder disease is one of the most common conditions that affects a significant portion of the worldwide population, and symptomatic cholelithiasis is responsible of a significant percentage of emergency department visit for abdominal pain.

The epidemiology and risk factors of cholelithiasis have been widely investigated over the last several decades. Gallstones formation is the result of a complex interaction of multiple factors, including increasing age, hormonal effects (female gender, parity, exogenous oestrogens) metabolic disorders (obesity, diabetes mellitus, dyslipidaemia), dietary factors (high cholesterol diets), liver disease (cirrhosis, HCV infection), gallbladder stasis (long-term parental nutrition, low physical activity), and also genetics factors [1].

Crystalline deposits in the gallbladder are classified by chemical composition: cholesterol stones (>70% of cholesterol content), the most common type in the Western world, formed by supersaturation of cholesterol and associated with a decrease in the quantity of bile salt and lecithin, and mixed stones (from 30 to 70% of cholesterol content) and pigmented stones (cholesterol <30%), further distinguished into black and brown stones. Black stones are formed from polymerized calcium bilirubinate and are associated with hemolytic disorders and cirrhosis; brown pigment stones are composed of unpolymerized calcium bilirubinate, are most common in Oriental population, and are correlated with recurrent pyogenic cholangitis and biliary parasite infections [2–4].

As well as their cause, the types of gallstone vary by the measures attempted to prevent their formation, their response to dissolution therapy, and their appearance on imaging procedures [5].

The prevalence of cholelithiasis in the developed countries varies between 5 and 25%, and most patients are asymptomatic. It was calculated that each year approximately 2–4% of people with gallstones develop symptoms [5, 6] with biliary colic being the most common symptom.

13.2 Biliary Tract Obstruction

13.2.1 Cholelithiasis and Biliary Colic

Biliary colic is typically steady in quality rather than "colicky" as the name implies, and it is described as a constant, dull right upper quadrant abdominal pain, sometimes radiating to the right back or the shoulder and not relieved or exacerbated by movement, position, or bowel function.

Electronic Supplementary Material The online version of this chapter (https://doi.org/10.1007/978-3-319-99822-0_13) contains supplementary material, which is available to authorized users.

B. Veronica · C. Francesca · L. Luigi
A. M. De Gaetano · M. Riccardo (✉)
Department of Radiology, Università Cattolica del Sacro Cuore, Rome, Italy
e-mail: riccardo.manfredi@unicatt.it

Typically, pain will last more than 30 min with the maximum time being 6 h [7, 8].

It results from gallbladder distention after acute and usually transient obstruction of the cystic duct by stones or sludge. When the stone falls back into the gallbladder or migrates into the common bile duct (CBD), the pain usually subsides; otherwise, gallstones can obstruct the cystic duct or gallbladder neck with an irritation of the gallbladder mucosa, a subsequent release of several inflammatory mediators, and progressive gallbladder wall inflammation, typically leading to an acute cholecystitis.

The presence of biliary stones into the choledochus defines the condition of choledocholithiasis.

This pathological entity is classified as primary or secondary according to stone origin: the primary form refers to stones formed directly within the biliary tree, while the secondary refers to stones ejected from the gallbladder. Primary choledocholithiasis is generally composed of brown stones and is rare in Western populations, while secondary choledocholithiasis is characterized by a stone composition analogous to that of cholelithiasis, with cholesterol as the most common type [9].

Once in the CBD, stones may reach the duodenum following the bile flow; otherwise, also owing to the smaller diameter of the distal duct caliber at the Vater papilla, they may remain in the choledochus. In this latter case, gallstones may be mostly asymptomatic or cause a variety of bile flow problems, including complete obstruction and jaundice. Bile stasis may be also responsible for bile infection and consequent ascending cholangitis, whereas bile/pancreatic juice flow obstruction may potentially trigger the intrapancreatic activation of pancreatic enzymes, causing acute biliary pancreatitis. Hepatic abscesses may also be a rarer infectious complication of choledocholithiasis, whereas chronic CBD obstruction may also cause biliary cirrhosis.

Extremely rarer is the condition of an obstruction of the common hepatic duct due to extrinsic compression by an impacted gallstone in the gallbladder neck, known as Mirizzi syndrome. Patients typically present with fever, right upper quadrant pain, and obstructive jaundice. Repeated bouts of recurrent cystic duct stone impaction and inflammation may lead to a cholecystobiliary fistula [10].

13.2.1.1 Imaging of Primary Condition

Since its advent in 1968, the endoscopic retrograde cholangiopancreatography (ERCP) has become the gold standard in the setting of biliary obstruction. It is an invasive procedure technique for the examination and intervention of the biliary tract, with a reported complication rate of 1 to 9% and a mortality rate from 0.2 to 0.5% [11].

Advances in biliary radiology with US, CT, and MRI technology have allowed an accurate, noninvasive imaging of the biliary tree and pancreas, in the setting of biliary obstruction and in the investigation of its causes and severity. In some cases, a multimodality imaging approach may be necessary.

US

Abdominal ultrasonography is the imaging of choice in patients with upper abdominal quadrant pain and is widely recommended as the initial imaging test in case of suspicion of biliary colic because of its high sensitivity and accuracy, noninvasiveness, lack of ionizing radiations, relatively low cost, and widely available.

Its accuracy for detecting gallbladder stones is more than 95%, and its sensitivity is comparable to that of MR cholangiopancreatography (MRCP) (97.7%), although it is less sensitive for the detection of microlithiasis and biliary sludge [12].

The characteristic findings of gallstones at US are a highly reflective echo from the anterior wall of the gallstone, gravitational mobility of the gallstone on repositioning the patient, and marked posterior acoustic shadowing (Fig. 13.1). This latter finding is extremely important in regard to the specificity of the technique and furthermore for the differential diagnosis of a gallbladder mass seen at US, because non-shadowing structures are considerably less likely than shadowing structures to represent gallstones.

When the gallbladder is completely filled with stones, the resulting appearance is termed the *wall-echo-shadow sign* (Fig. 13.2): the anterior

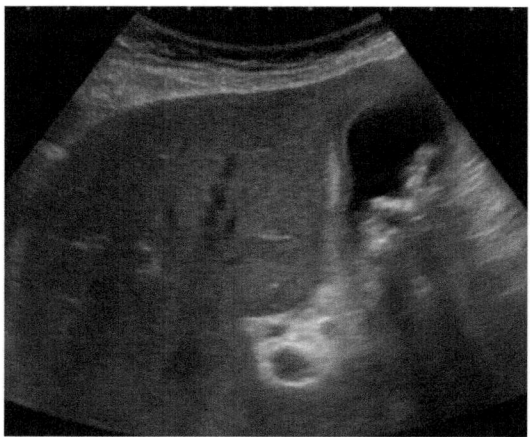

Fig. 13.1 Longitudinal scan on US exam showing multiple gallstones located on the posterior gallbladder wall

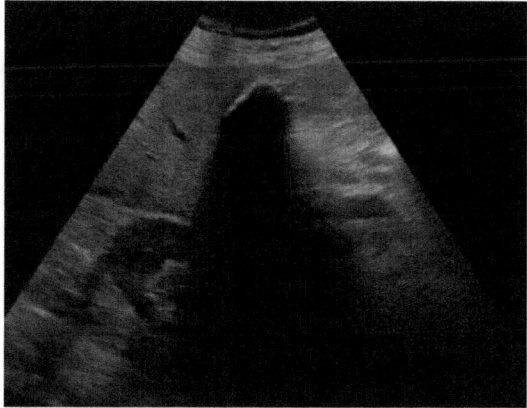

Fig. 13.2 *Wall-echo-shadow sign:* the gallbladder is completely filled with stones with intense acoustic shadow that obscures deeper structures

gallbladder wall is echogenic; a thin layer of bile immediately underneath the anterior wall is usually seen as a dark line; finally, the most superficial stones are seen as a highly echogenic layer beneath the bile with associated intense shadowing that obscures the deeper stones and the posterior gallbladder wall [12].

Even though US has a high specificity for choledocholithiasis, its sensitivity ranges from 22 to 33% for detecting CBD stones [13, 14].

The major limitation for US in detecting CBD stones is mostly represented by the presence of intestinal gas, which often obscures the distal common duct and the ampulla of Vater.

Operator experience also plays a major role: when the examination is performed by an expert operator, sensitivity is nearly double (77–90%) than that of an operator with little experience (37–47%) [15].

US, however, is able to detect indirect signs of obstruction, in particular the subsequent dilatation of the CBD and even of the intrahepatic biliary tree. Biliary dilatation greater than 6 mm in patients with an intact gallbladder and than 10 mm postcholecystectomy is suspected of biliary obstruction.

CT

Although ultrasonography (US) is the most useful imaging modality for initial evaluation of the biliary system, multidetector computed tomography (CT) is often ordered in the emergency department for patients who present with nonspecific abdominal complaints or in cases where US findings are equivocal.

The sensitivity of CT for detecting choledocholithiasis varies between 72 and 88%; however, sensitivities for direct depiction (excluding indirect signs like ductal dilatation from criteria) of CBD stones have not exceeded 75% [16–18].

The appearance of gallstones on CT imaging varies with their chemical composition; stones may be heterogeneous in appearance, ranging from being heavily calcified and radiopaque to being slightly less radiopaque than bile due to cholesterol and to having gas attenuation due to locules of nitrogen gas, and may vary in appearance even within the same patient [19] (Fig. 13.3).

Nitrogen gas accumulation within gallstone fissures is sometimes observed in a star-shaped pattern on CT, termed the "Mercedes-Benz" sign [12, 20].

Approximately 10 to 20% of gallstones is composed of pure cholesterol, which are low in density, and they appear isoattenuating with bile, resulting in being hard to see on CT images.

Detection of biliary stones depends in part on technologic factors and in part on the care taken by the interpreting physician.

In general, CBD stones at CT may be better evaluated using thin sections and multiplanar

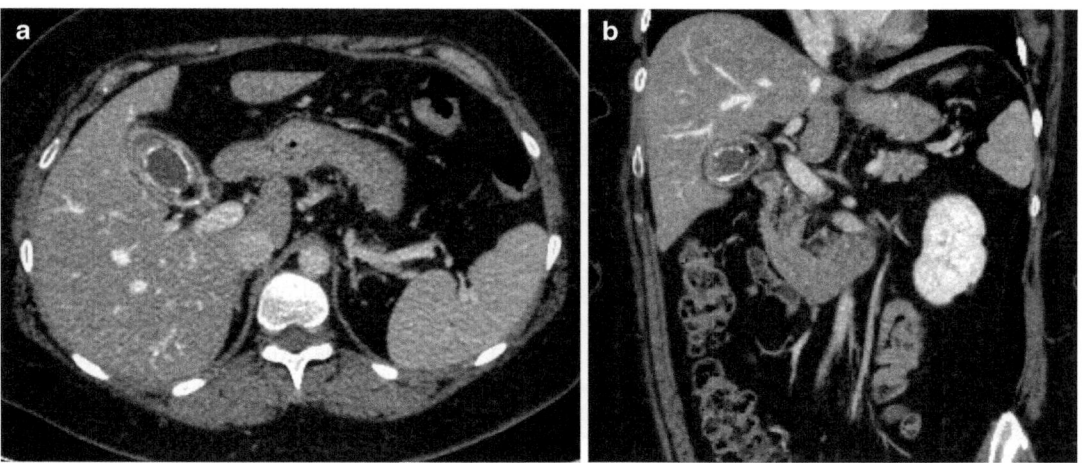

Fig. 13.3 Axial (**a**) and coronal (**b**) contrast-enhanced CT images show a voluminous mixed gallstone consisting in hypodense core and calcified shell with tiny peripheral gas collections

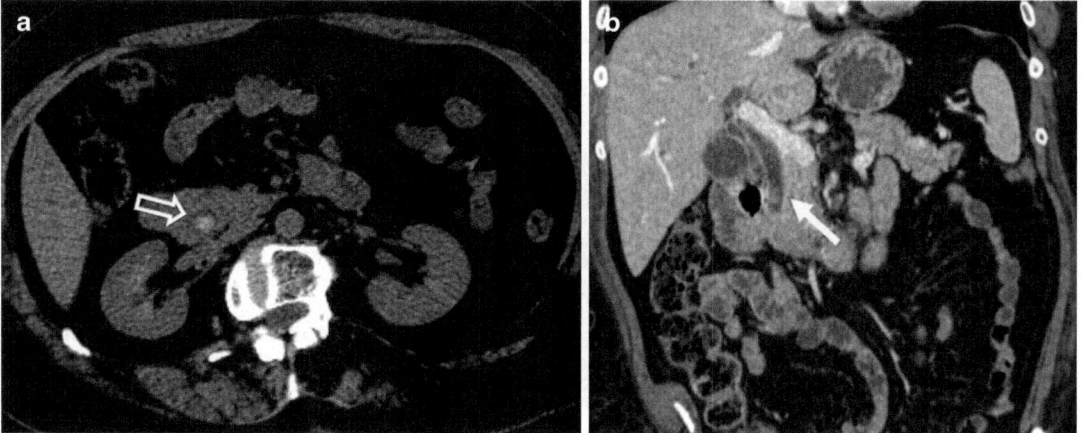

Fig. 13.4 A 66-year-old woman with choledocholithiasis. Axial (**a**) non-enhanced CT image with narrow window setting shows hyperdense sludge within the iuxtapapillary choledochus (empty arrow). Coronal (**b**) contrast-enhanced CT image confirm a dilated CBD with intraluminal sludge seen as mildly increased density (white arrow) in hypoattenuating bile

reconstructions; unenhanced CT to establish a baseline helps identify biliary stones and confirm their lack of contrast enhancement. The use of narrow window settings can accentuate the attenuation difference between the stone and adjacent bile or soft tissue, improving their detection [18] (Fig. 13.4).

Baron has recommended using the highest kilovoltage setting (140 kVp) to increase the chances of distinguishing stones from the bile [21].

A portal venous phase image, obtained through the abdomen 70–80 s after the intravenous injection of a 100–150-mL bolus of contrast material with a high iodine concentration (300–400 mg of iodine per millimeter), is required [17].

Traditionally, the presence or absence of bile duct stones can be determined through the criteria previously described by Baron, who illustrated the appearance of stones depending on a slice of examination [22]. In particular, the stone can be seen as a central density surrounded by hypoattenuating bile or ampullary soft tissue (target sign); otherwise, a faint rim of increased density can be visible along peripheral margin of low-density calculus (rim sign). Again, a calculus with increased density that is surrounded by a crescent of hypoattenuating bile is suggestive of the crescent sign.

When visible on CT images, biliary stones have a lamellated appearance and are angulated and geometric in shape and tend to be in a dependent posterior location in the biliary tract, with a crescent of bile outlining the anterior portion of the stone. Furthermore, signs of inflammation such as periductal edema, biliary epithelial thickening, and mural enhancement may point to local irritation caused by stones or to associated cholangitis or cholecystitis. However, mural enhancement has been reported to be frequently seen with malignancy and should prompt careful investigation [17].

A particular kind of CT imaging helpful for patients with suspected choledocholithiasis is the *CT cholangiography*, which provides a noninvasive opacification of the biliary tract and can be achieved with the administration of intravenous positive contrast materials, such as iopanoic acid, which are excreted into the bile. CT cholangiography is helpful for patients with suspected choledocholithiasis (sensitivity 86–93%, specificity 100%). It has also been shown to have sensitivity in diagnosing bile duct stones comparable with magnetic resonance cholangiography (>90%) and higher than unenhanced helical CT [23, 24].

However, this technique has some disadvantages that limit its use: a pre-imaging medication with antihistaminic drugs is required to prevent potentially life-threatening allergic reactions; a higher dose of radiation is needed, compared with conventional helical CT; and furthermore, the excretion of currently available biliary contrast materials is variable and is influenced by poorly understood factors. In particular, patients with liver insufficiency and high serum bilirubin levels (levels >3 mg/dl) often have CT cholangiographic images with insufficient opacification of bile ducts [25].

Definitely, CT imaging is better able to accurately demonstrate the location (97%) and cause (94%) of biliary obstruction, compared with US, but US is still more sensitive, specific, and accurate for diagnosis of cholelithiasis and has been shown to have a much higher positive predictive value (75% vs 50% for CT) and negative predictive value (97% vs 89% for CT) for diagnosing acute biliary disease [26].

MRI

In acute biliary disorders, MR imaging, including MR cholangiopancreatography (MRCP), can be a valuable complement to other imaging strategies in patients with severe symptoms and those suspected of having serious complications, especially when US and CT findings are inconclusive.

About 15–30% of patients who have acute biliary disorders are estimated to require MR imaging.

Because of its very high tissue contrast, multisequence MR imaging can provide a more comprehensive and detailed evaluation of the biliary tree and pancreatic duct, and because of its noninvasiveness and for the absence of the morbidity and mortality risk associated with ERCP, it has been widely adopted in the work-up of biliary obstruction [27].

On T1-weighted images, pigment gallstones appear to be hyperintense, while cholesterol gallstones are hypointense on the T1-weighted images; the reason of hyperintensity of pigment gallstones on T1-weighted images is in their composition, in particular in their metal ion content [28].

Gallstones are well depicted on MRCP, regardless of their location, and appear on T2-weighted images as foci of low signal intensity surrounded by bright bile (Fig. 13.5 and Fig. 13.6). Several studies have demonstrated that the sensitivity and specificity for MRCP in diagnosing choledocholithiasis are high (85–92% and 93–97%), with generally better results when sections with a thickness of 3 mm or less are acquired [29].

However, one important pitfall is represented by the reduced accuracy of MR cholangiography in the detection of small stones. Even with thin-section 3D imaging techniques, the sensitivity for stones that are 3 mm or smaller is substantially less than for larger calculi and may be less than 50%.

Additional limitations have also been reported, such as mistaking multiple impacted stones (with minimal surrounding bile) for a stricture or

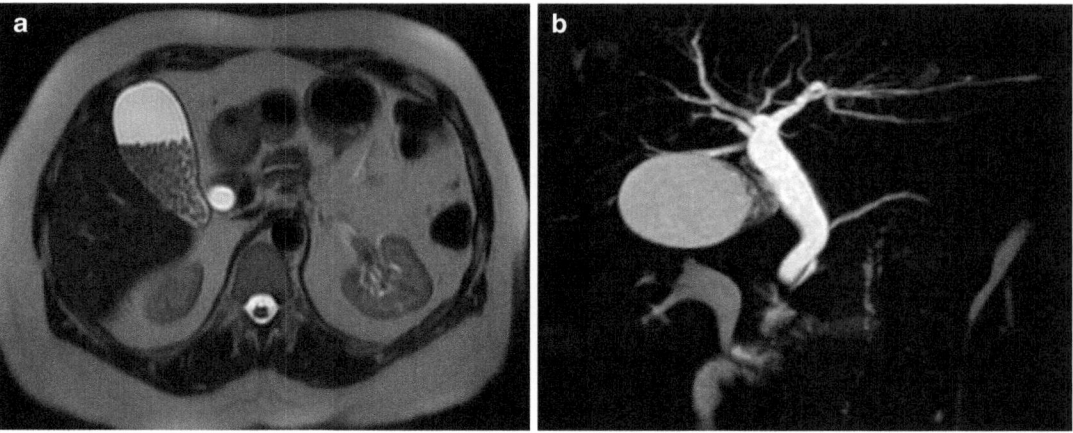

Fig. 13.5 (**a**) Axial T2-weighted MR image shows a distended gallbladder with several small stones layered in the lumen. (**b**) MR cholangiopancreatogram confirms the presence of numerous tiny stones in the gallbladder; the main bile duct and intrahepatic branches are dilated, but non-stones are clearly present in the lumen

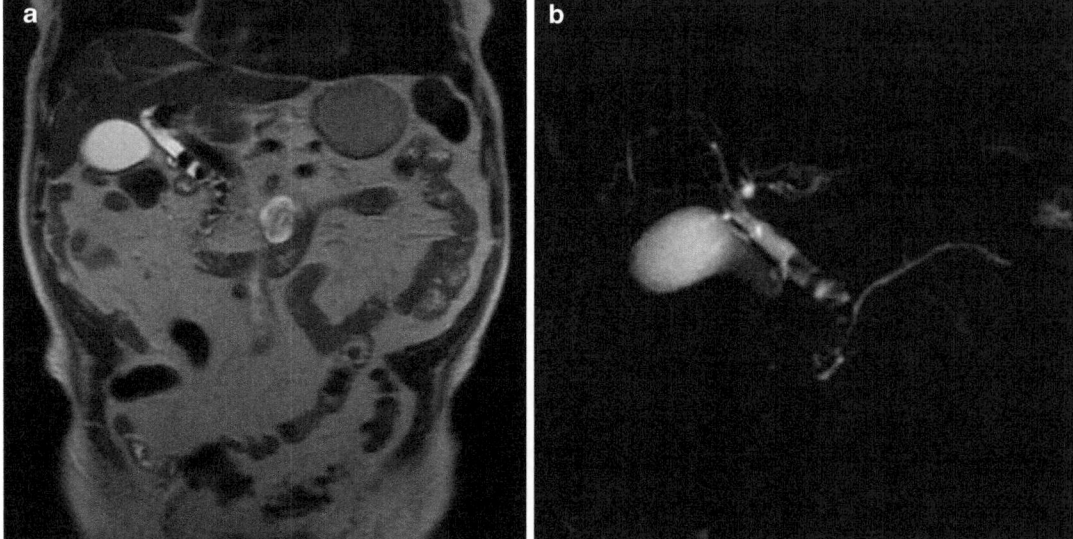

Fig. 13.6 Choledocholithiasis. Coronal T2-weighted image (**a**) and MRCP (**b**) show multiple filling defects in the CBD, related to numerous calculi

misidentifying pneumobilia, which manifests as signal voids with all sequences, for an intrabiliary stone [30].

When stones are not identified despite a high level of clinical suspicion, more invasive studies such as ERCP or endoscopic US may be pursued.

In particular, EUS is considered to have high sensitivity, especially for small CBD stones, seeming to be superior in the detection of CBD stones than 5 mm in diameter, compared to MRCP.

Endoscopic retrograde cholangiopancreatography (ERCP), despite its small but not negligible risk of complications, represents the most accurate diagnostic procedure for detecting CBD stones and also allowing their removal [31].

13.2.1.2 Imaging of Complications
The most frequent complications of choledocholithiasis are acute cholangitis and gallstone pancreatitis.

Acute cholangitis is a potentially life-threatening condition caused by partial or complete obstruction of the biliary tree with biliary stasis and increased intrabiliary pressure, which predisposes to bacterial overgrowth and ascending infection. Acute suppurative cholangitis refers to pus in the biliary tract, a condition that can lead to increased intraluminal pressure and precipitate biliary sepsis. Independent risk factors for this severe form of acute cholangitis include patient age older than 70 years, current smoker status, and an impacted biliary stone [32, 33].

The classical presentation is the "Charcot triad" of fever, right upper quadrant abdominal pain, and jaundice, which has however been reported to be present in 56–70% of patients. Patients can also present with "Reynold pentad", which is Charcot triad with shock and altered mental status [34].

The most common bacteria isolated in infected bile without prior instrumentation are *E. coli* (31%), *Klebsiella pneumoniae* (17%), *Enterococcus faecalis* (17%), and *Streptococcus* species (17%) [35].

Complications of acute cholangitis include pyogenic hepatic abscesses, portal vein thrombosis, and biliary peritonitis (Fig. 13.7).

The most common CT finding of acute cholangitis is biliary obstruction, with a diffuse and concentric thickening of the extrahepatic biliary duct with enhancement. Purulent bile may have increased CT attenuation. Transient hepatic attenuation differences (THADs), which appear as patchy, wedge-shaped, or geographic inhomogeneous hepatic parenchymal enhancement during the hepatic arterial phase on the CT, have been reported to be common in patients with acute cholangitis [36].

A recently described CT scoring system based on the extent of transient hepatic attenuation differences, degree of biliary dilatation, and presence of an obstructive lesion is highly sensitive (84–90%) and specific (84%) for the diagnosis of acute cholangitis [37].

There are no specific studies comparing multidetector CT with MR imaging in the setting of cholangitis. However, MR imaging seems to be more helpful than multidetector CT because of the higher signal-to-noise and contrast-to-noise ratios [38].

Enhancement of intrahepatic biliary duct walls is a common finding, reported in up to 92% of cases investigated with MR imaging, and it is best seen with gadolinium-enhanced delayed-phase fat-suppressed sequences.

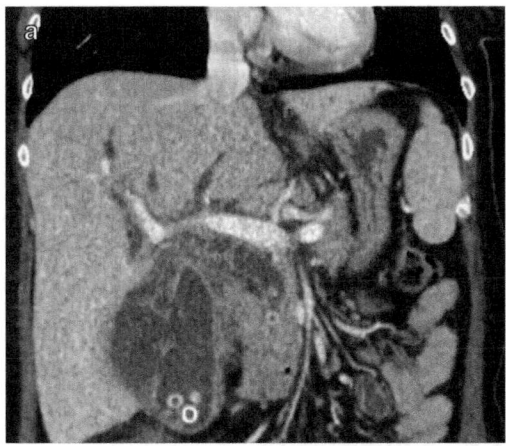
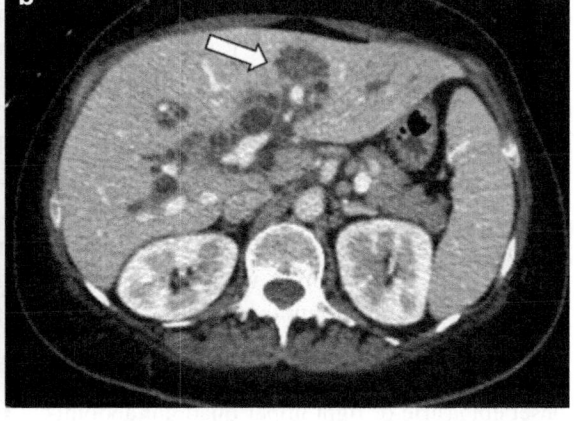

Fig. 13.7 Choledocholithiasis with acute cholangitis, gallbladder perforation, and hepatic abscess. Coronal contrast-enhanced CT image (**a**) shows obstructive gallstones in the distal CBD with marked proximal intra- and extrahepatic biliary ductal dilatation and a hydropic gallbladder with dependent stones, focal disruptions of the wall, and multiple loculated pericholecystic fluid collections. Axial (**b**) contrast-enhanced CT image shows an intrahepatic abscess, represented by a low-attenuation lesion with subtle peripheral enhancement in the left liver lobe (white arrow)

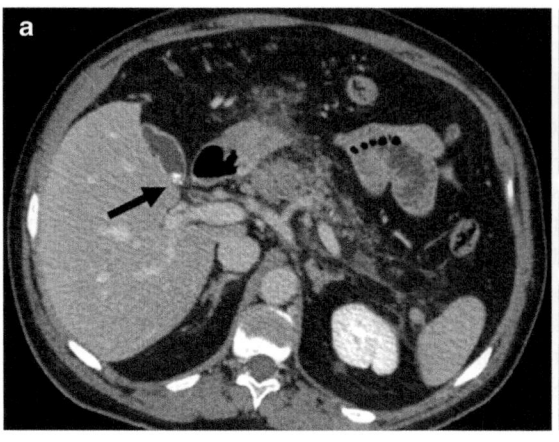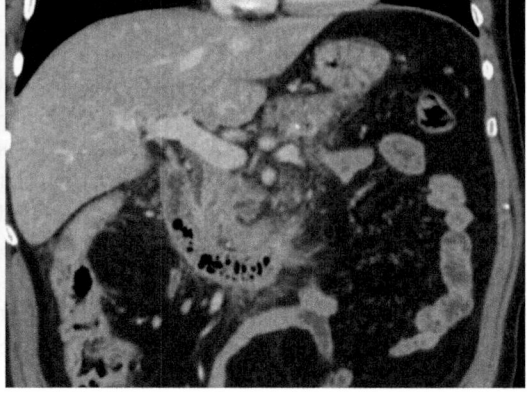

Fig. 13.8 Axial (**a**) and coronal (**b**) contrast-enhanced CT images show a diffuse pancreatic swelling with peripancreatic and retroperitoneal edema and fat stranding, extending to the pararenal space (thickened Gerota's fascia). Small calcified gallstones are present into the gallbladder lumen (black arrow)

Liver parenchymal changes, caused by an extension of the inflammatory process into the periportal tissues, with a dilatation of the peribiliary venous plexus and an increasing arterial flow, are seen in MR imaging as a high signal intensity on T2-weighted images and an inhomogeneous contrast enhancement with a wedge-shaped (72%), peripheral patchy (14%), or peribiliary (14%) pattern distribution [39].

Another potential complication of choledocholithiasis is represented by biliary pancreatitis.

Gallstone or biliary sludge impaction at the ampulla of Vater may cause ampullary spasm, pancreatico-biliary reflux, and obstruction of the common and pancreatic ducts, leading to acute pancreatitis (Fig. 13.8). Alternatively, biliary sludge may cause cholestasis or irritate the sphincter of Oddi, causing edema and biliopancreatic outflow obstruction. Anatomic variations such as a common pancreatico-biliary channel or pancreas divisum also raise the risk of acute pancreatitis [40, 41].

Most patients presenting with this complication present typical symptoms of pancreatitis, and fewer may also provide a history of biliary colic. The most common complaint is sudden-onset epigastric or right upper quadrant abdominal pain that is unrelenting and in 50% of cases radiates to the back [42].

Upper abdominal pain with amylase or lipase three times the upper normal limit is diagnostic of acute pancreatitis in many cases, and the addition of choledocholithiasis on imaging may sufficiently identify the cause as biliary. However, as previously said, ultrasonography may fail to detect stones smaller than 4 mm, and small stones are a known risk factor for biliary pancreatitis.

CT is often not an essential study in mild gallstone pancreatitis but provides more useful information in moderate to severe cases. The use of CT for stratification of severity and to direct management requires appropriate timing and technique because pancreatic involvement is best visualized on CT at a few days after the onset of symptoms. If an initial CT was obtained during diagnosis, it may need to be repeated if the patient's pain is persistent and laboratory values fail to trend toward normal.

Findings at contrast-enhanced CT include an obstructive stone in a dilated CBD, associated with an edematous hypoattenuating pancreas with surrounding peripancreatic inflammation and fluid. Severe cases of pancreatitis may include findings of pseudocyst formation and parenchymal necrosis.

13.3 Cholecystitis

13.3.1 Acute Cholecystitis

Acute cholecystitis is defined as inflammation of the gallbladder, generally caused by obstruction of the cystic duct. The most common causes of cystic duct obstruction are gallstones or biliary sludge (acute calculous cholecystitis), which represent over 90% of cases. Cholecystitis can also occur in the absence of gallstones and is known as acalculous cholecystitis, a much rarer condition which occurs in critically ill or injured patients (trauma, burns, sepsis), and it is generally the result of biliary stasis and/or gallbladder ischemia [43].

According to the World Society of Emergency Surgery (WSES) guidelines 2016, there is no single clinical or laboratory finding with sufficient diagnostic accuracy to establish or exclude acute cholecystitis (Level IIB); combination of detailed history, complete clinical examination, and laboratory tests may strongly support the diagnosis of acute cholecystitis (Level IVC) [44].

13.3.1.1 Imaging of Primary Condition

US

US exam is the first imaging modality performed in the suspect of acute cholecystitis according to guidelines [44], because of its high sensibility, sensitivity, and availability. US detects the presence of gallstones and the signs of acute cholecystitis and assesses the positivity of Murphy sign.

Typical findings of acute cholecystitis on US exam are distention of gallbladder (defined as diameter greater than 5 cm on axial scan and greater than 8 cm in longitudinal scan) due to cystic duct obstruction and homogeneous wall thickening (defined as thickness > than 4 mm), finding that must be differentiated from gallbladder wall thickening related to other causes (Table 13.1). Other typical findings are stratified

Table 13.1 Other causes of gallbladder wall thickening

Adenomyosis
Acute hepatitis
Hepatic cirrhosis
Gallbladder neoplasia
Congestive hepatic right failure
Secondary involvement in acute processes in upper abdomen

aspect of gallbladder wall related to submucosal edema (Fig. 13.9) and the presence of pericholecystic fluid. On Power Doppler hyperemia of the gallbladder wall could be demonstrated.

The detection of single or multiple obstructive stones or endoluminal sludge (Fig. 13.10) eventually confirms the underlying cause even though diagnostic performance of US in the diagnosis of inflammation of the gallbladder is not as good as its performance in the diagnosis of gallstones, as indicated in a recent meta-analysis [45]; moreover, it also presents several limitations related to body habitus.

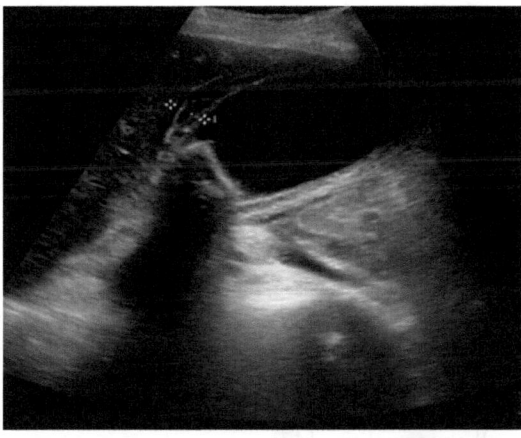

Fig. 13.9 Acute cholecystitis. Longitudinal US scan shows stratified aspect of gallbladder wall caused by submucosal edema and the presence of a single stone impacted in the infundibulum

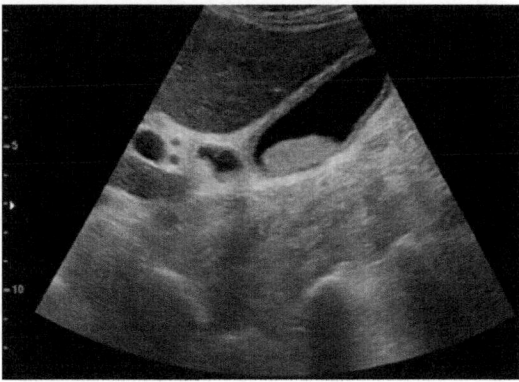

Fig. 13.10 Acute cholecystitis in a 76-year-old man with right upper quadrant pain. Longitudinal US scan shows a gallbladder wall thickening (>3 mm) with intraluminal bile sludge, forming a non-shadowing "sludge ball"

CT

As previously said, the main limitations of CT exam performed in patients with clinical suspicion of acute biliary disorders are represented by the detection of stones, which could be difficult to recognize—especially if they are small in size—and the radiation exposure. For these reasons, its use is limited to patients with atypical symptoms and signs or when complications are suspected.

Similarly to US exam, CT findings of acute cholecystitis include gallbladder distension with inhomogeneous bile attenuation and gallbladder wall thickening, with intense mucosal enhancement after endovenous injection of contrast media and ipo-attenuating submucosal edema (Fig. 13.11). In addition, the presence of pericholecystic fat stranding, pericholecystic fluid, and hyper-enhancement of liver parenchyma adjoining to gallbladder fossa (CT rim sign) could be detected [46].

MRI

When findings in previous exams are ambiguous, MR imaging may be helpful in detecting stones, especially in particular sites like gallbladder neck and cystic duct and the associated gallbladder wall abnormalities [47].

On T2-weighted images, the gallbladder wall may show increased signal intensity and

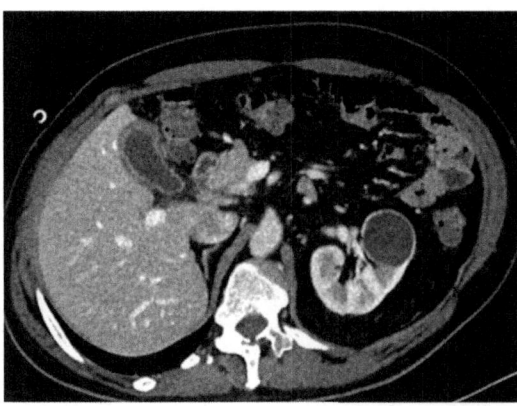

Fig. 13.11 Acute cholecystitis in a 51-year-old man with upper abdominal pain and fever, already treated by cholecystostomy. Axial contrast-enhanced CT image shows a gallbladder wall thickening, with intense mucosal enhancement and hypoattenuating submucosal edema

thickening. Pericholecystic fluid collections and edema of the surrounding liver tissue may be found. Periportal hyperintensity, although a nonspecific finding, may be observed on T2-weighted images. Although an inflammation-related increase in bile protein content may result in variable signal intensity of the bile on T1-weighted images, the bile usually appears markedly hypointense on T1-weighted sequences due to the impairment of gallbladder concentrating capability, a typical finding of the acute inflammatory phase. After administration of contrast media, gallbladder wall and surrounding fat show increased enhancement (Fig. 13.12). Similarly to CT exam, adjacent liver parenchyma can also show enhancement; this finding is due to a hyperemic response of the liver parenchyma related to acute inflammation of the gallbladder.

13.3.1.2 Complications

Emphysematous Cholecystitis

Emphysematous cholecystitis is a surgical emergency, prevalent in women and in diabetic population, and can occur as a complication of acalculous cholecystitis [48]. It is favored by hypoperfusion of cystic artery, and it carries a five times greater risk of perforation compared with uncomplicated acute cholecystitis [18].

It is typically caused by secondary infection of the gallbladder wall by gas-forming bacteria that infect the gallbladder wall producing intramural and intraluminal gas, such as *Clostridium welchii*, *C. perfringens*, *E. coli*, and *Bacteroides fragilis*.

On US exam it appears as inhomogeneous wall thickening, in which multiple hyperechoic, highly reflecting intramural spots can be detected ("dirty" shadowing). A more specific, though less common finding consists of small, non-shadowing echogenic foci rising up from the dependent portions of the gallbladder lumen, similar to effervescing bubbles in a glass of champagne ("champagne sign"). Also air in biliary ducts can be detected. The main limitations of ultrasound evaluation are represented by artifacts related to presence of gas within parietal wall or in the lumen of the

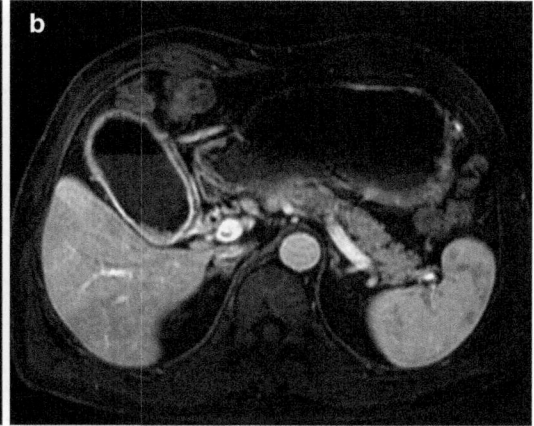

Fig. 13.12 Axial T1-weighted MR image before (**a**) and after gadolinium administration (**b**) in a 61-year-old man with persistent jaundice and biliary stent implantation. Gallbladder appears over-distended with a hyper-enhanced wall thickening and an intraluminal air-fluid level with hyperintense small stones in dependent position

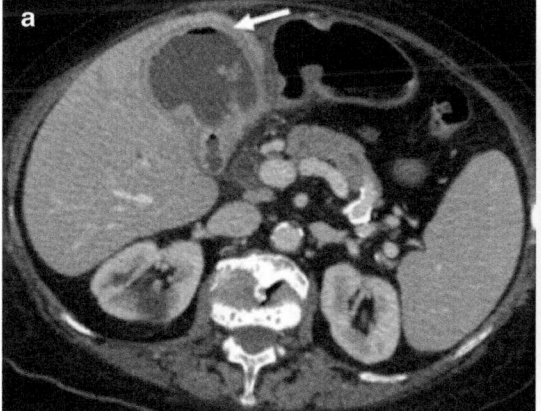 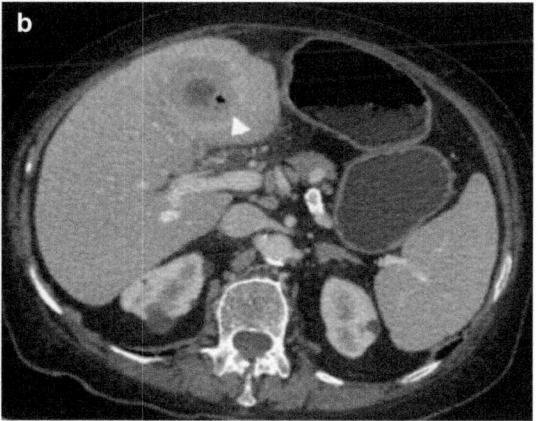

Fig. 13.13 (**a**, **b**) Emphysematous cholecystitis in an 86-year-old woman with upper abdominal pain and fever. Axial contrast-enhanced CT images show an over-distended gallbladder and an important wall thickening with intraluminal (arrow) and intramural air (arrow head)

gallbladder. For these reason CT (Fig. 13.13) is considered the most sensitive and specific imaging modality for identifying mural gas and for identifying complication like visceral perforation [49].

MR imaging has a supplementary role in providing information on intramural necrosis as well as intraluminal gas (Fig. 13.14). Gas in the gallbladder lumen and wall appears as signal void area, but it could be difficult to differentiate intramural gas from intramural stone. Susceptibility artifact at the air-tissue interface generates larger signal voids on fat-suppressed T1-w,

fat-suppressed T2-w, and black blood T2-w spin-echo echo-planar images than on heavily T2-w, because heavily T2-w images are less affected by susceptibility. This finding could help distinguish intramural gas from an intramural stone [27].

Gangrenous Cholecystitis

Gangrenous cholecystitis occurs in up to 39% of patients with acute calculous cholecystitis [50] as a consequence of ischemic injury of gallbladder wall related to inflammatory processes. The presence of focal mural defect can evolve into visceral perforation leading to loculated or freely

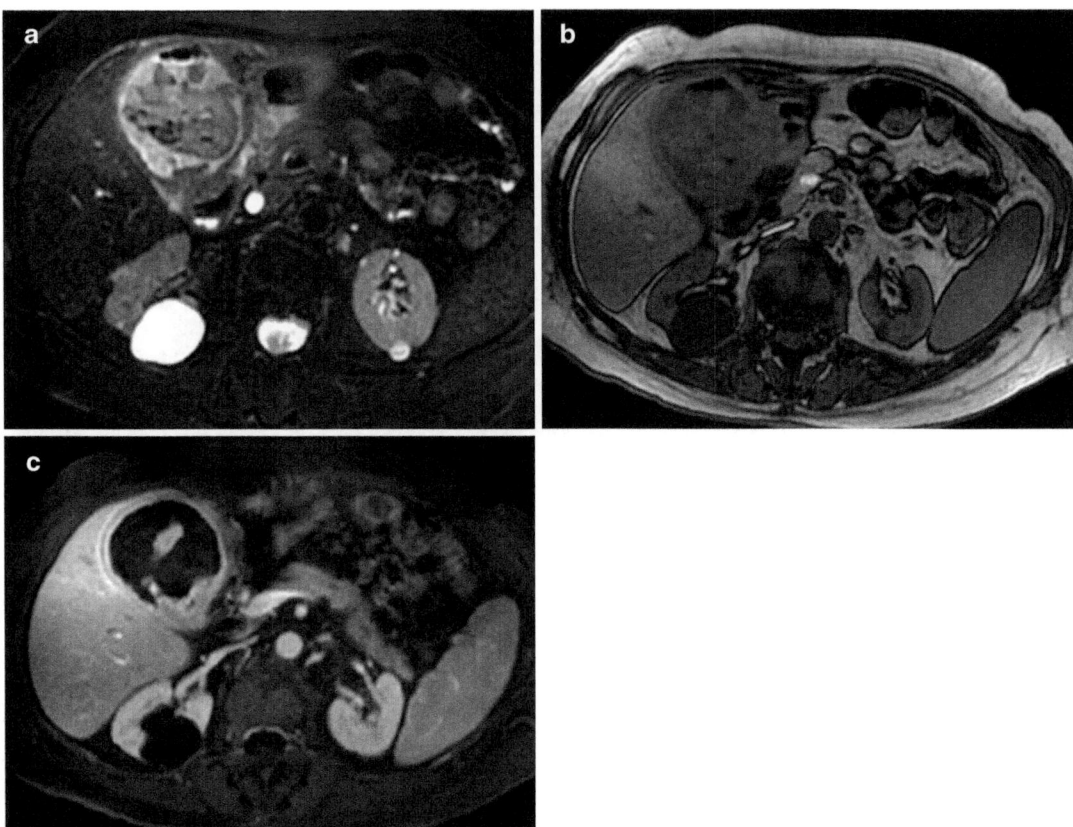

Fig. 13.14 Emphysematous cholecystitis in an 86-year-old woman: axial T2 fat-suppressed (**a**), T1 weighted out of phase (**b**), and contrast-enhanced (**c**). MR axial images show a marked gallbladder wall thickening with intense contrast enhancement. Inhomogeneous intraluminal material and void of signal areas due to air bubbles are also detected

flowing intraperitoneal bile [46], pericholecystic or intrahepatic abscess, and peritonitis, depending on the site of perforation [50].

Compared to not complicated cholecystitis, on US exam gangrenous cholecystitis appears as inhomogeneous, irregular hypoechoic wall thickening of gallbladder wall with hypoperfused areas on Doppler corresponding to necrosis with laminated intraluminal membrane.

Findings on CT exam are similar to US; in particular poorly enhancing wall with focal hypoattenuating defects in the gallbladder mucosa or sloughed intraluminal membranes suggests gangrene [46]. Pericholecystic abscesses, appearing as hypoattenuating areas rounded by tiny rim enhancement (Fig. 13.15), have been described in cases of gangrenous cholecystitis with specificity close to 90% [51].

On MRI, the "interrupted rim sign" (patchy enhancement of the gallbladder mucosa) represents areas of necrosis. Gangrenous cholecystitis may be suggested by asymmetric gallbladder wall thickening due to intramural microabscesses, intramural hemorrhage, and complex pericholecystic fluid collections containing debris.

Hemorrhagic Cholecystitis

Hemorrhagic cholecystitis is more prevalent in patients with alytiasic cholecystitis than lytiasic one. It can clinically present with hemobilia as a consequence of necrosis of the wall with subsequent rupture of small parietal vessels or bleeding of pseudoaneurysm of cystic artery.

In addition to the signs of acute inflammation, gallbladder appears distended by inhomogeneous hyperechoic finely corpusculated material

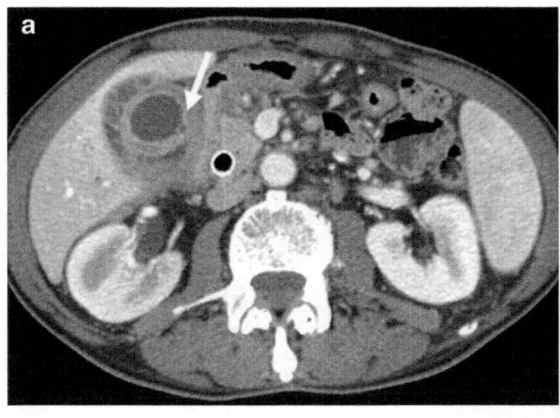

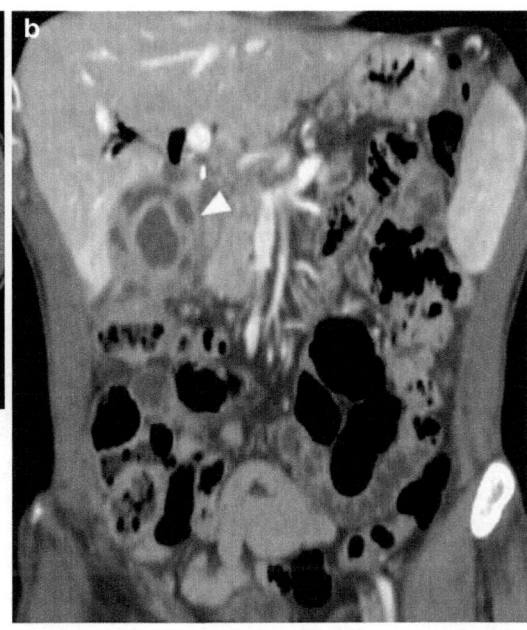

Fig. 13.15 Gangrenous cholecystitis in a 64-year-old woman with leukocytosis and abdominal pain and a clinical history of pancreatic adenocarcinoma. Axial (**a**) and coronal (**b**) contrast-enhanced CT images show gallbladder wall thickening with focal mucosal defects (arrow) without frank perforation and pericholecystic inflammation with multiple loculated fluid collections (arrow head)

suspended in the lumen or stratified in the declive position. Gallbladder wall can present irregular thickening with focal hypoechoic and hyperechoic areas related to underlying necrotic processes and focal hemorrhagic areas, respectively.

On CT exam, the gallbladder appears distended by hyperdense endoluminal material rounded by irregular thickening of the wall, which has patchy density before and after contrast media administration due to coexisting ischemic and hemorrhagic areas. Blood breakdown products in the gallbladder wall and lumen can be clearly identified on pre-contrast MRI sequences, detecting, according to their specific intensity of signal, the age of the hemorrhage [52].

Suppurative Cholecystitis

Suppurative cholecystitis (gallbladder empyema) typically occurs in diabetic patients as a consequence of infection by suppurative bacteria (Fig. 13.16). In addition to findings of acute non-complicated cholecystitis, gallbladder appears distended by corpusculated material that appears hyperechoic on US and hyperattenuating of CT exam, resembling sludge and without findings specific for empyema. At MRI imaging heavily T2-weighted imaging is sensitive enough to demonstrate purulent bile, which is dependent and has lower signal intensity. On other types of MR images, pus or purulent bile is difficult to demonstrate [27]. Only clinical signs and symptoms and percutaneous needle aspiration of the gallbladder can establish the diagnosis of empyema.

Cholecysto-Enteric Fistulas and Gallstones Ileus

Cholecysto-enteric fistulas are abnormal communications between gallbladder and gastrointestinal lumen via their wall and usually follow several episodes of acute or subacute cholecystitis.

Fistulas can occur between gallbladder and duodenum, in small bowel loops, or in colon (cholecysto-colic). When a gallstone greater than 2.5 cm in diameter passes through a fistula between the gallbladder and small bowel, the impacted gallstone on the ileocecal valve leads to a mechanical small bowel obstruction (*gallstones ileus*). Classical findings are defined in the "Rigler's

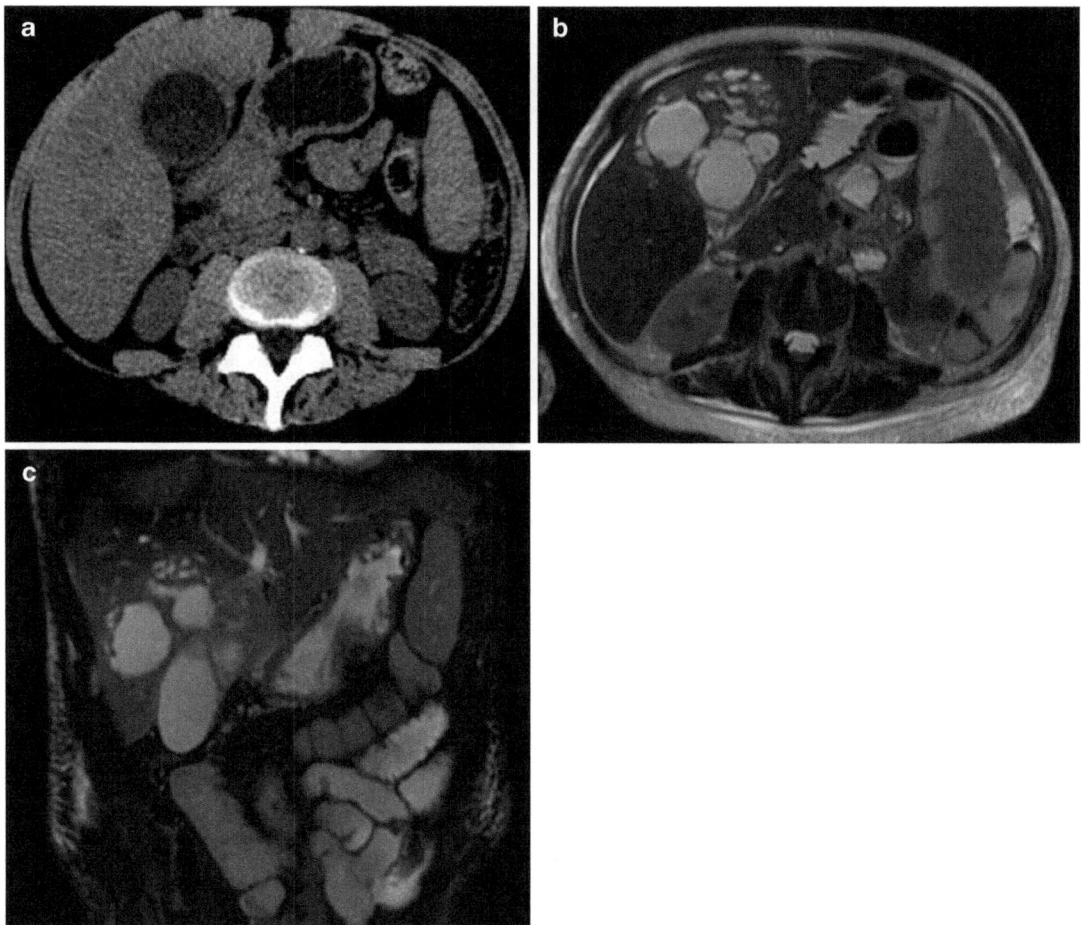

Fig. 13.16 Acute suppurative cholecystitis in a diabetic patient with abdominal pain and fever. Non-enhanced axial CT image (**a**) shows a distended gallbladder with moderate hypodense wall thickening and intraluminal high-attenuating corpusculated material resembling sludge. The MR images performed 1 week later (**b** and **c**) show gallbladder wall fissurations with multiple pericholecystic fluid collections. Percutaneous cholecystostomy was subsequently performed and purulent material was drained

triad": sign of small bowel mechanical obstruction, presence of gas in the lumen of gallbladder and/or in biliary tree (pneumobilia), and ectopic gallstone (usually in the right iliac fossa) (Fig. 13.17). The presence of two of the three signs of the Rigler's triad is considered diagnostic, and CT represents the imaging study of choice [53].

Bouveret syndrome consists in a gastric outlet obstruction produced by a gallstone impacted in the pylorus or proximal duodenum; it can be considered a very proximal form of gallstone ileus [54].

Pseudoaneurysms of Cholecystic Artery

Pseudoaneurysms of cholecystic artery are among the worst complications of acute cholecystitis because of their high risk of bleeding, and they are due to parietal artery damage as a consequence of acute inflammation. They could be asymptomatic when detected as incidental findings or can present as acute, massive upper abdomen bleeding. CT is the best effective instrument to detect the presence of pseudoaneurysms and to plan their best treatment.

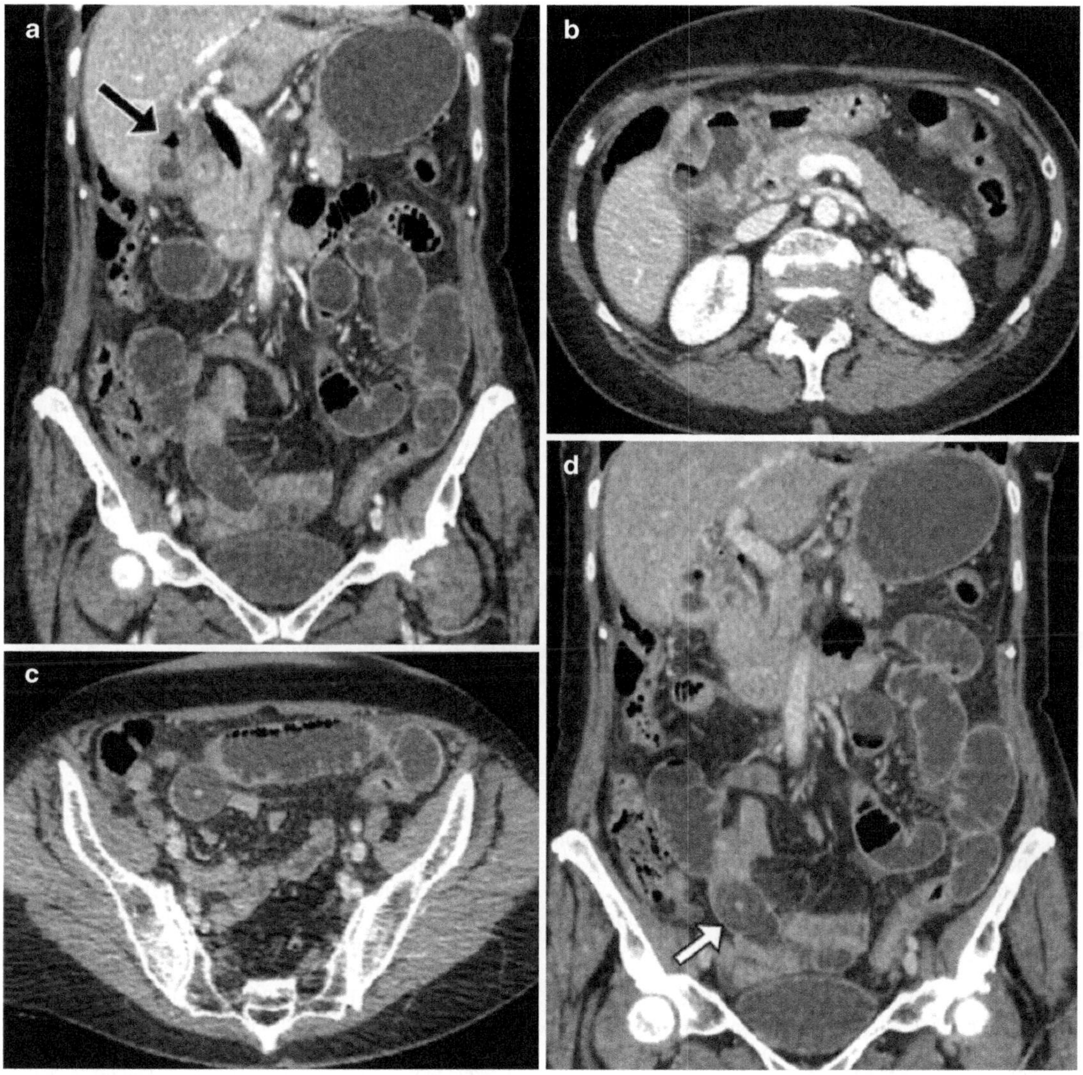

Fig. 13.17 Gallbladder perforation with an enterobiliary fistula in a 73-year-old woman with abdominal pain and high fever. Coronal (**a**) and axial (**b**) contrast-enhanced CT images show a collapsed gallbladder with an irregular wall thickening and inhomogeneous intense enhancement and a fistulous communication between the gallbladder wall and duodenum (black arrow). Axial and coronal CT images of the same patient (**c–d**) show dilated loops of small bowel up to the level of an obstructive gallstone, showing a hyperdense calcific core and a radiolucent peripheral component (white arrow)

References

1. Stinton LM, Shaffer EA. Epidemiology of gallbladder disease: cholelithiasis and cancer. Gut Liver. 2012;6:172–87.
2. Portincasa P, Moschetta A, Palasciano G. Cholesterol gallstone disease. Lancet. 2006;368:230–9.
3. Qiao T, Ma RH, Luo XB, Yang LQ, Luo ZL, Zheng PM. The systematic classification of gallbladder stones. PLoS One. 2013;8(10):e74887.
4. O'Connell K, Brasel K. Bile metabolism and lithogenesis. Surg Clin N Am. 2014;94:361–75.
5. Gurusamy KS, Davidson BR. Gallstones. BMJ. 2014;348:g2669.
6. Shaffer EA. Epidemiology of gallbladder stone disease. Best Pract Res Clin Gastroenterol. 2006;20(6):981–96.
7. Diehl AK, Sugarek NJ, Todd KH. Clinical evaluation for gallstone disease: usefulness of symptoms and signs in diagnosis. Am J Med. 1990;89(1):29–33.

8. Portincasa P, Moschetta A, Petruzzelli M, Palasciano G, Di Ciaula A, Pezzolla A. Symptoms and diagnosis of gallbladder stones. Best Pract Res Clin Gastroenterol. 2006;20:1017–29.

9. Molvar C, Glaenzer B. Choledocholithiasis: evaluation, treatment, and outcomes. Semin Intervent Radiol. 2016;33(4):268–76.

10. Csendes A, Diaz JC, Burdiles P, Maluenda F, Nava O. Mirizzi syndrome and cholecystobiliary fistula: a unifying classification. Br J Surg. 1989;76(11):1139–43.

11. Mallery JS, Baron TH, Dominitz JA, et al. Complications of ERCP. Gastrointest Endosc. 2003;57(6):633–8.

12. Bortoff GA, Chen MYM, Ott DJ, Wolfman NT, Routh WD. Gallbladder stones: imaging and intervention. Radiographics. 2000;20(3):751–66.

13. Einstein DM, Lapin SA, Ralls RW, Halls JM. The insensitivity of sonography in the detection of choledocholithiasis. Am J Roentgenol. 1984;142(4):725–8.

14. Blackbourne LH, Earnhardt RC, Sistrom CL, Abbitt P, Jones RS. The sensitivity and role of ultrasound in the evaluation of biliary obstruction. Am Surg. 1994;60(9):683–90.

15. Gandolfi L,v Torresan F, Solmi L, Puccetti A. The role of ultrasound in biliary and pancreatic diseases. Eur J Ultrasound. 2003;16:141–59.

16. Miller FH, Hwang CM, Gabriel H, Goodhartz LA, Omar AJ, Parsons WG. Contrast-enhanced helical CT of choledocholithiasis. Am J Roentgenol. 2003;181(1):125–30.

17. Yeh BM, Liu PS, Soto JA, Corvera CA, Hussain HK. MR imaging and CT of the biliary tract. Radiographics. 2009;29(6):1669–88.

18. Patel NB, Oto A, Thomas S. Multidetector CT of emergent biliary pathologic conditions. Radiographics. 2013;33(7):1867–88.

19. Chan WC, Joe BN, Coakley FV, Prien EL, Gould RG, Prevrhal S, et al. Gallstone detection at CT in vitro: effect of peak voltage setting. Radiology. 2006;241(2):546–53.

20. O'Connor OJ, Maher MM. Imaging of cholecystitis. Am J Roentgenol. 2011;196:W367–74.

21. Baron RL. Gallstone characterization: the role of imaging. Semin Roentgen. 1991;26:216–25.

22. Baron RL. Computed tomography of the bile ducts. Semin Roentgenol. 1997;32(3):172–87.

23. Soto JA, Velez SM, Guzmán J. Choledocholithiasis: diagnosis with oral-contrast-enhanced CT cholangiography. Am J Roentgenol. 1999;172(4):943–8.

24. Soto JA, Alvarez O, Munera F, Velez SM, Valencia J, Ramirez N. Diagnosing bile duct stones: comparison of unenhanced helical CT, oral contrast-enhanced CT cholangiography, and MR cholangiography. Am J Roentgenol. 2000;175(4):1127–34.

25. Cabada Giadás T, De Toledo LSO, Martínez-Berganza Asensio MT, Cozcolluela Cabrejas R, Alberdi Ibáñez I, Alvarez López A, et al. Helical CT cholangiography in the evaluation of the biliary tract: application to the

diagnosis of choledocholithiasis. Abdom Imaging. 2002;27(1):61–70.

26. Hou LA, Van Dam J. Pre-ERCP imaging of the bile duct and gallbladder. Gastrointest Endosc Clin N Am. 2013;23:185–97.

27. Watanabe Y, Nagayama M, Okumura A, Amoh Y, Katsube T, Suga T, et al. MR imaging of acute biliary disorders. Radiographics. 2007;27(2):477–95.

28. Hong-Ming T, Xi-Zhang L, Chiung-Yu C, Pin-Wen L, Jui-Che L. MRI of gallstones with different compositions. AJR Am J Roentgenol. 2004;182(6):1513–9.

29. Verma D, Kapadia A, Eisen GM, Adler DG. EUS vs MRCP for detection of choledocholithiasis. Gastrointest Endosc. 2006;64(2):248–54.

30. Irie H, Honda H, Kuroiwa T, Yoshimitsu K, Aibe H, Shinozaki K, et al. Pitfalls in MR cholangiopancreatographic interpretation. Radiographics. 2001;21:23–37.

31. Kondo S, Isayama H, Akahane M, Toda N, Sasahira N, Nakai Y, et al. Detection of common bile duct stones: comparison between endoscopic ultrasonography, magnetic resonance cholangiography, and helical-computed-tomographic cholangiography. Eur J Radiol. 2005;54:271–5.

32. Boey JH, Way LW. Acute cholangitis. Ann Surg. 1980;191(3):264–70.

33. Tsujino T, Sugita R, Yoshida H, Yagioka H, Kogure H, Sasaki T, et al. Risk factors for acute suppurative cholangitis caused by bile duct stones. Eur J Gastroenterol Hepatol. 2007;19(7):585–8.

34. Wada K, Takada T, Kawarada Y, Nimura Y, Miura F, Yoshida M, et al. Diagnostic criteria and severity assessment of acute cholangitis: Tokyo guidelines. J Hepato-Biliary-Pancreat Surg. 2007;14(1):52–8.

35. Flores C, Maguilnik I, Hadlich E, Goldani LZ. Microbiology of choledochal bile in patients with choledocholithiasis admitted to a tertiary hospital. J Gastroenterol Hepatol. 2003;18(3):333–6.

36. Pradella S, Centi N, La Villa G, Mazza E, Colagrande S. Transient hepatic attenuation difference (THAD) in biliary duct disease. Abdom Imaging. 2009;34(5):626–33.

37. Kim SW, Shin HC, Kim HC, Hong MJ, Kim IY. Diagnostic performance of multidetector CT for acute cholangitis: evaluation of a CT scoring method. Br J Radiol. 2012;85(1014):770–7.

38. Catalano O, Sahani DV, Forcione DG, Czermak B, Liu C-H, Soricelli A, et al. Biliary infections: spectrum of imaging findings and management. Radiographics. 2009;29(7):2059–80.

39. Bader TR, Braga L, Beavers KL, Semelka RC. MR imaging findings of infectious cholangitis. Magn Reson Imaging. 2001;19(6):781–8.

40. Testoni PA. Acute recurrent pancreatitis: etiopathogenesis, diagnosis and treatment. World J Gastroenterol. 2014;20:16891–901.

41. Cucher D, Kulvatunyou N, Green DJ, Jie T, Ong ES. Gallstone Pancreatitis. A review. Surg Clin N Am. 2014;94:257–80.

42. Attasaranya S, Fogel EL, Lehman GA. Choledocholithiasis, ascending cholangitis, and gallstone pancreatitis. Med Clin N Am. 2008;92:925–60.

43. Knab LM, Boller A-M, Mahvi DM. Cholecystitis. Surg Clin North Am. 2014;94(2):455–70.

44. Ansaloni L, Pisano M, Coccolini F, Peitzmann AB, Fingerhut A, Catena F, et al. WSES guidelines on acute calculous cholecystitis. World J Emerg Surg. 2016;11(16):2016.

45. Kiewiet JJS, Leeuwenburgh MMN, Bipat S, Bossuyt PMM, Stoker J, Boermeester MA. A systematic review and meta-analysis of diagnostic performance of imaging in acute cholecystitis. Radiology. 2012;264(3):708–20.

46. Shakespear JS, Shaaban AM, Rezvani M. CT findings of acute cholecystitis and its complications. AJR Am J Roentgenol. 2010;194(6):1523–9.

47. Catalano OA, Sahani DV, Kalva SP, Cushing MS, Hahn PF, Brown JJ, et al. MR imaging of the gallbladder: a pictorial essay. Radiographics. 2008;28(1):135–55.

48. Tellez LGS, Rodriguez-Montes JA, De Lis SF, Martin LGS. Acute emphysematous cholecystitis. Report of twenty cases. Hepatogastroenterology. 1999;46(28):2144–8.

49. Grayson DE, Abbott RM, Levy AD, Sherman PM. Emphysematous infections of the abdomen and pelvis: a pictorial review. Radiographics. 2002;22(3):543–61.

50. Chawla A, Bosco JI, Lim TC, Srinivasan S, Teh HS, Shenoy JN. Imaging of acute cholecystitis and cholecystitis-associated complications in the emergency setting. Singap Med J. 2015;56(8):438–44.

51. Bennett GL, Rusinek H, Lisi V, Israel GM, Krinsky GA, Slywotzky CM, et al. CT findings in acute gangrenous cholecystitis. Am J Roentgenol. 2002;178(2):275–81.

52. Elsayes KM, Oliveira EP, Narra VR, EL-Merhi FM, Brown JJ. Magnetic resonance imaging of the gallbladder: spectrum of abnormalities. Acta Radiol. 2007;48(5):476–82.

53. Ploneda-Valencia CF, Gallo-Morales M, Rinchon C, Navarro-Muñiz E, Bautista-López CA, de la Cerda-Trujillo LF, et al. Gallstone ileus: an overview of the literature. Rev Gastroenterol México (English Ed.) 2017;82(3):248–54.

54. Brennan GB, Rosenberg RD, Arora S. Bouveret syndrome. Radiographics. 2004;24:1171–5.

Imaging of Pancreatitis

Roberto Pozzi Mucelli, Riccardo Negrelli,
Matteo Catania, and Marco Chincarini

14.1 Introduction

Acute pancreatitis (AP) is an acute inflammatory process of the pancreatic gland that can involve pancreatic parenchyma or distant organs. In 80–85% of cases, AP is a self-limiting inflammatory process that can often cause even a multi-organ failure (MOF) [1, 2].

In Western countries the incidence of acute pancreatitis ranges from 5 to 70 cases per 100.000 adults, without a sex prevalence [3]. However, in the last decades, the incidence of AP has increased due to an increase of risk factors [4, 5]. AP remains one of the most common reasons for hospitalization, and its management is complex and requires a multidisciplinary team.

Acute pancreatitis has different etiologies; however, gallstones and alcohol abuse are the most frequent in adults. Gallstone pancreatitis accounts for about 35–40% [6, 7]. The stones cause an obstruction at the level of the papilla leading to increased pancreatic duct pressure and passage of bile into the pancreatic duct which lead to an acute inflammation of the pancreatic gland. Alcohol is the second most common cause

of AP, accounting for 30% of cases, and its effects seem to be dose related [4, 6]. Alcohol may cause a direct cytotoxic effect on acinar cells. Moreover, alcohol seems to cause transient contractions of the sphincter of Oddi and increases serum levels of triglycerides, both potentially independent causes of AP. Other rare causes of AP include hypertriglyceridemia, hypercalcemia, iatrogenic trauma during endoscopic retrograde cholangiopancreatography (ERCP), trauma, infections, and penetrating peptic ulcer. Genetic conditions, such as the mutation of PRSS1, SPINK1, and CFTR genes, are associated with AP due to a loss in control of pancreatic enzymes activation or in exocrine secretion. However, the cause of AP remains unknown in about 20% of cases [8].

Independently from etiology, the common final pathway for AP is the unregulated activation of the pancreatic enzymes within the pancreatic acinar cells, resulting in a damage of the pancreatic parenchyma and local inflammation (Table 14.1) [2, 5, 8].

Clinical manifestations of AP include a gradual or an acute onset of upper abdominal pain that sometimes extends to the back. The pain is often severe and constant and commonly lasts for several days in the absence of treatment. It is usually associated with fever, vomiting, tachycardia, and leukocytosis [5].

The management and study of acute pancreatitis remain complex [1, 6]. For this reason, in 1992 a group of experts introduced the

Electronic Supplementary Material The online version of this chapter (https://doi.org/10.1007/978-3-319-99822-0_14) contains supplementary material, which is available to authorized users.

R. P. Mucelli (✉) · R. Negrelli · M. Catania
M. Chincarini
Department of Radiology, Policlinico G. B. Rossi – University Hospital of Verona, Verona, Italy

M. A. Cova, F. Stacul (eds.), *Pain Imaging*, https://doi.org/10.1007/978-3-319-99822-0_14

Table 14.1 Causes of acute pancreatitis

Common causes	Rare causes
Biliary lithiasis	Pancreas divisum
Alcohol	Genetic
Hyperlipidemia	Infections
Hypercalcemia	Autoimmune disease
Drugs	Trauma
ERCP	Vasculitis
Sphincteric dysfunction	

Atlanta classification of AP. However, due to advances in knowledge in AP and the improvement in imaging studies, the 1992 Atlanta classification was considered outdated. For these reasons, an international panel of experts revised the first classification, and in 2012 the revised Atlanta classification was published [2, 4, 9, 10].

The role of this revision was to delineate a specific and standardized lexicon that allows the radiologist to be an effective member of the multidisciplinary team in the diagnosis and treatment of acute pancreatitis.

Chronic pancreatitis (CP) is an inflammatory disease characterized by progressive and irreversible distortion and destruction of the pancreatic parenchyma, with progressive loss of the endocrine and exocrine function of the gland [11, 12].

Several reports estimate a progressive increase in the incidence of CP, especially in emerging countries, as a result of availability of high-quality cross-sectional imaging techniques, rapid urbanization, and alcohol consumption. The annual incidence of CP ranges from 3.5 to 10/100.000 persons. The incidence of CP is higher in middle-aged men than in women (6.7 versus 3.2/100.000) [13–15].

The clinical diagnosis of chronic pancreatitis is usually achieved only in advanced disease. The clinical presentation of CP varies depending on the causal mechanism. Clinically CP is characterized by upper abdominal pain which sometimes may resemble an acute pancreatitis. In advanced disease, CP is associated with steatorrhea and diabetes, due to progressive loss of the exocrine and endocrine function of the pancreatic parenchyma [12, 16].

The etiology and the pathophysiology of chronic pancreatitis are not well defined. Several theories have been proposed: obstructive ductal involvement, oxidative stress of the parenchyma, fibrosis and necrosis of the pancreatic parenchyma secondary to acinar obstruction, autoimmune involvement, and multifactorial or idiopathic disease. Various systems have been proposed to classify pancreatitis on the basis of clinical presentation, radiological features, and etiology [11, 16, 17]. The "TIGAR-O" classification of chronic pancreatitis has been proposed to replace the previous Marseilles classification. The TIGAR-O risk factor system lists factors associated with chronic pancreatitis (Table 14.2) [12].

However, histologic alterations and clinical features of chronic pancreatitis are similar. It seems that CP results from an obstruction of the small or large pancreatic ducts leading to pancreatitis with the consequent precipitation of protein-rich plugs within the interlobular and intralobular ducts. Ductal obstruction results in inflammation, which subsequently leads to fibrosis of the pancreatic parenchyma. Moreover, obstruction of the pancreatic ducts leads to pancreatic ductal hypertension with the consequent hypoperfusion of the organ, with ischemic injury of the acinar cells. Furthermore the resulting reduction of pancreatic juice outflow is responsible for the increase of the precipitation of additional protein plugs and calcifications [12, 16].

Alcohol assumption is considered the leading cause of chronic pancreatitis, and it increases the risk of chronic disease in a dose-dependent manner. It is postulated that alcohol consumption is responsible for a direct injury of the acinar cells and it could interfere with mechanisms that protect against stress induced by reactive oxygen species and pancreatic enzymes. Other risk factors include smoke and genetic factors, such as mutations of genes *PRSS1* (cationic trypsin gene), *SPINK1* (serum protease inhibitor), and *CFTR* alteration [11, 14, 16–18].

Furthermore neoplasms, mass-forming pancreatitis (e.g., focal autoimmune pancreatitis, paraduodenal pancreatitis), sphincter of Oddi dysfunction, or anatomical variations of the pancreatic ductal system (pancreas divisum, annular

Table 14.2 Etiologic risk factors associated with chronic pancreatitis: TIGAR-O classification system

Toxic-metabolic
Alcoholic
Tobacco smoking
Hypercalcemia
Hyperparathyroidism
Hyperlipidemia (rare and controversial)
Chronic renal failure
Medications
Phenacetin abuse (possibly from chronic renal insufficiency)
Toxins
Organotin compounds (e.g., DBTC)
Idiopathic
Early onset
Late onset
Tropical
Tropical calcific pancreatitis
Fibrocalculous pancreatic diabetes
Other
Genetic
Autosomal dominant
Cationic trypsinogen (codon 29 and 122 mutations)
Autosomal recessive/modifier genes
CFTR mutations
SPINK1 mutations
Cationic trypsinogen (codon 16, 22, 23 mutations)
α1-Antitrypsin deficiency (possible)
Autoimmune
Isolated autoimmune chronic pancreatitis
Syndromic autoimmune chronic pancreatitis
Sjögren syndrome-associated chronic pancreatitis
Inflammatory bowel disease-associated chronic pancreatitis
Primary biliary cirrhosis-associated chronic pancreatitis
Recurrent and severe acute pancreatitis
Postnecrotic (severe acute pancreatitis)
Recurrent acute pancreatitis
Vascular diseases/ischemic
Postirradiation
Obstructive
Pancreas divisum
Sphincter of Oddi disorders (controversial)
Duct obstruction (e.g., tumor)
Periampullary duodenal wall cysts
Post-traumatic pancreatic duct scars

pancreas) are responsible for a stenosis of the main pancreatic duct or for an impaired pancreatic juice outflow in the duodenum. Moreover, it is demonstrated that recurrent episodes of acute pancreatitis could develop in chronic pancreatitis, as a disease continuum [19].

14.2 Acute Pancreatitis

14.2.1 Diagnostic Criteria

The revised Atlanta classification requires two of the three following conditions: (1) abdominal pain suggestive for AP; (2) serum amylase and/or lipase level greater than three or more times the upper limit of normal; and (3) characteristic imaging findings on contrast-enhanced computed tomography, magnetic resonance, or transabdominal ultrasonography [20].

AP is mainly a clinical diagnosis and CT or MR are usually performed to confirm the diagnosis. In most cases imaging should not be performed in the first days. The use of imaging early in the course of the disease may be useful when the cause is unclear or to find causative factors such as biliary stone disease. Diagnostic imaging is also appropriate when the biochemical criterion is not met but the clinical setting is highly suspicious for AP [4]. The onset of AP coincides with the first day of pain [20].

14.2.2 Clinical Classification

14.2.2.1 Phases of Acute Pancreatitis

The revised Atlanta classification divides acute pancreatitis into early and late phases [20].

The early phase occurs in the first week and is characterized by a systemic response to local inflammation, resulting in systemic complications. This phase is typically characterized by the presence of organ failure rather than morphological alterations. Moreover, imaging of local or systemic complications is usually not present.

The late phase starts after the first week, and it is characterized by persistent signs and symptoms and local or systemic complications such as infection of pancreatic necrosis or peripancreatic fluid collections. Moreover, the treatment is determined by the presence of symptoms due to

Table 14.3 Modified Marshall scoring system

Organ system	0	1	2	3	4
Respiratory (PaO$_2$/FiO$_2$)	>400	301–400	201–300	101–200	≤100
Renal: serum creatinine (mg/dL)	≤1.4	1.5–1.8	1.9–3.5	3.6–4.9	≥5
Cardiovascular: systolic blood pressure (mm Hg)	>90	<90, responding to fluid resuscitation	<90, not responding to fluid resuscitation	<90, with pH <7.3	<90, with pH <7.2

Based on Foster et al. [4]

Sources: [4, 20, 23, 24]

local complications, and thus, imaging plays a pivotal role in patient management. This phase usually occurs in patients with moderately severe and severe acute pancreatitis.

14.2.2.2 Severity of Acute Pancreatitis

The revised Atlanta classification defined three degrees of severity of acute pancreatitis, depending on the presence or absence of organ failure and local and systemic complications.

In *mild acute pancreatitis*, the inflammation does not lead to organ failure or complications. These patients are usually discharged within the first week with very low mortality. CT is usually not performed and imaging is useful to assess the cause of AP [21, 22].

Moderately severe acute pancreatitis is defined as the presence of transient organ failure lasting less than 48 h and/or the presence of local or systemic complications (not resulting in persistent organ failure). Local complications refer to pancreatic or peripancreatic collections that usually develop during the late phase and should be suspected in patients with unremitting pain, secondary peak in pancreatic enzymes, worsening of organ failure, or sepsis. In these cases, imaging studies (contrast-enhanced CT at first) should be performed [21]. This category of patients is characterized by high morbidity but very low mortality.

Severe acute pancreatitis is defined by organ failure that lasts more than 48 h.

An accurate evaluation of organ function is essential to define disease severity. For this reason, the modified Marshall scoring system is endorsed in the new Atlanta classification as the primary method for determining organ failure.

This scoring system evaluates the respiratory, cardiovascular, and renal functions [4, 23] (Table 14.3).

Two imaging-based scoring systems are the "CT severity index (CTSI)" and the "modified CTSI," which are based on morphological findings and correlate with morbidity and mortality [25, 26]. However often imaging is not able to define the presence of necrosis during the first days after onset of symptoms (early phase) and correlates poorly with clinical severity. Imaging becomes useful after 3–5 days after onset, when local complications have developed and pancreatic necrosis is clearly visible [4, 20].

14.2.3 Morphological Classification

Acute pancreatitis is morphologically classified into two types on the basis of imaging findings: interstitial edematous pancreatitis (IEP) and necrotizing pancreatitis [20, 40]. Imaging has the important role to assess the presence or absence of necrosis (necrotizing vs IEP), the site(s) of necrosis, and the presence or absence of infections (sterile vs infected necrosis).

IEP is the most common type of AP. At CT, IEP is characterized by a diffuse or focal enlargement of the pancreatic parenchyma. The pancreas may enhance normally, although sometimes, the enhancement can be reduced or heterogeneous because of the presence of edema. Peripancreatic and retroperitoneal tissues may be normal or show mild inflammatory changes, such as mild fat stranding or peripancreatic fluid-containing collections [4, 20] (Fig. 14.1). The presence of necrosis precludes the interstitial edematous subtype.

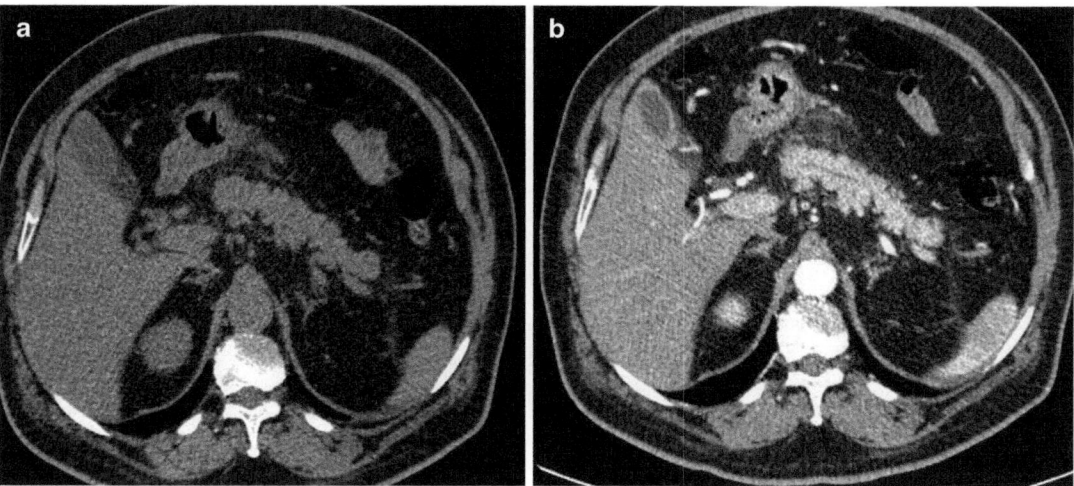

Fig. 14.1 Interstitial edematous pancreatitis (IEP). Axial CT images in the non-contrast (**a**) and in the arterial phase (**b**) show a pancreatic parenchyma with normal enhance-ment. Mild inflammatory changes (stranding of the peri-pancreatic fat tissues) are visible

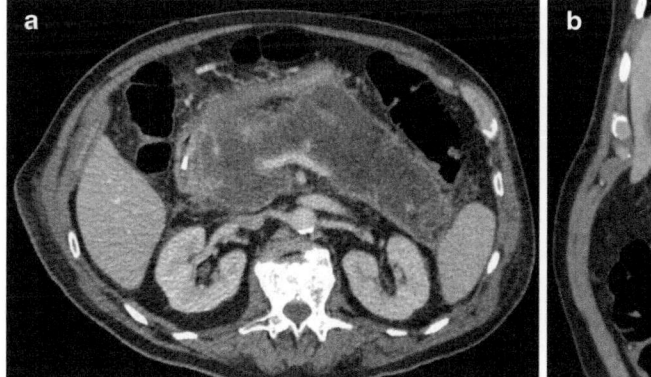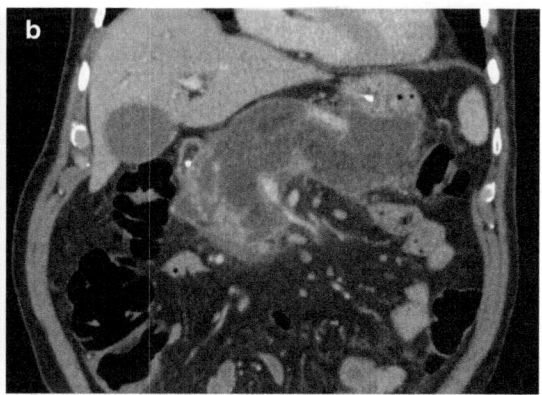

Fig. 14.2 Pancreatic necrosis only. Axial (**a**) and coronal curvilinear reformatted CT images (**b**) in the portal-venous phase show a diffuse inhomogeneous pancreatic parenchyma with lack of parenchymal contrast enhancement, due to necrosis of the pancreatic parenchyma

Necrotizing pancreatitis is defined as a focal or diffuse area of necrotic tissue due to vascular damage which leads to lack of contrast enhance-ment [1, 27]. Necrosis may involve the pancreatic parenchyma, the peripancreatic tissues, or both. Therefore, three subtypes of necrotizing pancre-atitis have been defined: (a) pancreatic parenchy-mal necrosis, (b) peripancreatic necrosis, and (c) combined pancreatic parenchymal necrosis and peripancreatic necrosis [20].

The first subtype is extremely rare, accounting for only 5% of cases, and it is characterized by necrotic tissue and lack of enhancement confined to the pancreatic parenchyma affected (Fig. 14.2). According to CTSI and m-CTSI, the extent of the necrosis can be quantified by <30%, 30–50%, >50%, or total pancreatic parenchyma [20].

The second subtype accounts for 20% of cases, and it is characterized by necrosis of peri-pancreatic fatty and connective tissue. The diag-nosis is based on the presence of heterogeneous density of the peripancreatic collections due to fat necrosis, fluid collections, and hemorrhagic components. This subtype has a better prognosis compared to pancreatic necrosis alone, but it has higher morbidity than IEP [20, 28].

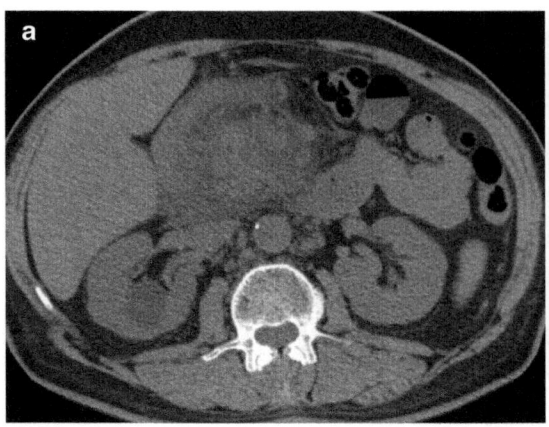
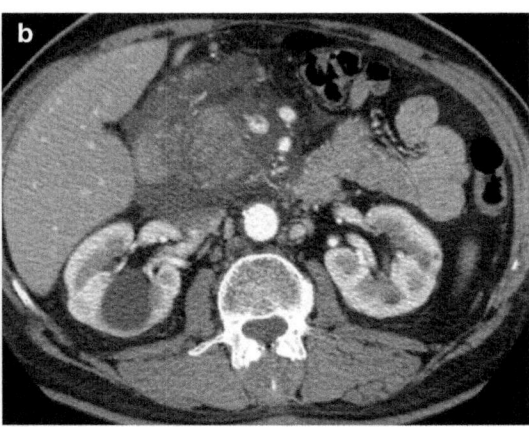

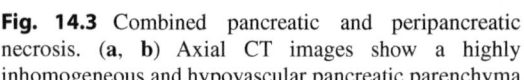

Fig. 14.3 Combined pancreatic and peripancreatic necrosis. (**a**, **b**) Axial CT images show a highly inhomogeneous and hypovascular pancreatic parenchyma of the head of the pancreas, with multiple hypodense areas due to necrosis that extend to the peripancreatic tissues

The combined subtype is the most common, accounting for 75% of cases (Fig. 14.3) [20].

14.2.4 Complications

According to the revised Atlanta classification system, complications from acute pancreatitis can be divided into organ failure, systemic complications, and local complications [20, 24].

14.2.4.1 Organ Failure
Three organ systems should be assessed to define organ failure: respiratory, cardiovascular, and renal. As discussed above, organ failure is usually primary assessed based on the modified Marshall scoring system (Table 14.3).

14.2.4.2 Systemic Complications
Systemic complications are events that are triggered by acute pancreatitis and represent acute exacerbations of preexisting comorbidities such as chronic lung disease and coronary artery disease.

14.2.4.3 Local Complications
In the revised Atlanta classification, the most important local complications are pancreatic and peripancreatic collections, and they may be sterile or infected. Other local complications caused by necrotizing pancreatitis include pseudoaneurysm, splenic or portal vein thrombo- sis, obstruction or ileus of the gastrointestinal tract, contiguous inflammation of the colon, biliary stones, cholecystitis, pancreatic duct strictures, involvement of neighboring solid organs, ascites, and pleural effusions.

Local complications should be suspected when there is a change in the clinical presentation, secondary increases in serum pancreatic enzyme activity, increasing organ dysfunction, and/or the development of clinical signs of sepsis, such as fever and leucocytosis. These developments usually prompt imaging to detect local complications.

Pancreatic and Peripancreatic Collections
The revised Atlanta classification introduces a distinction between purely fluid collections (seen in IEP) and collections that contain necrosis (seen in necrotizing pancreatitis). The new classification accurately distinguishes various types of collections: acute peripancreatic fluid collection (APFC), pseudocyst, acute necrotic collection (ANC), and walled-off necrosis (WON). The parameters for this classification are the time course (<4 weeks or >4 weeks) and the presence or absence of necrosis (Table 14.4) [4, 20].

14.2.4.4 Acute Peripancreatic Fluid Collection and Pseudocyst
APFCs usually develop in the first 4 weeks in patients with IEP. APFCs are inflammatory and

Table 14.4 Pancreatic and peripancreatic collections

	Time	Pancreatitis category	Location	Imaging
APFC	< 4 weeks	IEP	Peripancreatic	Fluid collection; homogeneous; no wall
ANC	< 4 weeks	Necrotizing pancreatitis	Intra- and/or extra-pancreatic	Inhomogeneous; debris; fat globules; no wall
Pseudocyst	> 4 weeks	IEP	Extra-pancreatic	Homogeneous, fluid filled, no debris; presence of wall
WON	> 4 weeks	Necrotizing pancreatitis	Intra- and/or extra-pancreatic	Inhomogeneous; debris; fat globules; blood; presence of a wall

Sources: [4, 24, 28]
APFC acute peripancreatic fluid collection, *ANC* acute necrotic collection, *WON* walled-off necrosis, *IEP* interstitial edematous pancreatitis

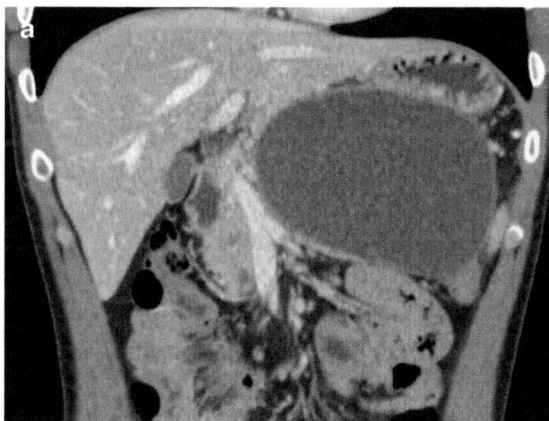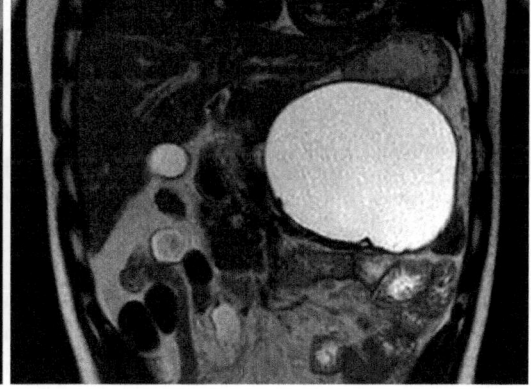

Fig. 14.4 Pancreatic pseudocyst. Coronal curvilinear reformatted CT image (**a**) shows a large, homogeneous fluid collection in the body-tail of the pancreas, 4 weeks after the first episode of acute pancreatitis. In the coronal T2-weighted image (**b**), the pseudocyst appears as a well-circumscribed collection, completely encapsulated, with no solid components

homogeneous nonencapsulated peripancreatic fluid collections (Fig. 14.1). If a collection with these characteristics is located within the pancreas, it becomes by definition an ANC, associated with necrotizing pancreatitis. APFCs tend to resolve spontaneously [29]. If they persist for more than 4 weeks, they become organized and develop an enhancing capsule. At this point, the collection is referred to as pseudocyst (Fig. 14.4). Pseudocysts contain only fluid without debris or areas of fat/soft tissues attenuation. Pseudocysts develop in less than 10% of cases of IEP [4, 29]. A pseudocyst is typically peripancreatic in location, although it can be intrapancreatic in case of prior necrosectomy. Pseudocyst can also be associated with necrotizing pancreatitis

in the setting of disconnected duct syndrome. In this case, the leakage of pancreatic juices flows into a fluid-containing cavity with the formation of a pseudocyst [4, 30].

Although CECT is the imaging modality used most commonly to describe pseudocysts, MRI or ultrasonography may be required to confirm the absence of solid content in the collection. Occasionally, a connection to the pancreatic duct can be visualized on CECT, particularly if a curvilinear reconstruction is obtained; however MR and endoscopic ultrasound are more accurate in performing this task. Ductal communication is not part of the revised Atlanta criteria for a pseudocyst, but it may be an important finding for deciding on the appropriate treatment.

14.2.4.5 Acute Necrotic Collection and Walled-Off Necrosis

ANCs develop in the first 4 weeks in patients with necrotizing pancreatitis and are ill-defined necrotic collections which are usually located in the retroperitoneum and in the anterior pararenal space. They can be in continuity with areas of pancreatic necrosis or extend inferiorly toward the pelvis. ANCs present often as multiple, loculated collections with variable amount of fluid and with non-liquefied debris within, represented by solid appearing components of fat globules (Figs. 14.2 and 14.3). Fat component inside a collection is highly suggestive for an ANC. It must be noted that in the presence of pancreatic necrosis, every peripancreatic collection should be defined as ANC, regardless of its appearance [4, 20]. It may be difficult to differentiate an APFC from ANC, especially in the first week. At CT both types may appear homogeneous with fluid density. However, during follow-up an ANC will frequently appear as a not fully encapsulated heterogeneous collection within the pancreatic parenchyma and/or peripancreatic areas. If a complete encapsulating wall is evident, which happens mostly after 4 weeks, the collection should be called walled-off necrosis (WON), which represents the late stage of an ANC (Fig. 14.5). WON contains heterogeneous components (fat and/or solid tissue), which are demonstrated at CT as non-liquefied debris. Like ANC, WON are most commonly located in both the pancreatic parenchyma and in the peripancreatic tissue [4, 20]. At CT, differentiation between WON and pancreatic pseudocyst may be difficult, and, therefore, an additional MRI, EUS, or US can better characterize the content of the collection. Management of WON is more invasive than management of pancreatic pseudocyst, since patients with WON may need interventional treatment by removing nonliquid material.

Infection

Any collection may become infected, although infection occurs more often in necrotic ones.

Independently from the subtype of necrosis, the presence of infected necrosis changes the natural history and prognosis of the disease, since it is associated with mortality rates of 30–40%, whereas in sterile necrosis mortality rates are between 0 and 10%. Infected necrosis has a peak incidence in the second-third week after onset of symptoms [27]. At contrast-enhanced CT, the infected area can show gas bubbles localized within the necrotic tissue (Fig. 14.6). However, this sign is reported to be present in only 20% of cases [27]. Wall enhancement is not reliable because it is usually present in mature collection (both pseudocysts and WON). Air bubbles may be present due to fistula formation between a collection and adjacent bowel (colon or duodenum) [31].

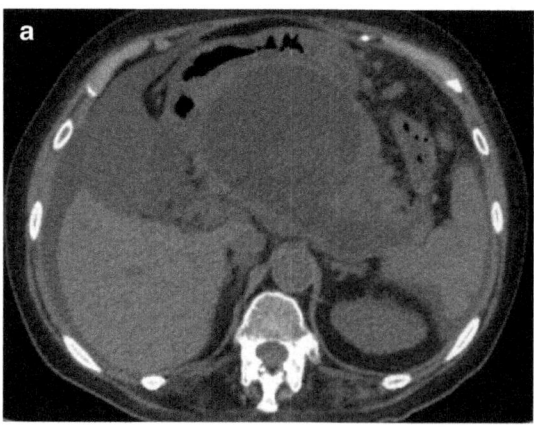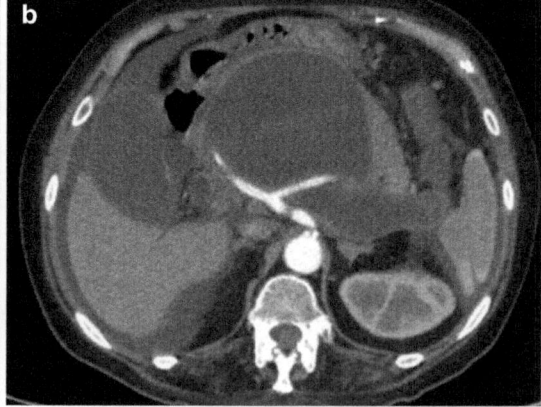

Fig. 14.5 WON. Axial CT images in the non-contrast (**a**) and in the arterial phase (**b**) show a heterogeneous collection with fluid components, non-liquefied debris, and fat globules inside. The collection has thick enhancing walls and it is by definition a WON

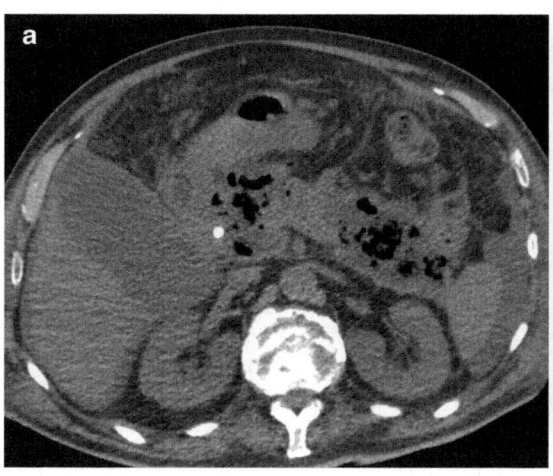
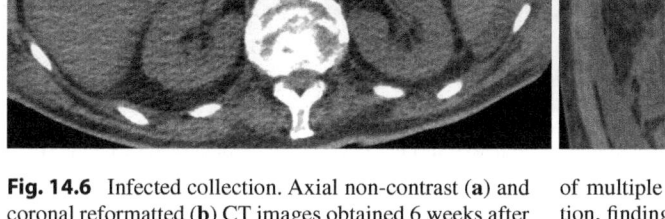
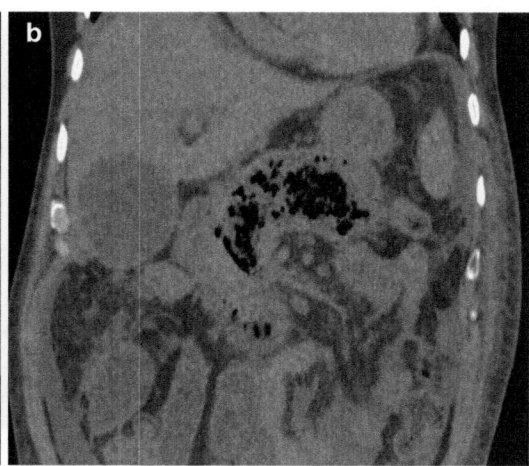

Fig. 14.6 Infected collection. Axial non-contrast (**a**) and coronal reformatted (**b**) CT images obtained 6 weeks after onset of acute necrotizing pancreatitis show the presence of multiple air bubbles within the heterogeneous collection, findings that are consistent with infected WON

The depiction of an infected necrotic area has a crucial role for the management of patients, since parenteral antibiotics combined with laparoscopic or endoscopic necrosectomy may be required.

Other Local Complications

Vascular complications are common, being encountered in 25% of patients with AP [4, 32]. The most frequent vascular complication is splenic vein thrombosis, while portal vein or superior mesenteric vein thrombosis is diagnosed less frequently [33]. Thrombosis is due to inflammatory reaction [34]. At CECT it is depicted as an increased vessel diameter, hyperdensity of the wall (enhancement of the vasa vasorum), and a central filling defect due to thrombosis [32].

The leakage of pancreatic enzymes can lead to arterial erosion with subsequent pseudoaneurysm formation. Pseudoaneurysms may also occur if a pseudocyst encases a visceral artery causing an erosion of the wall [35]. The most commonly involved arteries are the splenic artery (40%), the gastroduodenal artery (30%), the pancreaticoduodenal artery (20%), the gastric artery (5%), the hepatic artery (2%), and others (1–3%) [36]. Pseudoaneurysms may enlarge and eventually rupture leading to hemorrhage, which represents one of the most life-threatening complications of AP. CECT is the best diagnostic tool to depict the presence of a pseudoaneurysm and to detect active bleeding.

Other local complications include obstruction or ileus of the gastrointestinal tract, contiguous inflammation of the colon, biliary stones, cholecystitis, pancreatic duct strictures, involvement of neighboring solid organs, ascites, and pleural effusions [24] (Fig. 14.7).

14.2.4.6 Imaging

Radiography

Plain films of the abdomen are part of the initial diagnostic workup of acute abdominal pain. Findings on plain films are nonspecific but could be suggestive of acute pancreatitis. The most commonly recognized radiologic signs associated with acute inflammation of the pancreas include the following:

- Air in the duodenal C-loop
- The sentinel loop sign, which represents a focal dilated proximal jejunal loop in the left upper quadrant
- The colon cutoff sign, which represents distention of the colon to the transverse colon with a paucity of gas distal to the splenic flexure

Other findings include obscuration of the psoas margin, increased epigastric soft tissue

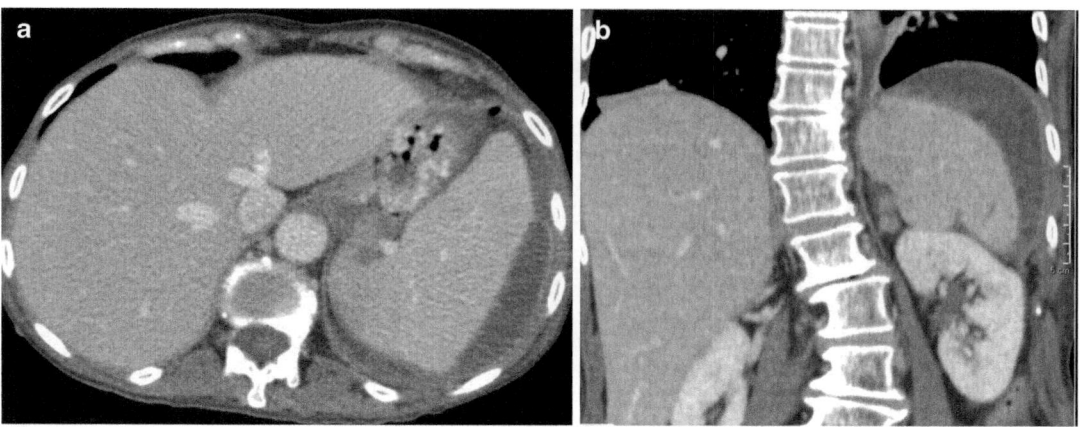

Fig. 14.7 Intrasplenic pseudocyst. Axial CT image in the portal-venous phase (**a**) and its coronal reconstruction (**b**) of a 56-year-old male 5 weeks after onset of acute pancreatitis show a fluid encapsulated subcapsular splenic collection

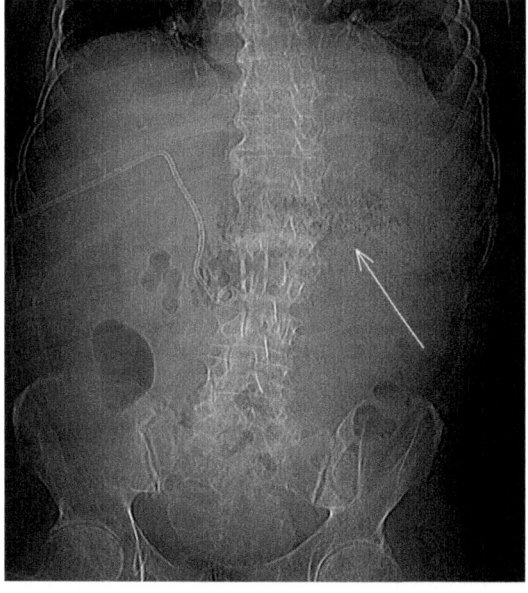

Fig. 14.8 Infected WON. Plain film of the abdomen, 5 weeks after onset of acute necrotizing pancreatitis, shows multiple air bubbles in a superinfected walled-off necrosis

Computed Tomography

Contrast-enhanced CT is the modality of choice for the evaluation of patients with acute pancreatitis because of its rapid acquisition, worldwide availability, and panoramic view which allows a complete visualization of local and distant complications.

As previously stated, not all patients with AP require CECT, since in case of mild pancreatitis, CT is not necessary; on the other hand, in patients with severe pancreatitis, a CECT study is mandatory [20].

A monophasic CT protocol after injection of contrast media is considered to be sufficient for the diagnosis and assessment of AP [4]. A multiphasic protocol can provide more information about pancreatic parenchyma (late-arterial phase) and about other abdominal structures or vessels (venous phase).

CT findings depend on the extent and severity of the disease. In mild pancreatitis, typically the pancreatic parenchyma appears diffusely enlarged, with normal enhancement, with or without fat stranding. In severe forms, parenchymal necrosis and necrotic collections may develop within the pancreatic parenchyma or in the peripancreatic region. Fluid or necrotic collections are usually located in the retroperitoneum, along the anterior pararenal fascia, at the base of the transverse mesocolon, and in the lesser sac [2].

density, increased gastrocolic separation, gastric curvature distortion, and pleural effusion (usually on the left). Rarely, in case of necrotizing pancreatitis and superinfected pancreatic collection, pancreatic emphysema may be visible (Fig. 14.8). However, it is noteworthy that in the majority of patients, the abdominal plain film can be completely normal in acute pancreatitis.

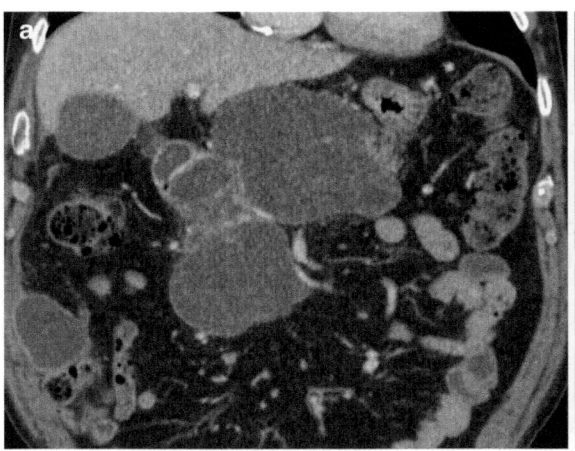 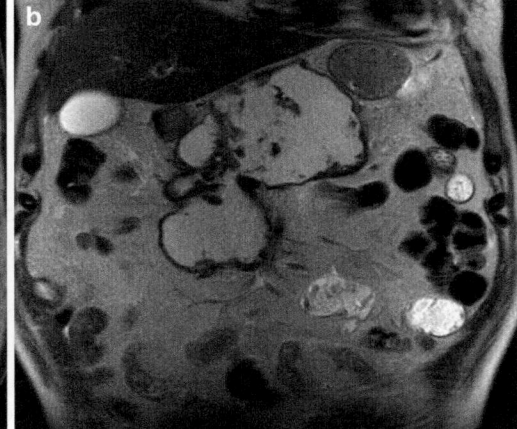

Fig. 14.9 Assessment of the composition of a pancreatic fluid collection. Coronal curvilinear reformatted CT image on portal-venous phase (**a**) shows an inhomogeneous pancreatic fluid collection in a 62-year-old. MRI coronal T2-weighted image (**b**) better demonstrates the presence of non-liquefied material suggestive for necrotic debris and permits an accurate diagnosis of WON

CT represents also an effective guidance tool for percutaneous interventional procedures, such as the placement of a percutaneous drainage catheter. Furthermore, in patients with complicated acute pancreatitis, CECT has an important role during the follow-up period to determine the success of treatment in patients who have undergone percutaneous drainage or other interventions including surgical debridement.

It is important to underline that imaging obtained during the first 3 days in patients with severe pancreatitis may underestimate or may not detect the presence or the extent of necrosis. The best time for scanning these patients by CECT is after 72 h from onset of symptoms.

CT has limited accuracy in biliary stone detection and in the early differentiation of fluid from nonliquid material within a collection. Finally, CECT is contraindicated in patients with allergy to iodinated contrast material or with renal failure.

Magnetic Resonance

MR is not considered the modality of choice for evaluating patients with acute pancreatitis; however it should be considered complementary to CT and also represents a useful tool in selected cases [24]. In particular MR is useful in patients with impaired renal function or allergies to iodinated contrast material, in pregnant women, and in patients with suspected choledocholithiasis not seen on CECT. Furthermore, because of its high contrast resolution, MR is able to assess the composition of a pancreatic fluid collection, in particular the presence or absence of non-liquefied material (necrotic debris) or superinfection (Fig. 14.9).

MR is more sensitive than CT for detecting pancreatic parenchymal alterations. In interstitial edematous pancreatitis, the pancreatic parenchyma is usually enlarged, and it changes its physiological intensity, with hypointensity on T1-weighted images and slight hyperintensity on T2-WI due to the presence of edema. In necrotizing pancreatitis, in the absence of hemorrhage, T1 signal intensity becomes more heterogeneous or decreased as compared to the hepatic parenchymal signal. T2 signal intensity of the pancreatic parenchyma and peripancreatic soft tissues can increase and become closer to fluid signal intensity. Hemorrhage and hemorrhagic fluid collections are better recognized on MR. Hemorrhage is usually hyperintense on T1-weighted images and should be differentiated from the physiological hyperintensity of the unaffected pancreatic parenchyma.

Contrast-enhanced MRI may be superior to contrast-enhanced CT in differentiating necrotic foci within the pancreas from intrapancreatic fluid or hemorrhagic regions [37]. Small areas of necrosis can be missed on CT or misinterpreted as intraparenchymal fluid collections, particularly when imaging is performed 72 h before the onset of symptoms.

Finally, MR with magnetic resonance cholangiopancreatography (MRCP) is able to assess ductal alterations, and it is considered a useful tool for demonstrating the communication of a fluid collection or a pseudocyst with the pancreatic ductal system. In selected cases this communication can be better evaluated after secretin stimulation.

Ultrasounds

Ultrasound examination is usually the first imaging modality which investigates the upper abdomen in patients with abdominal pain.

The standard evaluation consists in obtaining images of the pancreas and of the peripancreatic compartments, such as the lesser sac, anterior pararenal space, and transverse mesocolon, by scanning in the supine, longitudinal, transverse, semi-erect, and coronal planes.

The diagnosis of acute pancreatitis includes the increase in the volume of the pancreatic parenchyma, structural changes, and significant decrease in echoes. However, primary limitation of US is that sometimes the pancreas cannot be visualized due to overlying bowel gas; in these cases, the spleen can be used as an acoustic window to image the pancreatic tail. Moreover, the pancreatic parenchyma may appear completely normal in mild acute pancreatitis.

In patients with suspected acute pancreatitis, it is important to evaluate the common bile duct and its intrapancreatic portion to exclude an underlying biliary stone disease, since US is the most sensitive modality for evaluating the biliary tree/gallbladder [38].

US is also useful to assess the presence of local complications, such as peripancreatic fluid collections or pseudocyst. Furthermore, it could be used to clarify the presence or absence of non-liquefied components within a fluid collection whenever it cannot be distinguished at CECT (Fig. 14.10).

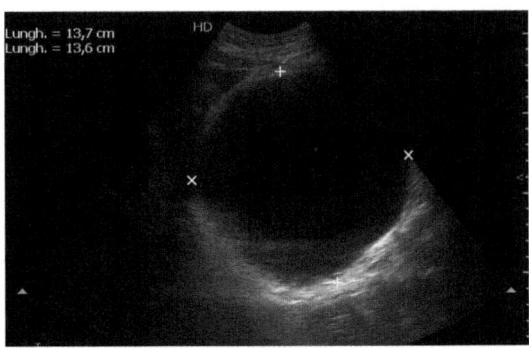

Fig. 14.10 Pancreatic pseudocyst. Ultrasound follow-up of a large pancreatic pseudocyst in a 32-year-old patient 5 weeks after onset of acute pancreatitis. The collection is completely anechoic due to the absence of solid material within the pseudocyst

Finally, US represents a useful tool to guide percutaneous interventional procedures in patients with complications such as needle aspirations and drainage of fluid collections and pseudocysts.

14.2.4.7   Differential Diagnosis

Usually, the clinical picture combined with laboratory data is strong enough to suggest the correct diagnosis of acute pancreatitis. Clinically, the differential diagnosis of abdominal pain that could be confused with acute pancreatitis includes peptic ulcer disease, intestinal obstruction, abdominal aortic aneurysm, cholangitis or cholecystitis, choledocholithiasis, viral gastroenteritis, mesenteric ischemia, hepatitis, or myocardial infarction [24]. In all these cases, additional clinical history and the fact that the lipase and amylase are normal should prevent a misdiagnosis. However, in all these cases, CECT should be performed and demonstrate a normal pancreas, except in rare instances:

- A perforated gastric or duodenal ulcer may be confused on CECT with pancreatitis because of stranding in the peripancreatic and duodenal areas but usually detection of even small pockets of free intraperitoneal air prevents such an error. Clinically, elevated amylase in these patients adds to the diagnostic dilemma; however the elevation is usually less marked than in acute pancreatitis.

- Similarly, severe peptic ulcer disease caused by *Helicobacter pylori*, nonsteroidal anti-inflammatory drug use, or Zollinger-Ellison syndrome can produce enough stranding near the pancreatic bed that could be confused with acute pancreatitis on CECT. Usually the gastric wall is thickened, the lipase and amylase are normal, and the epigastric pain does not generally radiate into the back, which should enable a correct diagnosis.
- Mesenteric ischemia can produce an elevation of the amylase with a normal lipase and also shows elevation of lactic acid. A history of atrial fibrillation or peripheral vascular disease in an elderly patient usually raises the index of suspicion for bowel ischemia, and CECT can be diagnostic without confusion with acute pancreatitis unless there is extensive mesenteric stranding in the upper abdomen.

Furthermore, resuscitation efforts with excessive rehydration can lead to generalized edema, ascites, and edema in the pancreas that are associated with stranding and fluid in the retroperitoneum, which mimics acute pancreatitis. The severity of the pancreatic manifestations depends on the degree of hydration. Similarly, hypoalbuminemia with ascites and generalized edema can mimic acute pancreatitis [24].

14.2.4.8 Pitfalls

In the early phase, mild acute pancreatitis can be missed on CECT if the patient is studied on the first day of onset of symptoms, because edema of the pancreatic tissue or stranding of the peripancreatic area is not yet evident. Furthermore, necrosis may be missed or misdiagnosed when CECT is performed in the first 72 h, since necrosis can be confused as an area of hypoperfusion of the pancreatic parenchyma due to edema [24].

In the late phase, infection can be suggested on CECT if gas bubbles are present within the pancreatic collection due to the presence of gas-forming organisms. An infected necrotic tissue could be confused with spontaneous drainage of the collection into the gastrointestinal tract. To avoid this diagnostic pitfall, the adjacent gastrointestinal walls need to be carefully analyzed. Similarly, marsupialization or other drainage procedures also can lead to the introduction of gas into a collection. Finally, an area of WON can be misinterpreted as a cystic neoplasm especially in cases in which a history of a previous pancreatitis cannot be elicited (Figs. 14.11 and 14.12) [24]. In these cases, MRI can demonstrate necrotic debris with or without loculations, which do not enhance after administration of contrast material, to confirm that the inhomogeneous cystic structure is related to a previous acute pancreatitis.

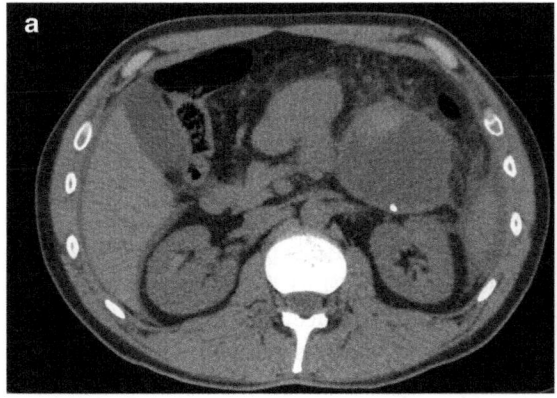
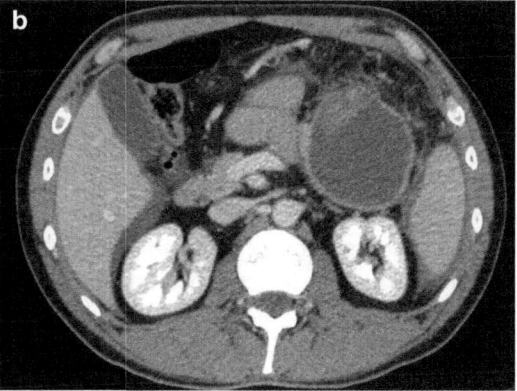
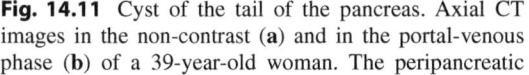

Fig. 14.11 Cyst of the tail of the pancreas. Axial CT images in the non-contrast (**a**) and in the portal-venous phase (**b**) of a 39-year-old woman. The peripancreatic collection has non-enhanced, non-viable solid tissue and refers to a walled-off necrosis

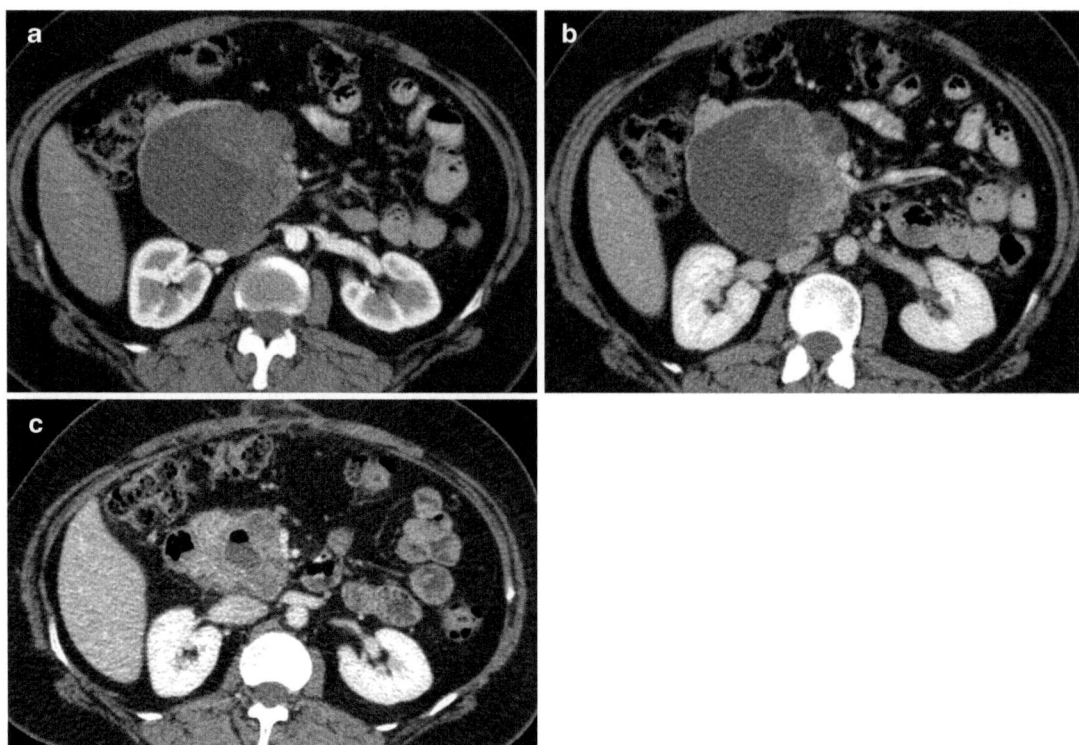

Fig. 14.12 Cyst of the head of the pancreas. Axial CT images in the arterial (**a**) and in the portal-venous phase (**b**) of a 35-year-old woman. The head of the pancreas shows a well-defined fluid collection with thickened and enhanced mural solid components. It was misinterpreted as a pancreatic pseudocyst and the patient underwent a pseudocyst-gastro-anastomosis. Axial CT image 6 months after the procedure (**c**) shows the reduction of the fluid component of the lesion; however, the thickened and enhanced areas are still visible. After US-guided biopsy, the lesion demonstrates the histological features suggestive for a solid pseudo-papillary tumor of the pancreas, which was confirmed at histological specimen after pancreaticoduodenectomy

14.2.4.9 Treatment

Mild and severe pancreatitis are both initially treated by conservative and supportive measures [39]. Prophylactic antibiotics in necrotizing pancreatitis are not recommended [28]. Mild and mild-severe pancreatitis usually do not require further therapies. In presence of necrotizing pancreatitis, any operative intervention is postponed as long as possible allowing collections to demarcate (3–4 weeks). Actually, operative treatment is usually reserved to infected necrotizing pancreatitis; in these cases, the treatment of choice is percutaneous drainage of the collection. Percutaneous drainage is also used if sterile collections are large enough to cause symptoms.

14.3 Chronic Pancreatitis

14.3.1 Imaging Techniques

A few decades ago, before the clinical introduction of cross-sectional imaging techniques, the imaging evaluation of CP was limited to plain radiography depicting calcifications (Fig. 14.13). Traditionally, the ductal morphology has been assessed with endoscopic retrograde cholangiopancreatography (ERCP), with severity assessed using the Cambridge classification [40]. Today routine imaging modalities in the evaluation of CP typically include computed tomography (CT) with one or more contrast-enhancement phases,

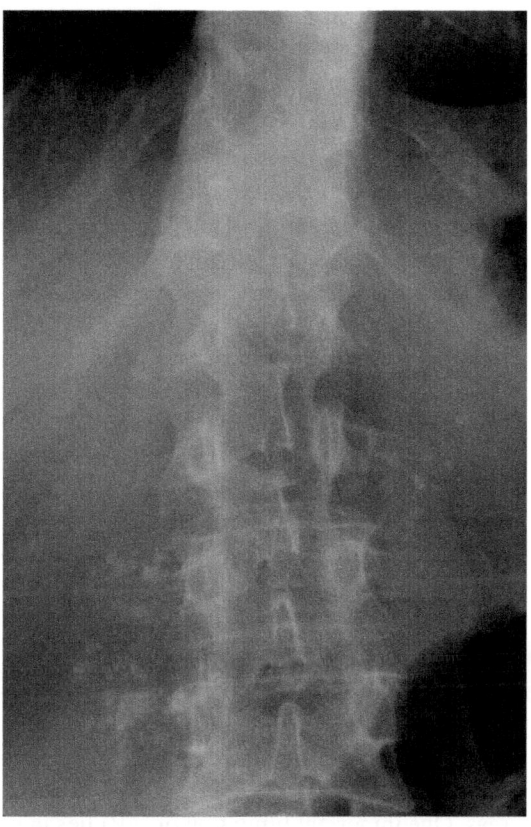

Fig. 14.13 Chronic pancreatitis. Plain radiography of the abdomen of a 60-year-old man shows multiple calcifications scattered through the entire pancreatic gland

MRI with magnetic resonance cholangiopancreatography (MRCP), and ultrasound with a transabdominal or endoscopic approach.

14.3.2 Computed Tomography: Examination Technique

Multidetector computed tomography (CT) represents the gold standard in pancreatic inflammatory and neoplastic diseases. The advantages of CT are the rapid image acquisition and the high spatial resolution, which permits multiplanar reconstructions, a useful tool in the evaluation of the pancreatic parenchyma and pancreatic ductal system.

A study protocol of the pancreas includes a non-contrast scan of the upper abdomen, to demonstrate the presence of intraductal filling defects, such as calculi or protein-dense plugs, followed by a contrast-enhanced acquisition in the late-arterial phase (pancreatic phase), in which normal pancreatic parenchyma is usually brightly enhanced. Finally a portal-venous phase scan of the entire abdomen should be acquired to exclude other organ involvement or abdominal complications (Figs. 14.14 and 14.15) [12].

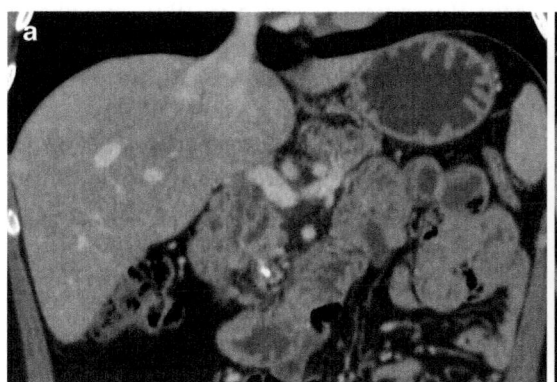
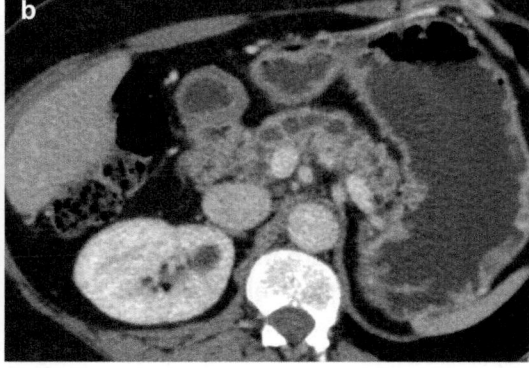

Fig. 14.14 Chronic pancreatitis. Coronal reconstructed image (**a**) and axial CT image (**b**) acquired in portal-venous phase show a calcification of the pancreatic head with marked dilation of the upstream main pancreatic duct which shows a tortuous path

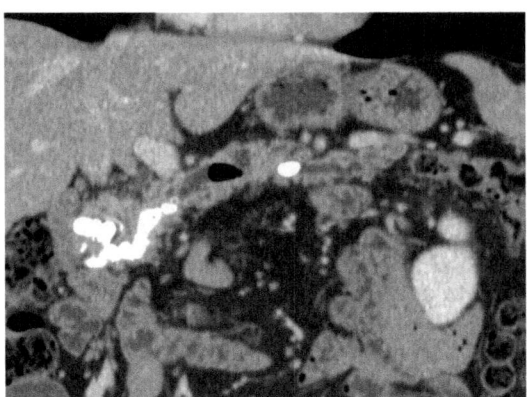

Fig. 14.15 Chronic pancreatitis. Coronal curvilinear reformatted CT image in the portal-venous phase shows multiple calcifications within the main pancreatic duct of the head and the tail of the pancreas. The MPD is diffusely dilated and irregular, with air within the lumen

14.3.3 Magnetic Resonance: Examination Technique

The development in imaging techniques, and especially in magnetic resonance imaging (MRI), has dramatically improved the information on both morphology and function of the pancreas. In the Mayo diagnostic criteria for CP, MRI is now an accepted method for assessing ductal and parenchymal alterations [41]. MRI has the unique capability of allowing noninvasive evaluation of the pancreatic parenchyma, pancreatic ductal system, peripancreatic soft tissue, and vascular network in a single examination. The concurrent use of secretin improved the diagnostic yield of MRCP in the evaluation of the pancreatic duct integrity and pancreatic exocrine function in cases of early pancreatitis [42–44].

14.3.3.1 Standard MR

The standard MR protocol includes T2-weighted images acquired at different planes and fat-suppressed 3D-GRE T1-weighted images, acquired before and after administrations of gadolinium chelates. The contrastographic phases include pancreatic, portal-venous, and delayed phases (3–10 min post-gadolinium). The recent advantages of these sequences include thinner sections (3 mm) and multiplanar imaging. Fat-suppressed T1-weighted images show high signal intensity in normal pancreas due to high aqueous protein content in the acini within the pancreatic parenchyma. Furthermore fat-suppressed T1-weighted images enhance the signal intensity of the pancreatic parenchyma in relation to the surrounding hypointense retroperitoneal fat, appearing typically hyperintense as compared to the liver parenchyma [45]. On gadolinium-enhanced images, the pancreas demonstrates a capillary blush on arterial pancreatic phase, which renders it markedly higher in signal intensity than the liver [46]. Echo-train spin-echo sequences such as T2-weighted half-Fourier acquisition snapshot turbo spin-echo (HASTE) provide a sharp anatomic delineation of the common bile duct (CBD) on coronal plane images and of the main pancreatic duct on transverse plane images. Furthermore, T2-weighted images provide information on the complexity of the fluid within pancreatic pseudocysts, which may reflect the presence of complications such as necrotic debris or infection. Standard MRI should be completed with MRCP to assess both parenchymal and ductal alterations of the pancreas. One important limitation of MRI lies in its inability to depict small parenchymal calcifications, which can be easily depicted with CT.

14.3.3.2 MRCP

MRCP was first described in 1991, providing a noninvasive alternative to ERCP, which relies on the endoscopic injection of contrast fluid into the common bile duct and main pancreatic duct [47, 48]. By applying either a single-shot breath-hold technique or a free-breathing technique with respiratory triggering, MRCP can provide both 2D and 3D images [49, 50]. Recent sequences allow faster image acquisition and better quality with more detailed images including 3D reconstructions. These advances benefit from a high signal-to-noise ratio. Additionally, the 3D free-breathing protocol makes it superior to 2D imaging in patients who are unable or unwilling to hold their breath for the duration of the scan [51]. MRCP sequences are heavily T2-weighted pulse sequences; therefore the pancreatobiliary tree is displayed as high signal intensity, and the pancreatic duct is clearly visualized in the normal pancreas. MRCP technique is relevant in detecting pancreatic ductal alterations, such as dilatations, filling defects, and stenoses. Furthermore, pseudocysts and other ductal congenital abnormalities and normal variants (such as pancreas divisum) can be visualized [52].

14.3.3.3 Secretin-Enhanced MRCP
Secretin is a polypeptide hormone secreted by the duodenum. Secretin stimulates the secretion of bicarbonate and a fluid rich in protons; moreover it increases the tone of the sphincter of Oddi. Consequently the main pancreatic duct distends by the accumulation of the pancreatic juice. The distention will be maximal in about 4–10 min with a better representation of pancreatic ductal anatomy [42, 43, 53]. It is recommended the administration of a negative oral contrast agent to remove high signal intensity from the fluid within the stomach and duodenum on MRCP images. If a commercial product is not available, pineapple juice or blueberry juice can be used as alternative negative MR contrast materials. Oral contrast agent should be given 30 min before the procedure.

Indications of secretin-enhanced MRCP include the evaluation of the pancreatic ductal system in patients with recurrent episodes of acute pancreatitis and to better analyze a stenosis of the main pancreatic duct, in particular to distinguish between stenoses due to neoplastic infiltration or strictures secondary to inflammatory compression. In these latter cases, it is often demonstrated a resolution of the stenotic tract after secretin injection, the so-called duct penetrating sign [54]. Furthermore exocrine function of the pancreas can be evaluated by a stratification in different grades (Matos' score) in secretin-enhanced MRCP according to the duodenal anatomic imaging findings: grade 1, pancreatic fluid is confined to the duodenal bulb; grade 2, fluid is seen as far as the second part of the duodenum; grade 3, when duodenal filling reaches the third part of the duodenum; and grade 4, fluid is seen at the fourth portion of the duodenum. Diminished estimated pancreatic exocrine function is suspected in the absence of duodenal fluid accumulation, or with grade 1 duodenal filling [55].

14.3.4 Imaging Features

In the **early stages** of chronic pancreatitis, pancreatic alterations are usually unspecific and inconclusive. Recurrent episodes of pancreatitis usually result in fine parenchymal alterations and ductal irregularities, which are rarely detected on CT [56]. In early chronic pancreatitis, the role of computed tomography is usually limited to rule out neoplastic disease or anatomical malformations. As parenchymal changes might be preceded by ductal changes in chronic pancreatitis, this makes MRCP alone more advantageous in suspected early chronic pancreatitis. MRI detects not only morphological characteristics but also early fibrotic changes. Fibrosis is shown by diminished signal intensity on fat-suppressed T1-weighted images and diminished parenchymal enhancement on immediate post-gadolinium images. Diminished pancreatic parenchymal enhancement on pancreatic phase reflects disruption of the normal capillary bed and increased chronic inflammation and fibrosis (Fig. 14.16). MRCP findings in early chronic pancreatitis often demonstrate normal main pancreatic duct with dilated and irregular side duct branches. Some authors reported that patients with abnormal MR imaging findings but normal MRCP might benefit from dynamic secretin-MRCP (S-MRCP), which may improve the visualization of the pancreatic ductal system.

In **advanced disease**, parenchymal and ductal alterations are irreversible and can be limited to the secondary ducts (*small-duct form*) or might extend to the main pancreatic duct (MPD) (*large-duct form*) (Table 14.5) [11]. The consequence of the obstruction of the pancreatic ductal system is the precipitation of dense protein plugs within the ducts, which gradually calcify in small or large calcifications [57].

The *macro-obstructive form* is secondary to a primary obstruction of the main pancreatic duct, with the consequent dilatation of the upstream pancreatic ductal system. The caliber of the MPD is usually larger than normal (4 mm in the head; 3 mm in the body-tail), resulting diffusely dilated with a tortuous path [58]. The impaired outflow can lead to dilation of the upstream secondary

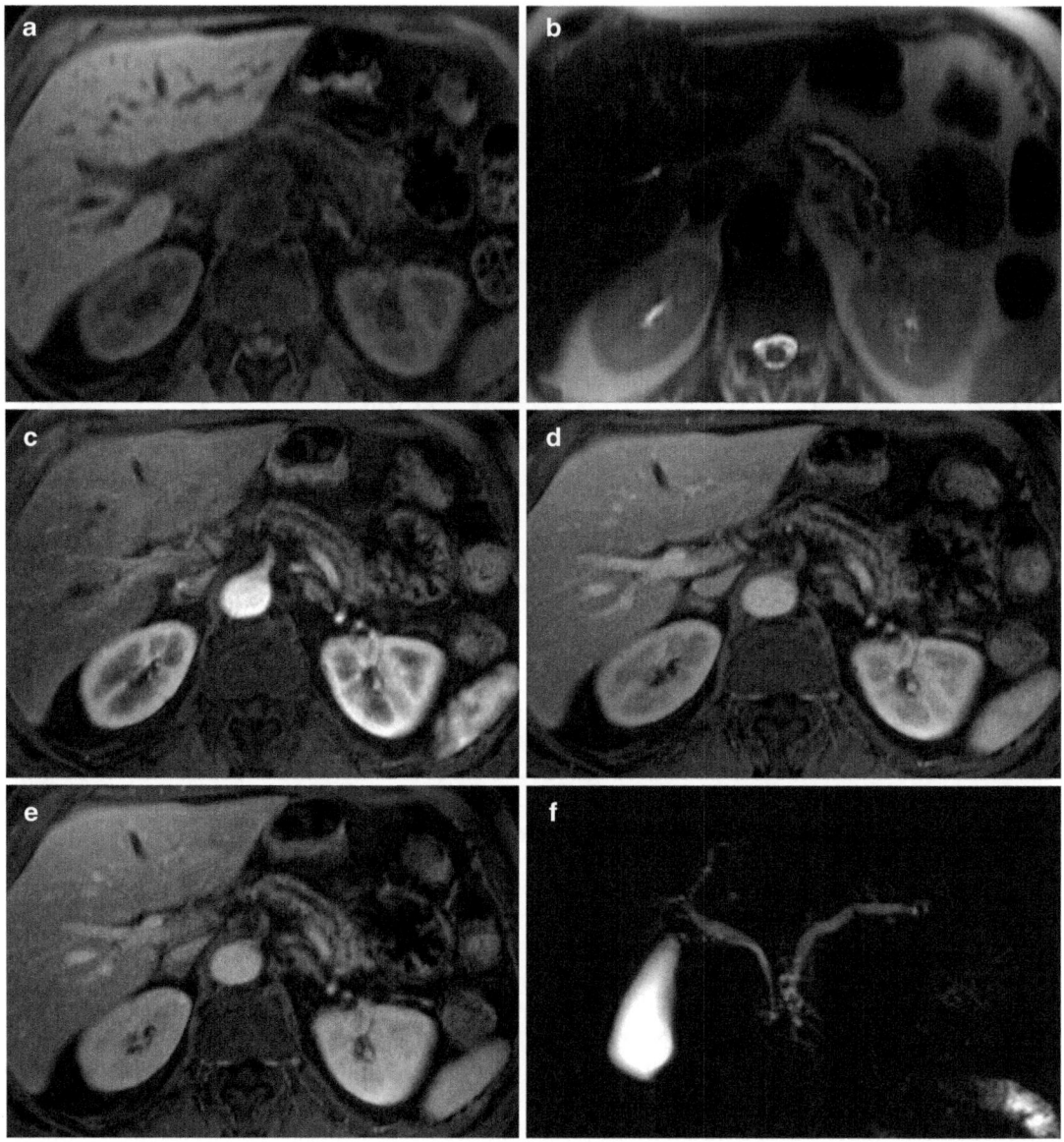

Fig. 14.16 Chronic pancreatitis. Axial fat-suppressed T1-weighted image (**a**) shows an atrophic pancreatic parenchyma, which appears hypointense as compared to the liver parenchyma. Axial T2-weighted image (**b**) shows an irregular dilatation of the main pancreatic duct. After contrast medium injection, the pancreatic parenchyma appears hypovascular during the pancreatic phase (**c**), with progressive delayed enhancement during the portal-venous and delayed phases (**d**, **e**). MRCP sequence (**f**) confirms the dilatation of the entire main pancreatic duct, with dilatation of multiple side branches

ducts (Fig. 14.17). On advanced disease, typically multiple small calculi precipitate within the secondary ducts, which can present cystic changes. The obstruction of the pancreatic ducts leads also to necrosis of the acinar cells with progressive substitution of the normal parenchyma by regions of fibrosis [12]. The affected parenchyma gradually reduces in size until complete atrophy of the gland.

CT non-contrast images are able to detect intraductal dense plugs or calcifications, which may be single or multiple and vary in size, limited to a portion of the pancreas or diffused throughout the whole extension of the gland. Usually these calcifications remain stable or increase in extent, although they can rarely decrease. After contrast media injection, the

Table 14.5 Morphological classification of chronic pancreatitis

Macro-obstructive form	Micro-obstructive form
• Sphincter of Oddi disease	• Autoimmune pancreatitis
Inflammatory	• Hereditary pancreatitis
Neoplastic	PRSS1
• Stenosis of the MPD	CFTR
Pseudocysts, trauma, slow tumors	SPINK1
• Alterations of the duodenal wall	
Paraduodenal pancreatitis	
• Congenital malformations	
• Pancreatic fibrosis (alcohol abuse)	
• Pancreatic lithiasis	
Of old age	
Hypercalcemia, dyslipidemia	
Drug-induced	
• Autoimmune pancreatitis (focal form)	

affected parenchyma appears hypovascular during the pancreatic phase, as compared to the unaffected parenchyma, as a result of the fibrotic infiltration. These fibro-inflammatory changes also lead to a delayed enhancement of the gland during the portal-venous and delayed phases, in which the parenchyma shows contrast retention and delayed washout (Figs. 14.16 and 14.17). These alterations are well demonstrated when chronic pancreatitis affects a focal region of the pancreas, in which normal aspects of the parenchyma coexist with chronic disease. During recurrent episodes of pancreatitis, edema of the peripancreatic fat or fluid collection of the anterior pararenal spaces can be rarely observed.

MRCP in advanced disease demonstrates dilatation and strictures of the main pancreatic duct with side branches dilated, giving a "chain of lakes appearance."

A benign condition involved in the obstructive disease is also the reduced pancreatic juice outflow in the duodenum secondary to sphincter of Oddi dysfunction or inflammatory stenosis of the major papilla. Sphincter of Oddi dysfunction (SOD) refers to benign obstruction of bile or pancreatic juice outflow, due to stenosis or dyskinesia of the sphincter of Oddi. The entity of the stenosis is often mild, and ductal alterations are

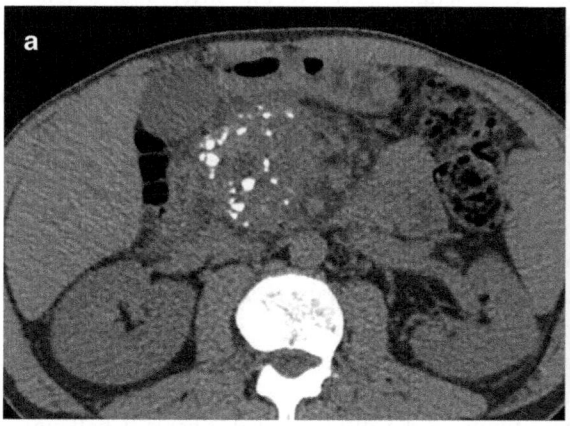
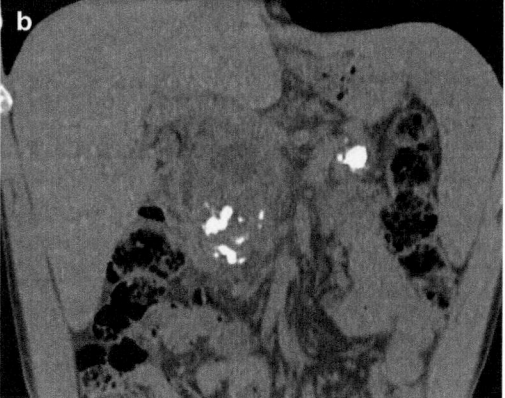
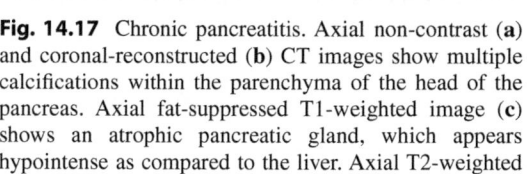

Fig. 14.17 Chronic pancreatitis. Axial non-contrast (**a**) and coronal-reconstructed (**b**) CT images show multiple calcifications within the parenchyma of the head of the pancreas. Axial fat-suppressed T1-weighted image (**c**) shows an atrophic pancreatic gland, which appears hypointense as compared to the liver. Axial T2-weighted image (**d**) shows a marked dilatation either of the main pancreatic duct and of multiple side branches. The pancreatic parenchyma is hypovascular during the portal-venous phase (**e**). MRCP sequence (**f**) confirms the diffuse dilatation of the MPD with multiple side branches dilated in a patient with a severe chronic pancreatitis

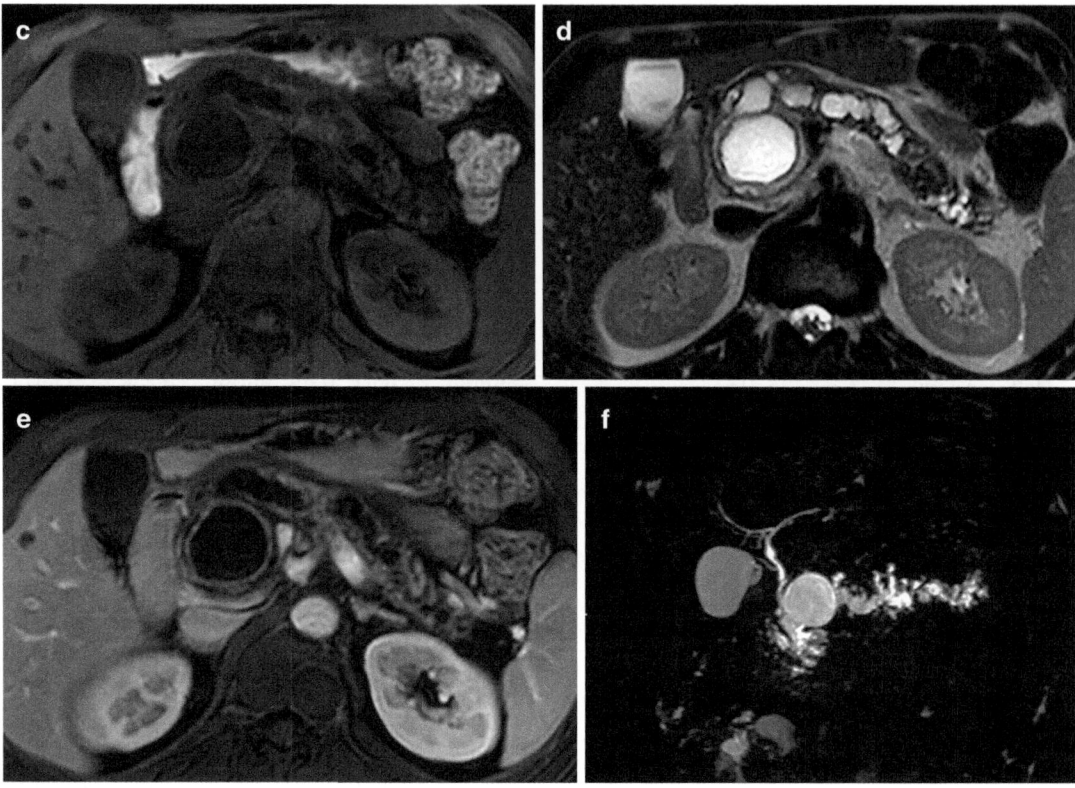

Fig. 14.17 (continued)

usually demonstrated only with secretin-enhanced magnetic resonance cholangiopancreatography (S-MRCP), in which a prolonged dilation of the MPD (at 10 min after secretin injection) with delayed recovery of the baseline diameter can be observed [54, 59, 60].

An important role of imaging is also to determine the cause of the obstruction of the pancreatic ductal system. Pancreatic solid slow-growing neoplasms (e.g., neuroendocrine tumors, ampullary tumors) or less commonly cystic neoplasms can determine a progressive extrinsic obstruction of the main pancreatic duct with secondary fibrosis and atrophy of the distal pancreatic parenchyma. Otherwise, aggressive neoplasms, as pancreatic adenocarcinoma, often infiltrate the ductal system with complete stenosis of the MPD. The most important differential diagnosis should be done between mass-forming pancreatitis and pancreatic cancer: chronic inflammatory process in chronic pancreatitis can produce a focal mass lesion that can mimic pancreatic adenocarcinoma. Both chronic pancreatitis and adenocarcinoma show similar imaging characteristics on MRI due to abundant fibrosis and ductal obstruction; therefore the differential diagnosis may be difficult. Both are generally seen as mildly hypointense on T1-weighted images and heterogeneously mildly hyperintense on T2-weighted images. Furthermore, both conditions may present with stenosis and dilation of the common bile duct and the main pancreatic duct dilation (double duct sign). Features favoring carcinoma include abrupt cutoff of pancreatic duct, with marked upstream dilation of the ductal system and pancreatic parenchyma atrophy. Finally, pancreatic adenocarcinoma can develop in patients with chronic pancreatitis, with further limits in the differential diagnosis. Challenging cases require histology for final diagnosis.

The *micro-obstructive form* includes rare conditions, which are involved in progressive acinar sclerosis and fibrotic changes of the pancreatic parenchyma, without a primary obstruction of the main pancreatic duct. In this type of chronic pancreatitis, the pancreatic ductal system is usually involved only in advanced disease. Genetic alterations, as mutation of genes *PRSS1*, *SPINK1*, and *CFTR* or inflammatory disease, such as autoimmune pancreatitis, are considered the leading causes of micro-obstructive chronic pancreatitis [18].

14.3.5 Complications of Chronic Pancreatitis

Complications of chronic pancreatitis include pseudocysts, pseudoaneurysms, splenic vein thrombosis, and biliary obstruction. Moreover gastrointestinal complications, such as gastric outlet obstruction or bowel ischemia, may be observed [61, 62]. These complications are well depicted on MRI and CT. MRI with MRCP may be superior to CT in detecting specific complications like pseudocysts, fistula formation, and distal common biliary dilatation. Vascular complications are better demonstrated with contrast-enhanced CT.

14.3.6 Treatment

The majority of the patients with chronic pancreatitis suffer from abdominal pain. The first goal is to slow chronic disease progression, starting from alcohol and smoke abstinence. Moreover, patients require analgesics. Supportive treatments for abdominal pain include administration of pancreatic enzymes, octreotide, and antioxidants [63, 64].

In patients with obstruction of the main pancreatic duct, endoscopic retrograde cholangiopancreatography (ERCP) can relieve the obstruction. Endoscopic therapy comprises endoscopic sphincterotomy of the major or minor papilla, stones extraction, dilation, and stenting of the inflammatory stenosis [57, 65].

Finally, surgery is recommended in patients who did not respond to medical or endoscopic treatment. Several surgical approaches have been described. The most common procedure is the lateral pancreaticojejunostomy (modified Puestow operation), which consists in a longitudinal incision of the anterior pancreas along the main pancreatic duct; ductal stones are removed and strictures are incised. Patients with a stenosis of the main pancreatic duct due to a mass localized in the pancreatic head need a pancreaticoduodenectomy (Whipple procedure) or duodenum-preserving pancreatic head resections (Frey, Berger, or Berne procedures), which have less postoperative complications than Whipple procedure [66, 67]. Distal pancreatectomy should be performed in patients with chronic pancreatitis localized in the tail of the pancreas. Finally, total pancreatectomy is rarely performed and is required in selected patients who failed to respond to medical treatments or more conservative surgery [64].

14.3.7 Other Forms of Chronic Pancreatitis

14.3.7.1 Paraduodenal Pancreatitis

Paraduodenal pancreatitis is a rare form of chronic pancreatitis affecting the "groove," which is an anatomical region located between the pancreatic head, the wall of the second portion of the duodenum, and the common bile duct [68].

The etiology is not yet known; however it has been demonstrated a strong association with long-term alcohol and smoke abuse [13, 69–71]. The most plausible hypothesis is the presence of a heterotopic pancreatic tissue, derived from the dorsal pancreatic bud, within the duodenal wall, near the region of the minor papilla. This heterotopic parenchyma could be more sensitive to exogenous factors, such as high alcohol intake or long-term cigarette smoke [72, 73].

Macroscopically, the duodenal mucosa of the "groove" is often thickened, with micro or macrocystic changes, as a result of inflammatory and fibrotic infiltration. Depending on the presence or absence of cystic components within the groove region, paraduodenal pancreatitis has been classified in *cystic* or *solid* type, respectively [13, 71, 74, 75]. In both the subtypes, the inflammatory infiltration can extend to the adjacent pancreatic parenchyma, with dilation of the main pancreatic duct as a result of functional obstruction of the

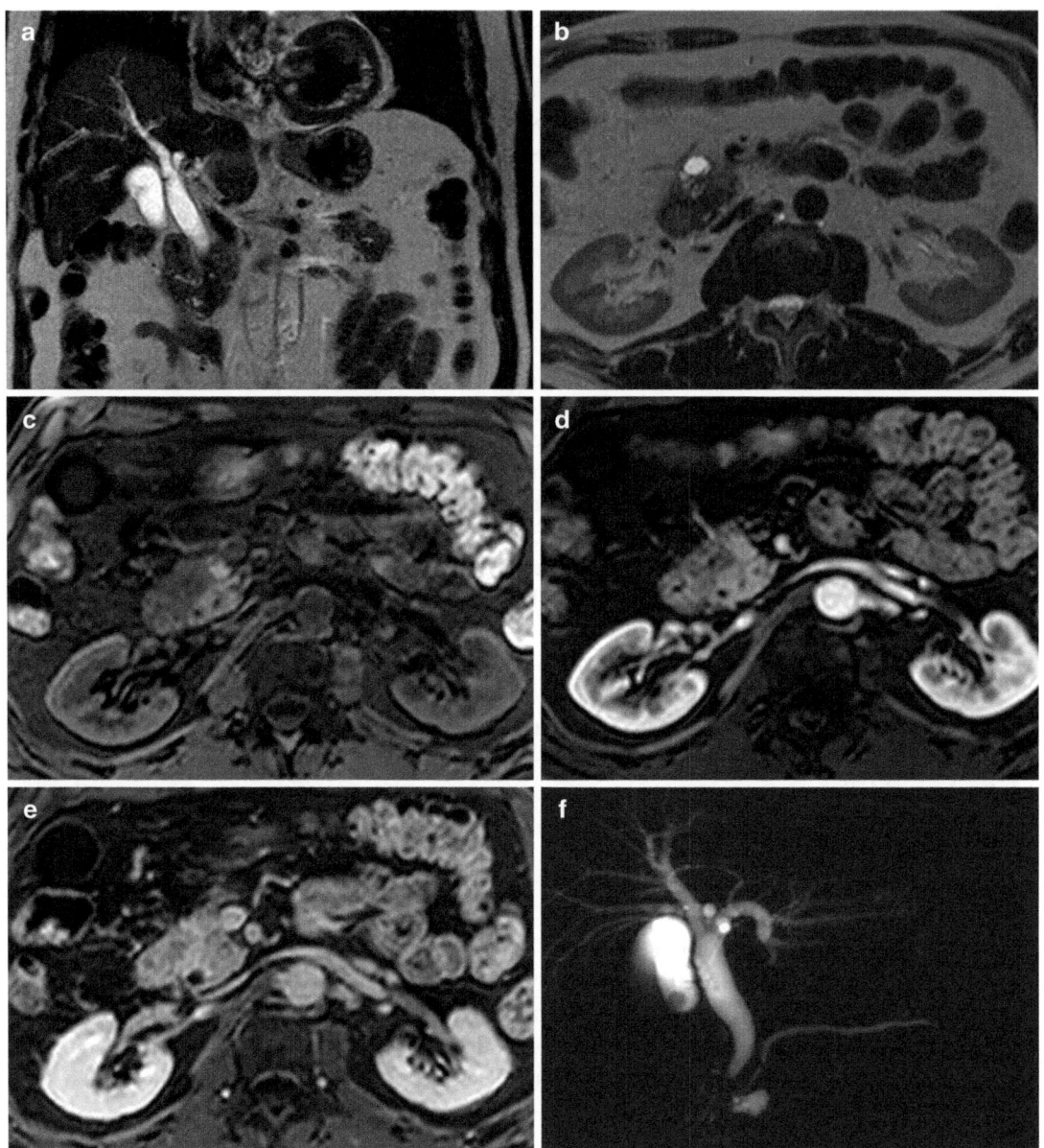

Fig. 14.18 Paraduodenal pancreatitis. Coronal T2-weighted image (**a**) shows a thickening of the wall of the "groove region." Axial T2-weighted image (**b**) demonstrates the presence of small cysts within the thickened area. The affected parenchyma appears hypointense as compared to the unaffected adjacent pancreatic parenchyma on fat-suppressed T1-weighted image (**c**), hypovascular during the arterial phase (**d**), with delayed enhancement during the delayed phase (**e**), due to the presence of fibrosis. MRCP sequence (**f**) confirms the presence of the small cysts near the pancreatic head; the main pancreatic duct is not dilated

minor or major papilla. On this basis, paraduodenal pancreatitis has been divided into two different forms: the *pure form*, which is limited to the "groove" region, and the *segmental form* that extends to the pancreatic head (Fig. 14.18).

Paraduodenal pancreatitis occurs predominantly in men; the incidence in women and young individuals is considerably lower.

At imaging, the wall of the second portion of the duodenum is thickened. On precontrastographic

CT images, the thickened wall appears iso-hypodense, as compared to the adjacent pancreatic parenchyma, with multiple micro- or macrocysts (3 mm–5 cm); calcifications are usually detected in advanced disease, especially in segmental forms. The most characteristic finding on MRI is a sheet-like mass between the head of the pancreas and duodenal C-loop. The mass demonstrates low signal on T1-weighted images compared to the rest of the pancreatic parenchymal tissue and variable signal on T2-weighted images. This variation in the T2 signal can be attributed to the time of onset of the disease, as subacute form of the disease shows brighter signal on T2-weighted images due to edema, while chronic form of the disease has a lower T2 signal due to fibrosis. Gadolinium-enhanced dynamic images show delayed and progressive heterogeneous enhancement, reflecting the fibrous nature of the tissue. Cystic lesions can also be well seen on T2-weighted images in the groove or duodenal wall. During the follow-up period, cysts can vary in size, even in a short time interval.

Paraduodenal pancreatitis may mimic a pancreatic adenocarcinoma, particularly in the solid variant. Findings at endoscopic ultrasonography (EUS) may help to confirm the sheet-like thickening of the duodenal wall, as well as intramural microcysts, which can be rarely identified on CT images. Some authors reported that the following three diagnostic criteria are suggestive for groove pancreatitis and can exclude pancreatic adenocarcinoma with a negative predictive value of 92.9%: [11] focal thickening of the second part of the duodenum, [12] abnormal increased enhancement of the second part of the duodenum, and [13] cystic changes in the region of the pancreatic accessory duct.

In advanced disease, patients may require surgery as a result of severe pancreatic insufficiency, weight loss, or pain [76]. These patients usually undergo either a classic or pylorus-sparing pancreaticoduodenectomy, although endoscopic drainage of the minor papilla has also been demonstrated to be effective [77].

14.3.7.2 Autoimmune Pancreatitis

Autoimmune pancreatitis (AIP) is a distinct form of chronic pancreatitis, in which an autoimmune mechanism has been postulated [78].

Histologically AIP consists of a dense periductal inflammatory infiltrate of neutrophils and plasma cells, with dense tumor-like regions of fibrosis. These changes are responsible for an increase in size of the pancreatic parenchyma, which can be either focal or diffused throughout the whole extension of the pancreatic gland [79–82]. For this reason, AIP has been morphologically classified in *focal* and *diffuse* forms [83].

AIP affects predominantly middle-aged males, with a wide age range (20–60 years). The symptoms are unspecific, including abdominal pain, obstructive jaundice, and occasionally weight loss. An elevation of IgG4 serum levels is often demonstrated. A typical feature of the disease is the dramatic remission of signs and symptoms after a short term of high-dosage steroid treatment [78, 84].

In 2011, the International Consensus Diagnostic Criteria distinguished two different subtypes with distinct histopathology and clinical profiles [78]: *type 1* AIP, which is considered an IgG4-related systemic disease, with pancreatic and extra-pancreatic involvement (e.g., autoimmune cholangitis, retroperitoneal fibrosis, interstitial nephritis), and *type 2* AIP, which has none or few IgG4-positive plasma cells and is considered an organ-specific disease, except for a rare association with inflammatory bowel diseases, especially ulcerative colitis.

The affected pancreatic parenchyma typically appears enlarged, with loss of the physiological lobular structure. Calcifications of the gland or peripancreatic fluid collections are unusual. After contrast media injection, the lesion appears hypovascular as compared to the unaffected adjacent parenchyma, in focal forms, or as compared to the liver parenchyma in diffuse forms. The affected parenchyma shows homogenous and progressive enhancement during the portal-venous phase and contrast retention with delayed washout in the delayed phase (Fig. 14.19) [85–88].

At MRI in diffuse AIP, the pancreas is typically swollen, with a sausage-like appearance with low T1 signal intensity, slight high T2 signal intensity, and delayed gadolinium enhancement. A capsule-like rim surrounding the affected

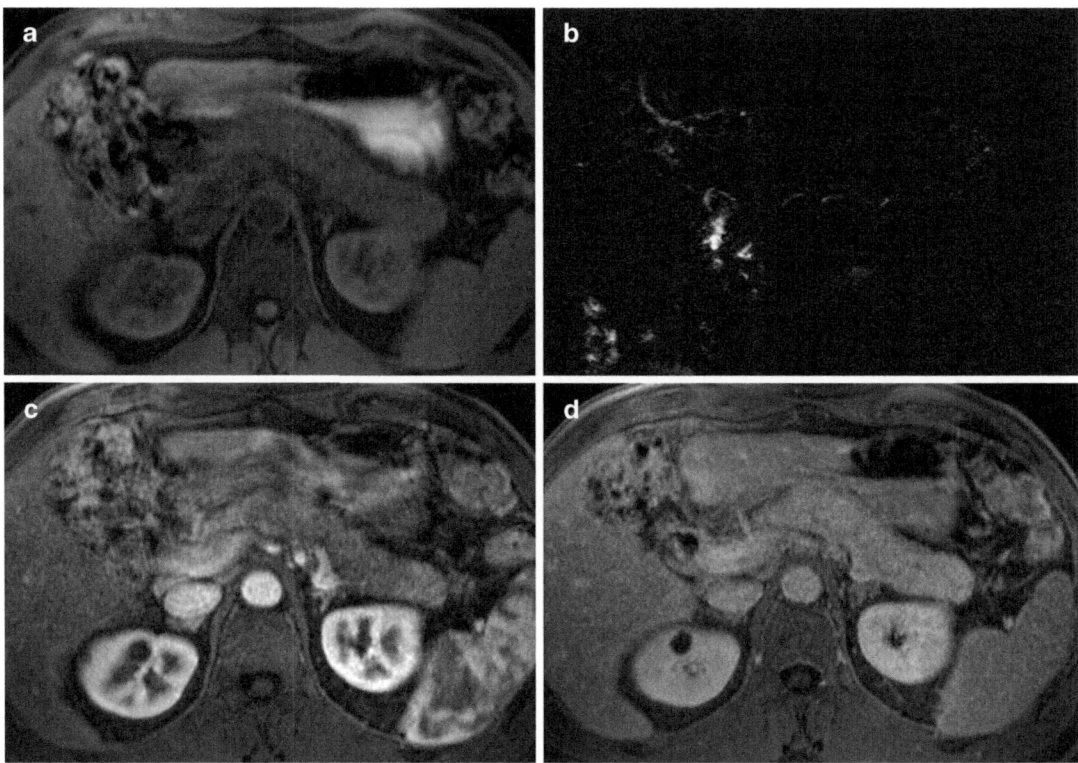

Fig. 14.19 Autoimmune pancreatitis. Axial T1-weighted (**a**) shows a diffuse "sausage-like" enlargement of the pancreatic parenchyma with loss of its lobular structure, which appears hypointense as compared to the liver. The inflammatory changes are responsible for an extrinsic compression of the main pancreatic duct which appears diffusely narrowed without dilatations at MRCP sequence (**b**). After contrast medium injection, the parenchyma affected results hypovascular during the arterial phase (**c**), with contrast retention in the delayed phase (**d**)

parenchyma on T2-weighted images and on delayed contrastographic sequences may be observed. The diffuse form of AIP may mimic diffuse disorders like lymphoma or interstitial edematous acute pancreatitis.

Focal disease is less common and manifests as a well-defined T1 hypointense lesion with delayed post-gadolinium enhancement, often mimicking pancreatic adenocarcinoma. The main pancreatic duct usually presents multiple skipped stenoses, even in focal involvement of the gland [87–89].

However extrinsic compression of the MPD may be focal with a marked dilation of the upstream MPD caliber, similarly to pancreatic adenocarcinoma. An early diagnosis of AIP is fundamental, since an unnecessary surgery can be avoided [84]. The dilation of the main pancreatic duct in focal AIP is usually milder than in pancreatic adenocarcinoma, in which the MPD is usually infiltrated in a single short stenosis with a marked dilatation of the upstream main pancreatic duct [68, 85–87, 90, 91]. However, in selected cases biopsy is mandatory [84, 92].

Furthermore, the periductal infiltrate can extend to the common bile duct leading to an inflammation that can mimic primary sclerosing cholangitis, with multiple dilations and strictures of the intrahepatic bile ducts and thickening of the wall of the common bile duct [85, 87]. Renal involvement represents the second most frequent extra-pancreatic site of AIP and resembles an interstitial nephritis. Renal lesions are usually multiple, bilateral, predominantly located within the renal cortex, with delayed contrast enhancement [93]. Finally, retroperitoneal fibrosis can be rarely demonstrated, especially in type 1 AIP.

High dosage of steroids represents the treatment of choice for recurrent AIP; however, some patients may require immunosuppressive drugs

[78, 84, 86, 94]. Recurrent disease has been well demonstrated, particularly in type 1 subtype.

14.3.7.3 Hereditary Chronic Pancreatitis

Hereditary chronic pancreatitis is a rare inherited form of pancreatitis associated to several gene mutations [12]. The most frequent involved mutations include the *CFTR* (cystic fibrosis transmembrane regulator) gene, the *SPINK1* (serine protease inhibitor, Kazal type 1) gene, and the *PRSS1* (cationic trypsin) gene [68, 95–99]. Patients are typically young and the disease is slowly progressive. The diagnosis and the follow-up of the patients affected by this form of chronic pancreatitis are crucial, since the risk of developing pancreatic adenocarcinoma is high. Hereditary form is characterized by the presence of multiple calcifications and dense plugs within the pancreatic ducts, with secondary dilation of the MPD. Several studies reported that a typical aspect of hereditary pancreatitis is the presence of numerous and large (>15 mm) pancreatic duct stones, which typically present dense peripheral margins and radiolucent, non-calcified, central core ("bull's-eye" pattern) (Fig. 14.20) [18, 100, 101].

CT should be used to identify large ductal stones with the typical bull's-eye pattern. In young patients with a history of chronic pancreatitis and who have no risks, CT may suggest a genetic etiology of the pancreatitis, which could subsequently be confirmed by genetic tests.

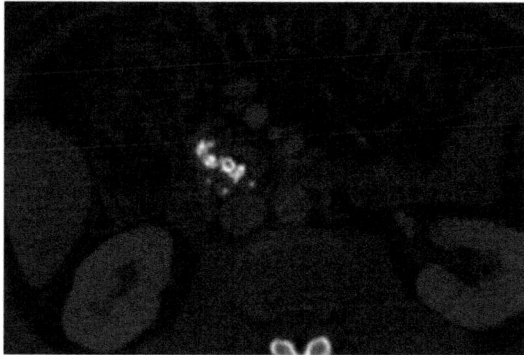

Fig. 14.20 Hereditary pancreatitis. Axial non-contrast CT image shows multiple calcifications of the pancreatic parenchyma of the head, with dense peripheral margins and radiolucent central core (typical "bulls-eye" appearance)

References

1. Bradley EL, 3rd. A clinically based classification system for acute pancreatitis. Summary of the International Symposium on Acute Pancreatitis, Atlanta, Ga, September 11 through 13, 1992. Arch Surg. 1993;128(5):586–90.
2. Bollen TL, van Santvoort HC, Besselink MG, van Es WH, Gooszen HG, van Leeuwen MS. Update on acute pancreatitis: ultrasound, computed tomography, and magnetic resonance imaging features. Semin Ultrasound CT MR. 2007;28(5):371–83.
3. Merkle EM, Gorich J. Imaging of acute pancreatitis. Eur Radiol. 2002;12(8):1979–92.
4. Foster BR, Jensen KK, Bakis G, Shaaban AM, Coakley FV. Revised Atlanta classification for acute pancreatitis: a pictorial essay. Radiographics. 2016;36(3):675–87.
5. Frossard JL, Steer ML, Pastor CM. Acute pancreatitis. Lancet. 2008;371(9607):143–52.
6. Zhao K, Adam SZ, Keswani RN, Horowitz JM, Miller FH. Acute pancreatitis: revised Atlanta classification and the role of cross-sectional imaging. AJR Am J Roentgenol. 2015;205(1):W32–41.
7. Forsmark CE, Baillie J. AGA Institute technical review on acute pancreatitis. Rev Gastroenterol Mex. 2007;72(3):257–85.
8. Whitcomb DC. Clinical practice. Acute pancreatitis. N Engl J Med. 2006;354(20):2142–50.
9. Dunnick NR, Langlotz CP. The radiology report of the future: a summary of the 2007 intersociety conference. J Am Coll Radiol. 2008;5(5):626–9.
10. Ellenbogen PH. BI-RADS: revised and replicated. J Am Coll Radiol. 2014;11(1):2.
11. Braganza JM, Lee SH, McCloy RF, McMahon MJ. Chronic pancreatitis. Lancet. 2011;377(9772):1184–97.
12. Etemad B, Whitcomb DC. Chronic pancreatitis: diagnosis, classification, and new genetic developments. Gastroenterology. 2001;120(3):682–707.
13. Adsay NV, Zamboni G. Paraduodenal pancreatitis: a clinico-pathologically distinct entity unifying "cystic dystrophy of heterotopic pancreas", "para-duodenal wall cyst", and "groove pancreatitis". Semin Diagn Pathol. 2004;21(4):247–54.
14. Levy P, Dominguez-Munoz E, Imrie C, Lohr M, Maisonneuve P. Epidemiology of chronic pancreatitis: burden of the disease and consequences. United Eur Gastroenterol J. 2014;2(5):345–54.
15. Yadav D, Lowenfels AB. The epidemiology of pancreatitis and pancreatic cancer. Gastroenterology. 2013;144(6):1252–61.
16. Majumder S, Chari ST. Chronic pancreatitis. Lancet. 2016;387(10031):1957–66.
17. Whitcomb DC, Frulloni L, Garg P, Greer JB, Schneider A, Yadav D, et al. Chronic pancreatitis: an international draft consensus proposal for a new mechanistic definition. Pancreatology. 2016;16(2):218–24.

18. Graziani R, Frulloni L, Cicero C, Manfredi R, Ambrosetti MC, Mautone S, et al. Bull's-eye pattern of pancreatic-duct stones on multidetector computed tomography and gene-mutation-associated pancreatitis (GMAP). Radiol Med. 2012;117(8):1275–86.

19. Sankaran SJ, Xiao AY, Wu LM, Windsor JA, Forsmark CE, Petrov MS. Frequency of progression from acute to chronic pancreatitis and risk factors: a meta-analysis. Gastroenterology. 2015;149(6):1490–500. e1.

20. Banks PA, Bollen TL, Dervenis C, Gooszen HG, Johnson CD, Sarr MG, et al. Classification of acute pancreatitis--2012: revision of the Atlanta classification and definitions by international consensus. Gut. 2013;62(1):102–11.

21. Baker ME, Nelson RC, Rosen MP, Blake MA, Cash BD, Hindman NM, et al. ACR Appropriateness Criteria(R) acute pancreatitis. Ultrasound Q. 2014;30(4):267–73.

22. Singh VK, Bollen TL, Wu BU, Repas K, Maurer R, Yu S, et al. An assessment of the severity of interstitial pancreatitis. Clin Gastroenterol Hepatol. 2011;9(12):1098–103.

23. Marshall JC, Cook DJ, Christou NV, Bernard GR, Sprung CL, Sibbald WJ. Multiple organ dysfunction score: a reliable descriptor of a complex clinical outcome. Crit Care Med. 1995;23(10):1638–52.

24. Thoeni RF. The revised Atlanta classification of acute pancreatitis: its importance for the radiologist and its effect on treatment. Radiology. 2012;262(3):751–64.

25. Balthazar EJ, Robinson DL, Megibow AJ, Ranson JH. Acute pancreatitis: value of CT in establishing prognosis. Radiology. 1990;174(2):331–6.

26. Mortele KJ, Wiesner W, Intriere L, Shankar S, Zou KH, Kalantari BN, et al. A modified CT severity index for evaluating acute pancreatitis: improved correlation with patient outcome. AJR Am J Roentgenol. 2004;183(5):1261–5.

27. Trout AT, Elsayes KM, Ellis JH, Francis IR. Imaging of acute pancreatitis: prognostic value of computed tomographic findings. J Comput Assist Tomogr. 2010;34(4):485–95.

28. Banks PA, Freeman ML. Practice guidelines in acute pancreatitis. Am J Gastroenterol. 2006;101(10):2379–400.

29. Lenhart DK, Balthazar EJ. MDCT of acute mild (nonnecrotizing) pancreatitis: abdominal complications and fate of fluid collections. AJR Am J Roentgenol. 2008;190(3):643–9.

30. Pelaez-Luna M, Vege SS, Petersen BT, Chari ST, Clain JE, Levy MJ, et al. Disconnected pancreatic duct syndrome in severe acute pancreatitis: clinical and imaging characteristics and outcomes in a cohort of 31 cases. Gastrointest Endosc. 2008;68(1):91–7.

31. Tuney D, Altun E, Barlas A, Yegen C. Pancreatico-colonic fistula after acute necrotizing pancreatitis. Diagnosis with spiral CT using rectal water soluble contrast media. Jop. 2008;9(1):26–9.

32. Scaglione M, Casciani E, Pinto A, Andreoli C, De Vargas M, Gualdi GF. Imaging assessment of acute pancreatitis: a review. Semin Ultrasound CT MR. 2008;29(5):322–40.

33. Bernades P, Baetz A, Levy P, Belghiti J, Menu Y, Fekete F. Splenic and portal venous obstruction in chronic pancreatitis. A prospective longitudinal study of a medical-surgical series of 266 patients. Dig Dis Sci. 1992;37(3):340–6.

34. Mortele KJ, Mergo PJ, Taylor HM, Wiesner W, Cantisani V, Ernst MD, et al. Peripancreatic vascular abnormalities complicating acute pancreatitis: contrast-enhanced helical CT findings. Eur J Radiol. 2004;52(1):67–72.

35. Bharwani N, Patel S, Prabhudesai S, Fotheringham T, Power N. Acute pancreatitis: the role of imaging in diagnosis and management. Clin Radiol. 2011;66(2):164–75.

36. Mallick IH, Winslet MC. Vascular complications of pancreatitis. Jop. 2004;5(5):328–37.

37. Hirota M, Kimura Y, Ishiko T, Beppu T, Yamashita Y, Ogawa M. Visualization of the heterogeneous internal structure of so-called "pancreatic necrosis" by magnetic resonance imaging in acute necrotizing pancreatitis. Pancreas. 2002;25(1):63–7.

38. Busireddy KK, AlObaidy M, Ramalho M, Kalubowila J, Baodong L, Santagostino I, et al. Pancreatitis-imaging approach. World J Gastrointest Pathophysiol. 2014;5(3):252–70.

39. Werner J, Feuerbach S, Uhl W, Buchler MW. Management of acute pancreatitis: from surgery to interventional intensive care. Gut. 2005;54(3):426–36.

40. Sarner M, Cotton PB. Classification of pancreatitis. Gut. 1984;25(7):756–9.

41. Layer P, Yamamoto H, Kalthoff L, Clain JE, Bakken LJ, DiMagno EP. The different courses of early- and late-onset idiopathic and alcoholic chronic pancreatitis. Gastroenterology. 1994;107(5):1481–7.

42. Tirkes T, Sandrasegaran K, Sanyal R, Sherman S, Schmidt CM, Cote GA, et al. Secretin-enhanced MR cholangiopancreatography: spectrum of findings. Radiographics. 2013;33(7):1889–906.

43. Carbognin G, Pinali L, Girardi V, Casarin A, Mansueto G, Mucelli RP. Collateral branches IPMTs: secretin-enhanced MRCP. Abdom Imaging. 2007;32(3):374–80.

44. Bian Y, Wang L, Chen C, Lu JP, Fan JB, Chen SY, et al. Quantification of pancreatic exocrine function of chronic pancreatitis with secretin-enhanced MRCP. World J Gastroenterol. 2013;19(41): 7177–82.

45. Balci C. MRI assessment of chronic pancreatitis. Diagn Interv Radiol. 2011;17(3):249–54.

46. Hamed MM, Hamm B, Ibrahim ME, Taupitz M, Mahfouz AE. Dynamic MR imaging of the abdomen with gadopentetate dimeglumine: normal enhancement patterns of the liver, spleen, stomach, and pancreas. AJR Am J Roentgenol. 1992;158(2): 303–7.

47. Wallner BK, Schumacher KA, Weidenmaier W, Friedrich JM. Dilated biliary tract: evaluation with MR cholangiography with a T2-weighted

contrast-enhanced fast sequence. Radiology. 1991;181(3):805–8.

48. Hansen TM, Nilsson M, Gram M, Frokjaer JB. Morphological and functional evaluation of chronic pancreatitis with magnetic resonance imaging. World J Gastroenterol. 2013;19(42):7241–6.

49. Takehara Y, Ichijo K, Tooyama N, Kodaira N, Yamamoto H, Tatami M, et al. Breath-hold MR cholangiopancreatography with a long-echo-train fast spin-echo sequence and a surface coil in chronic pancreatitis. Radiology. 1994;192(1):73–8.

50. Arish MA, Yucel EK, Soto JA, Chuttani R, Ferrucci JT. MR cholangiopancreatography: efficacy of three-dimensional turbo spin-echo technique. AJR Am J Roentgenol. 1995;165(2):295–300.

51. Kim JH, Hong SS, Eun HW, Han JK, Choi BI. Clinical usefulness of free-breathing navigator-triggered 3D MRCP in non-cooperative patients: comparison with conventional breath-hold 2D MRCP. Eur J Radiol. 2012;81(4):e513–8.

52. Kamisawa T, Tu Y, Egawa N, Tsuruta K, Okamoto A, Kamata N. MRCP of congenital pancreaticobiliary malformation. Abdom Imaging. 2007;32(1):129–33.

53. Boninsegna E, Manfredi R, Ventriglia A, Negrelli R, Pedrinolla B, Mehrabi S, et al. Santorinicele: secretin-enhanced magnetic resonance cholangiopancreatography findings before and after minor papilla sphincterotomy. Eur Radiol. 2015;25(8):2437–44.

54. Boninsegna E, Manfredi R, Negrelli R, Avesani G, Mehrabi S, Pozzi Mucelli R. Pancreatic duct stenosis: differential diagnosis between malignant and benign conditions at secretin-enhanced MRCP. Clin Imaging. 2017;41:137–43.

55. Cappeliez O, Delhaye M, Deviere J, Le Moine O, Metens T, Nicaise N, et al. Chronic pancreatitis: evaluation of pancreatic exocrine function with MR pancreatography after secretin stimulation. Radiology. 2000;215(2):358–64.

56. Kahl S, Glasbrenner B, Leodolter A, Pross M, Schulz HU, Malfertheiner P. EUS in the diagnosis of early chronic pancreatitis: a prospective follow-up study. Gastrointest Endosc. 2002;55(4):507–11.

57. Frulloni L, Falconi M, Gabbrielli A, Gaia E, Graziani R, Pezzilli R, et al. Italian consensus guidelines for chronic pancreatitis. Dig Liver Dis. 2010;42(Suppl 6):S381–406.

58. Manfredi R, Brizi MG, Masselli G, Gui B, Vecchioli A, Marano P. Imaging of chronic pancreatitis. Rays. 2001;26(2):143–9.

59. Matos C, Deviere J, Cremer M, Nicaise N, Struyven J, Metens T. Acinar filling during secretin-stimulated MR pancreatography. AJR Am J Roentgenol. 1998;171(1):165–9.

60. Matos C, Metens T, Deviere J, Nicaise N, Braude P, Van Yperen G, et al. Pancreatic duct: morphologic and functional evaluation with dynamic MR pancreatography after secretin stimulation. Radiology. 1997;203(2):435–41.

61. Manikkavasakar S, AlObaidy M, Busireddy KK, Ramalho M, Nilmini V, Alagiyawanna M, et al. Magnetic resonance imaging of pancreatitis: an update. World J Gastroenterol. 2014;20(40):14760–77.

62. Bollen TL. Imaging of acute pancreatitis: update of the revised Atlanta classification. Radiol Clin North Am. 2012;50(3):429–45.

63. Winstead NS, Wilcox CM. Clinical trials of pancreatic enzyme replacement for painful chronic pancreatitis--a review. Pancreatology. 2009;9(4):344–50.

64. Forsmark CE. Management of chronic pancreatitis. Gastroenterology. 2013;144(6):1282–91. e3.

65. Dite P, Ruzicka M, Zboril V, Novotny I. A prospective, randomized trial comparing endoscopic and surgical therapy for chronic pancreatitis. Endoscopy. 2003;35(7):553–8.

66. Diener MK, Rahbari NN, Fischer L, Antes G, Buchler MW, Seiler CM. Duodenum-preserving pancreatic head resection versus pancreatoduodenectomy for surgical treatment of chronic pancreatitis: a systematic review and meta-analysis. Ann Surg. 2008;247(6):950–61.

67. Buchler MW, Warshaw AL. Resection versus drainage in treatment of chronic pancreatitis. Gastroenterology. 2008;134(5):1605–7.

68. Shanbhogue AK, Fasih N, Surabhi VR, Doherty GP, Shanbhogue DK, Sethi SK. A clinical and radiologic review of uncommon types and causes of pancreatitis. Radiographics. 2009;29(4):1003–26.

69. Triantopoulou C, Dervenis C, Giannakou N, Papailiou J, Prassopoulos P. Groove pancreatitis: a diagnostic challenge. Eur Radiol. 2009;19(7):1736–43.

70. Kim JD, Han YS, Choi DL. Characteristic clinical and pathologic features for preoperative diagnosed groove pancreatitis. J Korean Surg Soc. 2011;80(5):342–7.

71. Arora A, Rajesh S, Mukund A, Patidar Y, Thapar S, Arora A, et al. Clinicoradiological appraisal of 'paraduodenal pancreatitis': Pancreatitis outside the pancreas! Indian J Radiol Imaging. 2015;25(3):303–14.

72. Shudo R, Obara T, Tanno S, Fujii T, Nishino N, Sagawa M, et al. Segmental groove pancreatitis accompanied by protein plugs in Santorini's duct. J Gastroenterol. 1998;33(2):289–94.

73. Hartwig W, Werner J, Ryschich E, Mayer H, Schmidt J, Gebhard MM, et al. Cigarette smoke enhances ethanol-induced pancreatic injury. Pancreas. 2000;21(3):272–8.

74. Procacci C, Graziani R, Zamboni G, Cavallini G, Pederzoli P, Guarise A, et al. Cystic dystrophy of the duodenal wall: radiologic findings. Radiology. 1997;205(3):741–7.

75. Arora A, Dev A, Mukund A, Patidar Y, Bhatia V, Sarin SK. Paraduodenal pancreatitis. Clin Radiol. 2014;69(3):299–306.

76. Kalb B, Martin DR, Sarmiento JM, Erickson SH, Gober D, Tapper EB, et al. Paraduodenal pancreatitis: clinical performance of MR imaging in distinguishing from carcinoma. Radiology. 2013;269(2):475–81.

77. Casetti L, Bassi C, Salvia R, Butturini G, Graziani R, Falconi M, et al. "Paraduodenal" pancreatitis: results of surgery on 58 consecutives patients from a single institution. World J Surg. 2009;33(12):2664–9.

78. Shimosegawa T, Chari ST, Frulloni L, Kamisawa T, Kawa S, Mino-Kenudson M, et al. International consensus diagnostic criteria for autoimmune pancreatitis: guidelines of the international association of pancreatology. Pancreas. 2011;40(3): 352–8.

79. Chari ST, Kloeppel G, Zhang L, Notohara K, Lerch MM, Shimosegawa T. Histopathologic and clinical subtypes of autoimmune pancreatitis: the honolulu consensus document. Pancreatology. 2010;10(6):664–72.

80. Kloppel G, Detlefsen S, Chari ST, Longnecker DS, Zamboni G. Autoimmune pancreatitis: the clinicopathological characteristics of the subtype with granulocytic epithelial lesions. J Gastroenterol. 2010;45(8):787–93.

81. Kloppel G, Sipos B, Zamboni G, Kojima M, Morohoshi T. Autoimmune pancreatitis: histo- and immunopathological features. J Gastroenterol. 2007;42(Suppl 18):28–31.

82. Zamboni G, Luttges J, Capelli P, Frulloni L, Cavallini G, Pederzoli P, et al. Histopathological features of diagnostic and clinical relevance in autoimmune pancreatitis: a study on 53 resection specimens and 9 biopsy specimens. Virchows Arch. 2004;445(6):552–63.

83. Frulloni L, Scattolini C, Falconi M, Zamboni G, Capelli P, Manfredi R, et al. Autoimmune pancreatitis: differences between the focal and diffuse forms in 87 patients. Am J Gastroenterol. 2009;104(9):2288–94.

84. Frulloni L, Amodio A, Katsotourchi AM, Vantini I. A practical approach to the diagnosis of autoimmune pancreatitis. World J Gastroenterol. 2011;17(16):2076–9.

85. Manfredi R, Frulloni L, Mantovani W, Bonatti M, Graziani R, Pozzi Mucelli R. Autoimmune pancreatitis: pancreatic and extrapancreatic MR imaging-MR cholangiopancreatography findings at diagnosis, after steroid therapy, and at recurrence. Radiology. 2011;260(2):428–36.

86. Manfredi R, Graziani R, Cicero C, Frulloni L, Carbognin G, Mantovani W, et al. Autoimmune pancreatitis: CT patterns and their changes after steroid treatment. Radiology. 2008;247(2):435–43.

87. Negrelli R, Manfredi R, Pedrinolla B, Boninsegna E, Ventriglia A, Mehrabi S, et al. Pancreatic duct abnormalities in focal autoimmune pancreatitis: MR/MRCP imaging findings. Eur Radiol. 2015;25(2):359–67.

88. Crosara S, D'Onofrio M, De Robertis R, Demozzi E, Canestrini S, Zamboni G, et al. Autoimmune pancreatitis: multimodality non-invasive imaging diagnosis. World J Gastroenterol. 2014;20(45): 16881–90.

89. Sugumar A, Levy MJ, Kamisawa T, Webster GJ, Kim MH, Enders F, et al. Endoscopic retrograde pancreatography criteria to diagnose autoimmune pancreatitis: an international multicentre study. Gut. 2011;60(5):666–70.

90. Graziani R, Frulloni L, Mantovani W, Ambrosetti MC, Mautone S, Re TJ, et al. Autoimmune pancreatitis and non-necrotizing acute pancreatitis: computed tomography pattern. Dig Liver Dis. 2012;44(9):759–66.

91. Graziani R, Mautone S, Ambrosetti MC, Manfredi R, Re TJ, Calculli L, et al. Autoimmune pancreatitis: multidetector-row computed tomography (MDCT) and magnetic resonance (MR) findings in the Italian experience. Radiol Med. 2014;119(8):558–71.

92. Ikeura T, Detlefsen S, Zamboni G, Manfredi R, Negrelli R, Amodio A, et al. Retrospective comparison between preoperative diagnosis by international consensus diagnostic criteria and histological diagnosis in patients with focal autoimmune pancreatitis who underwent surgery with suspicion of cancer. Pancreas. 2014;43(5):698–703.

93. Takahashi N, Kawashima A, Fletcher JG, Chari ST. Renal involvement in patients with autoimmune pancreatitis: CT and MR imaging findings. Radiology. 2007;242(3):791–801.

94. Kamisawa T, Chari ST, Giday SA, Kim MH, Chung JB, Lee KT, et al. Clinical profile of autoimmune pancreatitis and its histological subtypes: an international multicenter survey. Pancreas. 2011;40(6):809–14.

95. Whitcomb DC, Gorry MC, Preston RA, Furey W, Sossenheimer MJ, Ulrich CD, et al. Hereditary pancreatitis is caused by a mutation in the cationic trypsinogen gene. Nat Genet. 1996;14(2):141–5.

96. Cohn JA, Mitchell RM, Jowell PS. The impact of cystic fibrosis and PSTI/SPINK1 gene mutations on susceptibility to chronic pancreatitis. Clin Lab Med. 2005;25(1):79–100.

97. Durie PR. Pancreatitis and mutations of the cystic fibrosis gene. N Engl J Med. 1998;339(10):687–8.

98. Chen JM, Mercier B, Audrezet MP, Ferec C. Mutational analysis of the human pancreatic secretory trypsin inhibitor (PSTI) gene in hereditary and sporadic chronic pancreatitis. J Med Genet. 2000;37(1):67–9.

99. Kume K, Masamune A, Mizutamari H, Kaneko K, Kikuta K, Satoh M, et al. Mutations in the serine protease inhibitor Kazal Type 1 (SPINK1) gene in Japanese patients with pancreatitis. Pancreatology. 2005;5(4–5):354–60.

100. Rohrmann CA, Surawicz CM, Hutchinson D, Silverstein FE, White TT, Marchioro TL. The diagnosis of hereditary pancreatitis by pancreatography. Gastrointest Endosc. 1981;27(3):168–73.

101. Hoshina K, Kimura W, Ishiguro T, Tominaga O, Futakawa N, Bin Z, et al. Three generations of hereditary chronic pancreatitis. Hepatogastroenterology. 1999;46(26):1192–8.

Imaging of Renal Colic

15

Paola Martingano, Marco F. M. Cavallaro,
Fulvio Stacul, and Maria Assunta Cova

15.1 Introduction

Renal colic indicates a type of abdominal pain due to urinary tract obstruction, commonly caused by urinary stones. The pain is caused by stretching of mucosal and submucosal nerve endings of the ureter around the stones and by interstitial edema with distention of renal capsule.

The classic presentation of renal colic is the sudden onset of severe loin pain. The pain is colic; it means that it comes in waves of varying intensity, with completely pain-free periods between attacks. The patients are restless and often change position, by contrast with peritonitic conditions in which patients remain still. Symptoms such as nausea or emesis can accompany renal colic due to overstimulation of celiac ganglion. Depending on

the site of obstruction, the pain will radiate to the flank, groin, and testes or labia majora. Bladder irritability symptoms can be seen in stones located in ureterovesical junction. Microscopic or macroscopic hematuria is often present due to traumatizing effect of stones in the collecting system mucosa; however, the absence of hematuria does not rule out urinary stone disease [1–4].

Acute renal colic is a common problem in emergency care units, and up to 12% of the population will have a urinary stone in the lifetime, with a recurrence rate of 50% [4–7]. Unfortunately, symptoms due to many other abdominal diseases could be indistinguishable from renal colic because the kidney shares fibers transmitting sensation with other organs, and so there is a poor localization of pain, while physical examination could be nonspecific [8]. On the basis of this clinical overlap, up to 29% of the patients may have an alternative diagnosis; therefore, emergency imaging in patients with suspected renal colic is necessary to rule out other clinical conditions. Adnexal masses, pyelonephritis, appendicitis, and diverticulitis represent the most common alternative diagnosis, but also acute aortic conditions should be considered [4, 7, 9, 10].

Imaging is not only required to confirm diagnosis but also to guide patient management [11]. In fact on the basis of size, site, and composition of the stone, it is possible to stratify the likelihood of spontaneous passage or the need of a medical expulsive therapy, shock wave

Electronic Supplementary Material The online version of this chapter (https://doi.org/10.1007/978-3-319-99822-0_15) contains supplementary material, which is available to authorized users.

P. Martingano (✉) · M. A. Cova
Unità Clinico Operativa di Radiologia, Dipartimento Universitario Clinico di Scienze Mediche Chirurgiche e della Salute, Ospedale di Cattinara, Azienda Sanitaria Universitaria Integrata di Trieste, Università degli Studi di Trieste, Trieste, Italy
e-mail: paola.martingano@asuits.sanita.fvg.it; m.cova@fmc.units.it

M. F. M. Cavallaro · F. Stacul
Struttura Complessa di Radiologia, Ospedale Maggiore, Azienda Sanitaria Universitaria Integrata Trieste, Trieste, Italy
e-mail: fulvio.stacul@asuits.sanita.fvg.it

lithotripsy (SWL), percutaneous nephrolithotomy, or retrograde or percutaneous ureterorenoscopy (URS) [1].

Stone size is the major parameter determining the likelihood of spontaneous passage, with an almost linear relationship: passage rates of stones measuring 1, 4, 7, and 10 mm are, respectively, 87%, 72%, 47%, and 27%. In general stones less than 5 mm pass spontaneously in 71–100% of the cases, while just 25–46% of stones >5 mm will solve without therapy [12]. Stone size influences also the choice of active treatment modality because stone-free rate after extracorporeal SWL is significantly better for stones <10 mm (75–80% versus 44–60%), while stone size is not so significant for retrograde URS [13, 14].

Stone location helps to predict a spontaneous passage, since ureteral stones <5 mm pass in 71–100% of the cases if located in the distal part of the ureter, while the rate of spontaneous passage lowers to 22–81% if located in the proximal ureter [14]. Stone location has a role also in the choice of active therapy, because even if improving in recent times, retrograde URS has still higher successful rates for distal than proximal calculi, while extracorporeal SWL efficacy is not affected by stone location [13]. Furthermore in cases an extracorporeal SWL is planned, it is important to know the distance between the skin and the stone and to exclude the presence of vascular aneurism nearby or interposition of other organs [1, 15].

Stone composition knowledge is useful for patient management. There are five main types of urinary stones: calcium-based calculi (70–80%), due to hypercalciuria, hypercitraturia, and hyperoxaluria; magnesium ammonium phosphate calculi, known as struvite stones (15–20%), related to infections by urease-producing bacteria; uric acid calculi (5–10%), related to high body mass index, gout, and chronic diarrhea; cystine calculi (1–3%), due to genetic cystinuria; and medication-induced calculi, related to HIV protease inhibitors, but also herbal supplements and other drugs (triamterene, sulfonamides, amorphous silica) [2]. On the basis of stone composition, it is possible to predict treatment response; in fact pure uric acid stones could dissolute completely just by oral chemolysis, and calcium-based stones and uric acid stone could be fragmented by SWL, while cystine calculi are often refractory to SWL [1, 16].

Beside stone size, site, and composition, patient management is related to the identification of renal colic complications. An obstructing stone causes urinary tract dilation, hydroureter, and/or hydronephrosis, a serious clinical problem since it can produce a permanent deterioration of renal function if it lasts more than 4–5 weeks. Likelihood and grade of hydronephrosis generally depend on stone size, in fact stones ≤3 mm do not cause hydronephrosis, while stones of 4–5.5 mm usually cause just mild or moderate hydronephrosis, and a severe hydronephrosis is related to stones >10 mm. Urine leakage in the perinephric space, with development of an urinoma, is a sign of high pressure obstruction with consequent forniceal rupture, a condition which requires a prompt intervention. Urgent decompression is also required in case of infection, because if the filtration through the glomerulus is compromised, antibiotics could not reach the site of infection, and in case of an obstructing stone affecting a solitary or transplant kidney, to preserve renal function [8, 13].

Finally imaging plays a role in the follow-up of conservative management and in the evaluation of active treatment complications. Shock wave lithotripsy causes an acute ureteral obstruction in 4% of the patients, due to stone fragmentation, ureteral wall edema, or clots secondary to hematuria. With retrograde URS, the ureter could be injured directly in 2% of patients. With both modalities, the risk of infection is around 5%. Percutaneous URS brings a risk of hemorrhage, which requires transfusion in 3% of the patients, greater risk of infection (15%), and of ureteral injury (5%). Laparoscopic ureterolithotomy is the most invasive procedure and is related to higher incidence of complications, in particular urinary or surgical site infection (7%) and urinary extravasations with urinoma formation. Secondary ureteral strictures have been reported for all the procedures, with different incidence rates [13].

15.2 Imaging Modalities

15.2.1 Techniques

15.2.1.1 Plain Radiography

Abdominal plain films recognize a urinary stone for its opacity, but while most calculi are composed of calcium salts, many other (uric acid stones, some medication stones) are radiolucent. Furthermore, stone size, the presence of overlying fecal material or bowel gas, spinous vertebral processes, and bony pelvis may confound the image, and so only 48–63% of urinary stones are visible. Abdominal plain films sensitivity is affected by stone size; it is higher for stones >5 mm and located proximally, while it is poorer for little ones and for calculi located in distal ureter [1–3, 8].

Plain radiography is often used as first-step imaging in patients with abdominal pain, but since there are other imaging modalities more sensitive in urinary stone detection, it is not indicated in cases of suspected renal colic.

A kidney-ureter-bladder (KUB) radiography, as it is commonly indicated a radiography performed focusing on urinary tract, could be useful in planning extracorporeal SWL to confirm the possibility of localizing the stone with fluoroscopy during the treatment, and in some selected cases, it could be used to follow migration of stones recognized with other imaging modalities [1, 2].

15.2.1.2 Intravenous Urography

Intravenous urography (IVU) used to be the imaging modality of choice in renal colic in case of negative KUB, because of its higher sensitivity and specificity. IVU identifies the urinary tract dilation and the site of obstruction; it allows optimal anatomy depiction and offers physiologic information about renal function and the severity of obstruction. On the other hand, it requires contrast agent administration, which can be contraindicated in patients with renal impairment; it is time-consuming, especially in case of delay of excretion due to obstruction; and the contrast material could obscure some stones. Furthermore, a filling defect detected on IVU could represent a radiolucent calculus, but also a clot or a tumor. Nowadays, the advent of newer imaging modalities has changed its role, and IVU has been almost everywhere substituted by ultrasound or computed tomography [2, 3].

15.2.1.3 Ultrasonography

Ultrasonography (US) is often performed as an initial imaging modality in case of abdominal pain evaluation since it is safe, noninvasive, repeatable, and quite low expensive. Nevertheless, it requires expertise of dedicated operators and could be time-consuming, and its sensitiveness depends on body habitus and BMI of the patients [5, 8, 17].

In most cases, ultrasound examination allows the identification of calculi located in the renal calices and pelvis, in the pyelo-ureteral junction, and in the ureterovesical junction, and it recognizes also medication-induced stones, radiolucent both on KUB and on computed tomography (CT) [5, 18]. Nevertheless, US has a poor sensitivity in the identification of calculi located in the middle ureter due to bowel interposition, it has a lower capability in precise stone size evaluation when compared to CT [19], and it is not able to provide information on calcium content of the stones [1].

US could show indirect signs of obstruction consequent to stone disease depicting urinary tract dilation, the absence of ureteral jets within the bladder lumen, and elevated renal arterial resistive index; so its specificity and positive predictive value in the diagnosis of renal colic are comparable to CT without using of ionizing radiation [3, 20]. Unfortunately, it is to remember that not all symptomatic ureteral calculi cause hydronephrosis, which is present in 69–89% of patients, and that just mild hydronephrosis, more difficult to recognize, is present in 70% of the patients [7, 21].

Ultrasound could also demonstrate possible complications like urinary tract rupture, with development of an urinoma, and pyonephrosis, and it is quite sensitive in recognizing alternative diagnosis, such as subcapsular renal hematomas, pyelonephritis, hemorrhagic renal or ovarian cysts, renal or ovarian tumors, aortic aneurisms, appendicitis, or cholecystitis [5, 18, 22].

Although US certainly plays a role as first-line imaging test in the evaluation of flank pain, it is questioned if its use could be replaced by CT, since the latter gives more information needed for patient management, like direct visualization of the stone size and site, and seems to be more sensitive for alternative diagnosis [5, 18, 19].

15.2.1.4 Computed Tomography

Non-contrast-enhanced CT has been recognized as "the best imaging study to confirm the diagnosis of urinary stone in patient with acute flank pain" [7, 23]. The unenhanced CT study is rapid, independent of the operator, does not take risk of contrast medium injection (renal insufficiency and adverse reactions), and has a sensitivity of 94–98% and a specificity of 98–100% in recognition of urinary calculi [2, 3, 5, 18, 19]. It allows the direct visualization of the stone with the possibility to detect the number of stones and to perform an accurate measurement of calculus size, an important factor for patient management. In fact stones <5 mm in their maximum dimension pass spontaneously 68% of the times, while with a diameter of 5–10 mm, the likelihood lows to 47% and bigger stones usually need intervention [13, 24]. Furthermore, CT allows the exact localization of the calculus that is also of prognostic importance as proximal location of the stone is related to difficult spontaneous passage, and it depicts the exact distance between the stone and the skin, representing a limit to extracorporeal SWL.

Almost all stones are recognizable on CT by the meaning of their high density: calcium-based calculi can reach 1700–2800 Hounsfield Units (HU), struvite usually precipitate with calcium carbonate and form high density stones (600–900 HU), uric acid stones have lower density (200–500 HU), cystine calculi can have foci of low density with a density range of 600–1100 HU, while medication-induced calculi are radiolucent even on CT. Unfortunately, while in vitro characterization of stone composition on the basis of their density is quite accurate, differentiation in vivo is more complicated and less reliable [1, 2, 19].

In addition to direct calculus visualization, non-contrast-enhanced CT is able to recognize the severity of obstruction by indirect signs, such as hydronephrosis and perinephric or periureteral edema, and could depict signs of infection. Furthermore, it allows some anatomical considerations useful for treatment planning, like recognition of kidney abnormalities (solitary kidney, horseshoe kidney, pelvic or ectopic kidney), alteration of the urinary tract (duplication), and interposition of other anatomical structures, like colon or pleural reflection [1, 2, 4].

Even without contrast material administration, CT proved to be more accurate than US in the detection of alternative diagnosis, a condition reported in 10–29% of cases, and so in many centers, particularly in North America, unenhanced CT represents the first-line imaging for flank pain evaluation in emergency settings [19].

Nevertheless, the important radiation exposure represents a significant drawback to consider with attention, in particular in young patients [2]. A standard-dose unenhanced CT has a high sensitivity and specificity both in recognition of calculi <5 mm and in diagnosing alternative abdominal diseases but at cost of an estimated exposure of 9–12 mSv. Such exposure is thought to be related to a significant added malignancy risk, as high as 1 per 500 in a 20-year-old-woman [19, 25]. Moreover, renal colic recurs in 50–60% of patients, causing repeated CT scanning through years, with a sum of radiation exposure and relative risk [25]. For this reasons, many low-dose protocols have been described, in particular limiting scan range from upper kidney limit to bladder base, reducing tube voltage, using automatically modulated tube current on the basis of scout images, increasing slice thickness, and using adaptive statistical iterative reconstruction. Such protocols demonstrated, in patient with a BMI <30 kg/m^2, a reduction of radiation exposure as low as 1.5–2 mSv, at the cost of a reduced sensibility just for stones <3 mm, and so now they are recommended as the standard exam for renal colic studies [5, 19, 26]. Nevertheless, radiation exposure is still not negligible, in particular in case of repeated exams, and, despite the important rise in the use of CT for the diagnosis of urinary stones over the last two decades, it has been demonstrated that there had been change neither in frequency of diagnosis of urinary calculi or alternative diagnosis nor in hospitalization [7, 27]. For these reasons, the use of CT could probably be limited in emergency departments, leaving its role to the study of doubtful US exams and to patients selected by urologist for treatment planning (patients with persistent symptoms, renal failure, solitary or transplanted kidney, possible infection) [7].

Contrast medium administration is usually not indicated in a setting of renal colic, but in case of suspicious findings in the unenhanced scan, the study will be completed with tailored enhanced scans. The presence of a renal mass requires adequate characterization with a multiphasic study. If pyelonephritis and renal abscess are suspected, a nephrographic scan is indicated. The study of renal infarction or vascular aneurisms requires an angiographic phase; if a hematoma or other hemorrhagic conditions are present or suspected, the arterial and venous phases are necessary to recognize active bleeding. The presence of a considerable amount of free fluid around the kidney or in the retroperitoneal cavity is suspicious for an urinoma, and so an excretory phase is needed to confirm urinary tract rupture. If there are signs of obstruction without visible stones or in case of suspected urothelial malignancy, a CT urography (CTU) with an excretory phase is mandatory. A CTU could be occasionally required to obtain a picture of an aberrant urinary tract anatomy (duplicated system, ureteral strictures, and previous surgery) to guide the treatment.

With newer dual-energy and spectral CT systems, it is possible to characterize some renal calculi on the basis of different photoelectric absorptions of different materials at different tube potentials. In particular, the software algorithm can accurately differentiate pure uric acid stones from mixed uric acid ones and from calcified stones, information useful to decide for a chemolysis attempt. The software is also able to differentiate struvite stones from cystine stones, which are difficult to fragment at SWL. However,

double scanning with different tube potentials rises radiation exposure, but a substantial decrease could be obtained targeting the dual scanning to the stone, on the basis of a primary standard low-dose unenhanced scan [1, 2, 19, 28, 29].

15.2.1.5 Magnetic Resonance

Magnetic resonance (MR) imaging is not routinely performed in case of renal colic, because it is relatively expensive and time-consuming. Furthermore, there is generally less expertise in acute body MR imaging, and there is a restricted availability, in particular in an emergency setting and in off-hours. Nevertheless, the comprehensive evaluation of abdominal soft tissues granted by MR without exposure to ionizing radiation certainly reserves it a role in the evaluation of pediatric, pregnant, or serially imaged young patients [5, 30]. When US is not conclusive, MR imaging is recommended in pregnant patients since colic pain can induce a premature labor [31, 32].

MR of the urinary tract can be performed by using heavily T2-weighted sequences without contrast material administration to image the urinary tract as a static collection of fluid (static-fluid MRU) [33].

The static-fluid MRU performance depends on the grade of dilation. In fact, since protons are relatively absent in urinary stones, calculi are not directly visualized but are only recognizable as a signal void. For this reason, a calculus needs to be surrounded by a high signal to become recognizable, so small renal calculi (<10 mm) are easily missed in the absence of hydronephrosis [30].

On the other hand, ureteral stones are generally recognized on the basis of the obstruction they cause, and the presence of the signal void at that level confirms their nature, while the identification of soft tissue signal is suspicious for a tumor or a clot [34].

Static-fluid MRU not only clearly depicts the site of obstruction but shows also the grade of dilation of the urinary tract and the development of possible complications such as pyonephrosis, suspected in case of debris or a not homogeneously high signal inside the dilated renal pelvis [33].

The use of additional T2 sequences combined to a high-quality fat suppression offers a higher sensitivity for perirenal and periureteral edema or free fluid detection, to state severity of obstruction [30]. The sensitivity of these sequences allows recognizing edema related to inflammation in the kidney (pyelonephritis) or in other structures (like appendix, small bowel, gallbladder, adnexa) even in patients with small amount of intra-abdominal fat, usually difficult to evaluate on CT [31].

In case an infection is suspected, diffusion-weighted imaging (DWI) demonstrates with a high sensitivity pyelonephritis and pyonephrosis by the meaning of restricted proton diffusion [33].

Other useful sequences are True FISP or SSFP ones that allow uniform high signal intensity in vascular structures, which could be useful in recognizing adnexal vessels or vascular diseases at the basis of the symptoms, such as an aortic dissection [30].

Gadolinium-enhanced study is required in case of suspected neoplastic conditions. It allows the evaluation of enhancement pattern of the neoplastic lesion, and, in the excretory phase, it offers a depiction of the urinary tract similar to CTU but with less spatial resolution. Angiographic studies have higher sensitivity and specificity than non-contrast sequences in the study of vascular patency.

A dynamic contrast-enhanced study gives also information about time of excretion and, with dedicated software, permits to calculate glomerular filtration rate and renal blood flow of a single kidney, stating the severity of renal obstruction and the consequent need for a prompt intervention [30].

It is to remember that the use of gadolinium is not recommended during pregnancy since it crosses the placenta barrier, with unknown consequence for the fetus, but usually non-contrast sequences are sufficient to grant enough information for patient management [31].

15.2.2 Imaging Findings

15.2.2.1 Plain Radiography

Urinary stones are visible on plain radiography by the meaning of their radiopacity (Fig. 15.1), with cystine and struvite stones often poorly visible, and uric acid and matrix stones not visible at all. Usually stones appear as homogeneous and polymorphic radiopaque structures along the urinary tract. It is often difficult to distinguish them from other opacities like vessel calcifications or phleboliths, but the latter usually have a typical radiolucent center (Fig. 15.1 and Video 15.1).

15.2.2.2 Ultrasound

Stones typically appear on ultrasound imaging as hyperechoic structures with posterior shadowing (Figs. 15.2, 15.3, and 15.4), but the conspicuity of the latter depends on stone size and the use of spatial compound (Fig. 15.5) [7].

Renal calculi need to be 5 mm to be identified on US, but also calculi that are radiolucent on plain radiography are visible [2, 5]. Small renal calculi could be difficult to differentiate from vessel calcifications, but in these cases, a color Doppler artifact could be a useful tool. In fact the rough surface of the stone causes an irregular reflection of the signal, and so the software

Fig. 15.1 Elderly patient presenting in emergency room with acute abdominal pain. Plain radiography (**a**). Multiple urinary stones are visualized by the meaning of their size and radiopacity (arrows); in the pelvis differentiation between ureteral stones (empty arrow) and phleboliths (arrowhead) is quite difficult, but the latter show more regular shape and a typical radiolucent center. Unenhanced CT, MPR reconstruction (**b**), shows incomplete duplication with multiple renal stones and dilation.

A lumbar ureteral stone is located in the upper system, cranial to ureteral fusion (arrow), and multiple stones are impacted in the single pelvic ureter (empty arrow). Unenhanced CT, axial image (**c**), depicts the impacted pelvic ureteral stone with the typical "soft tissue rim sign" (arrow). At lower level, axial image with soft tissue window setting (**d**) shows phlebolith with the "comet tail sign" (arrow), while the bone window setting (**e**) recognizes the radiolucent center of a phlebolith

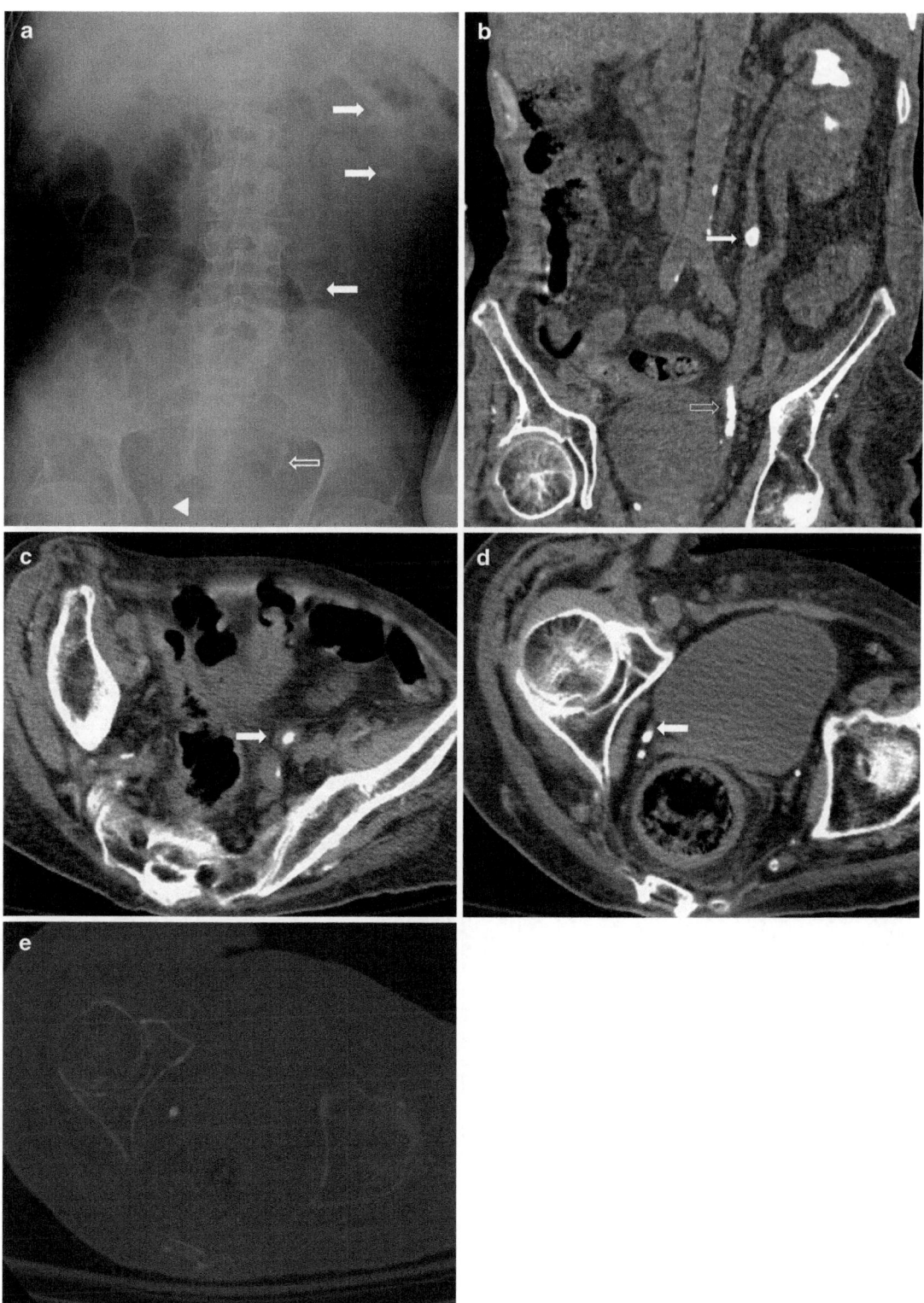

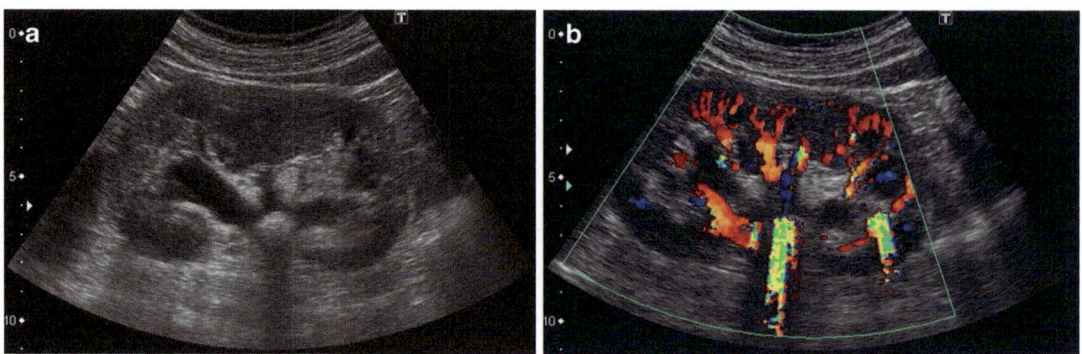

Fig. 15.2 US stone features. Urinary stones appear as hyperechoic formations with posterior shadowing (**a**); on color Doppler the rough surface of the stones causes an irregular reflection of the signal, the "twinkling artifact" (**b**)

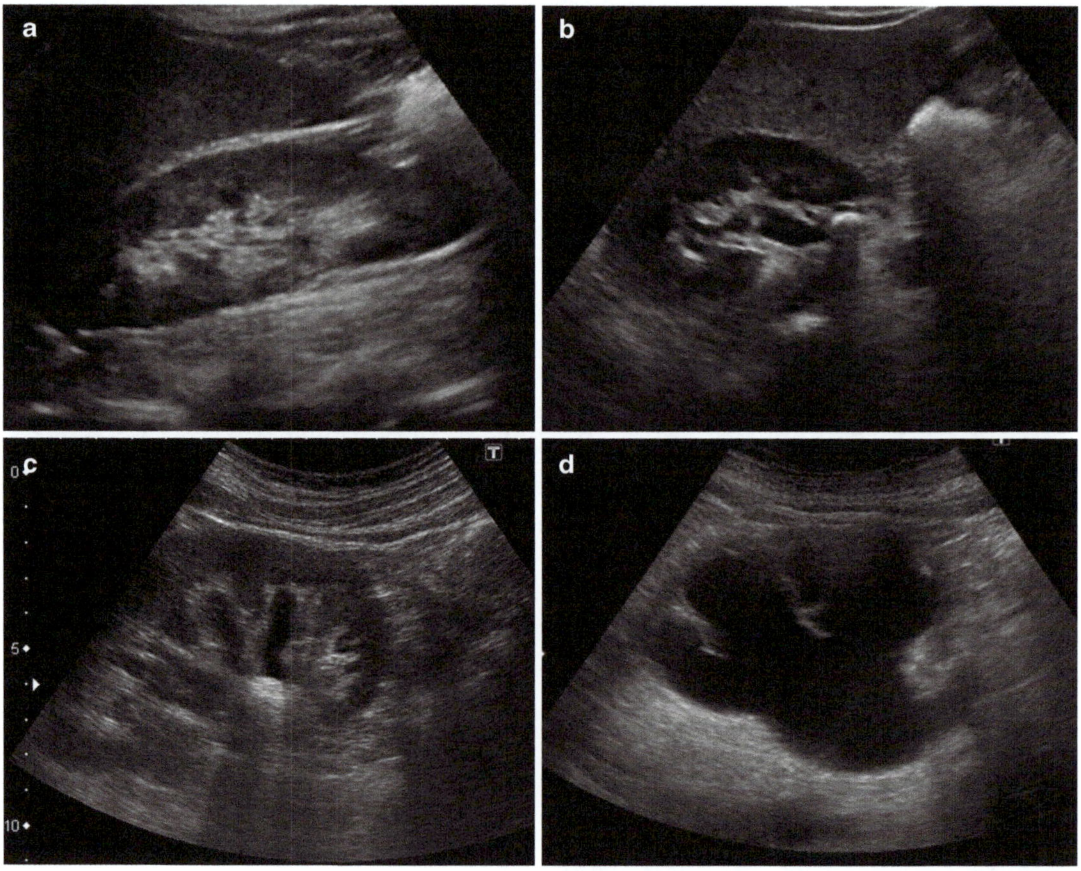

Fig. 15.3 Grade of hydronephrosis on US. Normal kidney: the collecting system is empty (**a**). Mild hydronephrosis: renal pelvis and calices are filled with urine, and the renal papillae are preserved (**b**); note the hyperechoic stone with posterior shadowing in the pyelo-ureteral junction. Moderate hydronephrosis: renal pelvis is ample, calyces are open with blunt aspect, and renal papillae are obliterated (**c**); note the hyperechoic stone with posterior shadowing in the renal pelvis. Severe hydronephrosis: pelvis and calyces are wide open with caliceal ballooning, obliteration of medulla, and cortical thinning (**d**)

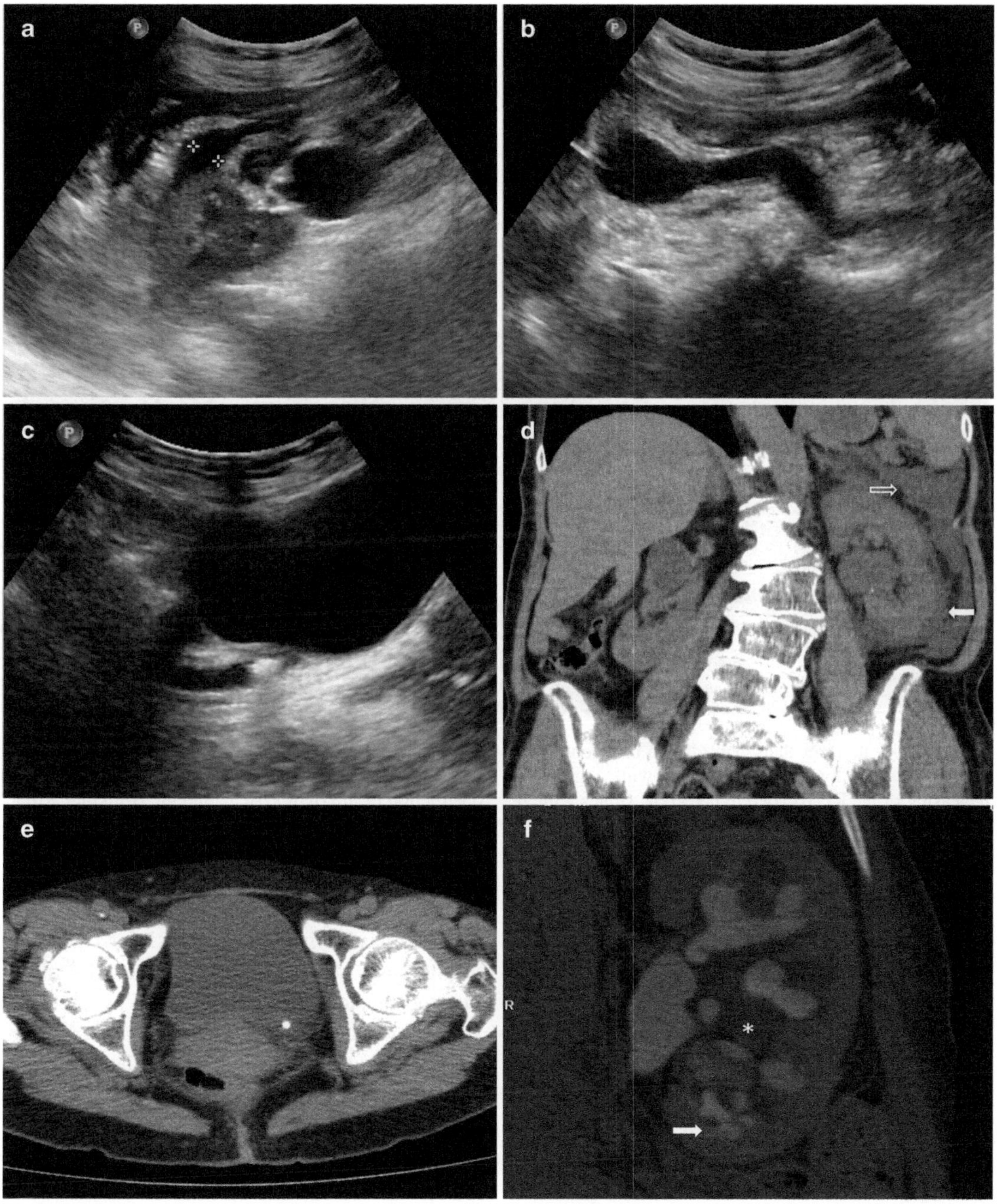

Fig. 15.4 Acute left flank pain due to renal colic with urine leakage. US shows a mild hydronephrosis accompanied by free fluid around the kidney (between calipers in **a**), a significant hydroureter (**b**) and a hyperechoic stone with posterior shadowing at the ureterovesical junction (**c**). Unenhanced CT, coronal image (**d**), depicts the presence of a great amount of free fluid in the perinephric (arrow) and retroperitoneal space (empty arrow); axial image (**e**) confirms stone location. In a different patient CT urography, coronal reconstruction (**f**), demonstrates hydronephrosis in the left kidney, the presence of parapelvic cysts (*), and a forniceal rupture with urine leakage (arrow)

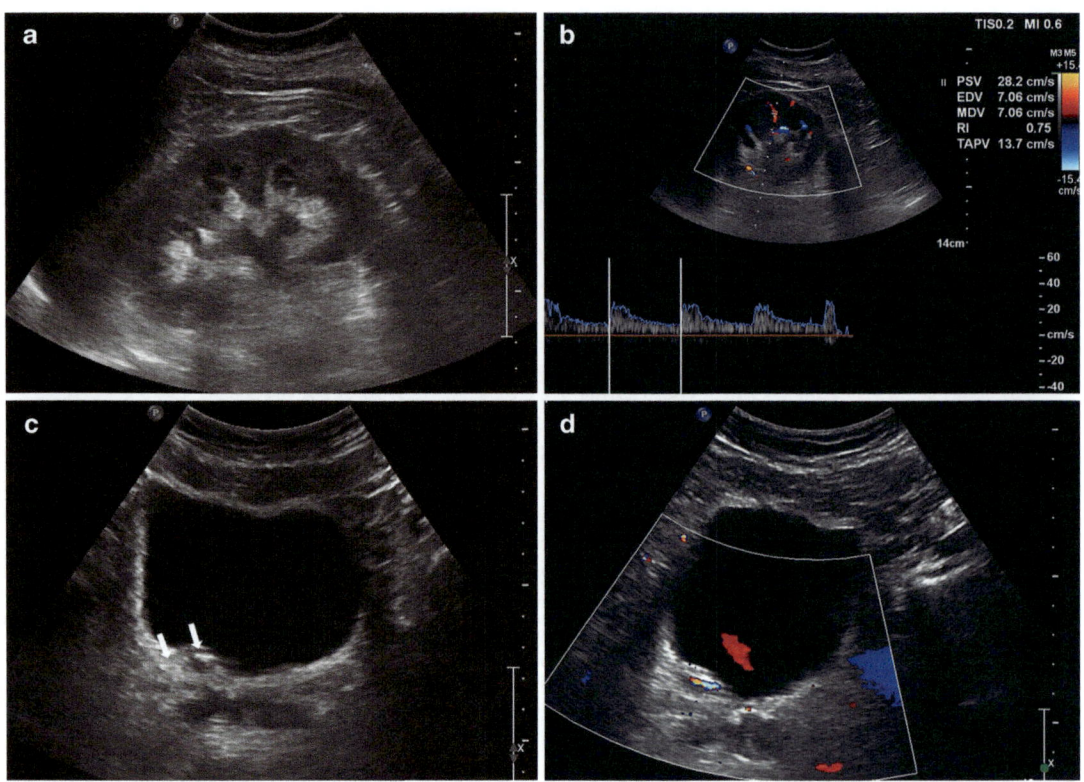

Fig. 15.5 Acute right flank pain due to renal colic. US shows a mild hydronephrosis (**a**) with significant increasing of the RI (**b**). Two hyperechoic stones without posterior shadowing are visible at the level of the ureterovesical junction (arrows in **c**). Color Doppler depicts only the left ureteral jet, indicative of a complete obstruction of the right system, and the twinkling artifact deep to ureteral calculi (**d**)

shows a tail of aliasing colors posterior to the stone, a phenomenon indicated as "twinkling artifact" (Fig. 15.2) [7, 35].

Beside the direct visualization of the stone, US identifies secondary signs of obstruction, such as pelvi-calyceal and ureteric dilation, subcapsular fluid collection, impairment of renal arterial resistive index, and the absence of ureteral jet. These signs prove particularly useful when the stone is not directly visible, generally middle ureter one.

The hydronephrosis is graded on US as mild, moderate, or severe (Fig. 15.3), and it is easily recognizable, as well as the presence of free fluid around the kidney, a finding suspicious for a urinary tract rupture with urinoma development (Fig. 15.4) [7]. However dilation could be absent in the first hours after symptoms onset, especially in case of poor hydrated patients, so it is important to complete the examination with color

Doppler imaging and measurement of the renal arterial resistive index (RI). The RI is calculated on the basis of the peak systolic velocity minus the end-diastolic velocity divided by the peak systolic velocity, measured between the interlobar and arcuate arteries of the kidney. It represents an indirect estimate of the pressure inside the collecting system, since it directly affected pressure into intrarenal vessels. A RI >0.70 is indicative of obstruction, but since the presence of diabetes or hypertension could influence this index, it is important to recognize also a difference >0.04 between the normal and affected kidney (Fig. 15.5) [20]. The RI is a useful tool in distinguishing renal obstruction from physiologic hydronephrosis during pregnancy, because the latter does not affect renal resistances [33]. Unfortunately, sensitivity and specificity of RI varies in cases of partial obstruction and decreases substantially 48 h after obstruction onset [20].

Normally, the contraction of ureters causes a urinary jet into the bladder clearly visible on color Doppler imaging, but in case of obstruction, it will be absent or diminished compared to the not affected side (Fig. 15.5). Nevertheless, the presence of the ureteral jet does not rule out partial obstruction to the urinary flow [17].

US examination has to be focused also on the evaluation of stone complications to guarantee a prompt treatment. The presence of echoic material inside an obstructed and dilated renal pelvis is indicative of pyonephrosis (Fig. 15.6), especially in the presence of hypervascularization of nearby structures on color Doppler imaging. The presence of total or partial renal enlargement, with inhomogeneous parenchyma and blurring of the cortical sinus, is suspicious for pyelonephritis.

Reporting has to indicate the presence, site, and size of stones, if directly visualized, or the presence and the conspicuity of secondary signs.

15.2.2.3 Computed Tomography

Computed tomography generally visualizes urinary calculi, even <3 mm, as high attenuating formations inside urinary tract (Figs. 15.1, 15.4, and 15.7) [36]. The use of an abdominal window-level setting allows recognition of stones independently to their composition, since their density is >200 HU, and just medication-induced calculi are radiolucent on CT because of their soft tissue attenuation (15–30 HU). Some stones present low attenuating foci inside, and this could predict the susceptibility to fragmentation, so it is a data to add to the report [37, 38].

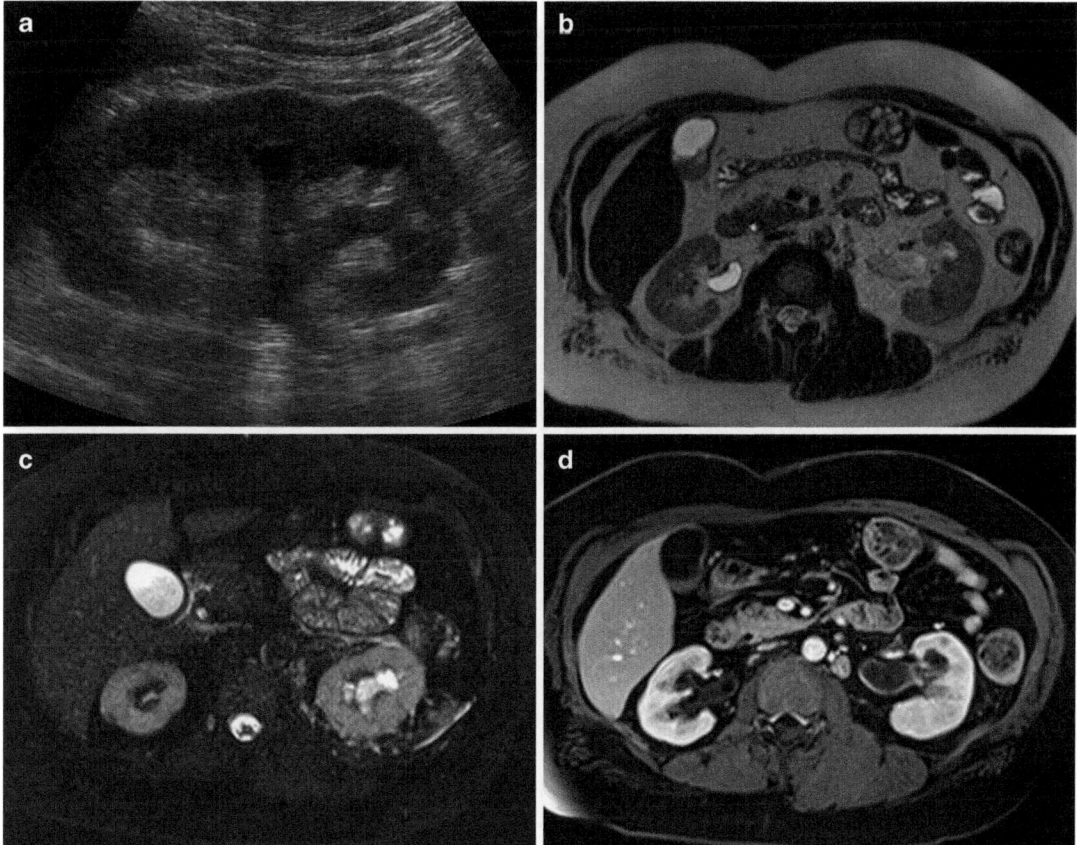

Fig. 15.6 Ureteral obstruction complicated by pyonephrosis. US (**a**) shows echoic material inside the dilated renal pelvis. MR, T2-weighted axial image (**b**), shows not homogeneously high signal inside left renal pelvis; T2-weighted image with fat suppression (**c**) recognizes perinephric fluid and edema; T1-weighted image after contrast medium administration (**d**) depicts the thickened urothelial wall; DWI (**e**) demonstrates pyonephrosis by its high signal inside renal pelvis

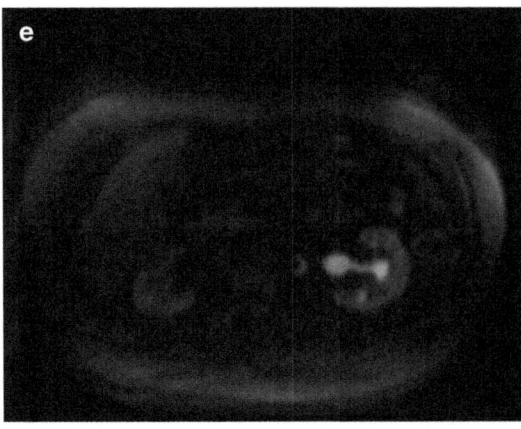

Images should be visualized both on axial and coronal/sagittal reconstructions to perform the best possible measurement of the stone dimension, an important information to select therapeutic strategy, since the transverse diameter alone often underestimates calculus size (Fig. 15.7 and Videos 15.2 and 15.3) [1, 24, 39]. Furthermore, it has been proven that a bone window setting is more accurate than the soft tissue one to measure stones (Fig. 15.7) [40].

In case of renal calculi, CT allows to recognize anomalous anatomy (Fig. 15.8), which can change therapeutic approach [2], and the precise stone location, since calculi located in

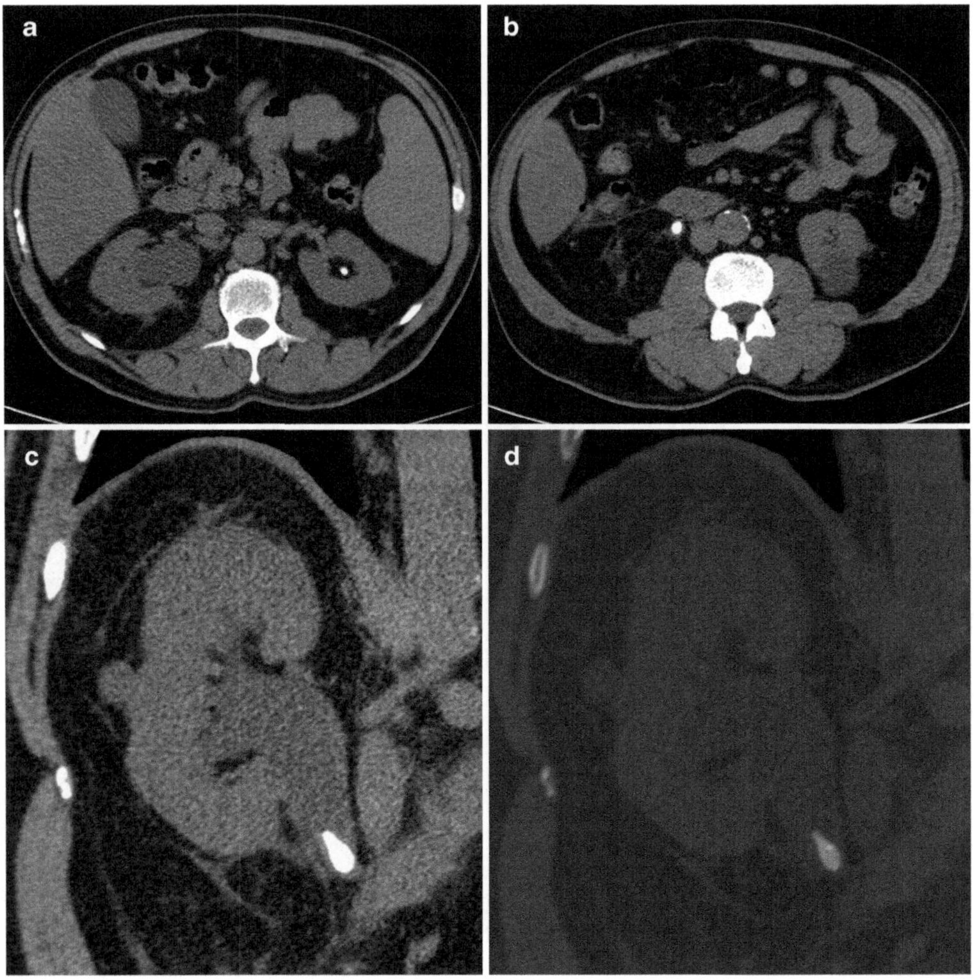

Fig.15.6 (continued)

Fig. 15.7 Stone size evaluation. Unenhanced CT, axial image (**a**), shows moderate right hydronephrosis with fat stranding and perinephric edema; note a nonobstructing stone in the left kidney. Axial image, at lower level (**b**), identifies a right obstructing stone. Coronal reconstruction (**c**) clearly demonstrates a larger stone diameter in the longitudinal axis, and the same reconstruction visualized with a bone window setting (**d**) depicts more precisely stone shape and structure

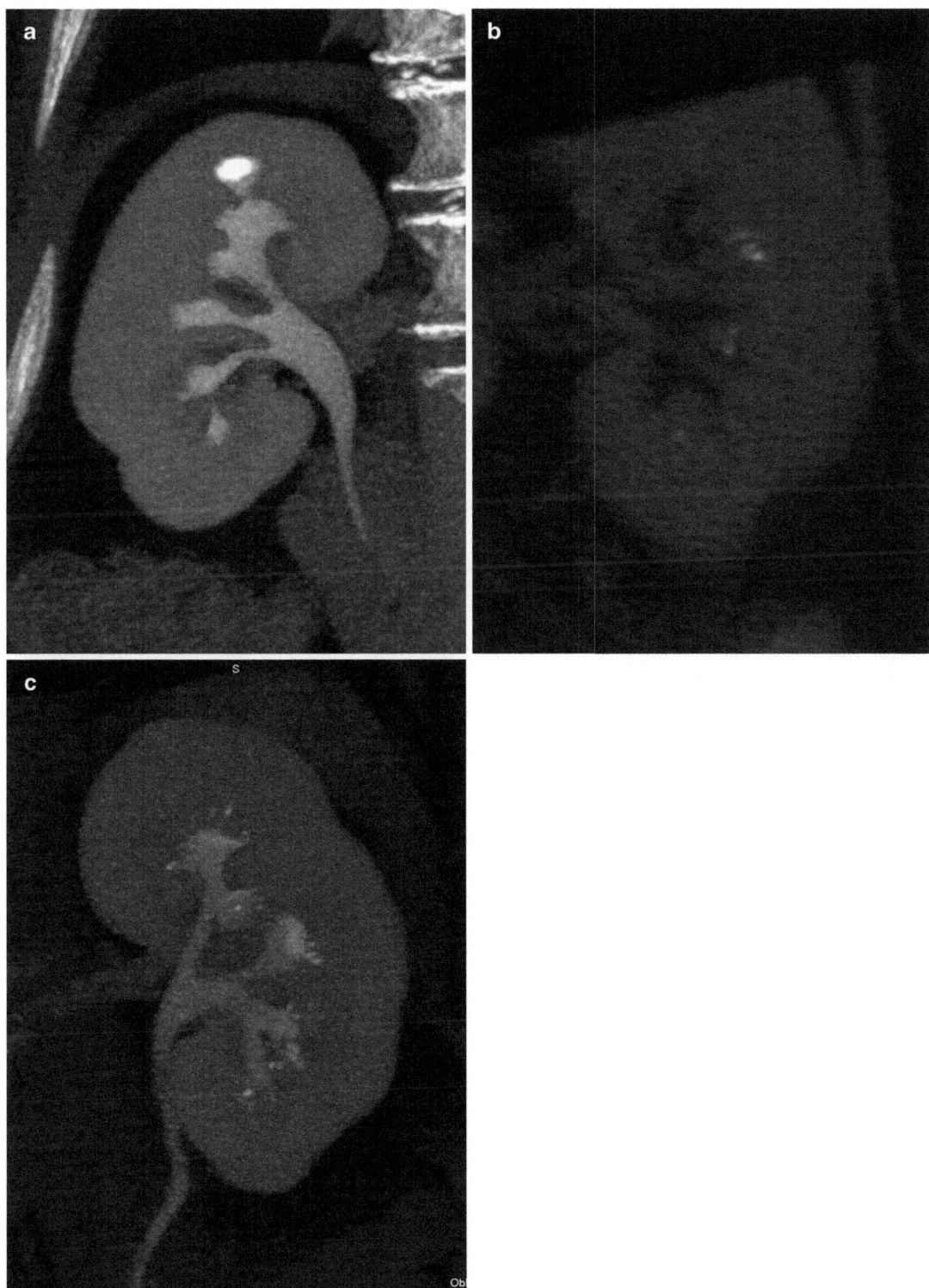

Fig. 15.8 Abnormal location of renal stones. CT urography, coronal reconstruction (**a**), depicts a stone inside a caliceal diverticulum. In a different patient unenhanced CT, coronal reconstruction (**b**), shows tiny stones located in pyramids, indicative for a medullary sponge kidney. CT urography, coronal reconstruction (**c**), demonstrates the presence of dilation of distal tubules confirming medullary sponge kidney diagnosis

the pyramids are indicative of medullary sponge kidney (Fig 15.8), a disease associated with an increased incidence of nephrolithiasis [24]. CT easily recognizes not only obstructing stones but also nonobstructing ones, which could be in some cases responsible of a renal colic pain [24].

In case of ureteral calculi, the best diagnostic clue on CT is the demonstration of a stone within the ureteral lumen, associated to dilation of the urinary tract proximal to the stone and normal caliber below [1, 41]. Unfortunately, dilation is not always present, and so ureteral calculi have to be distinguished from other calcifications, most commonly vascular calcifications and phleboliths. In these cases, the use of coronal images usually helps tracking the ureteral course, confirming intraureteral location [36]. In particularly difficult cases, like patients with small amount of intra-abdominal fat, contrast medium administration with imaging in the excretory phase allows the recognition of the entire ureter, but usually it is not necessary, since some secondary signs could help diagnosis [1, 24].

The presence of the "soft tissue rim sign" confirms the stone nature of the calcification. It is a rim of soft tissue density of 1–2 mm surrounding the high attenuation structure, representing the edema of the ureteric wall at the level of the impacted stone (Fig. 15.1). The rim sign is quite specific, but unfortunately not always present, in particular in case of larger calculi which stretch the ureteral wall. Phleboliths represent the most common calcifications in the pelvis [1, 24, 42]. On CT imaging, the radiolucent center described on plain radiography is usually nondistinguishable [43], but it is possible to recognize a tail of eccentric tapering soft tissue, known as "comet tail sign", representing the noncalcified portion of the vein (Fig. 15.1). Again this sign has a high positive predictive value in differentiating phleboliths from stones but has a very low sensitivity [1, 24, 44].

CT is very sensitive in recognizing even mild hydronephrosis and hydroureter, signs which have high positive and negative predictive values [36]. If hydronephrosis and/or hydroureter are present but no calcification is visible, the recent passage of a stone has to be considered [36]. The presence of the renal pelvic wall thickening in an obstructed kidney is suspicious for pyonephrosis, but it is generally not possible to distinguish it from simple hydronephrosis on the basis of the fluid attenuation.

Hydronephrosis has to be distinguished from extrarenal pelvis, an anatomical variant with normal caliceal morphology (Fig. 15.9), and from parapelvic cysts, which are not in continuity with the caliceal structures (Fig. 15.9).

Perinephric edema in a renal colic setting is a sign of increased lymphatic flow and reabsorbed urine due to obstruction, and it can be easily demonstrated on CT by the presence of fat stranding (Fig. 15.7 and Video 15.2 and 15.3) [36]. Furthermore, a certain degree of periureteral edema could be present at the level of the impacted stone. The degree of fat stranding is related to the severity of obstruction and the time passed from obstruction onset, with a peak after 8 h from symptoms appearance. However it is not a specific sign, since a perinephric edema is often present bilaterally in older patients or in case of impaired renal function, while unilateral edema can be recognized also in case of inflammation and malignancy. So if a stone is not visible, but there is mild hydronephrosis associated with fat stranding, differential diagnosis must include the recent passage of a stone, but also pyelonephritis and tumors [4, 36].

An impacted stone may determinate a high pressure obstruction with consequent forniceal rupture and urine leakage in the perinephric space. This complication can be suspected on the bases of fluid amount, with relatively low grade of urinary tract dilation, and confirmed in the excretory phase after contrast medium administration (Fig. 15.4) [36].

CT is also a useful imaging modality to evaluate active treatment complications, like hemorrhages, infections, and ureteral injuries. Depending on the kind of suspected lesion, CT scans have to be performed in different phases: an arterial phase is indicated to identify active bleeding in case of hemorrhage, a nephrographic

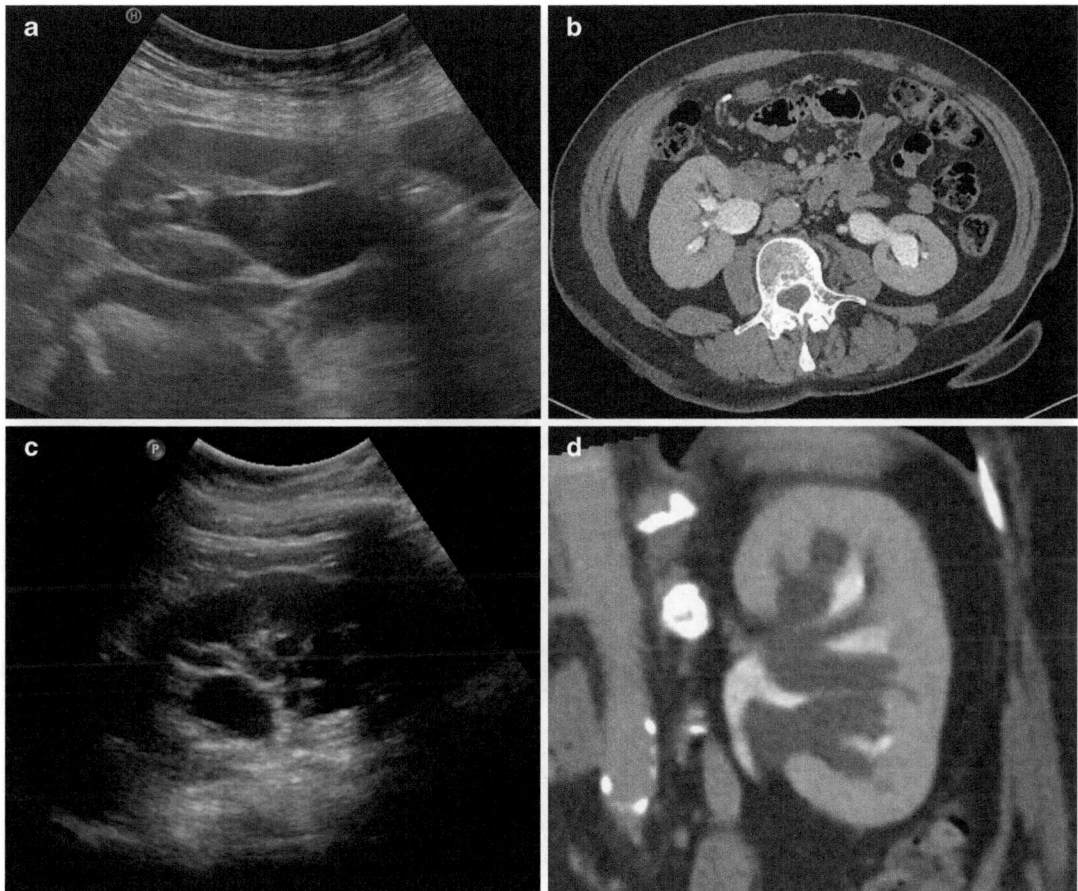

Fig. 15.9 Mimics of hydronephrosis. US (**a**) and CT urography (**b**) show a large right renal pelvis located in the extrarenal space, with no dilation of the caliceal structures. In a different patient US (**c**) depicts fluid cysts in the renal pelvis, with no dilation of the excretory system; CT Urography, coronal reconstruction (**d**), confirms diagnosis depicting multiple parapelvic cysts, not in continuity with opacified caliceal structures

phase for infection recognition, or an excretory phase to prove urinary tract damage (Fig. 15.10).

Reporting has to indicate the number and precise size of obstructing and nonobstructing stones, signs of obstruction or infection since they change need and time of active treatment, and the presence of any abnormal urinary or extra-urinary anatomy (Figs. 15.1 and 15.8).

15.2.2.4 Magnetic Resonance

Stones are not directly visualized on magnetic resonance, since protons are relatively absent in urinary calculi, and they become recognizable only as a signal void inside the urinary tract. The T2-weighted sequences are the best ones to highlight this signal void because the high signal intensity of urine delineates stones, but the lack of direct visualization results in a low sensitivity in detecting little renal calculi (<10 mm) and in a poor accuracy in stone measurement. Furthermore, a signal void artifact may be seen in urine within a dilated collecting system, with possible misdiagnosis, but while this artifact is centrally located, the stone typically lays dependently (Fig. 15.11) or is impacted in a ureteral stricture [30].

Although there is a not optimal visualization of calculi, MR clearly depicts the secondary signs of an obstructing stone, even a partially obstructing one. T2-weighted images show urinary tract

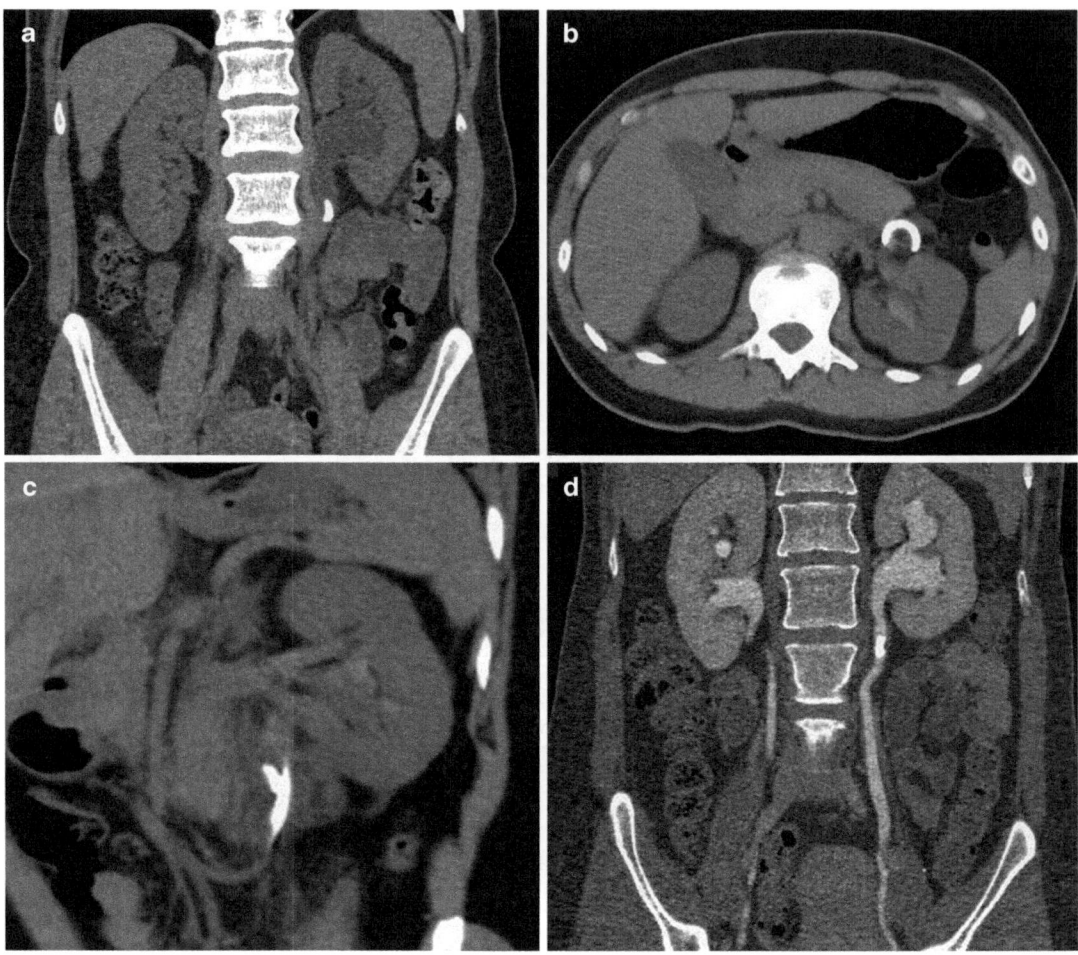

Fig. 15.10 Active treatment complication. Unenhanced CT, coronal image (**a**), shows a lumbar obstructing stone. After positioning of a ureteral double J stent repeated CT depicts the proximal stent end located outside the urinary tract, axial image (**b**), and the ureteral injury at the stone level, coronal image (**c**). CT urography performed after stent removal, MPR reconstruction (**d**), demonstrates complete healing of the ureteral wall, with no leakage of contrast medium, and the stone persistence

dilation and allow accurate grading of hydrone-phrosis. The recognition of a signal void at the level of obstruction confirms urolithiasis, while the presence of soft tissue signal is suspicious for a tumor or a clot and requires further evaluation [31, 33, 34]. Analogously to CT imaging, T2-weighted sequences allow the recognition of ureteral wall thickening around the stone.

The presence of debris or a not homogeneously high signal inside the dilated renal pelvis, especially if associated to a thickened urothelial wall, is suspicious for pyonephrosis (Fig. 15.6).

T2-weighted images with fat suppression are really sensitive for perinephric fluid and edema identification, even of low grade and in patients with small amount of intra-abdominal fat (Fig. 15.6). These sequences allow recognition of edema not only in the retroperitoneal fat but also inflammatory changes into kidney and other organs, helping differential diagnosis.

In case an infection is suspected, DWI has a high sensitivity in recognizing pyelonephritis and pyonephrosis, by the meaning of restricted proton diffusion and consequent hyperintense signal on high b-value (Fig. 15.6) [33].

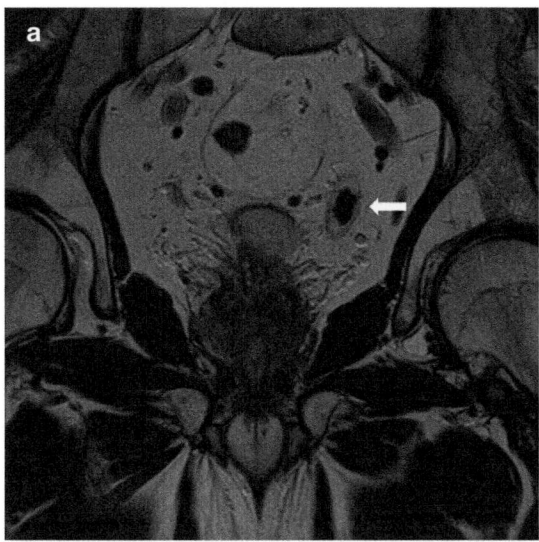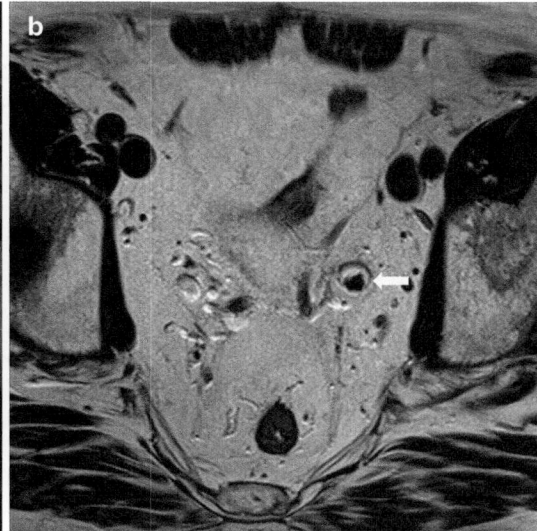

Fig. 15.11 Stone features on MR imaging. Coronal T2-weighted image (**a**) shows the flow void signal circumscribed by fluid of a nonobstructing stone inside the distal left ureter (arrow). On the axial image (**b**) the stone lays dependently in the ureteral lumen (arrow)

Stone disease reporting has to indicate the number, average size, and location of recognizable calculi. The severity of obstruction has to be underlined, on the basis of dilation and edema recognizable, and it is important to point out any sign of secondary infection.

15.3   Differential Diagnosis

On the basis of clinical evaluation, up to 29% of the patients presenting with renal colic may not have urolithiasis. Alternative diseases could affect the kidney, but also other organs [10].

15.3.1 Renal Diseases

Inflammatory Conditions Urinary tract infections are quite common, representing the second urologic disease in emergency department. Infection may involve the kidney or urinary tract, the latter generally complicating a urinary obstruction.

Pyonephrosis could be recognized on US by the presence of echoic material inside an obstructed and dilated renal pelvis, especially if hypervascularization of nearby structures is present on color Doppler imaging [22, 45]. MR shows debris or a not homogeneously high signal inside the dilated renal pelvis, with thickened urothelial wall, and restricted proton diffusion, together with perirenal edema (Fig. 15.6). CT evaluation is not diagnostic for pyonephrosis, but it has to be suspected by the presence of thickening of renal pelvic wall and perirenal edema [4, 46].

Pyelonephritis could be suspected on US examination when a total or partial renal enlargement is recognized, with inhomogeneous parenchyma and blurring of the cortical sinus. Vascular representation on power Doppler could be heterogeneous, and imaging after contrast medium administration reveals hypovascular areas [22, 45]. On unenhanced CT, unilateral renal enlargement with perinephric stranding, without sign of obstruction or stones, is suspicious for pyelonephritis, but mild disease could have no findings at all; contrast medium administration confirms diagnosis demonstrating wedge-shaped hypodense areas on nephrographic phase, or typical striated nephrogram on delayed phase [4, 46]. MR imaging is very sensitive due to its high contrast resolution. The T2-weighted sequences with fat suppression demonstrate even small degree of parenchymal edema, and diffusion imaging confirms diagnosis. The presence of a fluid collection inside the affected kidney, easily recognizable with all techniques, is indicative of an abscess formation [47].

Vascular Conditions Many vascular diseases could affect the kidney mimicking a renal colic [4].

An acute renal infarction occurs in case of aortic dissection or isolated renal artery dissection but most commonly is due to renal embolism. It could be initially misdiagnosed because

US, generally performed as the first imaging modality, is not sensitive since some vascular structures could be recognized on color Doppler even in the affected kidney. Contrast-enhanced ultrasound improves diagnostic performance showing areas of absent vascularization in renal parenchyma. Unenhanced CT may show just unilateral renal enlargement without signs of obstruction, and contrast medium administration is necessary to confirm diagnosis demonstrating the absence of enhancement of the entire kidney or parts of it (Fig. 15.12). In these cases, angiographic scan is needed to search for artery dissection [10, 48].

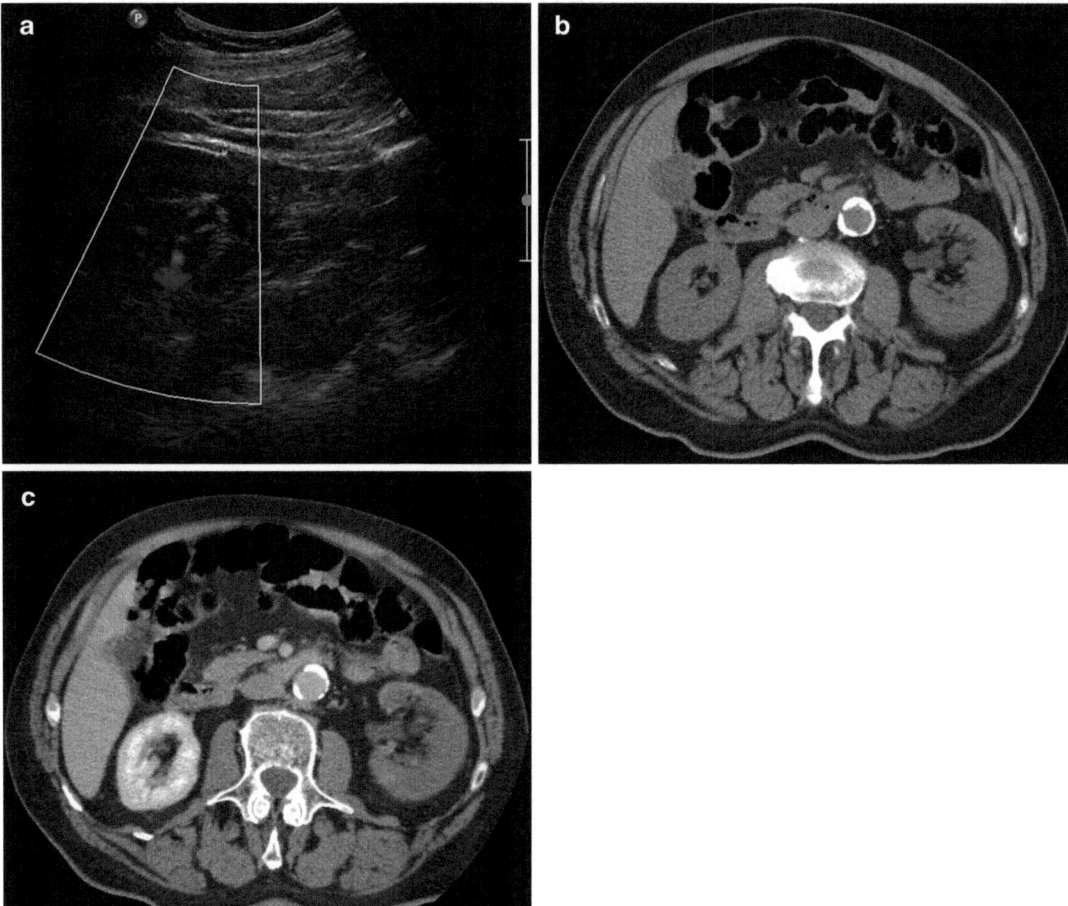

Fig. 15.12 Renal infarct in a patient with atrial fibrillation and acute left flank pain. Color Doppler US shows an apparent normal left kidney with some vascular structures at the hilum (**a**). Unenhanced CT, axial image (**b**), shows just a mild enlargement and blurring of renal margins; CT scan after contrast medium administration (**c**) demonstrates an almost complete absence of enhancement indicative of renal infarct

In renal vein thrombosis, symptoms depend on the speed with which it occurs: usually neoplastic thrombosis is silent, while acute thrombosis, most commonly in case of membranous glomerulonephritis, causes flank pain and hematuria. US and unenhanced CT show renal enlargement and perinephric fluid, while contrast-enhanced CT demonstrates diminished nephrogram and filling defect in the renal vein [4, 46].

Hemorrhagic Conditions Nontraumatic bleeding may involve perinephric or subcapsular space, renal parenchyma (most commonly into renal cysts or tumors), or collecting system. Acute pain is usually secondary to renal capsule distention or urinary tract obstruction due to clots.

A subcapsular hematoma appears on US as iso- or hypoechoic material around the kidney, with no vascular sign on color Doppler evaluation. CT demonstrates high attenuation material inside renal capsule, and contrast medium administration permits to recognize the presence of active bleeding or an underlying solid or cystic mass (Figs. 15.13 and 15.14) [4, 10, 46].

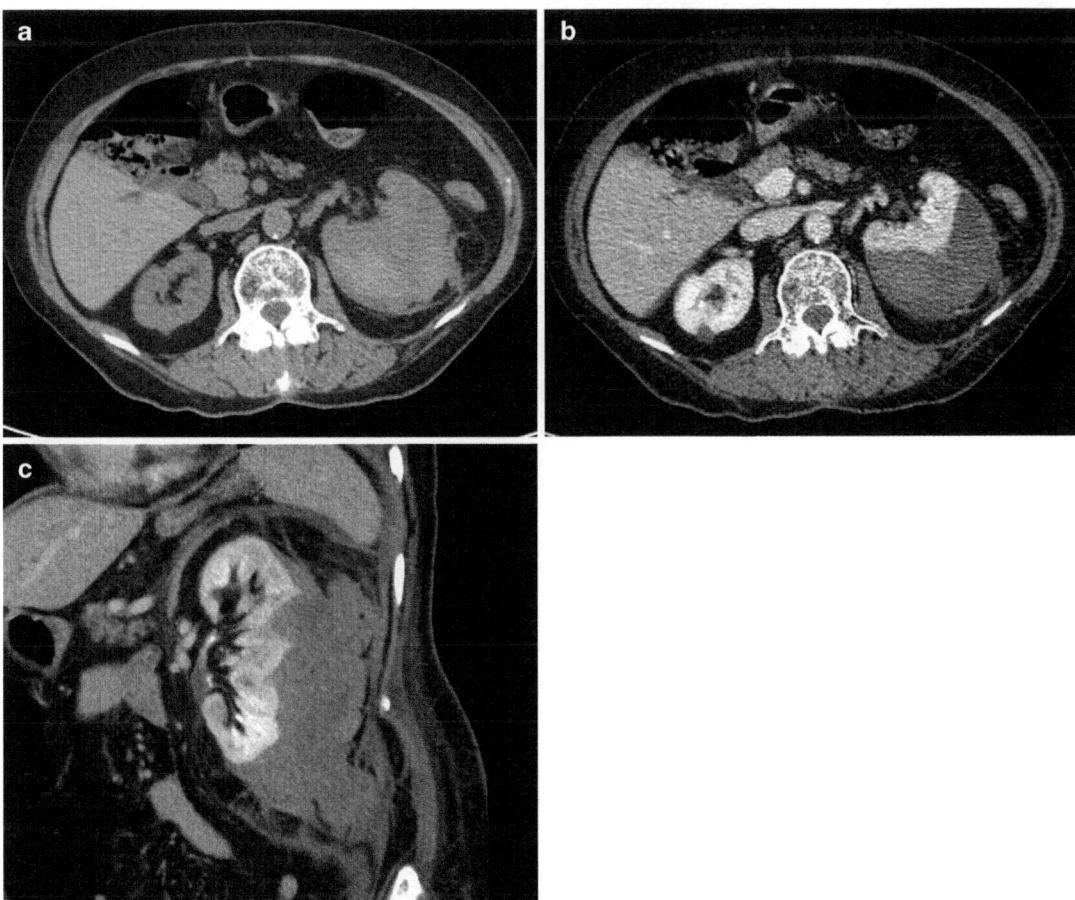

Fig. 15.13 Spontaneous subcapsular hematoma in a patient with right renal colic and in anticoagulants treatment. Unenhanced CT, axial image (**a**), shows renal enlargement with perinephric fat stranding and the presence of a subcapsular collection with high attenuation density. Contrast-enhanced CT, axial image (**b**), shows no enhancement of the lesion and excludes signs of active bleeding; coronal image (**c**) better depicts the extension of the subcapsular hematoma with partial extension to the perinephric space

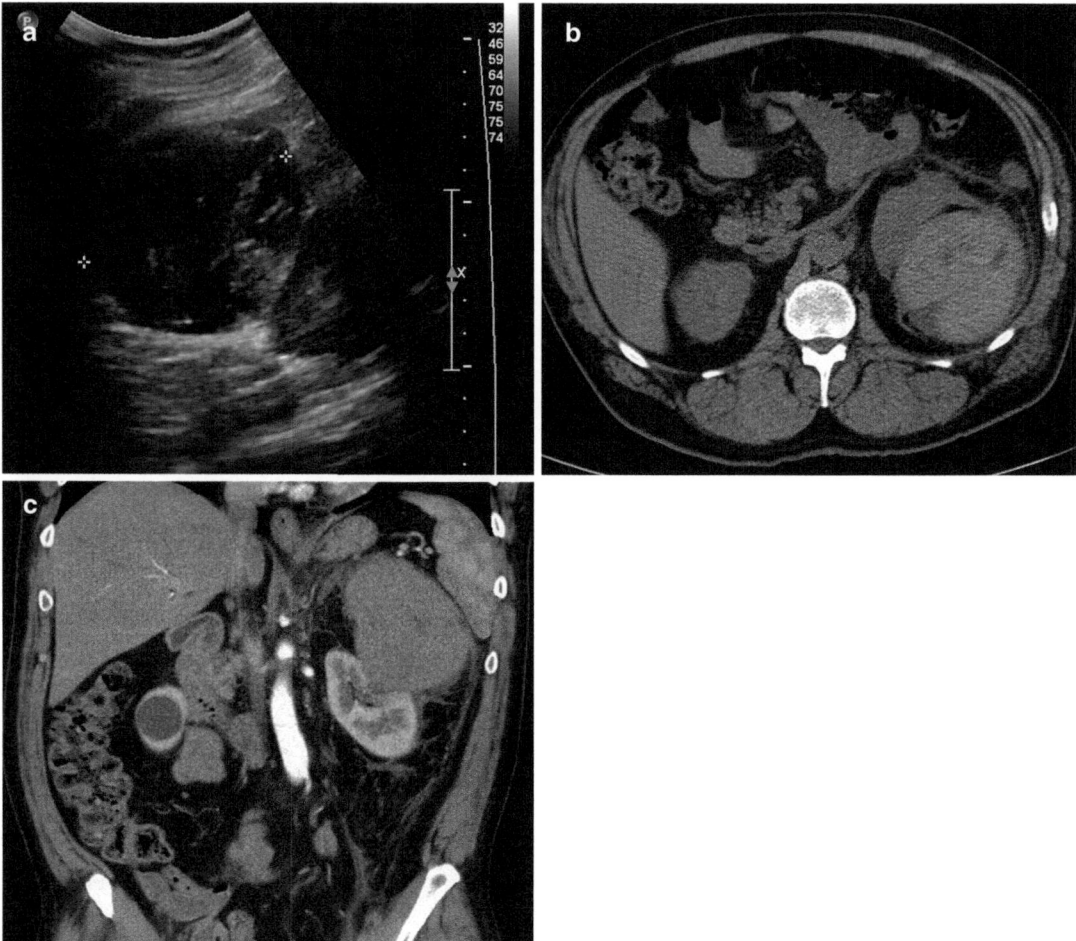

Fig. 15.14 Hemorrhagic cyst in a patient with left renal colic and in anticoagulants treatment. US of the left kidney (**a**) shows large cyst with echoic material at the upper pole, consistent with recent bleeding inside a known cyst. Unenhanced CT, axial image (**b**), depicts a hemorrhagic mass, appearing as a not homogeneous hyperattenuating lesion with perinephric fat stranding; enhanced scan, coronal image (**c**), demonstrates the absence of pathological enhancement and excludes signs of active bleeding

Neoplastic Conditions Transitional cell carcinoma could cause acute flank pain due to hematuria with clots formation and secondary occlusion, while dilation due to the mass itself generally occurs over time and so remains silent. The presence of a soft tissue lesion, with abnormalities of the urinary tract contours both on US and CT, requires further imaging with CT urography (Fig. 15.15). Renal solid or complex cystic neoplasm may cause hemorrhage or hematuria, with consequent renal colic pain. The neoplastic lesion could be recognized both on US and unenhanced CT, but it has to be studied with contrast-enhanced CT or MR for a better characterization [10, 46].

15.3.2 Extrarenal Diseases

15.3.2.1 Gynecologic Conditions

Gynecologic disorders frequently manifest as abdominal and flank pain, and they represent one of the most common alternative diagnoses (about 10%) on unenhanced CT performed for urolithiasis.

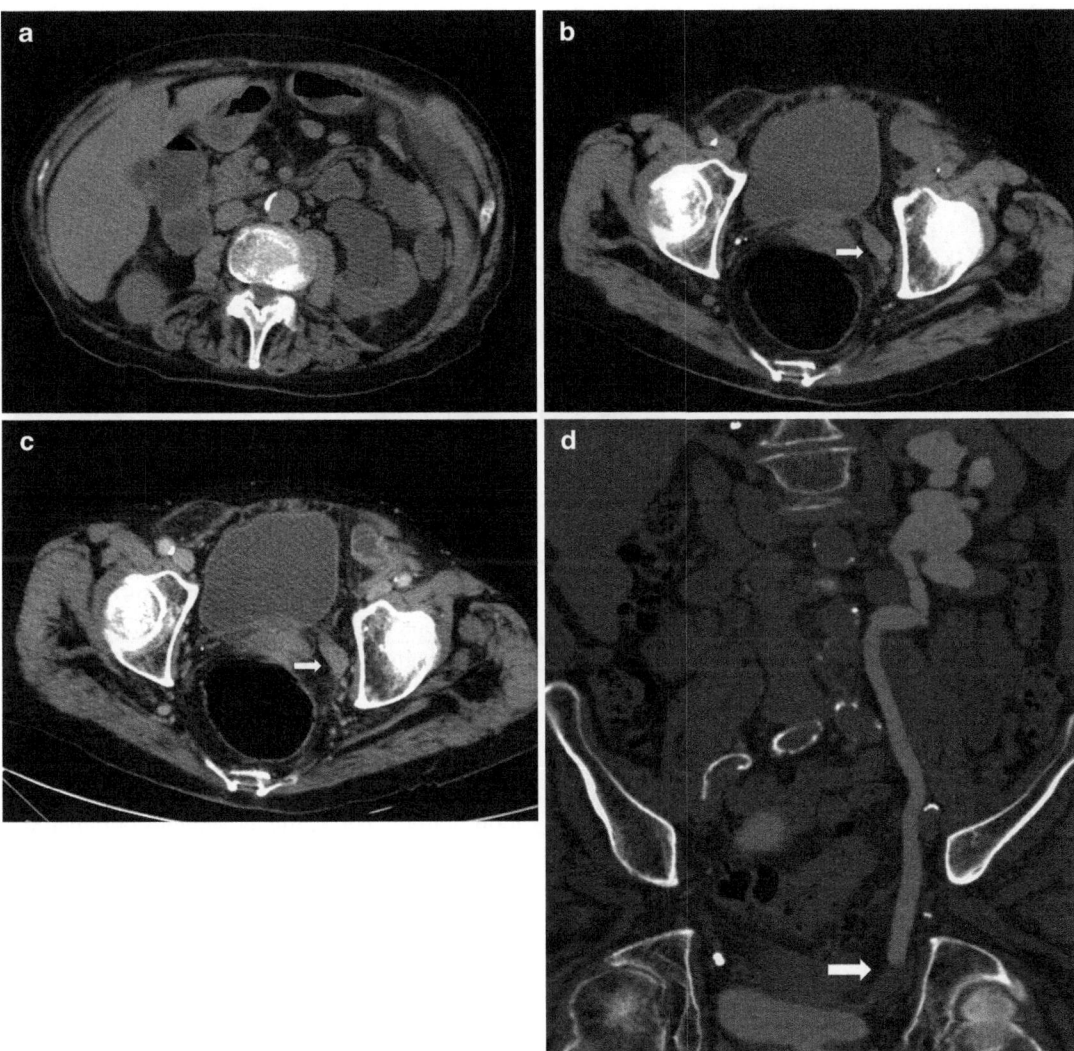

Fig. 15.15 Ureteral obstructing transitional cell carcinoma in a patient with left flank pain. Unenhanced CT, axial image (**a**), depicts hydronephrosis with perinephric fat stranding and, at a lower level (**b**), shows soft tissue in the site of obstruction (arrow). Nephrographic scan, axial image (**c**), demonstrates soft tissue enhancement (arrow), and CT urography, MPR coronal reconstruction (**d**), shows the filling defected (arrow) inside the dilated urinary tract

Ovarian hemorrhagic cyst is frequently encountered, but also tubo-ovarian abscess, hemorrhagic neoplasm, adnexal torsion, and ectopic pregnancy may be found [31]. Proper diagnosis is best made on US studies or MR imaging but could be reached also on CT. On unenhanced CT, the presence of pelvic fat haziness, stranding of pelvic fat, free pelvic fluid, and the evidence of an adnexal mass are indicative of a gynecologic disease [46].

On US the presence of echoic content may indicate a hemorrhagic cyst; hyperemic and dilated tube with or without fluid-debris level indicates hydro- or pyosalpinx; and a complex cyst with solid component and destruction of ovarian structure indicates a tubo-ovarian abscess (Fig. 15.16) but also a neoplastic mass. Ovarian torsion causes a severe pelvic pain, and it appears as an enlarged ovary in an abnormal location, with twisted pedicle; the absence of venous flow

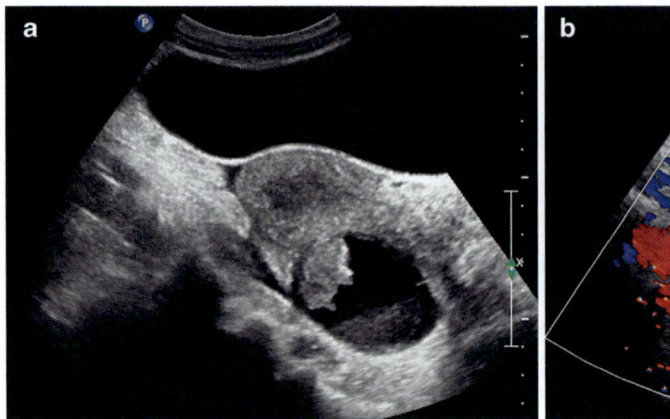

Fig. 15.16 Tubo-ovarian abscess in a patient with low right flank pain and fever. US (**a**) shows a complex cyst with solid component and fluid-fluid level in the right adnexa, and free fluid in cul-de-sac. Color Doppler image (**b**) demonstrates hypervascularization of nearby structures

on color Doppler examination or the absence of enhancement on CT confirms diagnosis. An adnexal hemorrhagic mass associated with hemoperitoneum usually represents a ruptured ectopic pregnancy [22, 45, 49].

15.3.2.2 Gastrointestinal Conditions

Gastrointestinal disorders, especially appendicitis and diverticulitis but even bowel occlusion or perforation, represent the other most common alternative diagnosis (about 10–12%) on unenhanced CT performed for urolithiasis [10].

Appendix has to be looked for in every US or CT examination performed for flank pain but negative for ureteral calculi. Various radiological signs are indicative of appendicitis: a width more than 6 mm, the presence of hyperemic walls or free fluid nearby, and the stranding or haziness of the pericecal fat [22, 46].

An inflammatory bowel disease may be confused for urolithiasis, especially at its first presentation. In these cases, the thickening of the terminal ileum bowel wall, the presence of inflammation of abdominal fat, and the evidence of enlarged lymph nodes have to guide radiological diagnosis [45].

Diverticulitis is more commonly located in left and sigmoid colon but could involve also other portions. Recognizing a diverticulitis on US examination could be more challenging, but the tenderness at probe compression helps to focus on a thickened colonic wall, possibly surrounded by hyperechoic inflammatory fat. Unenhanced CT is easily diagnostic for the presence of diverticula associated with focal wall thickening, haziness, and stranding of perivisceral fat (Fig. 15.17) [46].

Bowel occlusion could be suspected on US imaging when there is a dilation of small bowel loops without peristaltic movements or hyperperistalsis; in these cases, CT confirms diagnosis and reveals degree, site, and cause of occlusion. Perforation is not commonly recognizable on US examination, but free peritoneal air is clearly depicted on CT images [45, 46].

15.3.2.3 Pancreatic and Hepatobiliary Conditions

The most common hepatobiliary conditions responsible for acute flank pain are cholecystitis and choledocholithiasis. US is the imaging modality of choice for gallstone evaluation and clearly depicts biliary duct dilation and the presence of intraductal stones. It also easily demonstrates signs of cholecystitis such as gallbladder distention with thickened and hyperemic walls and pericholecystic fluid [22, 31, 45]. CT imaging is less sensitive in gallstone recognition, but, even on unenhanced CT, it is possible to demonstrate biliary ductal dilation or gallbladder distension with pericholecystic fat haziness or fluid; in these cases, contrast medium administration or further imaging with US or MR may be warranted (Fig. 15.18).

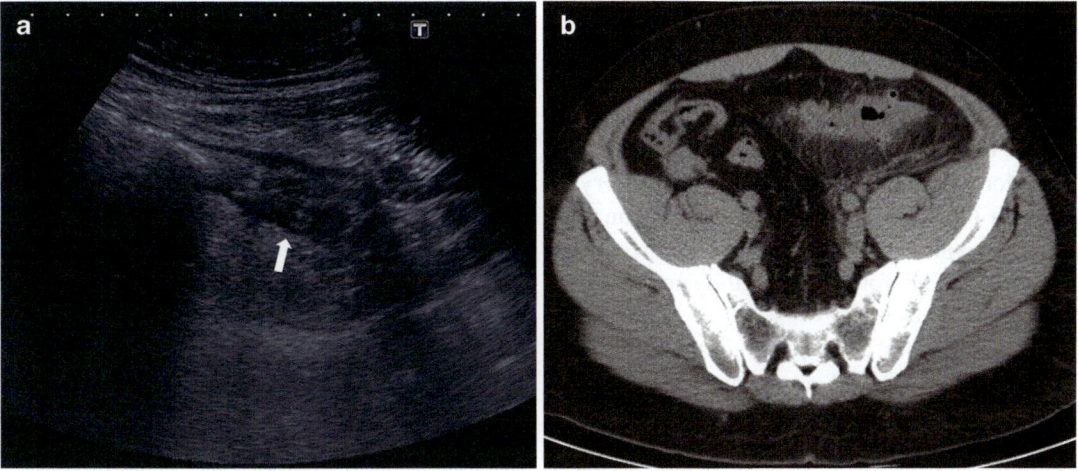

Fig. 15.17 Diverticulitis in a patient with low left flank pain and fever. US (**a**) shows colonic wall thickening (arrow) in the site of probe tenderness. Unenhanced CT, axial image (**b**), depicts diverticula and focal bowel wall thickening, associated to pericolonic fat stranding and thickening of the adjacent fascia

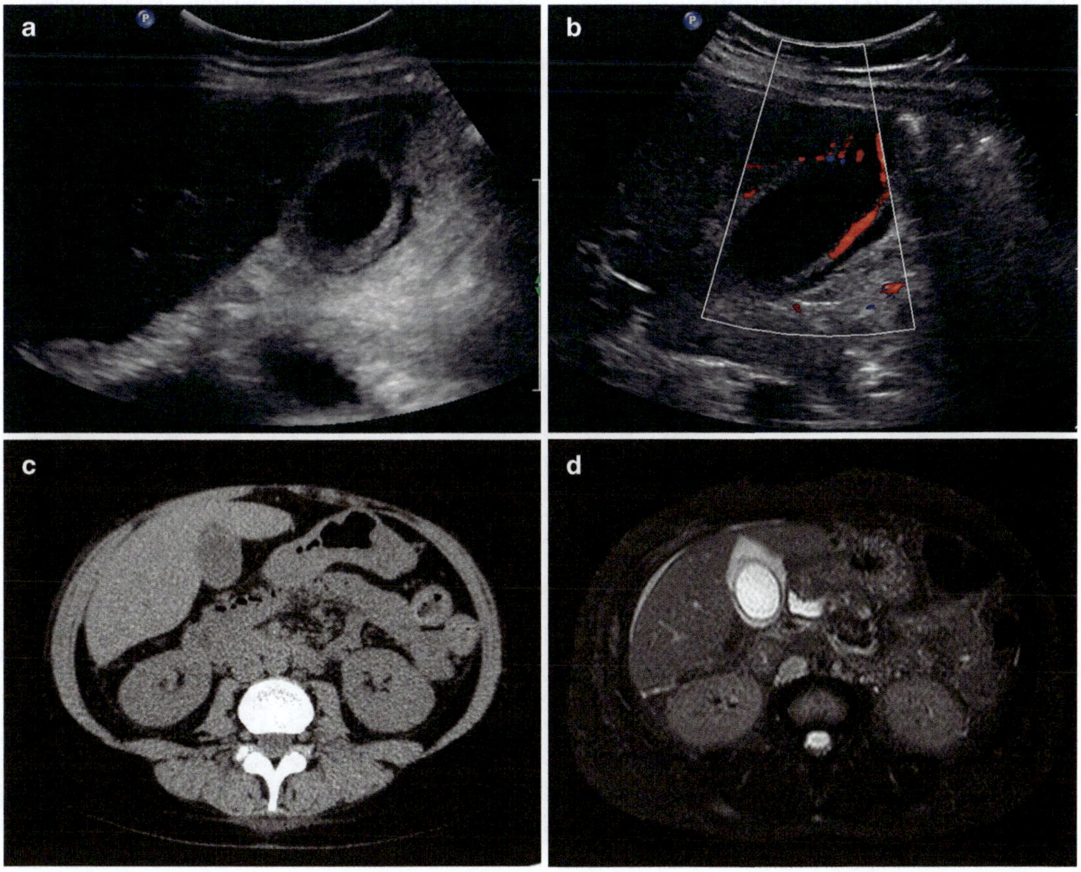

Fig. 15.18 Acute cholecystitis in a patient with right flank pain and nausea. US (**a**) shows important gallbladder wall thickening and pericholecystic fluid. Color Doppler image (**b**) depicts hypervascularization of gallbladder wall and nearby structures. On Unenhanced CT (**c**) pericholecystic fluid is difficult to identify. MR, T2-weighted image with fat suppression (**d**), clearly recognizes pericholecystic fluid and wall edema

Liver subcapsular hematoma causes an acute flank pain secondary to hepatic capsule distention due to bleeding in subcapsular space, even in nontraumatic patients. It appears as echoic material around the liver on US, with no vascular sign on color Doppler evaluation. CT is necessary to confirm diagnosis, recognizing high attenuation material without enhancement under liver capsule, and to look for active bleeding and underlying solid masses [46].

In some cases acute pancreatitis may cause left flank pain. On CT, the pancreas appears to be enlarged, with inhomogeneous parenchyma and blurring of peripancreatic fat or free fluid. CT imaging after contrast medium administration is helpful in recognizing possible complications [46].

15.3.2.4 Vascular Conditions

Acute vascular diseases could be very difficult to recognize on US and unenhanced CT imaging, but they represent the most life-threatening diagnosis.

A ruptured aortic or iliac aneurism presents as an aneurism with inhomogeneous thrombus and perivascular fat stranding or hemorrhage both on US and CT (Fig. 15.19) [45].

Aortic dissection is recognizable for the presence of an intramural hematoma or a displacement of the intimal flap inside the lumen, the latter recognizable on unenhanced CT only in the presence of intimal calcifications.

In both cases, contrast medium administration is mandatory to delineate the severity of disease [46].

15.3.2.5 Musculoskeletal Conditions

Low mechanical back pain is a common complaint in emergency department, and it may be easily confound with renal colic. Nevertheless in some cases more important skeletal conditions could cause flank and back pain, and they are to be ruled out by imaging. So it is important to search all unenhanced CT negative for urolithiasis to recognize spontaneous vertebral fractures in elderly or osteopenic patients and for vertebral metastases. In patients receiving anticoagulant agents, another cause of flank tenderness is spontaneous iliac psoas muscle hematoma; this diagnosis may sometimes be reached by US, but CT and MR provide a better visualization of the iliac psoas compartment, and imaging in the arterial phase is needed to rule out active bleeding (Fig. 15.20) [35, 46, 50].

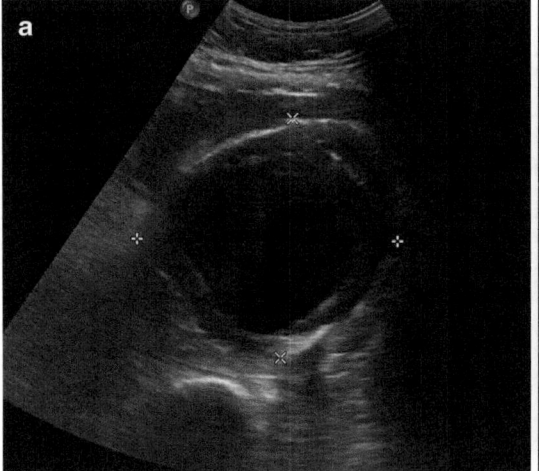
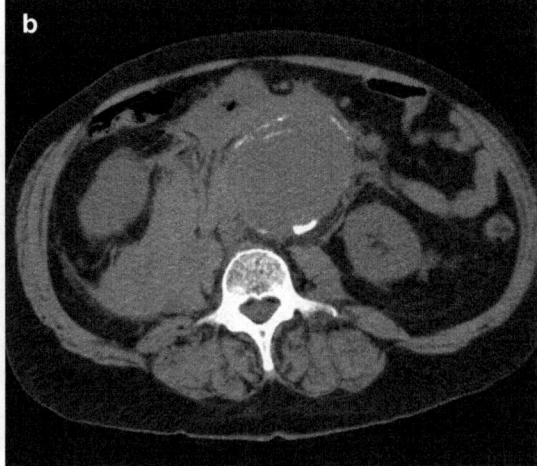
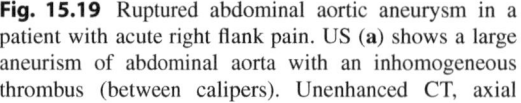

Fig. 15.19 Ruptured abdominal aortic aneurysm in a patient with acute right flank pain. US (**a**) shows a large aneurism of abdominal aorta with an inhomogeneous thrombus (between calipers). Unenhanced CT, axial image (**b**), depicts the ruptured aortic aneurism with a large retroperitoneal hematoma extending in the renal space; enhanced CT, angiographic phase (**c**), shows aneurism features, useful for treatment planning

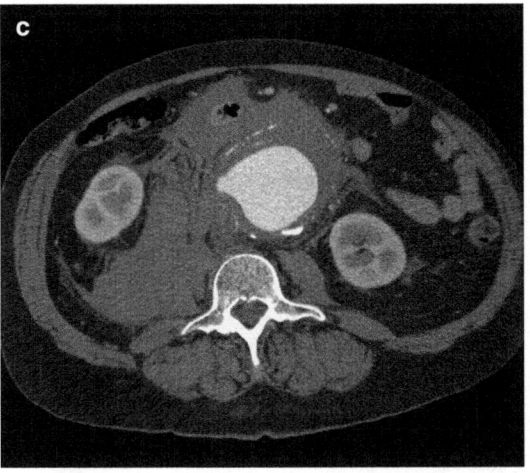

Fig. 15.19   (continued)

15.3.3 Diagnostic Algorithm

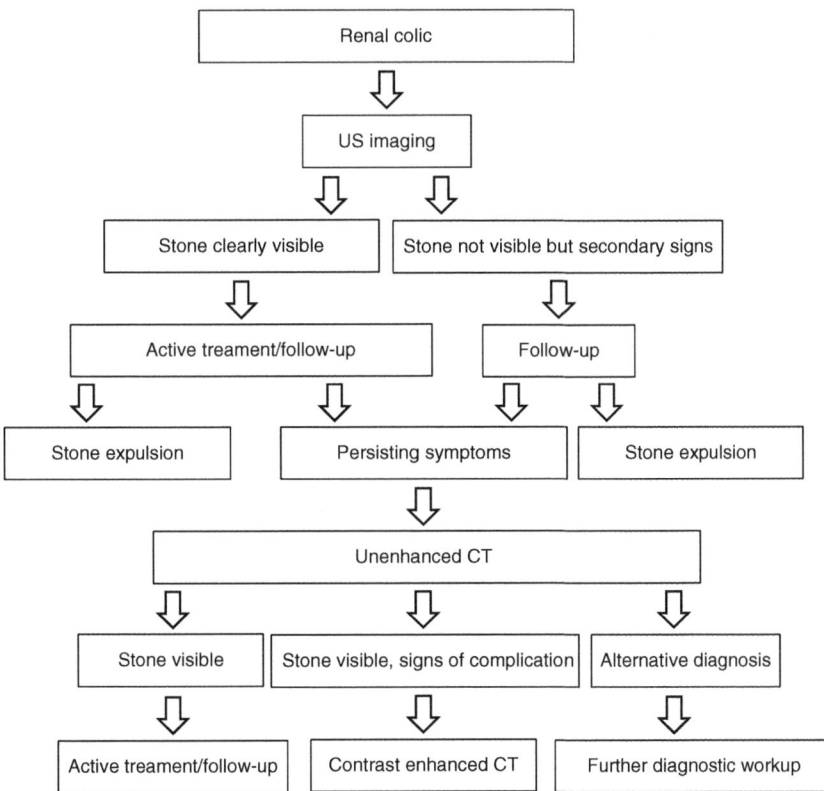

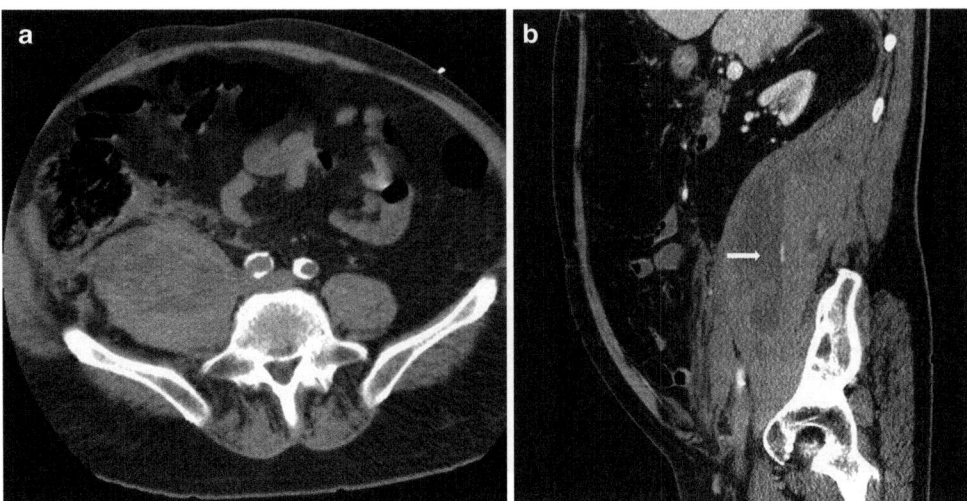

Fig. 15.20 Spontaneous psoas hematoma in a patient with right renal colic and in anticoagulants treatment. Unenhanced CT, axial image (**a**), shows an enlarged and hyperattenuating psoas muscle with stranding of retroperitoneal fat. Enhanced CT, sagittal image (**b**), depicts the extension of the spontaneous hematoma in the psoas compartment with fluid-fluid level and signs of active bleeding (arrow)

Imaging is an essential component in the evaluation of patients presenting with renal colic, both to confirm diagnosis and to decide patient management.

Although unenhanced CT provides highest sensitivity and specificity both for urolithiasis and for alternative diagnosis, the ALARA (as low as reasonably achievable) principles compel to keep radiation exposure as low as possible, preferring an alternative imaging modality. In this perspective, US certainly represents the imaging modality of choice as first step in renal colic evaluation. US is quite sensitive and specific in recognizing urinary stones or secondary signs of obstruction. In case of visible stone, it is possible to know the likelihood of spontaneous passage and consequently the necessity of an active treatment. Evaluation could be completed with CT for treatment planning, if required by the urologist. If the stone is not visible but there are secondary signs of obstruction, it is possible to decide for follow-up, awaiting for spontaneous passage. In case of symptoms persistence, important hydronephrosis, or signs of complications imaging will be completed with unenhanced CT to better decide patient management. If signs of complications of other diseases are recognized, it is recommended to complete evaluation with contrast-enhanced scans or further appropriate diagnostic workup.

The low availability of MR in emergency setting does not allow its routine use in renal colic workup, but evaluation of pregnant and pediatric patients after not conclusive US imaging has to be completed with MR, whenever it is possible.

References

1. Kambadakone AR, et al. New and evolving concepts in the imaging and management of urolithiasis: urologists' perspective. Radiographics. 2010;30(3):603–23.
2. Cheng PM, et al. What the radiologist needs to know about urolithiasis: part 1--pathogenesis, types, assessment, and variant anatomy. AJR Am J Roentgenol. 2012;198(6):W540–7.
3. Heidenreich A, Desgrandschamps F, Terrier F. Modern approach of diagnosis and management of acute flank pain: review of all imaging modalities. Eur Urol. 2002;41(4):351–62.
4. Taourel P, et al. Computed tomography in the nontraumatic renal causes of acute Flank pain. Semin Ultrasound CT MRI. 2008;29(5):341–52.
5. Jha P, et al. Imaging of flank pain: readdressing state-of-the-art. Emerg Radiol. 2017;24(1):81–6.
6. Stamatelou KK, et al. Time trends in reported prevalence of kidney stones in the United States: 1976–1994. Kidney Int. 2003;63(5):1817–23.
7. Samim M, et al. Incidental findings on CT for suspected renal colic in emergency department patients:

prevalence and types in 5,383 consecutive examinations. J Am Coll Radiol. 2015;12(1):63–9.

8. Leveridge M, et al. Renal colic: current protocols for emergency presentations. Eur J Emerg Med. 2016;23(1):2–7.

9. Tirotta D, et al. Abdominal pain: a synthesis of recommendations for its correct management. Ital J Med. 2015;9(2):193–202.

10. Jindal G, Ramchandani P. Acute flank pain secondary to urolithiasis: radiologic evaluation and alternate diagnoses. Radiol Clin North Am. 2007;45(3):395–410. vii.

11. Moore CL, Scoutt L. Sonography first for acute flank pain? J Ultrasound Med. 2012;31(11):1703–11.

12. Wolf JS. Treatment selection and outcomes: Ureteral calculi. Urol Clin North Am. 2007;34(3):421.

13. Preminger GM, et al. 2007 guideline for the management of ureteral calculi. Eur Urol. 2007;52(6):1610–31.

14. Coll DM, Varanelli MJ, Smith RC. Relationship of spontaneous passage of ureteral calculi to stone size and location as revealed by unenhanced helical CT. Am J Roentgenol. 2002;178(1):101–3.

15. Wen CC, Nakada SY. Treatment selection and outcomes: Renal calculi. Urol Clin North Am. 2007;34(3):409.

16. Perks AE, et al. Stone attenuation and skin-to-stone distance on computed tomography predicts for stone fragmentation by shock wave lithotripsy. Urology. 2008;72(4):765–9.

17. Nicolau C, et al. Imaging patients with renal colic-consider ultrasound first. Insights Imaging. 2015;6(4):441–7.

18. Ather MH, et al. Alternate and incidental diagnoses on noncontrast-enhanced spiral computed tomography for acute flank pain. Urol J. 2009;6(1):14–8.

19. Villa L, et al. Imaging for urinary stones: update in 2015. Eur Urol Focus. 2016;2(2):122–9.

20. Piazzese EM, et al. The renal resistive index as a predictor of acute hydronephrosis in patients with renal colic. J Ultrasound. 2012;15(4):239–46.

21. Song Y, et al. Can ureteral stones cause pain without causing hydronephrosis? World J Urol. 2016;34(9):1285–8.

22. Tomizawa M, et al. Abdominal ultrasonography for patients with abdominal pain as a first-line diagnostic imaging modality. Exp Ther Med. 2017;13(5):1932–6.

23. Moore CL, et al. Prevalence and clinical importance of alternative causes of symptoms using a renal colic computed tomography protocol in patients with flank or back pain and absence of pyuria. Acad Emerg Med. 2013;20(5):470–8.

24. Cheng PM, et al. What the radiologist needs to know about urolithiasis: part 2--CT findings, reporting, and treatment. AJR Am J Roentgenol. 2012;198(6):W548–54.

25. Elkoushy MA, Andonian S. Lifetime radiation exposure in patients with recurrent nephrolithiasis. Curr Urol Rep. 2017;18(11):85.

26. Jellison FC, et al. Effect of low dose radiation computerized tomography protocols on distal ureteral calculus detection. J Urol. 2009;182(6):2762–7.

27. Westphalen AC, et al. Radiological imaging of patients with suspected urinary tract stones: national trends, diagnoses, and predictors. Acad Emer Med. 2011;18(7):700–7.

28. Chaytor RJ, et al. Determining the composition of urinary tract calculi using stone-targeted dual-energy CT: evaluation of a low-dose scanning protocol in a clinical environment. Br J Radiol. 2016;89(1067):20160408.

29. Franken A, et al. In Vivo differentiation of uric acid versus non-uric acid urinary calculi with third-generation dual-source dual-energy CT at reduced radiation dose. Am J Roentgenol. 2018;210(2):358–63.

30. Kalb B, et al. Acute abdominal pain: is there a potential role for MRI in the setting of the emergency department in a patient with renal calculi? J Magn Reson Imaging. 2010;32(5):1012–23.

31. Spalluto LB, et al. MR imaging evaluation of abdominal pain during pregnancy: appendicitis and other non-obstetric causes. Radiographics. 2012;32(2):317–34.

32. Masselli G, et al. Stone disease in pregnancy: imaging-guided therapy. Insights Imaging. 2014;5(6):691–6.

33. Masselli G, et al. Imaging of stone disease in pregnancy. Abdom Imaging. 2013;38(6):1409–14.

34. Semins MJ, et al. Evaluation of acute renal colic: a comparison of non-contrast CT versus 3-T non-contrast HASTE MR urography. Urolithiasis. 2013;41(1):43–6.

35. Ripolles T, et al. Sonographic diagnosis of symptomatic ureteral calculi: usefulness of the twinkling artifact. Abdom Imaging. 2013;38(4):863–9.

36. Kennish SJ, Wah TM, Irving HC. Unenhanced CT for the evaluation of acute ureteric colic: the essential pictorial guide. Postgrad Med J. 2010;86(1017):428–36.

37. Zarse CA, et al. CT visible internal stone structure, but not Hounsfield unit value, of calcium oxalate monohydrate (COM) calculi predicts lithotripsy fragility in vitro. Urol Res. 2007;35(4):201–6.

38. Christiansen FE, et al. Internal structure of kidney calculi as a predictor for shockwave lithotripsy success. J Endourol. 2016;30(3):323–6.

39. Hiller N, et al. The relationship between ureteral stone characteristics and secondary signs in renal colic. Clin Imaging. 2012;36(6):768–72.

40. Eisner BH, et al. Computerized tomography magnified bone windows are superior to standard soft tissue windows for accurate measurement of stone size: an in vitro and clinical study. J Urol. 2009;181(4):1710–5.

41. Dalla Palma L, Pozzi-Mucelli R, Stacul F. Present-day imaging of patients with renal colic. Eur Radiol. 2001;11(1):4–17.

42. Heneghan JP, et al. Soft-tissue "rim" sign in the diagnosis of ureteral calculi with use of unenhanced helical CT. Radiology. 1997;202(3):709–11.

43. Traubici J, Neitlich JD, Smith RC. Distinguishing pelvic phleboliths from distal ureteral stones on routine unenhanced helical CT: is there a radiolucent center? Am J Roentgenol. 1999;172(1):13–7.

44. Bell TV, et al. Unenhanced helical CT criteria to differentiate distal ureteral calculi from pelvic phleboliths. Radiology. 1998;207(2):363–7.
45. Kameda T, Taniguchi N. Overview of point-of-care abdominal ultrasound in emergency and critical care. J Intensive Care. 2016;4:53.
46. Rucker CM, Menias CO, Bhalla S. Mimics of renal colic: alternative diagnoses at unenhanced helical CT. Radiographics. 2004;24:S11–28.
47. Stunell H, et al. Imaging of acute pyelonephritis in the adult. Eur Radiol. 2007;17(7):1820–8.
48. Gun C, et al. What do we miss without contrast in patients with flank pain? Am J Emer Med. 2016;34(4):765.e3–5.
49. Revzin MV, et al. Pelvic inflammatory disease: multimodality imaging approach with clinical-pathologic correlation. Radiographics. 2016;36(5): 1579–96.
50. Marquardt G, et al. Spontaneous haematoma of the iliac psoas muscle: a case report and review of the literature. Arch Orthop Trauma Surg. 2002;122(2): 109–11.

Imaging of Pyelonephritis

16

Raymond Oyen

16.1 General

Pyelonephritis encompasses a range of infectious conditions and disease processes that affect the kidney's tubulointerstitial parenchyma and collecting system. It is a frequently encountered condition in daily practice. Its course can be either acute or chronic, and severity can range from mild to life-threatening.

Acute pyelonephritis (APN) is a sudden onset and painful, commonly bacterial, infection ascending from the urethra and bladder (lower urinary tract). Usually it is multifocal, and it may involve the entire kidney or even be bilateral. Typically it occurs in young, otherwise healthy, (nonpregnant) women and responds to treatment within 72 h, in which case the disease is called uncomplicated.

In any other case, the course of APN is considered complicated. Then, further investigation with diagnostic imaging is required, especially in children which are more prone to irreversible renal damage. In addition, imaging is required in the elderly, diabetics, and immunocompromised patients, in particular when symptoms persist under appropriate antibiotic therapy.

16.1.1 Epidemiology

Urinary tract infection (UTI) is a frequent cause of a medical consult in general practices as well as in the emergency department (ED). An estimated 10.5 million office visits in the USA were related to UTI in 2007, or about 0.9% of all ambulatory visits. In addition, 2–3 million visits were made for UTI at the emergency department [1–3]. About 11.5% of people visiting the ED with abdominal pain in 2013 in the USA were diagnosed with UTI [4]. Worldwide an estimated 150 million people are affected each year [5].

Urologic infections are differentiated into lower (bladder, urethra) and upper (kidney, collecting system, ureter) UTIs. Acute uncomplicated pyelonephritis is much less common than cystitis (28 cases of cystitis per case of pyelonephritis), with a peak annual incidence of 25 cases per 10,000 women 15–34 years of age [6].

APN is common among diabetics with an incidence of 51.4 and 147.9/1000 person-years for men and women, respectively [7].

Although the problem of renal abscesses is underestimated in the literature, the frequency is high: in the USA, they are responsible for 1–10/10,000 hospitalizations yearly with a mortality rate of 0.7–1.6% [8].

Electronic Supplementary Material The online version of this chapter (https://doi.org/10.1007/978-3-319-99822-0_16) contains supplementary material, which is available to authorized users.

R. Oyen (✉)
Department of Radiology, Catholic University of Leuven, Leuven, Belgium
e-mail: raymond.oyen@uzleuven.be

16.1.2 Etiology and Pathophysiology

UTIs are caused by both gram-negative and gram-positive bacteria, less frequent by certain fungi. The most common causative agent for both uncomplicated and complicated UTIs is the uropathogenic *Escherichia coli* (in 85–90%) [9, 10].

Various other bacteria are identified that less frequently cause community-acquired UTIs (*Klebsiella*, *Proteus*, *Enterococcus*). Their common characteristic is the ability to propagate from the urethra up to the kidney by use of pili or flagella. These are specifically accommodated to attach to the uroepithelium. Propagation is facilitated further because of the production of bacterial endotoxins, which inhibit ureteric peristalsis. The infection typically starts with periurethral contamination by a uropathogen residing in the gut, followed by colonization of the urethra and subsequent migration of the pathogen to the bladder. This explains why pyelonephritis is frequently associated with symptoms of lower UTI.

About 30% of all nosocomial infections are urinary tract infections. Residing catheters make patients more prone to infection. Most of these hospital-acquired infections are caused by more virulent or multiresistant agents such as *Pseudomonas aeruginosa* [10].

Bacteria like *Staphylococcus aureus* can reach the kidney by hematogenous dissemination. In contrast to the ascending route infections, these septic localizations originate in the renal cortex first and can extent to the medulla, mostly within 24–48 h. The lesions are more peripheral and rounded and may mimic infarction or even a neoplasm (pseudotumor). This can be challenging for diagnosis, in particular when there is no communication with the collecting system and urinalysis is negative [11, 12].

16.2 Renal Pain Pathophysiology

The kidney is a highly innervated organ. The afferent sensory nerve fibers are located primarily in the pelvic walls and renal capsule.

Flank pain from the urogenital tract is usually caused by acute distention of the ureter, renal pelvis, or renal capsule. The magnitude of the pain is linked to the rapidness of disease onset. Acute renal obstruction, as is seen with obstruction due to lithiasis, elicits an excruciating pain (renal colic). Inflammation is mostly slower in onset, because dilatation is caused by endotoxins which inhibit peristaltic function rather than acute obstruction. Therefore pain is perceived less severe. Furthermore, pelvic dilatation or kidney enlargement is mostly less prominent in infection and causes a continuous pain, whereas obstruction causes undulating/colicky pain.

Finally, local inflammatory mediators irritate both slow-type A and fast-type C fibers and create afferent impulses. These travel to the spinal cord at the T11-L1 levels, thus triggering flank pain in infectious and inflammatory disease [13].

Pain originating from the kidney or the renal capsule is perceived in the costovertebral angle lateral to the erector spinae muscle. Kidney pain may be associated with gastrointestinal symptoms due to autonomic reflexes. Furthermore, other abdominal organs may cause pain in the costovertebral angle as may pain originate from the shoulder. This may obscure correct diagnosis, and imaging can be an aid in characterizing the correct cause of pain [14, 15].

16.3 Diagnosis

Uncomplicated UTIs typically affect individuals who are otherwise healthy and have no structural or neurological urinary tract abnormalities, generally premenopausal women. These patients do not require diagnostic imaging and can be diagnosed by typical symptoms and laboratory tests. An exception to this is the pediatric population where it is mandatory for early detection and follow-up. Precaution should be taken as well with diabetic and immunocompromised patients.

16.3.1 Clinical Features

Typical clinical symptoms are an abrupt onset of high-grade fever (>39 °C) and chills and uni-

or bilateral flank pain. In combination with nausea and/or vomiting, these complete the typical clinical triad of symptoms. Clinical signs of associated cystitis include urinary frequency and urgency, dysuria, and suprapubic tenderness [16, 17].

16.3.2 Laboratory Test

Blood samples may show signs of inflammation: elevated C-reactive protein, leukocytosis with a predominance of neutrophils, and elevated erythrocyte sedimentation rate. Blood cultures may occasionally grow the pathogen. Blood cultures are positive in about 20% of cases [18]. In some cases, the renal function is impaired with elevated creatinine levels.

Urinalysis may show typically pyuria, bacteriuria, chains of cocci, and large numbers of leukocyte casts. Samples can be used to perform an antibiogram to tailor the antibiotic therapy in more complicated cases.

Clinical tests alone are not sufficient to detect all cases of APN. In the study of Rollino et al. [19], only 23.5% of patients, with findings on CT/NMR for APN, had positive urine cultures, only 15.3% had positive blood culture, and 7.6% had both (Fig. 16.1). Furthermore, no differences were found between patients with or without abscesses with regard to these parameters and risk factors. Pyuria and bacteriuria may be absent if the infection is not communicating with the urinary tract or if an obstruction is present [20, 21].

16.3.3 Imaging

Imaging is not routinely required in uncomplicated cases of APN. It may be desirable to obtain an US evaluation within 24 h to exclude obstruction [11].

More extensive imaging is needed when appropriate therapy fails, an underlying cause or complication is suspected, and also for evaluating disease extent or differential diagnosis when clinical and laboratory tests are not sufficient. These are refered to as complicated UTIs. The objective is to visualize emergencies or complications that would change treatment management, for example, urinary obstruction which may require direct intervention for drainage or abscess formation which needs a longer antibiotic treatment and follow-up imaging.

CT is the modality of choice in evaluation of acute pyelonephritis, although ultrasound is often the first imaging study performed because of its known practical advantages (Box 16.1).

Box 16.1 Advantages of US

- Readily available
- Quick
- Portable
- Noninvasive
- Low cost
- No radiation
- No iv contrast
- Vascular evaluation with color Doppler
- High spatial resolution

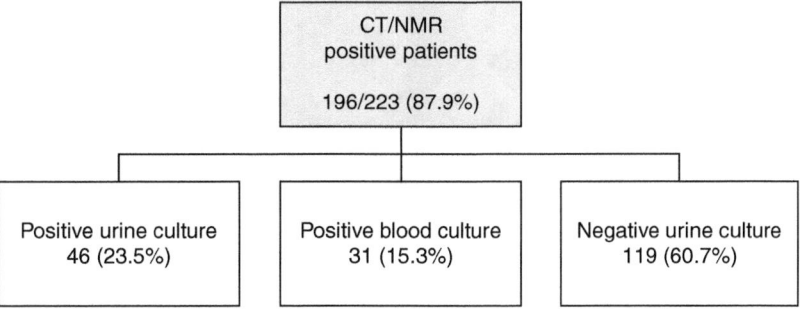

Fig. 16.1 Rate of positive laboratory test in patients with CT/MR positive for APN [19]

16.4 Imaging Modalities

16.4.1 Abdominal Plain Film and IVU

Plain abdominal film is not very useful as an imaging tool for renal infection. For the detection of calculi, a low-dose CT more and more is performed as imaging modality of choice because of its higher sensitivity and specificity as well as higher negative predictive value compared to abdominal plain film combined with an ultrasound examination [22, 23].

Intravenous urography (IVU) is completely replaced by CT urography. It was commonly performed in the past for evaluation of acute pyelonephritis. According to several studies, in up to 75% of the cases of uncomplicated acute pyelonephritis IVU was normal [24–26]. In the remaining, the IVU findings seen in cases of acute renal infections include diffuse renal enlargement (due to edema), delayed nephrogram (occasionally with striated appearance), delayed opacification of the renal collecting system, and dilatation or effacement of the collecting system (Fig. 16.2).

IVU is not sensitive enough to demonstrate parenchymal abnormalities, renal abscesses, and perirenal involvement [26]. For the detection of urinary tract obstruction, alternatives are available. According to recent literature, IVU should be abandoned for the evaluation of acute pyelonephritis.

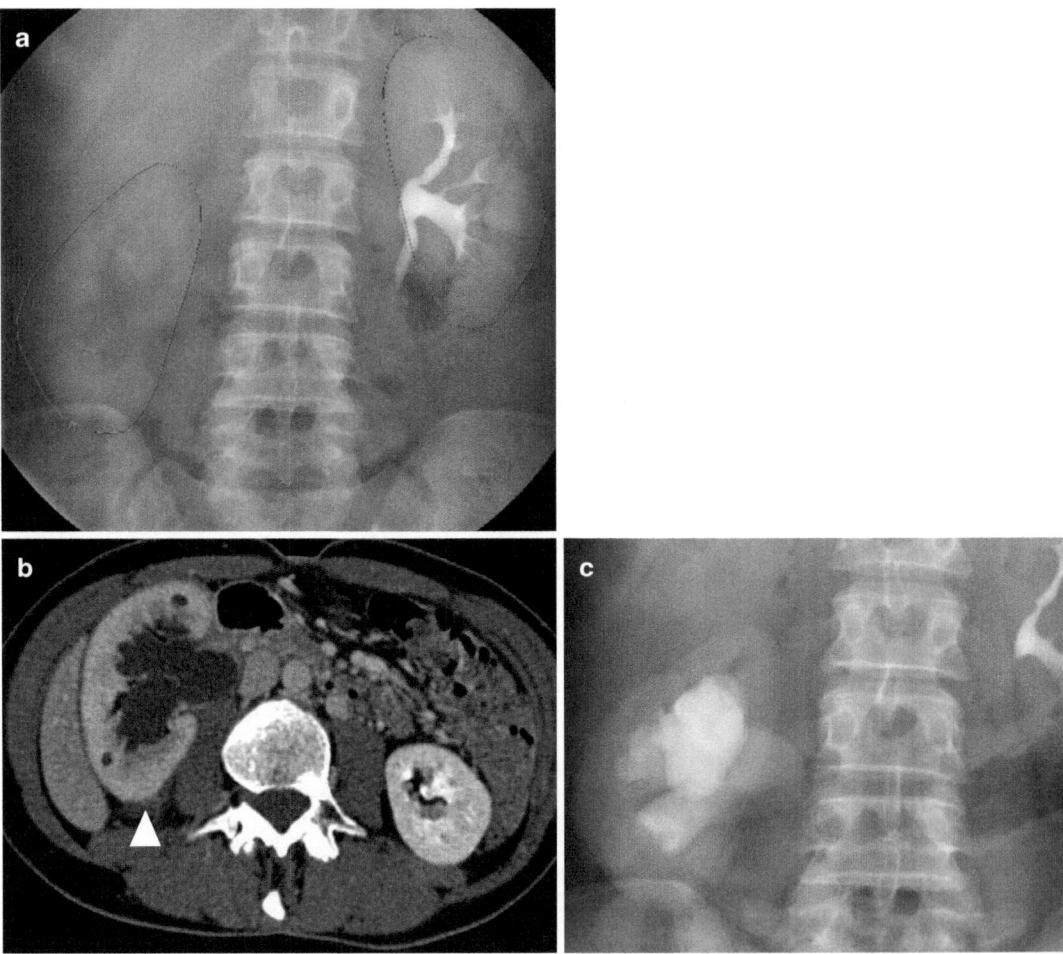

Fig. 16.2 (**a**, **b**, **c**) IVU in APN. (**a**) IVU image in a patient with right-sided diffuse APN. The right kidney has a swollen appearance and delayed opacification of the collecting system. (**b**) Enlarged, hypo-enhancing right kidney. Dilatation of the collecting system and perinephric infiltration can be depicted. (**c**) Dilatation of the collecting system in the right kidney at IVU

16.4.2 Cystography

When vesicoureteral reflux (VUR) is suspected or needs to be excluded, a cystogram is still indicated. Also in patients with signs of chronic pyelonephritis, it is necessary to evaluate the presence of vesicoureteral reflux. In children, contrast-enhanced ultrasound, the bladder filled with ultrasound contrast agent, offers a valid alternative for the exploration of vesicoureteral reflux [27].

Retrograde urethrocystography and micturition urethrography are useful when lower urinary tract obstruction is suspected, e.g., urethral stricture in men.

16.4.3 Ultrasound/Doppler Sonography

The use of ultrasound has been widely debated in the context of clinical suspicion of APN. The sensitivity is largely operator dependent. Low sensitivity has been reported in various studies, ranging as low as 33% [28]. Color Doppler ultrasound finding can increase the sensitivity and obviate the need for further imaging [29]. In addition, when combined with concomitant laboratory findings, sensitivity and specificity can be improved, and results correlate with those of DMSA findings [30]. It has, therefore, taken into account that a "negative" ultrasound study does not rule out the diagnosis of (uncomplicated) APN.

Mitterberger et al. showed that intravenous contrast-enhanced ultrasound (CEUS) may improve the sensitivity to 98% (Fig. 16.3) [31]. CEUS is however not routinely used in clinical practice and in some countries not reimbursed for this indication.

Ultrasound still remains a first-line screening tool in assessing local complications such as hydronephrosis, renal abscess formation, renal infarction, and perinephric collections and thus may guide therapeutic management.

Signs that can be detected with US include generalized renal edema attributed to inflammation and congestion. The renal parenchyma may be hypoechoic or attenuated, and a length of more than 15 cm or at least 1.5 cm longer than the unaffected side is indicative [33]. Farmer et al. [34] suggest that an US appearance of increased

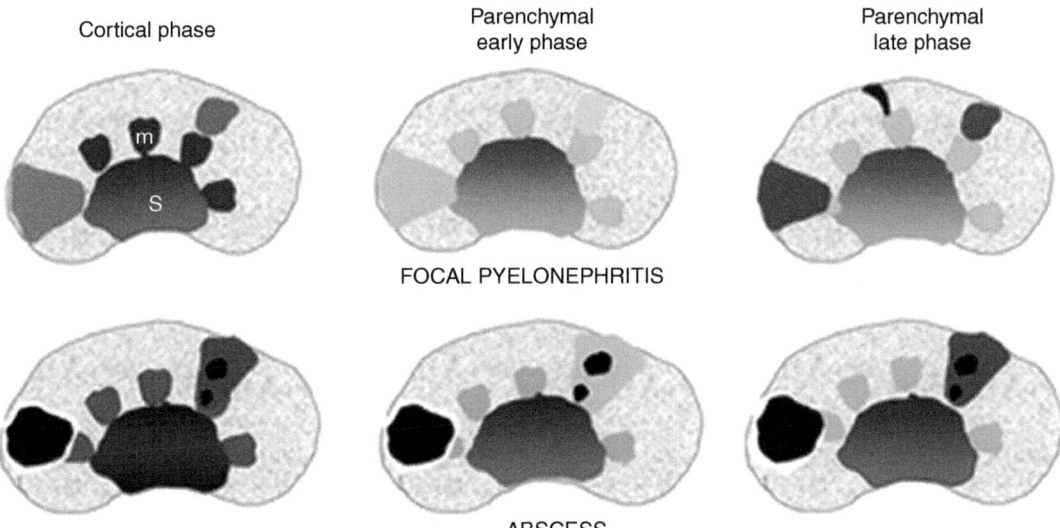

Cortical phase   Parenchymal   Parenchymal
                      early phase   late phase

FOCAL PYELONEPHRITIS

ABSCESS

Fig. 16.3 Contrast-enhanced ultrasound [32]. Focal pyelonephritis and abscess are shown in the different phases of CEUS. m, medullae; s sinus. Pyelonephritis areas are always most conspicuous during the parenchymal late phase, as round- or wedge-shaped cortical or corticomedullar hypoechoic areas (shown in the drawing as *gray areas*). These areas may be seen also during the cortical phase and are less conspicuous during parenchymal early phase. Abscesses are always seen as anechoic areas (shown in the drawing as *black areas*), with or without rim or septal enhancement, alone or within areas of pyelonephritis

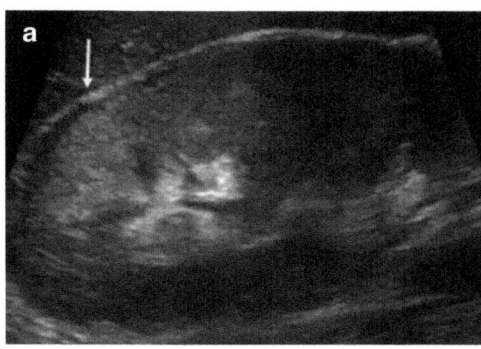
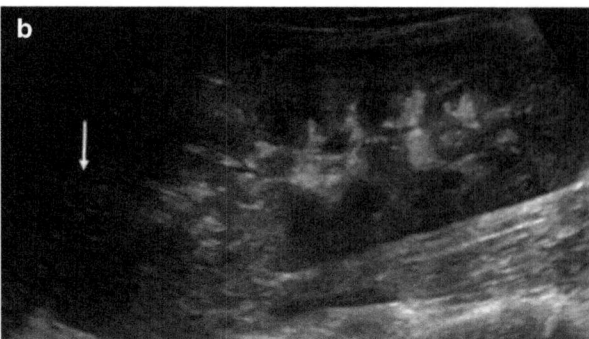

Fig. 16.4 (**a**, **b**) Longitudinal US of a 15-year-old boy with a focal wedge-shaped hyperechoic region of pyelonephritis in the upper pole of the right kidney (arrow in **a**). A US sagittal scan of an 18-year-old girl with a hypoechoic area in the upper pole of the right kidney, suggestive for acute pyelonephritis (arrow in **b**) [36]

echogenicity, rather than sonolucent areas, may be commonly seen in focal nephritis, i.e., "hemorrhagic-like acute pyelonephritis" (Fig. 16.4). With appropriate low velocity scales, affected areas definitely show decreased vascularity on color Doppler US, compared to the unaffected renal cortex. Dilatation of the collecting system in the absence of appreciable obstructive cause may also be seen. Parallel lucent streaks in the renal pelvis and ureter, which are most likely caused by mucosal edema, may occasionally be detected.

In cases of fungal infection, US may demonstrate evidence of fungal debris in the collecting system, such as a bezoar and consequent obstruction. Furthermore, US can detect collections of air in the bladder or collecting system as the fungus may be gas forming [35].

The US should be complemented with a CT evaluation, which is more sensitive in detecting focal pyelonephritis and evaluation of disease extent. Perirenal infiltration or abscess is often missed with US.

16.4.4 CT

CT is not routinely performed in the setting of pyelonephritis but is the modality of choice in the evaluation of complicated cases. On unenhanced CT, the affected kidney can appear normal; sometimes diffuse (or rarely focal) enlargement can be observed [37, 38]. Contrast-enhanced CT should be performed for complete evaluation, if no contraindication for i.v. contrast administration is present.

Focal pyelonephritis is characterized by an ill-defined wedge-shaped or rounded mass-like area of decreased enhancement. On delayed scans, 4–6 h after intravenous administration of contrast, inversion of the attenuation of the lesions can be expected: the sites of inflammatory involvement that were initially hypodense become hyperdense. The affected areas typically have a striated appearance: an area of alternating hypoattenuating and hyperattenuating rays, radiating from the papilla to the cortex following the direction of the excretory tubules. This reflects the decreased flow and consequent hyperconcentration of the contrast in the infected tubules, which is due to obstruction of the tubules by inflammatory debris, external compression by the inflammatory process in the interstitium, and the impaired function due to tubular ischemia. The striated nephrogram is not pathognomonic for APN, however. It can also be seen in other conditions such as renal vein thrombosis, ureteric obstruction, and contusion [39]. Occasionally, focal pyelonephritis can mimic a neoplasm.

Diffuse pyelonephritis may cause a global enlargement of the kidney and a poor enhancement of the whole parenchyma, with absent excretion of contrast. Other nonspecific radiological signs include perinephric stranding, thickening and mucosal enhancement of the urothelium, inflammatory changes in Gerota's fascia and/or the renal sinus, and fluid collections/effusions [12].

Also infarction can have a similar aspect on CT with multifocal hypoattenuating areas, but some features may contribute in differentiating from inflammatory disease (Fig. 16.5).

16.4.5 Scan Protocol

A three- or four-phase CT examination is no routine practice. If renal colic is suspected, an unenhanced CT scan with lower dose allows the detection of renal calculi. Clinical information may guide the decision for using one or more contrast phases; a single venous phase (60–90 s post-contrast) in most cases. If renal ischemia is a possible differential diagnosis, then an arterial scan (15–25 s) is ideal to assess perfusion. When still in doubt, after venous phase CT or when there is a mismatch between imaging and clinical features, a delayed scan (after 4–6 h) can be obtained. An excretory phase with opacification of the ureters (urography) can be obtained with or without i.v. administration of a diuretic agent.

16.4.6 MRI

MR imaging offers inherently high soft-tissue contrast, is independent of excretory function, and allows multiplanar imaging. MRI will provide similar diagnostic information as CT, with similar high sensitivity and specificity, and is also able to perform urography (MRU).

However, the lack of readily available scan time in many institutions and the costs make MRI a less suitable modality for imaging of pyelonephritis, especially in emergency stetting. It is useful in cases where CT scan is contraindicated, e.g., allergy to iodinated contrast agents or when ionizing radiation should be avoided (e.g., in pregnancy).

The cortical phase of contrast-enhanced MRI is likely the best sequence to detect and differentiate pyelonephritis from cortical defects [40]. MRU can distinguish among acute pyelonephritis, renal scarring, and renal tumor [41]. MRU is also useful for detecting and characterizing congenital anomalies of the kidneys

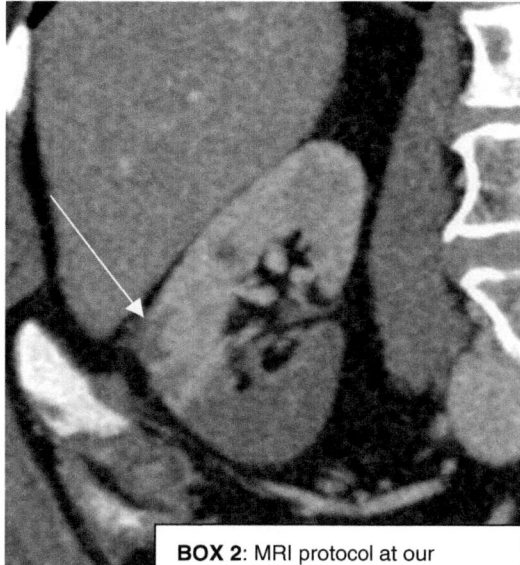

BOX 2: MRI protocol at our institution.

- Localizer
- T2 HASTE C
- T2 HASTE T (TE 82/360)
- T1in/opposed phase T
- T1VIBE fs C
- T1 VIBE fs T
- T2 TRUFI S localizer
- FLASH 3D

I.V. Gadolinium+ Lasix
- T1 VIBE fs C (arterial)
- T1 VIBE fs C (venous)
- T1 VIBE fs T (late venous)
- FLASH 3D
- EPI 2D diffusion

T: transverse, C: coronal, S: sagittal, fs: fat saturation,
HASTE: Half-Fourier Acquisition Single-shot Turbo spin
Echo, VIBE: volumetric interpolated breath-hold examination,
TRUFI: true fast imaging with steady-state free precession, EPI: Echo Planar Imaging.

Fig. 16.5 Infarct in the lower pole of the right kidney and in a lesser degree of the left interpolar area. Renal infarct can mimic (multi-) focal APN, although absence of renal enlargement and signs of pyelitis as well as the subcapsular distribution with "cortical rim sign" (arrow) and more sharply delineated hypodense areas may be helpful in distinguishing between these two entities. The clinical presentation of the patient and additional laboratory findings contribute to the differential diagnosis

and genitourinary tract in the pediatric and adult population [42]. The use of diffusion-weighted sequences is certainly promising, assisting in the differentiation between pyonephrosis and hydronephrosis, which may be particularly helpful for pregnant patients in their second and third trimesters [43]. Early studies have shown diffusion-weighted sequences to provide reproducible information regarding renal function [44]. A potential disadvantage of MRI is its inability to detect smaller calculi, especially when the stones are not fully surrounded by urine [42].

16.4.7 Scan Protocol

The imaging protocol for evaluation of the kidney on a 1.5-Tesla (T) MRI system should at least consist of the following sequences (Box 16.2). Multiplanar T2-weighted TSE (HASTE) for detailed T2-weighted anatomic information and also transverse T1-weighted gradient echo sequence in-phase and opposed-phase and transverse T1-weighted images before and after i.v. gadolinium should be acquired. Lesion perfusional assessment could be done but is more useful for differentiation of solid lesions when tumor is in the differential diagnosis.

The T2-weighted sequence is especially helpful in characterizing cysts and abscesses and in evaluating hydronephrosis. Furthermore, the T2-weighted sequence is helpful in detecting solid lesions.

Lesions with hemorrhage, lesions with macroscopic fat, melanin-containing lesions, and cysts with high protein content may show hyperintense signal on T1. Opposed-phase T1-weighted gradient echo sequences can be used to prove the presence of small amounts of fat, which can be useful in cases of XGP, a disease characterized by lipid-laden macrophages [45]. FLASH sequence can be used to make volumetric scans and 3D reconstruction as well as maximal intensity projection images comparable to urography [46].

Diffusion-weighted MRI is very sensitive for the noninvasive detection of focal areas of pyelonephritis [11].

Box 16.2 MRI Protocol at Our Institution
- Localizer
- T2 HASTE C
- T2 HASTE T (TE 82/360)
- T1 in/opposed-phase T
- T1 VIBE fs C
- T1 VIBE fs T
- T2 TRUFI S localizer
- FLASH 3D

I.V. Gadolinium+ Lasix

- T1 VIBE fs C (arterial)
- T1 VIBE fs C (venous)
- T1 VIBE fs T (late venous)
- FLASH 3D
- EPI 2D diffusion

T transverse, *C* coronal, *S* sagittal, *fs* fat saturation, *HASTE* half-Fourier acquisition single-shot turbo spin echo, *VIBE* volumetric interpolated breath-hold examination, *TRUFI* true fast imaging with steady-state-free precession, *EPI* echo planar imaging

---

16.4.8 Tc-99m DMSA Scan

Tc-99m DMSA (dimercaptosuccinic acid) is a technetium radiopharmaceutical used in renal imaging to evaluate renal structure and morphology, particularly in pediatric imaging for detection of scarring and pyelonephritis [47].

In the pediatric population, where a missed diagnosis can mean irreversible damage, with hypertension or chronic kidney failure as a consequence, Tc-99m DMSA scintigraphy is still considered the gold standard of imaging (Fig. 16.6) [48].

Fig. 16.6 (**a, b**): Tc-99m DMSA scan of the same 7-year-old boy. (**a**) Initial DMSA scan reveals a negligible difference in renal excretion: 46% in the left kidney and 54% in the right one. It does however show a photopenic zone in the interpolar area of the left kidney: location of the abscess. (**b**) Follow-up exam after 8 months. The location of the former abscess in the left kidney is still faintly photopenic. There is still a symmetrical excretory function: 47% left and 53% right

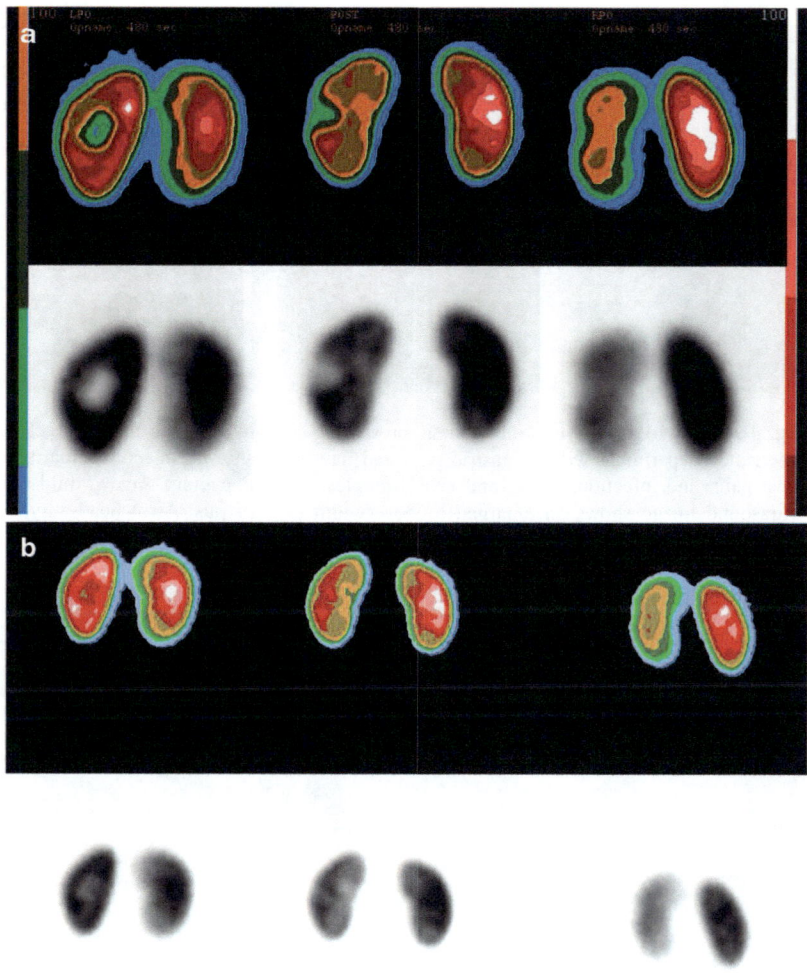

16.5   Imaging of Inflammatory Renal Disease

16.5.1   Acute Pyelonephritis

Acute pyelonephritis can be unilateral or bilateral; unifocal, multifocal, or diffuse; and uncomplicated or complicated. Ultrasound can show enlargement due to edema and areas of hypo- or hyperechogenicity in the parenchyma with decreased vascularity on color Doppler imaging in the corresponding areas (Fig. 16.7).

Parenchymal phase CT typically shows decreased enhancement within (wedge-shaped) areas of affected tissue or in the entire kidney in case of diffuse APN (Fig. 16.8). Other signs include thickening and hypervascular urothelium of the collecting system and perinephric infiltration (Fig. 16.9). The striated nephrogram can be seen on delayed scan phases (after 4–6h), but it is not necessary to perform this late phase in all patients (Fig. 16.10).

MRI can show similar characteristics as CT (Fig. 16.11).

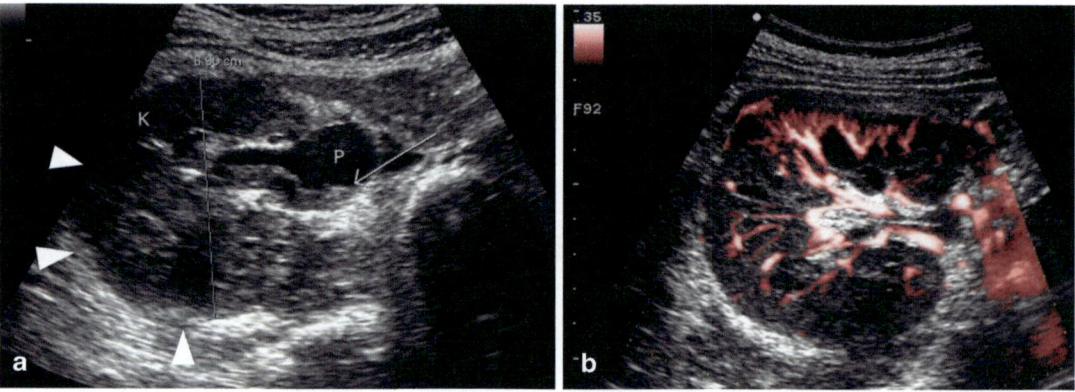

Fig. 16.7 (**a**, **b**) A 41-year-old woman presenting at emergency department with epigastric pain and nausea, renal pain, and infectious blood and urine samples. (**a**) Ultrasound image shows an enlarged kidney (width of 6,9 cm) with heterogeneous parenchyma with multifocal hypoechoic and hyperechoic areas. (**b**) Power Doppler US shows reduced vascularity in the affected areas. K, kidney; P, pyelum. Arrow: fluid-fluid level by urine and sediment of pus. Arrowheads: hypoechoic areas compatible with nephritis

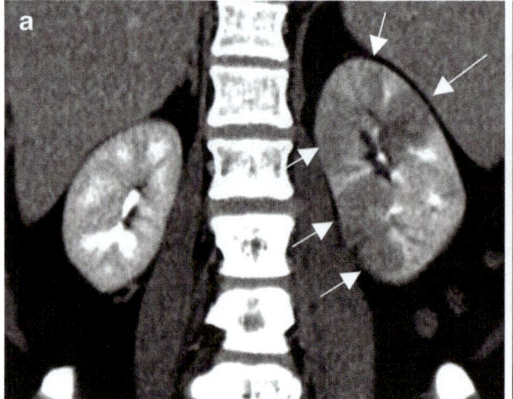

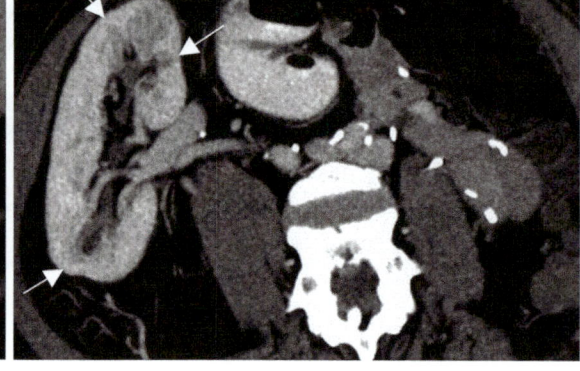

Fig. 16.8 (**a**, **b**) Two cases of multifocal acute pyelonephritis. (**a**) Coronal contrast-enhanced CT shows an edematous left kidney with multiple wedge-shaped hypodense areas (arrows) in the native left kidney in a 35-year-old woman in postpartum. Urine and blood cultures yielded *E. coli*. (**b**) Reformatted contrast-enhanced CT study of a renal graft showing some subtle wedge-shaped hypodense areas (arrows) in the lower and upper pole

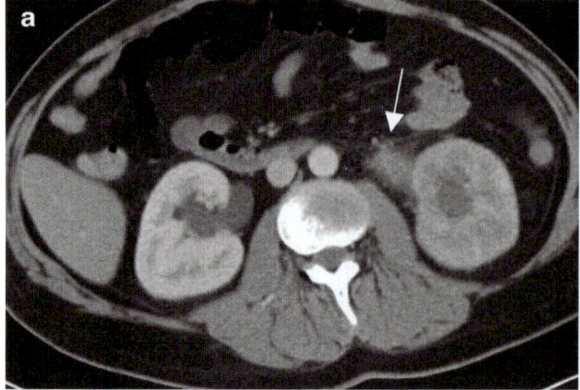

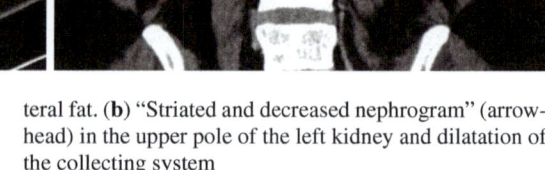

Fig. 16.9 (**a**, **b**) CT images of two different patients with diffuse APN on the left side. The kidney is swollen and hypo-enhancing after i.v. contrast injection. (**a**) Extensive pyelitis (arrow) is present with infiltration of the periureteral fat. (**b**) "Striated and decreased nephrogram" (arrowhead) in the upper pole of the left kidney and dilatation of the collecting system

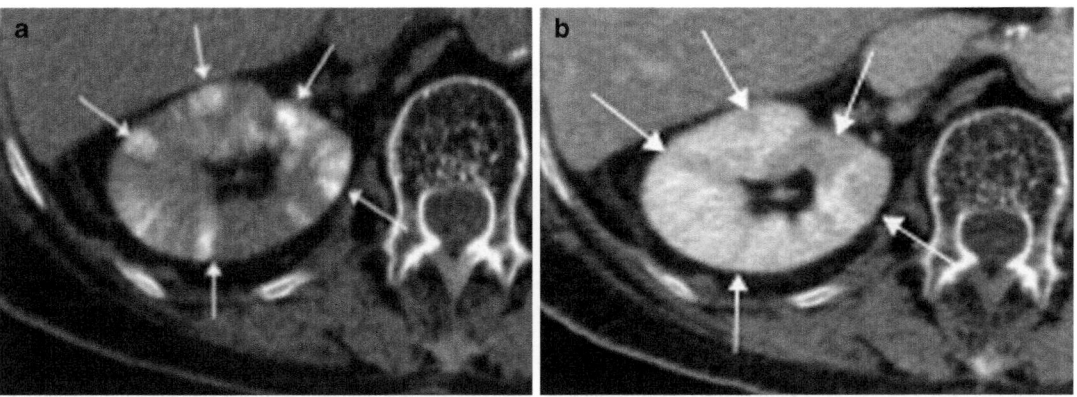

Fig. 16.10 (**a, b**) Delayed phase CT scan (**a**) taken 6 h later without further injection of contrast material show retained contrast material (arrows in **a**) in the area of poor enhancement (arrows in **b**) at initial parenchymal phase CT (**b**) [12]

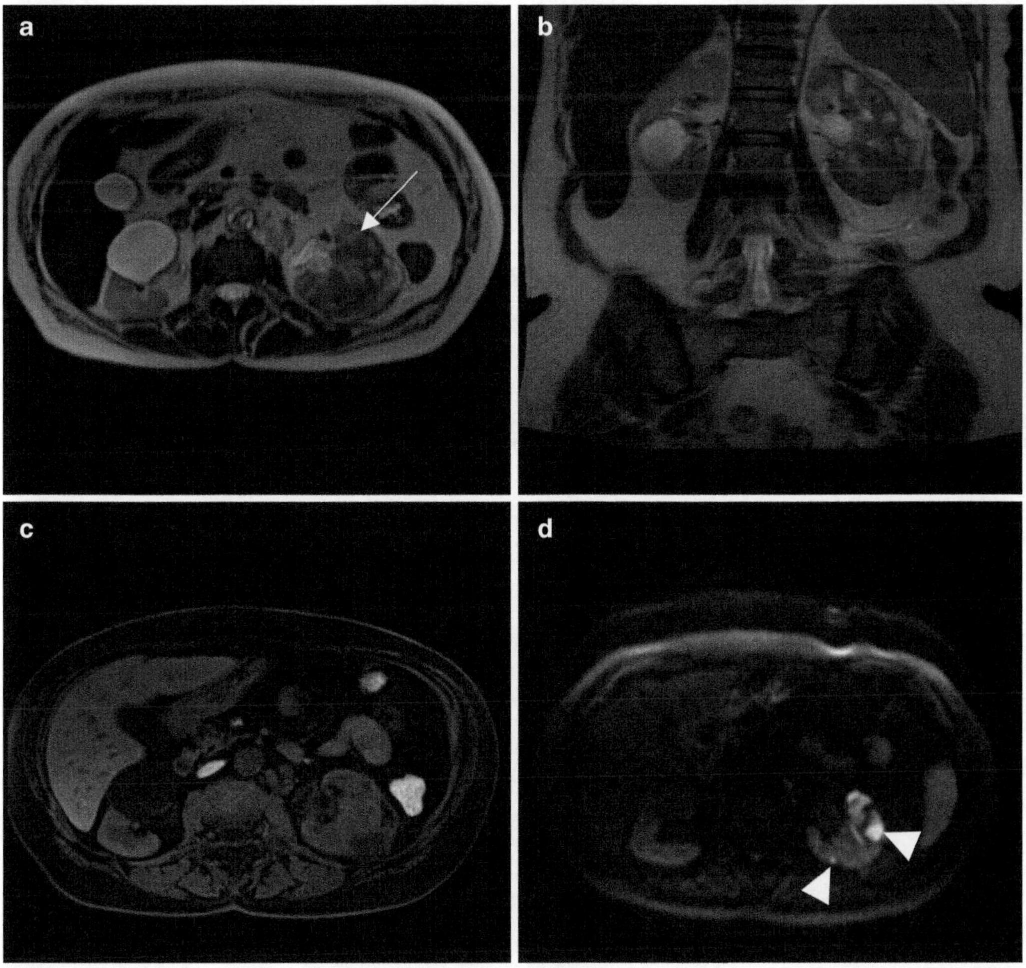

Fig. 16.11 (**a, b, c, d**) MRI of 67-year-old (diabetic) female with acute multifocal pyelonephritis. (**a** and **b**) axial and coronal T2-weighted MR-images, respectively. The left kidney is diffusely enlarged with hypointense wedge-shaped areas as well as somewhat striated appearance in the anterior hilar lip (arrow). There is perinephric infiltration at the posterolateral edge of the kidney. T1 VIBE pre-contrast (**c**) shows hypointensity in the areas of T2 hyperintensity due to edema. No i.v. contrast was administered because of acute renal failure. Diffusion restriction is seen (**d**) as hyperintense signal in the left kidney due to the inflammatory process (arrowheads)

16.5.2 Renal/Perirenal Abscess

In cases of severe infection, inappropriate antibiotic therapy, diabetics, and immunosuppressed patients, an abscess may develop. It is an underestimated complication of APN.

CT is more sensitive in detection of renal abscesses than US. A hypoechoic mass with a thick and hypervascular wall on color Doppler and internal echoes with or without fluid-fluid level is highly suggestive of a renal abscess (Fig. 16.12). However occasionally an abscess presents as an echogenic mass, and CT is required for final diagnosis. CT shows a peripheral enhancing lesion with thick irregular outer wall and centrally non-enhancing liquid with varying attenuation numbers between 0 and 40 Hounsfield units (Fig. 16.13). Delayed scan can show rim or striated nephrogram as in APN surrounding the abscess, similar to the typical CT features of APN. MRI can be used and has similar findings as CT. T1 hypointensity and T2 hyperintensity are seen inside the abscess due to the fluid content which is enveloped by a hypointense outer wall. Because of the viscous content of the pus, diffusion restriction can be

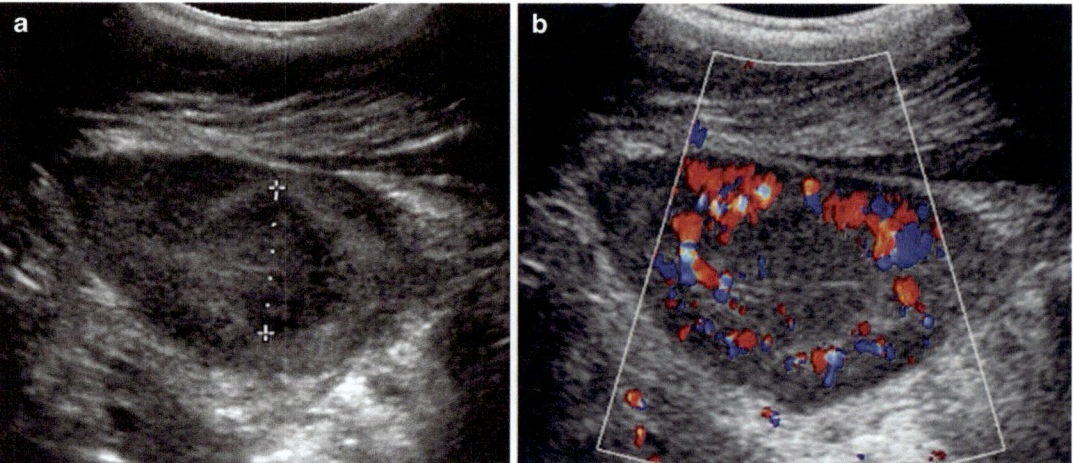

Fig. 16.12 (a, b) Gray scale US (a) and color Doppler US (b) of a 7-year-old boy showing a nodular lesion in the midpole area of the left kidney. A typical renal abscess is heterogeneous, slightly hypoechoic with a thick outer wall and without internal vascularity

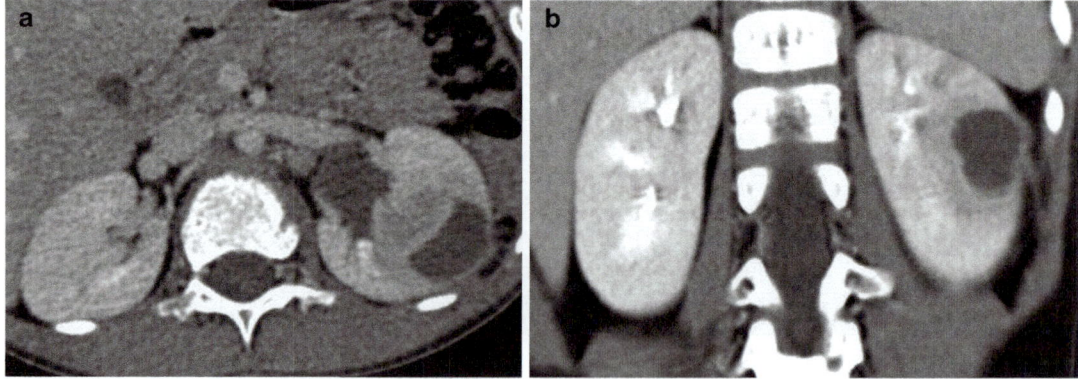

Fig. 16.13 (a, b) Axial (a) and coronal (b) CT image of the same 7-year-old with renal abscess in the left kidney. Typical renal abscess: thick vascularized wall and adjacent striated nephrogram. Some perirenal stranding

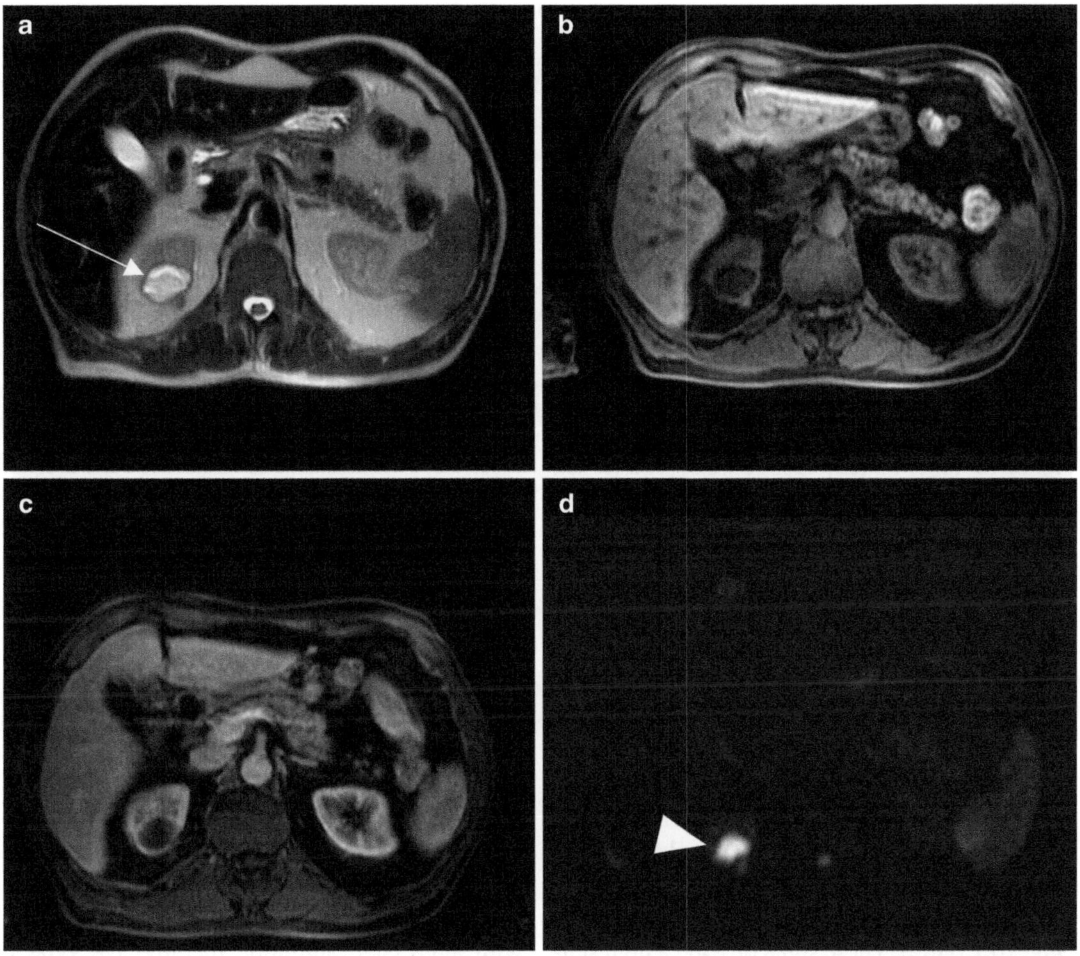

Fig. 16.14 (a–d) MRI of renal abscess. (a) T2 image shows hyperintense lesion in the upper pole of the right kidney with a hypointense surrounding wall (arrow). (b) The lesion is hypointense on T1-weighted images (WI).

(c) T1 WI after i.v. contrast injection shows only a slight peripheral rim enhancement. (d) high *b*-value diffusion-weighted image (*b*-1000) shows a central hyperintense area in the lesion due to diffusion restriction (arrowhead)

expected (Fig. 16.14) [49]. The main differential diagnoses are diverticula, complicated cysts, or necrotic tumor.

When left untreated, the abscess may involve the perinephric space to become a perinephric abscess.

When the abscesses become larger than 4–5 cm in diameter, percutaneous aspiration under imaging guidance may be performed to fasten recovery under antibiotic treatment [50]. Perinephric abscesses with minor extension may require partial nephrectomy. Nephrectomy must be considered if the abscess reaches the perirenal fat [51].

16.5.3 Pyonephrosis

Pyonephrosis is a suppurative infection in the setting of obstructive hydronephrosis. Accumulation of pus is distending the renal pelvis and calyces even further, but due to the obstruction, bacteriuria can be absent.

The "pus under pressure" state associated with pyonephrosis is one of the few urological emergencies. It is imperative to relieve the obstruction by means of nephrostomy or ureteral stenting. If left untreated, this condition can cause parenchymal destruction, irreversible loss of renal function, and even sepsis.

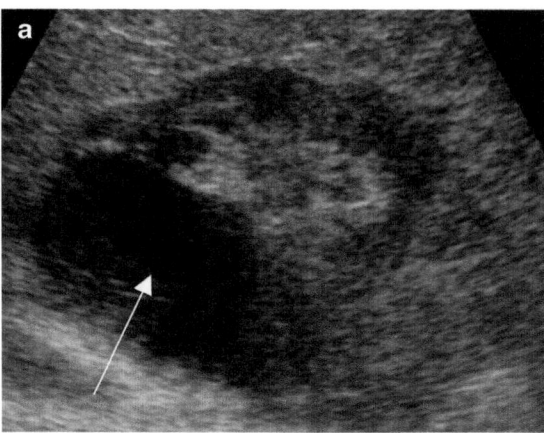 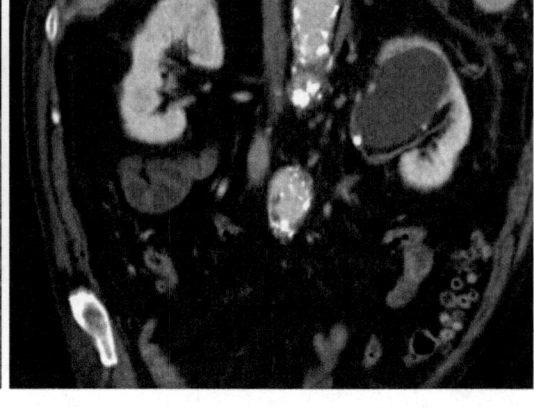

Fig. 16.15 (**a**, **b**) 81-year-old male with obstructed left upper pole duplex system by lithiasis. (**a**) US image shows the dilated upper system with internal echoic material in the posterior part (arrow: fluid-fluid level). (**b**) Obstructing lithiasis is clearly depicted at CT with distention of the upper calyx. Attenuation numbers of the content of the posterior part of the calyx were 65 HU caused by pus and the infectious debris. Note decreased contrast enhancement of the renal parenchyma in the upper pole compared to the lower pole

Differentiation between pyonephrosis and simple hydronephrosis is not always easy. There are however a few signs that are indicative of superimposed infection. These include thickening of the pyelum wall, gas in the collecting system (without history of recent catheterization), or a fluid-fluid level. Bulging of the renal contour in the setting of hydronephrosis as well as an abnormal nephrogram are suggestive as well (Fig. 16.15) [52]. These signs provide a high sensitivity (90%) and specificity for diagnosis of pyonephrosis [53].

16.5.4 Emphysematous Pyelonephritis

Emphysematous pyelonephritis is a rare but possible life-threatening entity most commonly seen in diabetic patients. This necrotizing infection is characterized by gas formation within the renal parenchyma, perirenal tissue, and/or collecting system. The gas develops by fermentation of glucose into carbon dioxide and hydrogen [12].

Emphysematous pyelonephritis can be classified into two types. Type I is the classic form characterized by renal parenchymal destruction that manifests with streaky/mottled areas of gas (Fig. 16.16). Intra- or perirenal fluid collections are notably absent. Type II is characterized by renal or perirenal fluid collections that are directly associated with bubbly or loculated gas or by gas within the renal collecting system (Fig. 16.17). The importance of this classification lays in the different therapeutic approaches. When extensive, the type I lesions should be treated by emergent nephrectomy, and milder type I cases could still be treated successfully with aggressive antibiotic therapy. The type II lesion may be treated with percutaneous drainage, as they are to be considered a form of renal/perirenal abscess, in combination with appropriate antibiotic therapy [37].

Emphysematous pyelitis is a less aggressive form of emphysematous infection of the upper urinary tract. The gas is confined to the renal collecting system, and overall mortality rate is significantly less than that for emphysematous pyelonephritis [12].

16.5.5 Chronic Pyelonephritis

Chronic pyelonephritis is a form of pyelonephritis where there are long-standing sequelae of recurrent renal infections. Usually fibrosing nephritis develops in the case of occult vesico-ureteral reflux.

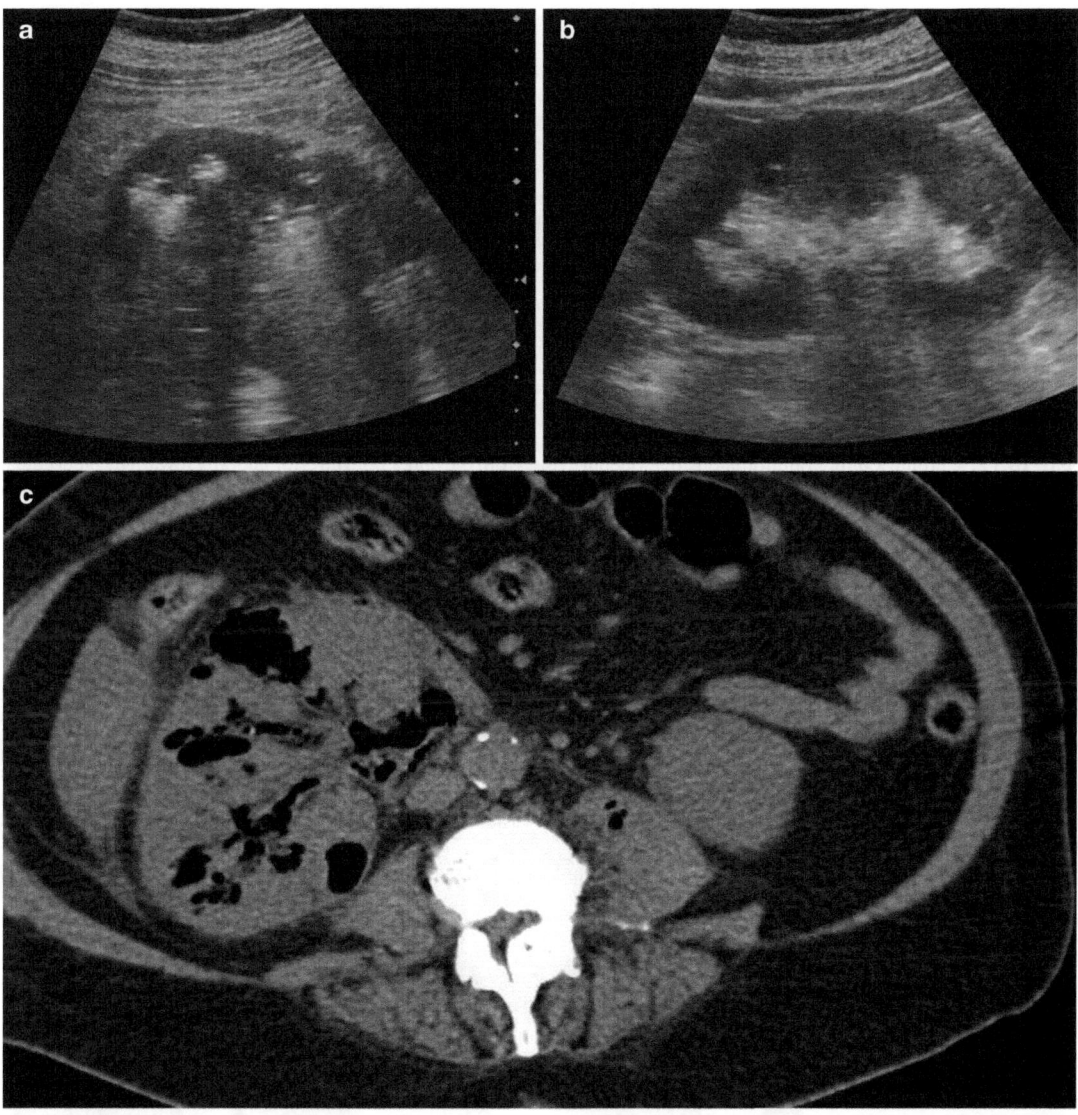

Fig. 16.16 (**a**, **b**, **c**) Emphysematous pyelonephritis—type 1. US shows multiple hyperechoic streaks in the right kidney due to intraparenchymal air with ring-down artifacts in (**a**), compared to the normal left kidney in (**b**). (**c**) Unenhanced CT image of the same patient shows diffuse enlarged right streaky and mottled gas in the renal parenchyma and collecting system. There are also some gas bubbles in the left psoas muscle

In general, (repeated) bacterial infection results in focal thinning, scarring, and atrophy in the renal cortex overlying a calyx and is usually associated with some calyceal distortion. Other signs may be compensatory hypertrophy of residual normal tissue (which may mimic a mass lesion), calyceal clubbing secondary to retraction of the papilla from overlying scar, thickening and dilatation of the calyceal system, and overall renal asymmetry. Sometimes dystrophic calculi form [37].

On ultrasound the small kidney size, contour alterations, and corticomedullary dedifferentiation can be depicted. Contrast-enhanced CT may illustrate the full picture, if at least the renal function allows administration of contrast (Fig. 16.18). A retrograde cystography should be performed to evaluate vesicoureteral reflux.

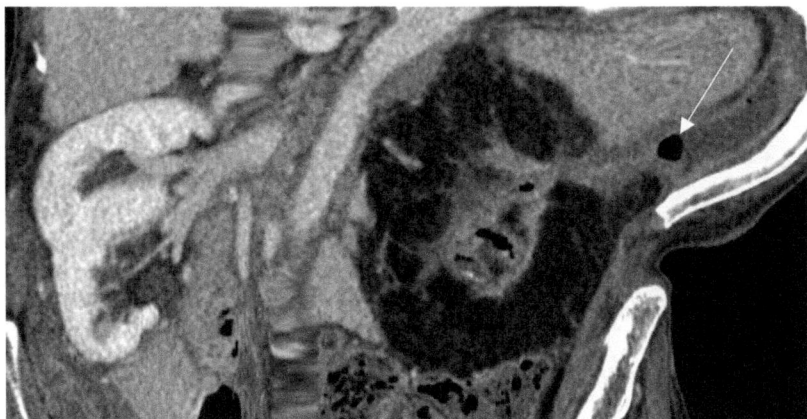

Fig. 16.17 Chronic xanthogranulomatous pyelonephritis superimposed with type 2 emphysematous infection. Coronal CT showing streaky gas within the completely destructed left kidney. A perirenal collection is spreading from the upper pole inferior laterally toward the abdominal wall, with some gas bubbles in the perirenal collection (arrow). Note the extensive perirenal fibro-fatty replacement as can be seen with XGP

Fig. 16.18 (a, b) Coronal CT scan of patient with multiple cysts in the kidneys and had a cystectomy with an orthotopic bladder pouch. (a) Slight hypo-enhancing left kidney and dilatation of the collecting system due to chronic reflux and obstruction of the ureterointestinal anastomosis. (b) CT study of the same patient 11 years later shows a decreased volume of left kidney and retracted renal contour predominately centered on dilated and distorted calyces. Some renal parenchyma is preserved and hypertrophic with a nodular appearance, which should not be mistaken for tumor. Cortical cysts in the right kidney are enlarged over time

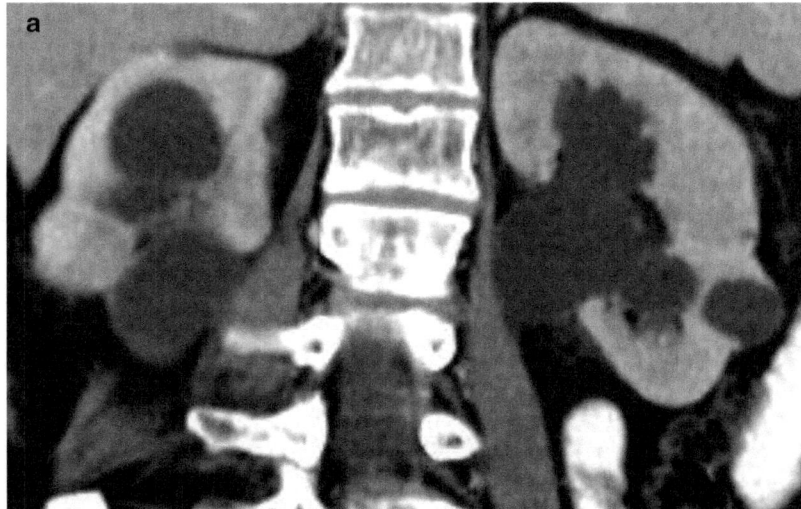

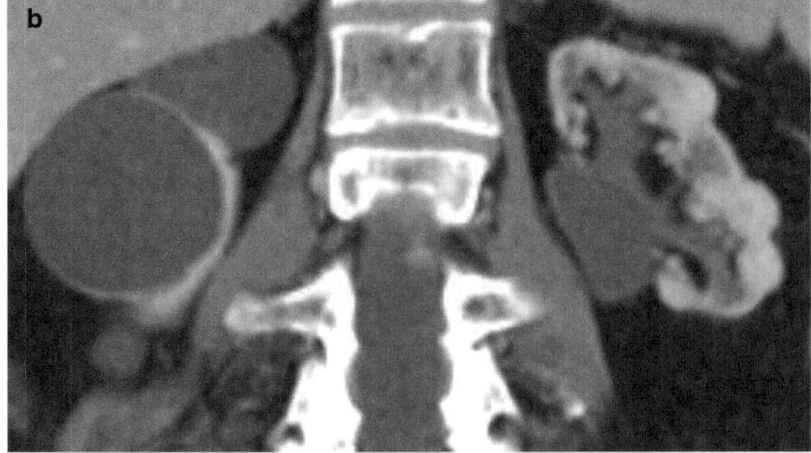

Repeated imaging is unlikely to provide evidence of new findings once the chronic state had been established [37].

These patients usually have a well-known urologic disease history or present with decreased renal function and hypertension [54].

16.5.6 Xanthogranulomatous Pyelonephritis

Xanthogranulomatous pyelonephritis is a rare form of chronic renal infection. It can be identified histologically by the presence of granulomatous material containing lipid-laden foamy macrophages and histiocytes, in combination with the same characteristic appearance of chronic infection, including scarring and contraction of the renal pelvis and renal parenchymal destruction.

The main cause is chronic renal obstruction, and lithiasis is present in 80% of cases, staghorn shaped. Stenosis can also be a cause of obstruction, either post-infectious, congenital, or after surgery, as seen in ureteropelvic junction stenosis, or even more rarely a tumor of the collecting system. No specific risk factor is known, although diabetes mellitus is present in approximately 10% of patients.

XGP can manifest in two different types, the most common being diffuse involvement of the kidney (up to 85% of cases) or as a focal process, at times with pseudotumoral features [12].

Symptoms are nonspecific and in the diffuse form mimic those of pyonephrosis including fever, chills, hematuria, pyuria, and flank pain. The majority of the cases have extensive perirenal inflammation.

Abdominal plain film can depict the faintly calcified, struvite stone with staghorn appearance (Fig. 16.19). US demonstrates a globally enlarged and hypoechoic kidney with calculi and thick debris in the dilated collecting system (Fig. 16.20a). Differentiation from tuberculosis can be difficult.

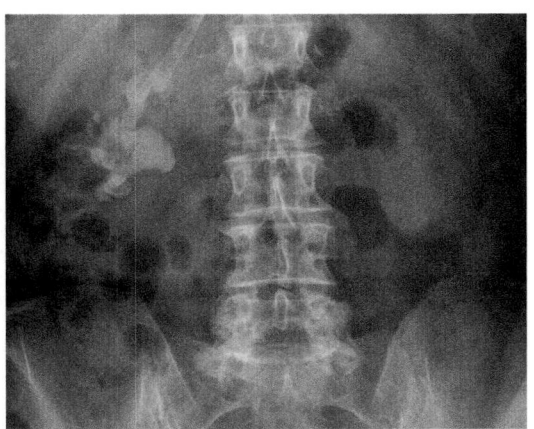

Fig. 16.19 Abdominal plain film showing a typical staghorn calculus in the right kidney

The kidney is enlarged, and mild enhancement of the inflamed but nonfunctioning parenchyma surrounding the dilated calyces is seen on CT, as well as thickening of the renal fascia. Calculi are readily seen. CT is especially useful for assessment of perirenal spread and fistulae formation to adjacent organs or the abdominal wall. Dilated calyces opposed to a contracted pelvis have been compared to the paw print of a bear (bear's paw sign) (Figs. 16.20b and 16.21a) [55]. The localized form may mimic a hypovascular tumor, as it may have features of a minimally enhancing renal mass (Fig. 16.21b).

MRI shows heterogeneous lesions on all sequences due to cystic, solid, and calcified components.

16.5.7 Summary: ACR Guidelines

The latest ACR appropriateness criteria related to imaging of acute pyelonephritis are helpful to select patients for imaging studies [56].

- Otherwise healthy patients with uncomplicated pyelonephritis will typically need no radiologic workup if they respond to antibiotic therapy within 72 h.

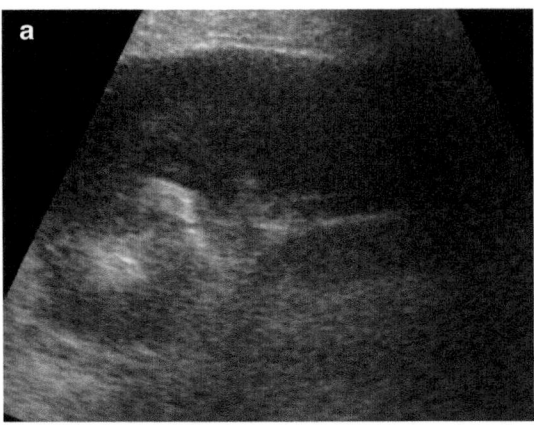
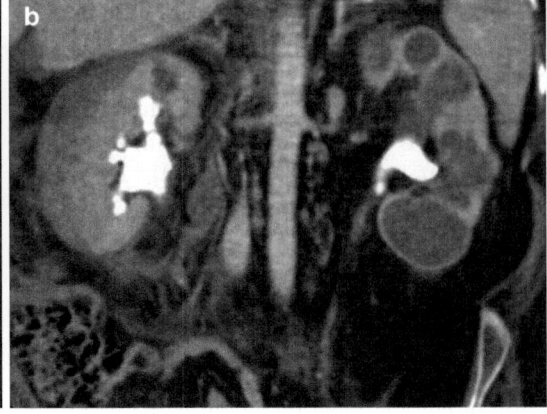

Fig. 16.20 (**a, b**) Case of xanthogranulomatous pyelonephritis. (**a**) Ultrasound of 39-year-old man with bilateral XGP shows diffuse enlargement and hypoechogenic aspect of the right kidney with staghorn calculus. (**b**) CT of this patient shows bilateral XGP and staghorn calculi. Perinephric infiltration on the right side and the typical "bear's paw sign" in the left kidney

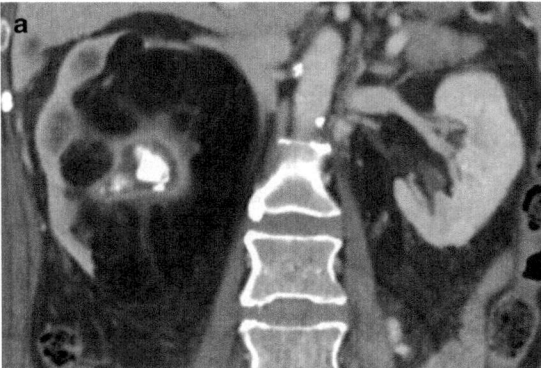
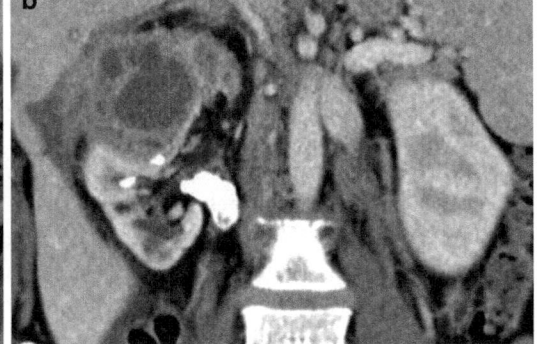

Fig. 16.21 (**a, b**) Two cases of xanthogranulomatous pyelonephritis. (**a**) Severely affected right kidney, with extensive replacement lipomatosis in the hilum. Staghorn calculus is present. (**b**) Case of focal XGP in the upper pole of the right kidney, with perirenal involvement. Focal XGP should not be mistaken for a renal tumor

- If there is no response to therapy, CT of the abdomen and pelvis is the study of choice.
- Diabetics or other immunocompromised patients should be evaluated with pre-contrast and post-contrast CT within 24 h of diagnosis, if response to therapy is not prompt.
- US should be reserved for patients in whom pyonephrosis is suspected and those patients for whom exposure to contrast or radiation is hazardous.
- All other complicated adult patients (e.g., patients with a history of stones or other urologic conditions, prior urologic surgery, repeated episodes of pyelonephritis) probably deserve early evaluation with CT.
- For patients in whom contrast-enhanced CT is contraindicated, MRI could be considered as an alternative to CT.

References

1. Schappert SM, Rechtsteiner EA. Ambulatory medical care utilization estimates for 2007. Vital Health Stat. 2011;13:1–38.
2. Foxman B. Urinary tract infection syndromes: occurrence, recurrence, bacteriology, risk factors, and disease burden. Infect Dis Clin North Am. 2014;28:1–13.
3. Foxman B. The epidemiology of urinary tract infection. Nature Rev Urol. 2010;7:653–60.
4. Meltzer AC, Pines JM, Richards LM, Mullins P, Pharm MM. US emergency department visits for

adults with abdominal and pelvic pain (2007–13): trends in demographics, resource utilization and medication usage. Am J Emerg Med. 2017;35(12):1966–9.

5. Stamm WE, Norrby SR. Urinary tract infections: disease panorama and challenges. J Infect Dis. 2001;183(Suppl 1):S1–4.

6. Hooton TM. Uncomplicated urinary tract infection. N Engl J Med. 2012;366(11):1028–37.

7. Hooton T, Gupta K. Recurrent urinary tract infection in women. 2014. https://www.uptodate.com/contents/recurrent-simple-cystitis-in-women

8. Fowler JE Jr, Perkins T. Presentation, diagnosis and treatment of renal abscesses: 1972–1988. J Urol. 1994;151:847–52.

9. Flores-Mireles AL, Walker JN, Caparon M, Hultgren SJ. Urinary tract infections: epidemiology, mechanisms of infection and treatment options. Nat Rev Microbiol. 2015;13(5):269–84.

10. Collège des universitaires de maladies infectieuses et tropicales. Infections urinaires. In: E. Pilly: Vivactis Plus Ed. 2010. p. 211–4.

11. Ifergan J, Pommier R, Brion MC, Glas L, Rocher L, Billin MF. Imaging of upper urinary tract infections. Diagnostic and interventional imaging, vol. 9. France: Elsevier; 2012. p. 509–19.

12. Cho JY. Renal infection. In: Kim SH, editor. Radiology illustrated: uroradiology. Heidelberg: Springer; 2012. p. 393–24.

13. Forster TH, Bonkat G, Wyler S, Ruszat R, Ebinger N, Gasser TC, et al. Diagnosis and therapy of acute ureteral colic. Wien Klin Wochenschr. 2008;120(11–12):325–34.

14. Manski D. Abdominal pain and Flank pain. 2017. http://www.urology-textbook.com/abdominal-pain.html.

15. Shokeir AA. Renal colic: new concepts related to pathophysiology, diagnosis and treatment. Curr Opin Urol. 2002;12(4):263–9.

16. Blandino A, Mazziotti S, Minutoli F, Ascenti G, Gaeta M. Acute renal infections. In: Quaia E, editor. Radiological imaging of the kidney. Heidelberg: Springer; 2011. p. 417–44.

17. Fulop T. Acute Pyelonephritis: clinical presentation. 2017. https://emedicine.medscape.com/article/245559-clinical.

18. Rollino C, Sandrone M, Peruzzi L, De Marchi A, Beltrame G, Ferro M, et al. Direct bacterial infection of the renal parenchyma: pyelonephritis in native kidneys. In: Satoskar AA, editor. Bacterial infections of the kidney. Cham: Springer; 2017. p. 161–95.

19. Rollino C, Beltrame G, Ferro M, Quattrocchiono G, Sandrone M, Quarello F. Acute pyelonephritis in adults: a case series of 223 patients. Nephrol Dial Transplant. 2012;27:3488–93.

20. Gupta K, Hooton TM, Naber KG, et al. International clinical practice guidelines for the treatment of acute uncomplicated cystitis and pyelonephritis in women: a 2010 update by the Infectious Diseases Society of America and the European society for micro-biology and infectious diseases. Clin Infect Dis. 2011;52:e103–20.

21. Hooton TM, Roberts PL, Cox M, et al. Voided midstream urine culture and acute cystitis in premenopausal women. N Engl J Med. 2013;14(369):1883–91.

22. Soenen O, Balliauw C, Oyen R, Zanca F. Dose and image quality in low-dose CT for urinary stone disease: added value of automatic tube current modulation and iterative reconstruction techniques. Radiat Prot Dosim. 2017;174(2):242–9.

23. Niemann T, Kollmann T, Bongartz G. Diagnostic performance of low-dose CT for the detection of urolithiasis: a meta-analysis. AJR Am. J. Roentgenol. 2008;191:396–401.

24. Webb JAW. The role of imaging in adult acute urinary tract infection. Eur Radiol. 1997;7:837–43.

25. Baumgarten DA, Baumgarten BR. Imaging and radiologic management of upper urinary tract infections. Urol Clin North Am. 1997;24:545–69.

26. Browne RFJ, Zwirewich C, Torreggiani WC. Imaging of urinary tract infection in the adult. Eur Radiol. 2004;14:168–83.

27. Wong LS, Tse KS, Fan TW, et al. Voiding urosonography with second-generation ultrasound contrast versus micturating cystourethrography in the diagnosis of vesicoureteric reflux. Eur J Pediatr. 2014;173:1095.

28. Yoo JM, Koh JS, Han CH, et al. Diagnosing acute pyelonephritis with CT, ^{99m}Tc-DMSA SPECT, and Doppler ultrasound: a comparative study. Korean J Urol. 2010;51:260–5.

29. Bykov S, Chervinsky L, Smolkin V, et al. Power Doppler sonography versus Tc-99m DMSA scintigraphy for diagnosing acute pyelonephritis in children: are these two methods comparable? Clin Nucl Med. 2003;28(3):198–203.

30. Wang YT, Chiu NY, Chen MJ, et al. Correlation of renal ultrasonographic findings with inflammatory volume from dimercaptosuccinic acid renal scans in children with acute pyelonephritis. J Urol. 2005;173(1):190–4.

31. Mitterberger M, Pinggera GM, Colleselli D, Bartsch G, Strasser H, Steppan I, Pallwein L, Friedrich A, Gradl J, Frauscher F. Acute pyelonephritis: comparison of diagnosis with computed tomography and contrast-enhanced ultrasonography. BJU International. 2008;101:341–4.

32. Fontanilla T, Minaya J, Cortés C, et al. Abdom Imaging. 2012;37:639.

33. Schaeffer AJ. Urinary tract infection. In: Gillenwater JY, Grayhack JT, Howards SS, Mitchell ME, editors. Adult and pediatric urology. 4th ed. Philadelphia: Lippincott Williams & Wilkins; 2002. p. 211–72.

34. Farmer KD, Gellet LR, Dubbins PA. The sonographic appearance of acute focal pyelonephritis 8 years' experience. Clin Radiol. 2002;57(6):483–7.

35. Wise G. Fungal and actinomycotic infections of the genitourinary system. In: Walsh PC, Retik AB, Vaugh ED, editors. Campbell's urology. 8th ed. Philadelphia: Elsevier; 2002. p. 797–827.

36. Scionti A, Rossi P, Gulino P, Semeraro A, Defilippi C, Tonerini M. Acute pyelonephritis. In: Miele V, Trinci M, editors. Imaging non-traumatic abdominal emergencies in pediatric patients. Cham: Springer; 2016.

37. Craig WD, Wagner BF, Travis MD. Pyelonephritis: radiologic-pathologic review. Radiographics. 2008;28:255–76.

38. DAS CJ, et al. Multimodality imaging of the renal inflammatory lesions. World J radiol. 2014;6:865–73.

39. Quaia E, et al. Computed tomography. In: Quaia E, editor. Radiological Imaging of the kidney. Medical radiology. Berlin: Springer; 2010.

40. Cerwinka WH, Kirsch AJ. Magnetic resonance urography in pediatric urology. Curr Opin Urol. 2010;20(4):323–9.

41. Grattan-Smith JD, Little SB, Jones RA. Evaluation of reflux nephropathy, pyelonephritis and renal dysplasia. Pediatr Radiol. 2008;38(1):S83–105.

42. Leyendecker JR, Gianini JW. Magnetic resonance urography. Abdom Imaging. 2009;34(4):527–40.

43. Chan JH, Tsui EY, Luk SH, et al. MR diffusion-weighted imaging of kidney: differentiation between hydronephrosis and pyonephrosis. Clin Imaging. 2001;25(2):110–3.

44. Thoeny HC, De Keyzer F, Oyen RH, Peeters RR. Diffusion-weighted MR imaging of kidneys in healthy volunteers and patients with parenchymal diseases: initial experience. Radiology. 2005;235(3):911–7.

45. Cova MA, Cavallaro M, Martingano P, Ukmar M. In: Quaia E, editor. Radiological imaging of the kidney. Medical radiology. Berlin: Springer; 2010.

46. Nikken JJ, Krestin GP. MRI of the kidney - state of the art. Eur Radiol. 2007;17(11):2780–93.

47. Ziessman HA, O'Malley JP, Thrall JH. Nuclear medicine. Saunders. ISBN:0323082998.

48. Johansen TE. The role of imaging in urinary tract infections. World J Urol. 2004;22(5):392–8.

49. Oto A, Schmid-Tannwald C, Agrawal G, et al. Diffusion-weighted MR imaging of abdominopelvic abscesses. Emerg Radiol. 2011;18:515.

50. Siegel JF, Smith A, Moldwin R. Minimally invasive treatment of renal abscess. J Urol. 1996;155:52–5.

51. Dembry LM, Andriole VT. Renal and perirenal abscesses. Infect Dis Clin North Am. 1997;11:663–8.

52. Demertzis J, Menias CO. State of the art: imaging of renal infections. Emerg Radiol. 2007;14:13–22.

53. Subramanyan BR, Raghavendra BN, Bosniak MA, Lefleur RS, Rosen RJ, Horii GC. Sonography of pyonephrosis: a prospective study. AJR Am J Roentgenol. 1983;40:991–3.

54. Schreir RW. Infections of the upper urinary tract. In: Diseases of the kidney end urinary tract. Philadelphia: Williams and Wilkins; 2001. p. 847–69.

55. Tan WP, Papagiannopoulos D, Elterman L. Bear's paw sign: a classic presentation of xanthogranulomatous pyelonephritis. Urology. 2015;86:e5–6.

56. Nikolaidis P et al. ACR appropriateness criteria: acute pyelonephritis. 2012. https://acsearch.acr.org/docs/69489/Narrative/.

Francesca Iacobellis, Ettore Laccetti,
Federica Romano, Michele Altiero,
and Mariano Scaglione

17.1 Bowel Obstruction

Bowel obstruction is one of the most common causes of acute abdominal pain [1, 2]; small bowel obstruction (SBO) accounts for about 15% of hospital admissions for the evaluation of acute abdominal pain, whereas large bowel obstruction has a prevalence of about 2–4% [3, 4].

The diagnosis can be challenging because clinical presentation may be insidious and results of physical examination and laboratory values are often nonspecific and nondiagnostic [4].

Bowel obstruction may occur due to functional or organic etiology [5, 6].

Paralytic ileus represents an acute functional alteration of the intestinal canalization, due to a sudden impairment of the intestinal peristalsis in absence of an organic obstruction.

It can be determined in response to:

– An inflammatory intra-abdominal condition (e.g., pancreatitis, renal colic), limited to an intestinal segment (sentinel loop) or involving more loops
– Some drugs: opioids, neuroleptics
– Metabolic alterations: hypocalcemia or diabetes
– Vascular causes: altered perfusion [7]

A specific form of paralytic ileus involving the colon is the Ogilvie syndrome or acute colonic pseudo-obstruction (ACPO). Risk factors include drugs that decrease motility, infection, recent surgery, and debilitation associated with severe medical or traumatic illness [2, 6].

It is characterized by the signs, symptoms, and radiological pattern of a large-bowel obstruction but without a detectable organic cause. It is due to an altered autonomic innervation of the colon. Unlike in a dynamic ileus, perforation may occur with ACPO; if perforation occurs, ACPO may raise a mortality rate as high as 40% [8].

Francesca Iacobellis and Ettore Laccetti are equal contributors.

Electronic Supplementary Material The online version of this chapter (https://doi.org/10.1007/978-3-319-99822-0_17) contains supplementary material, which is available to authorized users.

F. Iacobellis
Department of Diagnostic Imaging, "Pineta Grande" Hospital, Castel Volturno (CE), Italy

Department of General and Emergency Radiology, "A. Cardarelli" Hospital, Naples, Italy

E. Laccetti · F. Romano · M. Altiero
Department of Diagnostic Imaging, "Pineta Grande" Hospital, Castel Volturno (CE), Italy

M. Scaglione (✉)
Department of Diagnostic Imaging, "Pineta Grande" Hospital, Castel Volturno (CE), Italy

Department of Radiology, Sunderland Royal Hospital, NHS, Sunderland, UK

Mechanical ileus recognizes an organic cause leading to the interruption of the lumen patency.

This may depend on several causes:

– Occupation of the intestinal lumen: alimentary bolus, gallstone migration, foreign body, polypoid masses, intussusception
– Pathological thickening of the bowel wall: intramural pathological processes (inflammatory bowel disease, acute diverticulitis, neoplasms)
– Extrinsic compression: adhesional bands, perivisceritis, abdominal masses causing compression, hernias
– Complex mechanisms in which there is involvement of the loop-mesentery complex (e.g., strangulation) and vascular and nervous impairment are added to those of canalization interruption [9, 10]

SBO is more common than LBO. The most frequent causes of SBO in Western countries are represented by adhesions (60–70% of the cases), hernias (10–15%), and neoplasms (5–10%). Other etiologies are Crohn's disease, intussusceptions, volvulus, gallstone ileus, foreign bodies, bezoar, trauma, and iatrogenic problems [9–13].

LBO is four to five times less frequent than SBO, and the causes of LBO and SBO differ substantially. The causes most frequently responsible are represented by neoplasms (60%), volvulus (10–15%), diverticulitis (less than 10%), and adhesions [8].

The main clinical and radiological problem consists in differentiating the obstruction from a purely occlusive risk from the obstruction in which vascular risk is added [9].

The radiological evaluation in patient with bowel obstruction should point out firstly if the obstruction is present and if it is mechanical or functional in nature: in case of mechanical obstruction, what is the level, what is the cause of the obstruction, what is its severity, if it is simple or closed-loop, and if signs of ischemia or perforation are present.

Basing on pathophysiologic, imaging, and surgical findings, mechanic ileus can be differentiated in:

– Simple
– Decompensated
– Complicated [9, 10]

Simple mechanical ileus is the initial phase of the obstructive condition, in which the loops proximal to the site of obstruction show an increase in the peristalsis with an increase in the representation of conniventes valvulae attempting to force the obstruction, whereas the loops distal to the obstruction collapse. In this phase, the parietal thickness of the loops is normal, and no free fluid is observed in the peritoneal cavity.

If the occlusive status persists, the increase of intraluminal pressure in the loops proximal to the obstruction, due to gas-fluid mixed stasis, leads to loop dilation and consequent drop of the neuromuscular tone. Furthermore, the increase of intraluminal pressure, greater than the pressure into parietal capillary vessels, causes a change of parietal microcirculation, impairing bowel capability to reabsorb and causing transudative loss of fluid into the peritoneal cavity. In this stage, *decompensated mechanic ileus*, the bowel wall is stretched and thin.

The further persistence of the occlusive cause leads to the *complicated mechanical ileus*, which represents an occlusive state with vascular impairment of the loop leading to ischemia, necrosis, and perforation [4].

This complication may derive from "fight," in response to a significant slowing of the intramural venous drainage in the loop proximal to the obstruction, whose walls become thickened as congested, or by strangulation, with an axial rotation mechanism of the loop-mesentery complex, in which the vascular impairment first affects the venous outflow, due to its lower pressure, and, subsequently, the arterial one, with the persistence and worsening of strangulation [9, 10].

Usually the diagnostic approach begins with an abdominal radiograph and with ultrasound

(US) examination and continues with CT which constitutes the examination of choice to obtain an adequate diagnostic assessment [14].

17.1.1 Abdominal Radiograph

Abdominal radiograph is still the first diagnostic procedure adopted in a patient with acute abdominal pain because it was able to provide useful informations for the correct assessment of the patient, if correctly performed and carefully interpreted.

The examination is indicated in the clinical suspicion of occlusive syndromes and in their follow-up [13, 15, 16]. It can also help to differentiate LBO from SBO and in detecting pneumoperitoneum [4, 11].

The reported accuracy of radiography for the diagnosis of SBO varies from 50% to 86% [11], whereas the reported sensitivity and specificity for LBO are of 84% and 72%, respectively [4].

This range of sensitivity is related to the variability of the findings and their timing of appearance, in fact the sensitivity increases in high-grade obstruction [17].

The examination is differently performed depending on the patient cooperation. If the patient is uncooperative, two overview radiographs of the abdomen, with the patient in the supine position, are taken: one anteroposterior (AP) radiograph and one latero-lateral (LL) radiograph with the X-ray tube parallel to the floor. The abdominal plain films should be completed with a chest radiograph (AP radiograph in the supine position) in the anterior-posterior (AP) projection [18]. The delivered radiation dose from abdominal radiographs is limited (0.1–1.0 mSv) compared to that of computed tomography (CT) of the abdomen and pelvis (10–15 mSv) [2].

In cooperative patients both the chest and the abdominal radiographs should be acquired in the upright position in posteroanterior (PA) and latero-lateral (LL) projections.

The latero-lateral (LL) radiograph with the X-ray tube parallel to the floor and the upright abdominal radiograph shift the gas-fluid stasis creating air-fluid levels and facilitate the detection of free air [18].

Signs of bowel occlusion are altered distribution of intestinal air with small bowel loop dilation larger than 3 cm or large bowel dilation greater than 6 cm (greater than 9 cm for the cecum), stomach dilation, presence of gas-fluid level due to mixed stasis proximal to the transition point, and possible thickening of the intestinal walls. The slow reabsorption of the endoluminal gas in the small bowel is responsible for the *"string of pearls"* sign in which small air bobbles remain trapped between the folds of the valvulae conniventes [17, 19]. The absence of rectal gas may be also a sign of obstruction [11].

An additional finding that may occur in SBO is the gasless abdomen; it consists in paucity of small-bowel gas. There are several causes that may be responsible for the gasless abdomen; when it is detected in obstruction syndromes, it usually indicates high-grade bowel obstruction with fluid-filled dilated bowel or an obstruction complicated by a closed-loop obstruction [11].

Plain abdominal X-ray also allows to hypothesize the functional or organic nature of the ileus: in the mechanical ileus, the loops proximal to the obstruction show a hyper-representation of the valvulae in response to the increase of peristaltic movements attempting to overcome the obstruction. In this case, the loops appear arcuate, and unlike in the paralytic ileus, the loops have a horizontalized appearance without representation of the valvular pattern due to the fall in the neuromuscular tone [20].

In the advanced phases of mechanical ileus, however, it is no longer possible to make a clear differentiation between the functional or organic etiology basing on X-ray findings, as the persistence of the organic stenosis also leads to the loss of neuromuscular tone and the consequent flattening of the loops proximal to the obstructive site with a radiological picture similar to that of the paralytic ileus [20].

Look at the gas usually present in the rectum is useful in distinguishing ACPO from mechanical obstruction. If ACPO is suspected, rectal gas may be more easily seen on a prone lateral or right lateral decubitus view [8].

17.1.2 Abdominal Ultrasound

In the clinical suspicion of intestinal obstruction, abdominal US is indicated as it offers important additional findings to those obtained with the plain X-ray and helps in the overall diagnostic confidence. It would be appropriate for the same radiologist to perform both the abdominal radiograph and the US.

Abdominal US is usually performed with a convex probe; the additional use of a superficial linear probe may improve the examination of the bowel.

With US it is possible to evaluate the caliper of the bowel loops, but above all, their movements in real time appreciating an increased peristalsis in case of mechanical ileus and a diffuse bowel distension with reduction of the kinetic tone in the paralytic ileus and in the advanced phases of the mechanical ileus.

Moreover, it is possible to define alterations in the wall thickness, suggestive of an associated vascular impairment and, therefore, of greater surgical urgency, and the presence of free fluid in the peritoneal recesses is also indicative of a condition of greater severity.

Sometimes it is also possible to define the exact cause of the occlusion, for example, in cases of bowel intussusception, acute appendicitis without (Fig. 17.1) or with perforation (Fig. 17.2, Video 17.1) responsible for reflex paralytic ileus, extensive bowel wall thickening due to inflammatory disease (Fig. 17.3) or diverticulitis (Fig. 17.4), and bowel involvement in abdominal wall hernias [21–23].

17.1.3 Computed Tomography

CT examination is suggested as first imaging modality in case of acute abdomen clinical presentation. CT is the gold standard for the diagnostic confirmation and differential diagnosis, to identify the etiology, the location of the occlusion site, and the timing of the surgical approach [4, 9, 10, 13]. Once the diagnosis of bowel obstruction is made, the crucial point is to define if surgery is necessary. Indeed, in the absence of signs of ischemia, many patients can be conservatively treated, up to 72 h, by decompression with a nasogastric tube and hydro-electrolytic rebalancing [3].

CT should be routinely performed with intravenous (iv) contrast media (cm) unless there is a specific contraindication; the administration of oral or rectal contrast medium is not indicated. The administration of iv cm is particularly useful to assess for the presence of signs of inflammation and ischemia.

CT, acquired from the dome of the diaphragm to the symphysis pubis, consists in a biphasic

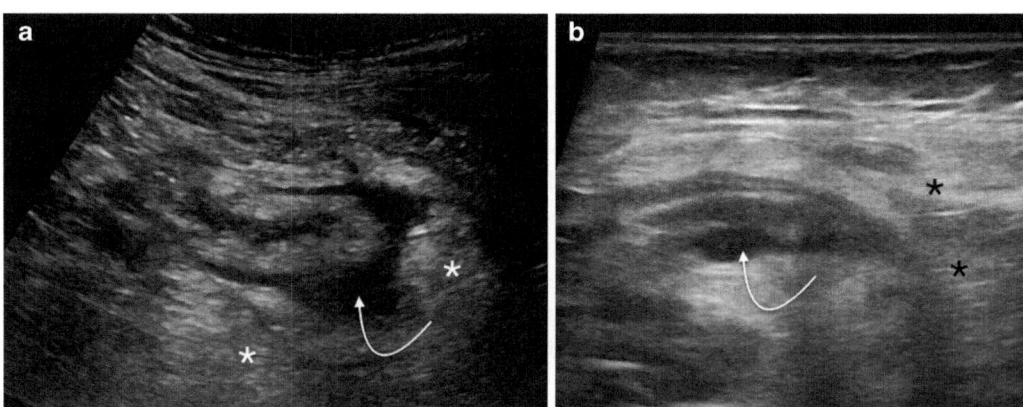

Fig. 17.1 US showing two different cases of acute appendicitis. Note the thickened appendix with surrounding fluid (**a, b,** curved arrows) and hyper-echoic fat due to inflammation (**a, b,** asterisks)

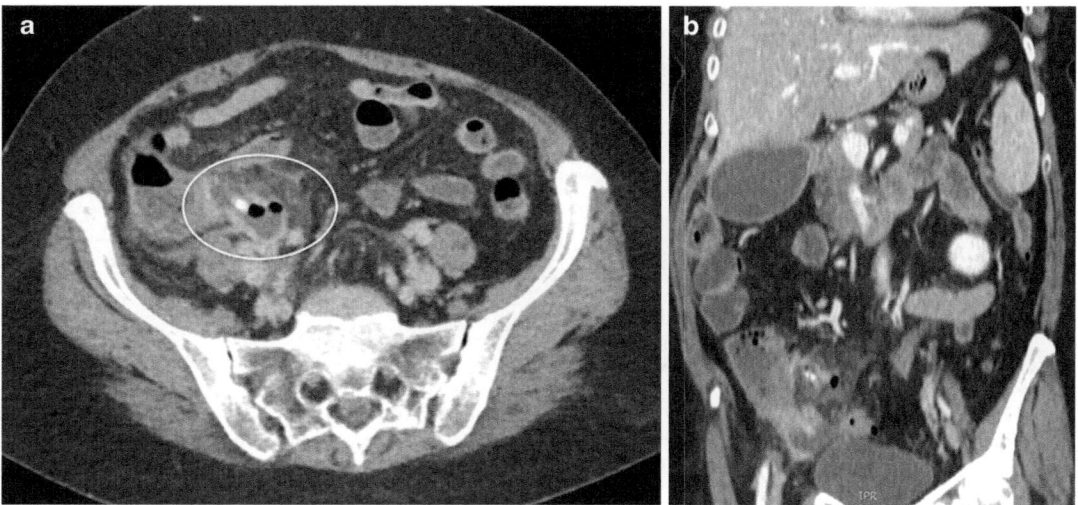

Fig. 17.2 Female, 64 years old, presenting with acute abdominal pain in the right iliac fossa. Fluid distended appendix with wall discontinuity and adjacent abscess consistent with a complicated appendicitis (**a**, circle; **b**, coronal view)

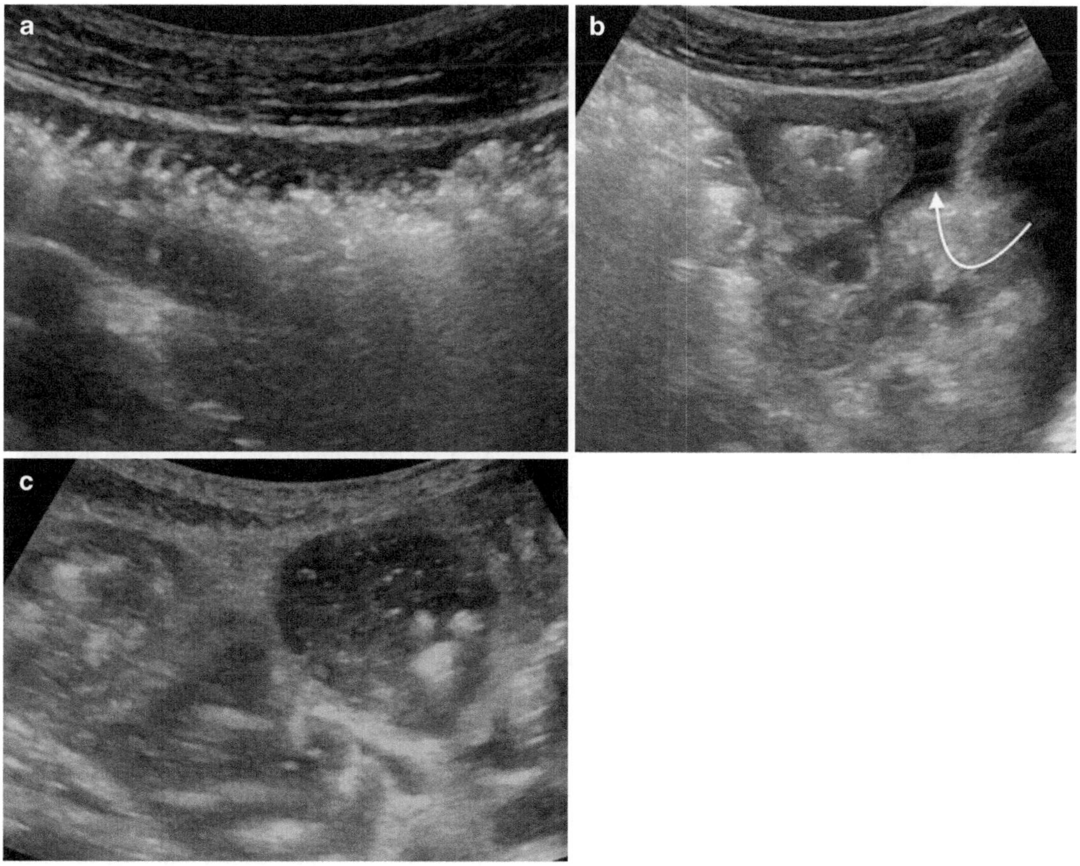

Fig. 17.3 Male, 35 years old, presenting with acute abdominal pain and bowel obstruction. US demonstrate an extensive inflammatory involvement of the small bowel with wall thickening (**a**) and perivisceral fluid (**b**, arrow). The proximal loop are dilated with increased representation of conniventes valves (**c**)

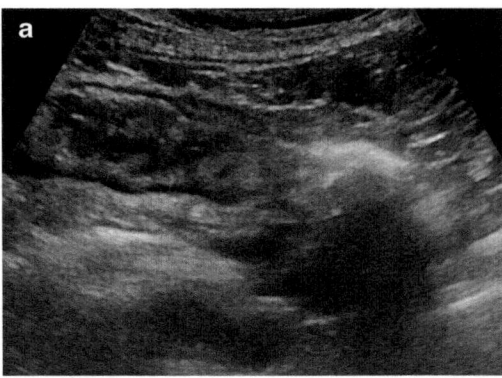 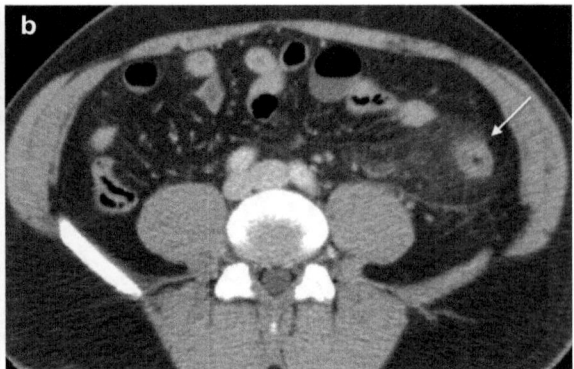

Fig. 17.4 Male, 52 years old, presenting with acute abdominal pain and constipation. US demonstrate an inflammatory involvement of the descending-sigmoid colon with edematous thickening of the bowel wall and hyper-echoic aspect of the surrounding fat (**a**). CT shows colonic wall thickening with pericolic stranding (**b**, arrow)

study with one or two acquisitions after the administration of the iv cm obtaining an evaluation on both arterial and portal venous phases. The pre-contrast images may be obtained by subtraction with the new available CT scanner. Coronal and/or sagittal multiplanar reconstructions (MPR) are helpful to identify the transition point and to assess for evidence of a volvulus or closed-loop obstruction [11].

The CT findings to be investigated in the clinical suspicion of intestinal obstruction are:

– Loop. The loop caliber is the first to change with a progressive increase in the loops proximal to the obstruction with gas-fluid mixed stasis and collapse of the loops distal to the obstruction.

  This helps in the identification of the *transition point*, that is, the site where the variation in caliber is observed due to the presence of the obstructive cause. When identified, it should always be indicated as it helps in the surgical approach. The appearance of the transition point may change depending on the cause. On CT scans, the adhesion is generally not identified. Their presence is inferred when there is an abrupt transition from dilated to collapsed bowel without an identifiable cause at the transition zone (Fig. 17.5, Video 17.2). As adhesions compress the bowel extrinsically, they often cause an abrupt tapering or "beak" at the site of obstruction [11]. Signs of bowel obstruction due to hernia are the presence of dilated bowel up to the hernia sac followed by decompressed bowel exiting from the sac (Fig. 17.6, Video 17.3). In bowel obstruction due to intestinal cancer, more common in the large bowel, loop findings consist in short-segment colonic wall thickening or an enhancing soft-tissue mass centered in the colon that narrows the colonic lumen with or without findings of ischemia and perforation [8] (Fig. 17.7, Video 17.4). In patients with known primary tumors and SBO, the most likely cause is peritoneal carcinomatosis either involving bowel or peritoneum. Closed-loop obstruction implies a segment of bowel that is obstructed at two points along its course; in this condition, the sites of obstruction are adjacent to each other, often the result of a single constricting lesion that occludes the bowel and affects adjacent mesentery. The CT findings of a closed-loop obstruction depend in part on the orientation of the loop relative to the plane of imaging. If the loop is within the plane of imaging, the lesions often appear as a "U," "C," or "coffee bean" configuration.

Normal wall thickness of the bowel loops usually does not exceed 2 mm; an increase in the parietal thickness may be indicative of an impairment of the venous drainage or of the arterial supply, and therefore it must be carefully researched and reported. Furthermore, it is important to evaluate the enhancement of the wall, which will appear reduced when the arte-

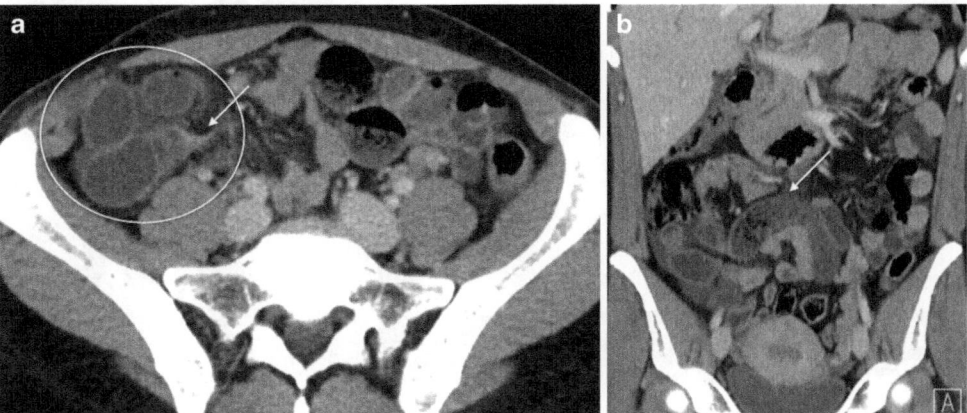

Fig. 17.5 Female, 37 years old, appendectomy 3 years before, presenting with acute abdominal pain in right iliac fossa. There is a cluster of fluid distended small bowel loops in the right iliac fossa showing thickened bowel walls with decreased enhancement (**a**, circle), consistent with closed-loop obstruction complicated with ischemic changes due to adhesions. Note the presence of intraluminal fecaloid content (**b**, arrow) in the dilated bowel loops proximal to the obstruction

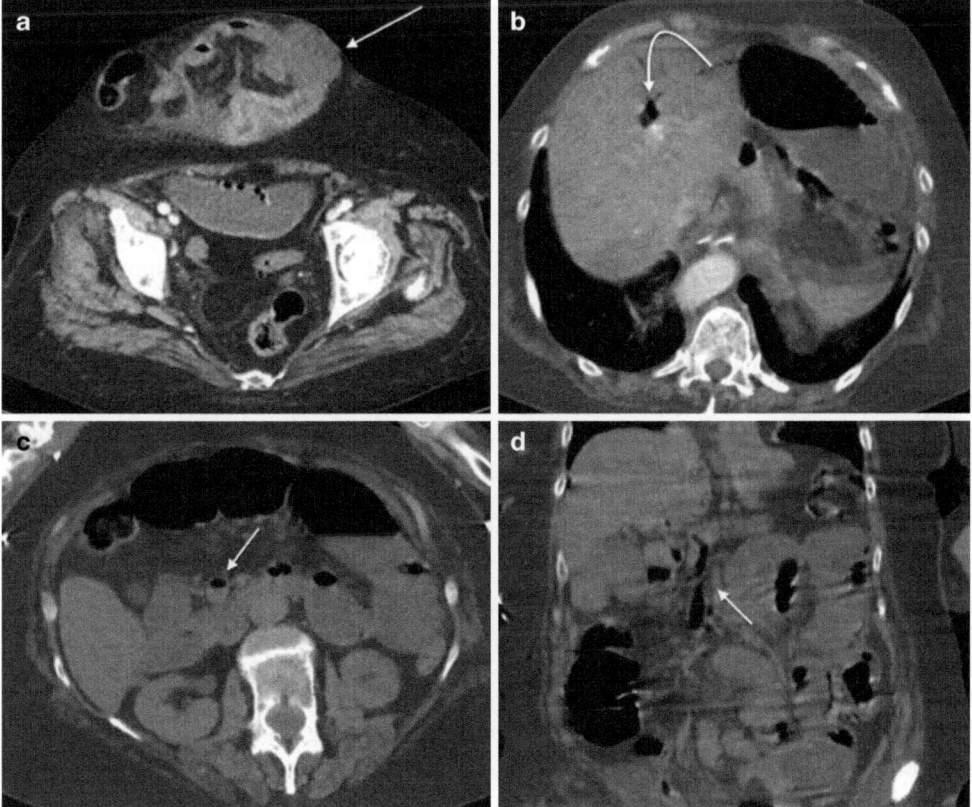

Fig. 17.6 Female, 65 years old, presenting with incarcerated laparocele (**a**, arrow). There is no enhancement in the herniated loops (**a**, arrow) with small amount of fluid in the herniated sac. Note also the presence of gas within the superior mesenteric vein (**c, d** straight arrow) and in intrahepatic portal system (**b**, curved arrow) in keeping with pneumatosis

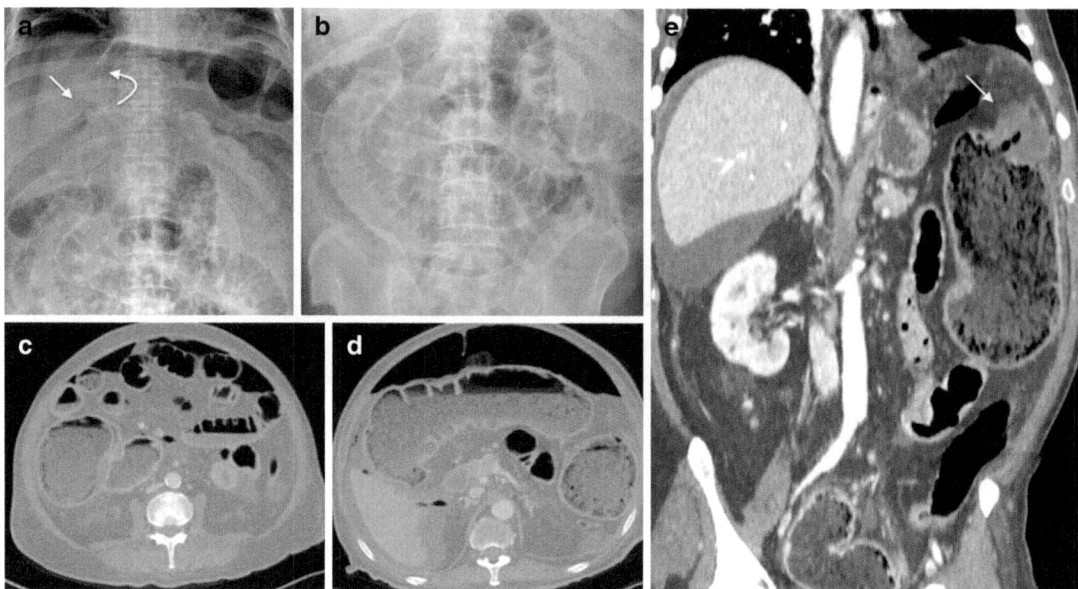

Fig. 17.7 Male, 65 years old, presenting with diffuse abdominal pain, swelling, and fever. Plain film (**a**, **b**) shows large pneumoperitoneum with "Doge cap sign" (**a**, straight arrow), the "bright liver sign," the "falciform ligament sign" (**a**, curved arrow), and the "Rigler sign"(**b**). Contrast-enhanced CT images (**c**, **d**, **e**) confirm pneumoperitoneum and demonstrate dolichocolon with abnormal lumen distension and tortuosity due to an obstructing stenotizing mass of the splenic flexure (**e**, arrow)

rial vascular supply is compromised (Fig. 17.7, Video 17.4 and Fig. 17.8, Video 17.5) or increased and persistent if there is an impairment of the venous drainage [9] and the presence of pneumatosis with or without associated gas in mesenteric or portal veins [11] (Fig. 17.6, Video 17.3).

- Mesentery. The mesentery changes its appearance depending on its involvement. It will appear transparent with preserved vascular appearance in the initial phases of the mechanical ileus and when an endoluminal obstruction occurs (Fig. 17.9, Video 17.6); otherwise it assumes a congested appearance with tortuosity of the vessels in the complicated mechanical ileus and particularly in strangulation, volvulus, or closed-loop mechanisms [9, 24–26].
- Vessels. The detection of an altered course of the main mesenteric vessels may help in the identification of an abnormal disposition of the intestinal loops as it happens in internal hernia or volvulus; the torsion of the loop-mesentery complex generates the so-called whirl sign; it consists in the appearance of spiraled loops of collapsed bowel with enhancing engorged ves-

sels radiating from the twisted bowel [8] (Fig. 17.10, Video 17.7). The occurrence of the volvulus does not necessarily imply the strangulation of the vascular pedicle, which occurs only if the obstruction is tightened [27].

- Cavity. Depending on both the mechanism and the entity of the occlusive state, it is possible to detect any fluid effusion in the peritoneal cavity, simple mechanical ileus, to detect a variable amount of fluid, decompensated mechanic ileus, or a larger quantity with hematic components in complicated mechanic ileus. If perforation occurs, peritoneal free air will be also detected [9, 28, 29].

17.1.4 Magnetic Resonance

MR is playing an increasing role in the emergency setting, both in primary diagnosis and for differential diagnosis purposes.

Its properties as high-resolution, multiparametric imaging and multiplanar capability, in the absence of ionizing radiations, are the major advantages of MR. Gastrointestinal peristalsis

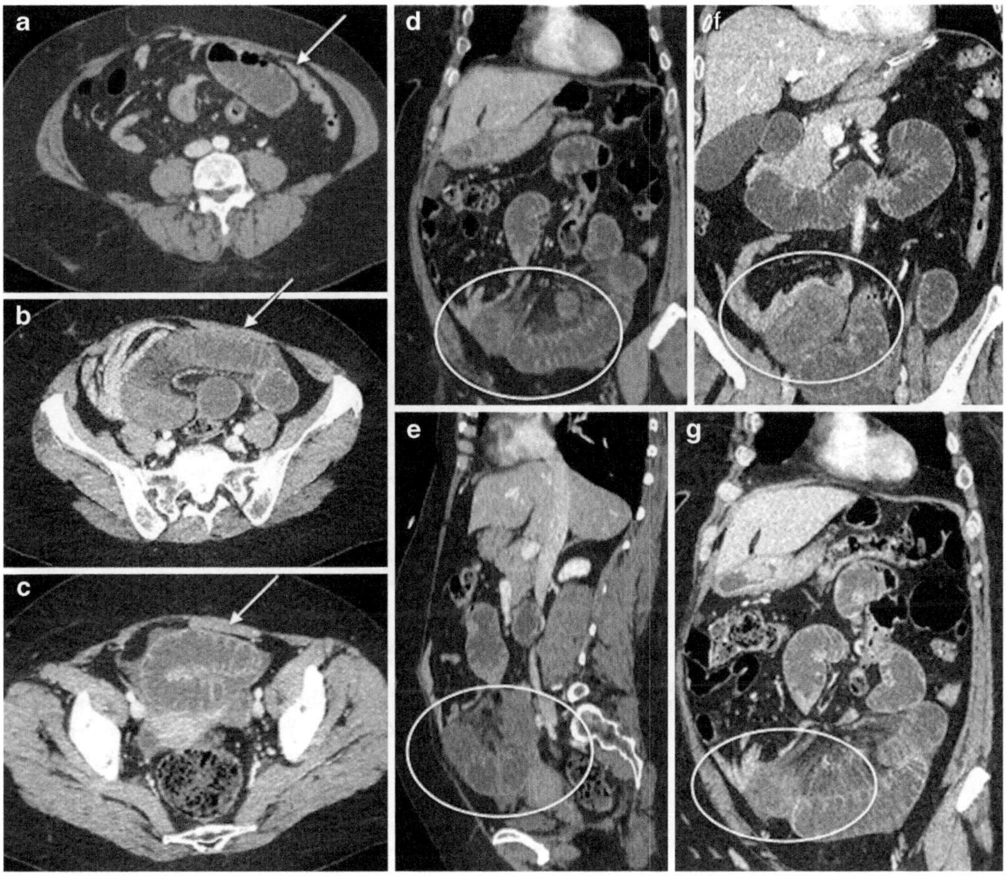

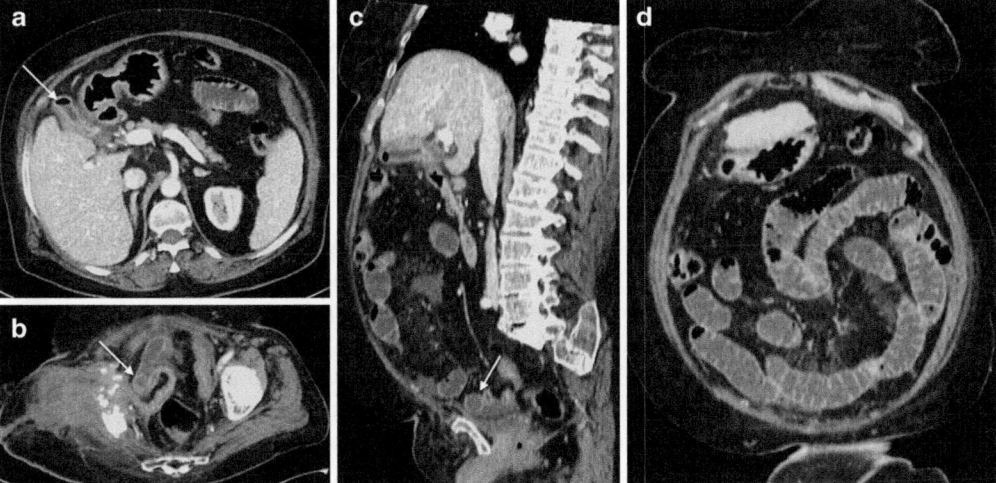

Fig. 17.8 Female, 57 years old, presenting with acute abdominal pain and previous history of right hemicolectomy. Contrast-enhanced CT images show dilated small bowel loops with multiple valvulae conniventes in keeping with obstruction (**a**, **b**, **c**, arrows). Note also a decreased wall enhancement due to ischemic bowel changes (**d**, **e**, **f**, **g**, circles)

Fig. 17.9 Female, 78 years old, presenting with acute abdominal pain, biliary vomiting, and previous history of cholelithiasis. The gallbladder shows thickened walls and air bubbles in its lumen (**a**, arrow). A gallstone in the small bowel lumen is shown (**b**, **c** arrows) which determines dilation of the proximal bowel loops with an increased representation of conniventes valvulae (**d**) consistent with mechanical ileum (gallstone ileus)

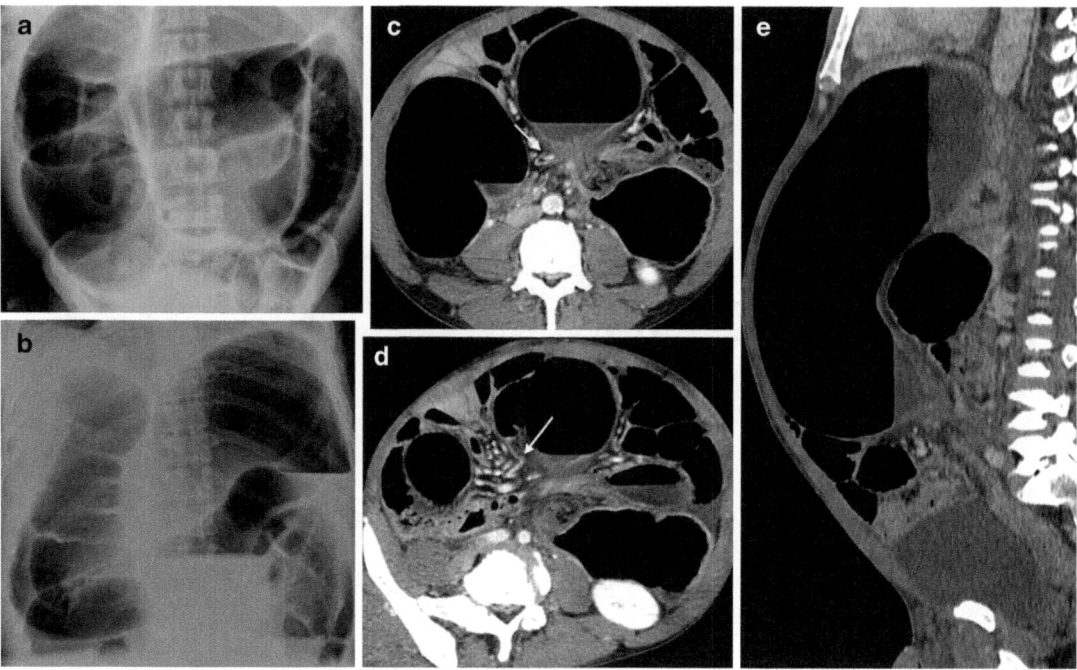

Fig. 17.10 Male, 65 years old, presenting with acute abdominal pain and abdominal distension. Plain film in supine (**a**) and upright (**b**) position show abnormal dilated colonic loops with large air-fluid levels. Contrast-enhanced CT (**c**, **d**, **e**) shows twisted mesenteric vessel (**c**, **d**, arrows) and sigmoid narrowing due to colonic volvulus

may be considered a limit, but the availability of fast MR sequences allows to obtain an accurate depiction of many acute gastrointestinal conditions.

MR plays a particular role in women in child-bearing age, in patients who already undergone a significant radiation dose due to their underlying pathological conditions, in infants, and pregnant women.

According to the literature data, MRI has a high sensitivity (95%) and specificity (100%) in detecting bowel obstruction, and the site responsible for the obstruction can be accurately depicted up to 92.6% of cases [30].

17.2 Bowel Perforations

Perforation of the alimentary tract is a surgical emergency and life-threatening condition, requiring a prompt diagnosis to address a tailored surgical management [31]. In the assessment of patients with clinical suspicion of perforation,

imaging plays a major role, not only in confirming or excluding the perforation but also in defining its level and etiology [32, 33]. This information is essential to plan the right surgical approach. Clinical evaluation may be unreliable in such cases and often difficult, as symptoms rely on the cause and the site of the perforation, so they are extremely variable, especially in the early stage. The most common symptom is acute abdominal pain, which is persistent, progressive, and unremitting, initially located in the site of perforation and then diffuse, poorly localized, expression of a peritonitic status ("acute abdomen") [34, 35]. Associated symptoms include fever, nausea, and vomiting [36]. Alimentary tract perforations recognize different etiology: spontaneous, traumatic, or iatrogenic. In supramesocolic tract, the most frequent site of perforation is gastroduodenal, and the peptic ulcers are the main cause [31, 32, 35, 37, 38]; other etiologies are iatrogenic, neoplastic, and traumatic (penetrating or blunt), for example, in a blunt trauma, perforation may be caused by a sudden increase in intra-abdominal pressure in an over-filled bowel lumen [39, 40]. In sottomesocolic tract the most frequent site of perforation is the colon, with diverticular and neoplastic disease as major etiologies, while the small bowel perforations are more often inflammatory, infectious, and ischemic [31, 41–45]. Surgery represents the treatment of choice, and, if delayed, there is a high probability of sepsis and multi-organ failure with a mortality reaching 30% of cases [31, 46]. Diagnostic imaging allows the radiologists to determine the presence of the perforation even in early stages addressing the best surgical approach. Abdominal radiograph remains the first imaging modality requested in the emergency department, although its sensitivity may be low in the early stages. US and CT offer more panoramic and specific informations becoming necessary in the diagnostic workup of patients with acute abdominal pain. MR is not suggested in the clinical suspicion of bowel perforation, but it may be useful in the differential diagnosis of acute abdominal pain in children, in young female, and in pregnant patients [33].

17.2.1 Abdominal Radiograph

As mentioned above, in the assessment of patients who present with acute abdominal pain to the emergency department, abdominal radiograph is still now the most frequently requested examination performed as initial imaging, as it is cost-effective, widely available, and easily reported [47]. However, the American College of Radiology (ACR) appropriateness criteria [48] suggest the use of enhanced CT of the abdomen and pelvis as the most appropriate examination for patients with fever, nonlocalized abdominal pain, and no recent surgery [20, 34, 49–51] as plain radiography presents low sensitivity and specificity in the detection of intraperitoneal gas with reported specificity ranging from 50 to 89% according to different authors [35, 52, 53]. Moreover, the site of perforation is never depicted on plain films, and this information is crucial to guide the surgeon to the best approach. Furthermore, it is important to consider that a

hollow viscus may be perforated even in the absence of pneumoperitoneum if filled with fluid or if perforation is "covered" by the adjacent mesenteric fat. Abdominal radiograph depends on a rigorous technique and is not always possible to correctly perform it in bedridden patients. Even if some investigators [54] have shown that on upright chest film it is possible to detect as little as 1 ml of gas below the right hemidiaphragm [55], in critically ill patients it is not possible to perform an upright acquisition, and the only supine abdominal radiograph can detect only a large amount of free air, and so, in the early phases, perforation may be overlooked [49]. Small amount of free air may be obscured on upright abdominal radiographs as the X-ray beam is centered on the mid-abdomen with high exposure, so abdominal radiograph needs to be integrated with chest radiograph in posteroanterior and latero-lateral projections. Small air collection may be demonstrated on lateral chest radiograph as the long axis of X-ray beam can depict air trapped anterior to the liver [35, 49, 55–57].

In the era of pre-CT, a lot of signs on upright and supine plain film have been individuated to help radiologists in the difficult diagnosis of free air in the abdomen [47, 58, 59]. Briefly, a summary of these signs is reported as they become crucial in some cases. The most famous and known sign on upright posteroanterior chest radiography is a translucent crescent area below the diaphragm (Fig. 17.11, Video 17.8); different signs have been also described on supine abdominal radiograph as free peritoneal air may present various shapes and sizes.

These free air signs can be categorized into four groups: bowel-related signs, right upper quadrant signs, peritoneal ligament-related signs, and other signs [47, 60].

Bowel-related signs include the following:

- The Rigler sign, also known as the bas-relief sign or the double-wall sign on a supine abdomen plain film; in the presence of a large amount of free air, it becomes possible to visualize both sides of the bowel wall and to distinctly appreciate the bowel loops as separated from each other [61] (Fig. 17.7).

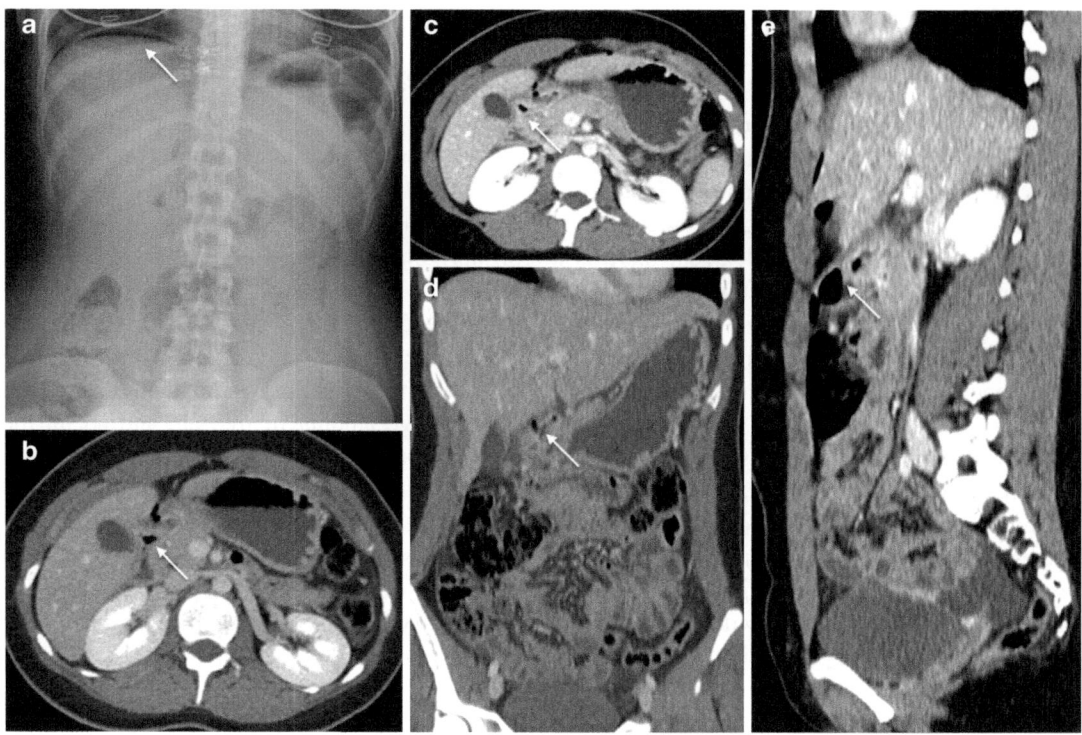

Fig. 17.11 Female, 49 years old, presenting with abdominal pain in mesogastrium. Plain film shows air under the right hemidiaphragmatic dome (**a**, arrow). Contrast-enhanced CT images confirm the presence of pneumoperitoneum, due to perforation of the ventral wall of the first duodenal loop (**b, c, d, e**, arrows)

- Triangle sign is a triangular radiolucency created from free intraperitoneal air accumulation among three contiguous bowel loops or two bowel loops and the parietal peritoneum [62].

Right upper quadrant signs include the following:

- Hyperlucent liver sign is visible on the supine radiographs when free gas covers anteriorly the ventral hepatic surface replacing the brightness of the hepatic shadow [62] (Fig. 17.7).
- Fissure for ligamentum teres sign refers to an elongated hyperlucent area reflecting the free air entrapped within the fissure for the ligamentum teres [63].
- The visible gallbladder refers to a hyperlucent gallbladder due to the surrounding free air on supine abdominal radiograph [64].

- Doge cap sign is a triangle-shaped right translucent area reflecting free air accumulated in Morison pouch on supine abdominal films [62, 65] (Fig. 17.7).
- Hepatic edge sign is a visible liver hyperlucent contour saucer or cigar shaped created from free air collected in the subhepatic space [62, 66].
- Dolphin sign. The undersurface of the long costal muscle slips of the diaphragm that indented the adjacent air-filled space in the right upper quadrant on supine films is a sign of pneumoperitoneum [67].

Peritoneal ligament-related signs include the following:

- Falciform ligament sign is created from the intraperitoneal free air outlining the falciform ligament that appears as a hyperlucent linear density within the right upper abdomen [62, 68] (Fig. 17.7).

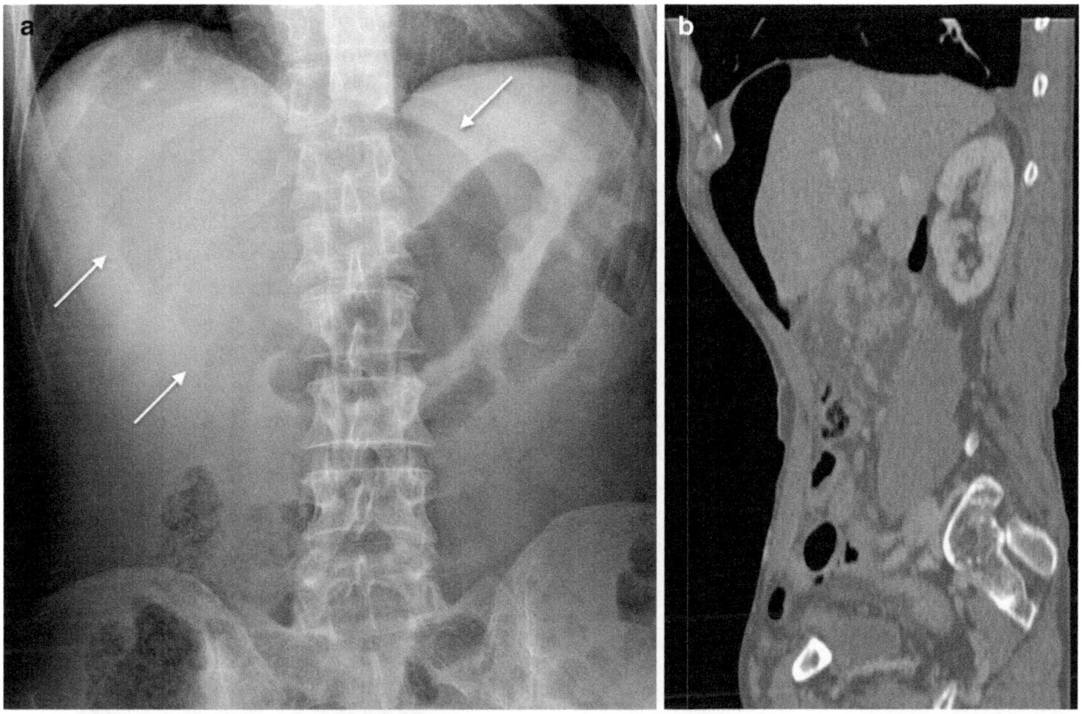

Fig. 17.12 Male, 40 years old, presenting with acute abdominal pain. Plain film (**a**) demonstrates an area or lucency in the upper abdominal quadrant with a shape on an American football ("football sign") (arrows). CT with MPR reconstruction in sagittal view (**b**) confirm the plain film finding and allow to depict the site of perforation located at the pyloroduodenal junction

- Extrahepatic ligamentum teres sign refers to an elongated translucent image outlined from free air entrapped in the ligament teres [69].
- The "inverted V" sign is created by free air contouring the lateral umbilical ligaments in the lower abdomen [60].
- Urachus sign is a visible midline lucent urachus created by free air in the lower abdomen [70].
- The transverse mesocolon and root of small bowel mesentery signs are visible when free air outlines the transverse mesocolon and the root of the small bowel mesentery on plain abdominal radiographs obtained in the supine and in the prone position [71].
- The mesoappendix sign is visible when there is a large amount of free air creating a visible linear mesoappendix directed from the cecum to the middle of abdomen on the supine radiograph.

Other signs of pneumoperitoneum are the following:

- Football sign is visible on supine radiograph as a large oval radiolucent with the shape of an American football producing a sharp interface with the parietal peritoneum [72, 73] (Fig. 17.12, Video 17.9).
- Cupola sign is visible as an arcuate lucency anterior to the lower thoracic spine and projecting lower to the heart on supine radiograph [74].
- Left-sided anterior superior oval sign was described by Chiu et al. [60] as single or multiple oval, round, or pear-shaped free air projected over the left upper quadrant abdomen.
- Subphrenic radiolucency is visible on the supine chest radiographs as a lucent area beneath the diaphragm, right or left sided [60].
- Focal radiolucency is a sign of exclusion, when the free air creates abnormal gas pattern on the supine films without fitting any sign mentioned above [60].

Even if it is difficult, sometime it is possible to differentiate pneumoperitoneum from pneumoretroperitoneum with plain film: according to some AA., retroperitoneal air is usually crescentic, with curvilinear upper and lower borders positioned more inferiorly and laterally with respect to intraperitoneal free air that usually rises to the peak of the diaphragmatic dome [35, 75]. Furthermore, free air in the retroperitoneum may assume an aspect similar to "breadcrumb" due to its diffusion in the retroperitoneal fat [59] (Fig. 17.13, Video 17.10). Another sign indicative of pneumoretroperitoneum on supine abdominal radiographs is the lack of left psoas muscle shadow [59, 76].

A rare cause of perforation is ingestion of foreign bodies; in this suspicion plain film is the first examination required that allows not only to identify free air but also to detect the presence and the site of radiopaque foreign body [75].

With the advent of CT, patients with positive finding in plain films or with high suspicion of bowel perforation undergo CT with iv cm administration to clarify the site and the etiology of perforation [77, 78].

The use of plain film with oral contrast administration has recently increased particularly in the evaluation and follow-up of patients who underwent bariatric surgery (gastric bypass and sleeve

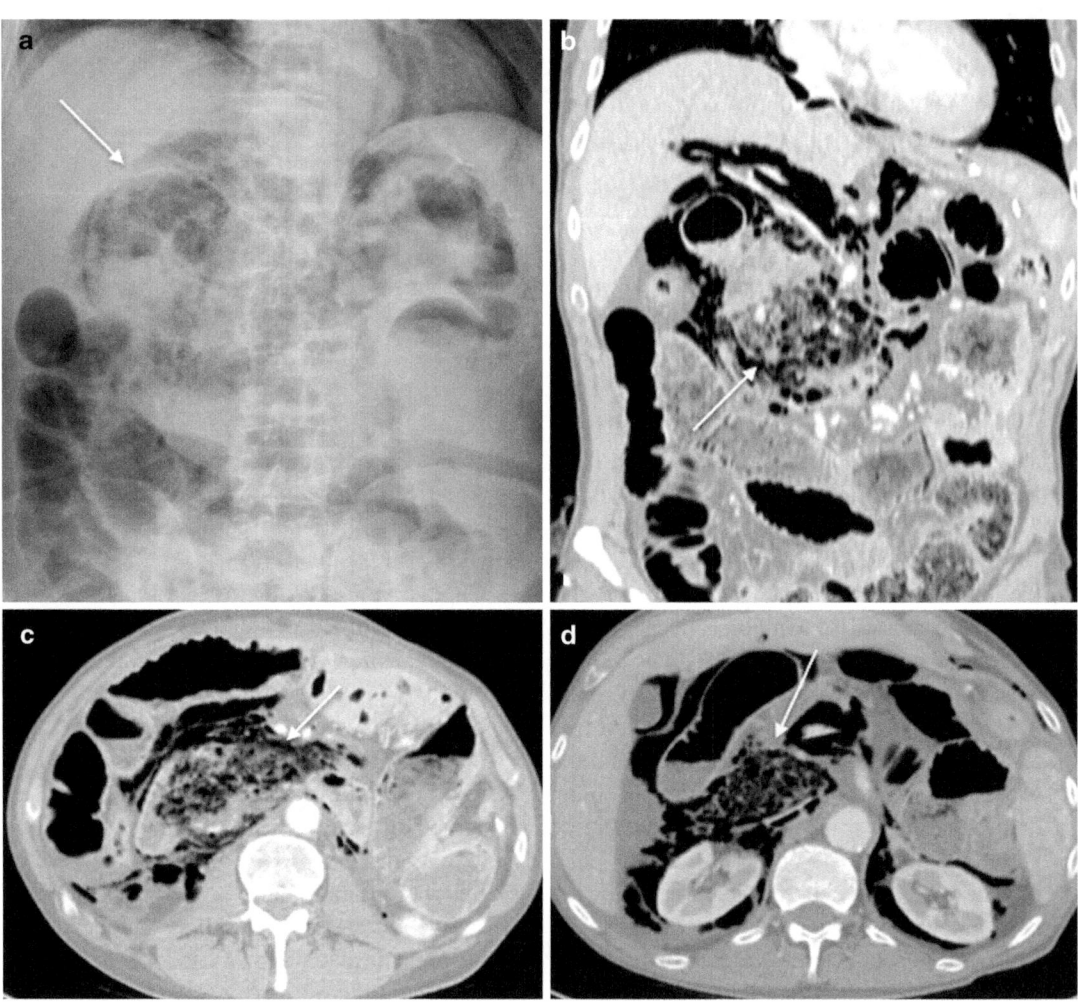

Fig. 17.13 Male, 63 year old, complaining for abdominal pain 3 days after gastrectomy. There is a "dirty mass" around the III portion of the duodenum (**a, b, c, d**, arrows).

Note also massive free air in the retro- and intraperitoneal spaces tracking into the mediastinum

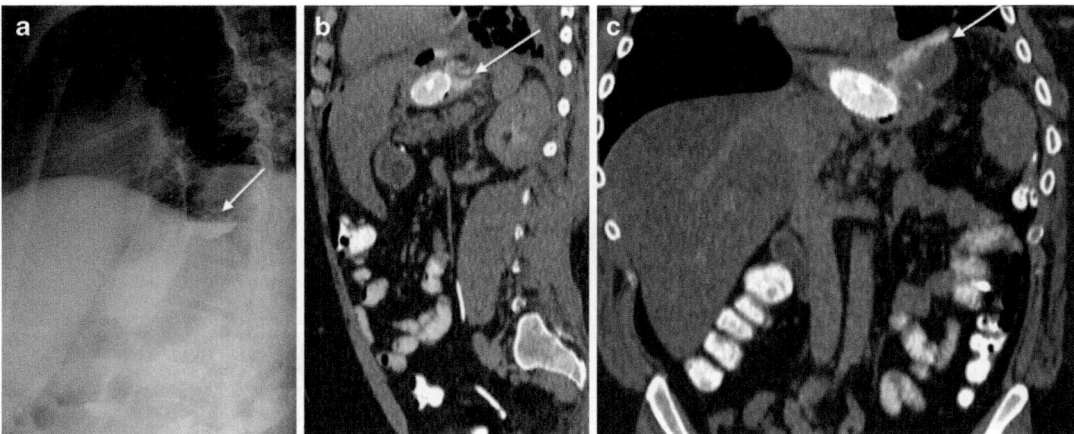

Fig. 17.14 Male, 33 years old, with previous history of gastric bypass 5 months before an esophageal endoprosthesis. There are multiple small air bubbles in the upper abdominal cavity and an extravasation of oral contrast at the level of the anastomosis in the surrounding tissue, due to dehiscence (**a, b, c,** arrows)

gastrectomy) for radiation dose-related issue. It may allow to detect oral contrast extravasation, dehiscence, or fistulas (Fig. 17.14, Video 17.11). However, sometimes this study is poor for different reasons (patient's habitus, noncooperative patients, plain films, and clinical evidence correlation); CT results are more useful and accurate in detecting complications of bowel or gastric wall (the size and location of anastomotic or staple line dehiscence) (Fig. 17.14, Video 17.11) and surrounding tissue (abscess cavity) or guiding percutaneous drainage of abscess collection.

17.2.2   Abdominal Ultrasound

US is routinely performed to investigate patients with abdominal pain and, thanks to the absence of ionizing radiations, the low cost, and its availability, it is the first imaging modality [79].

US examination allows the radiologist to examine the entire abdominal cavity, including bowel and mesentery. US has emerged as a useful technique also to study patients with suspicion of pneumoperitoneum; in fact, an expert radiologist can quickly identify also the artifacts due to free intra-abdominal air eventually present [80, 81] (Fig. 17.15).

Linear array transducers (10–12 MHz) may be more sensitive than convex transducers (2–5 MHz) to detect intraperitoneal free air [81]. With patient in the supine position and slightly elevated chest (10–20° inclination) or in a semilateral decubitus position, the best place to look for pneumoperitoneum is in the right hypochondrium, superficial to the liver [82].

Direct and indirect signs were described.

US direct signs of pneumoperitoneum are [81]:

- Strong reverberation anterior to the liver surface, represented by echogenic lines or spots with comet-tail reverberation artifacts adjacent to the abdominal wall; this sign is the result of air resistance and impermeability to ultrasound waves, making it a strong reflector, which hides the information below.
- Shifting phenomenon, consisting in the "shifting" of free air in the abdominal cavity, particularly in the space between the peritoneum and liver or in the hepatorenal space, after repositioning the patient on the left semilateral decubitus; the reverberation anterior to the liver surface alone is not specific for pneumoperitoneum if it is not possible to identify the shifting phenomenon.

As some pathological conditions can mimic the shifting phenomenon, Karahan and colleagues suggested an alternative method for the US detection of pneumoperitoneum: once the reverberation artifact is visible, it becomes

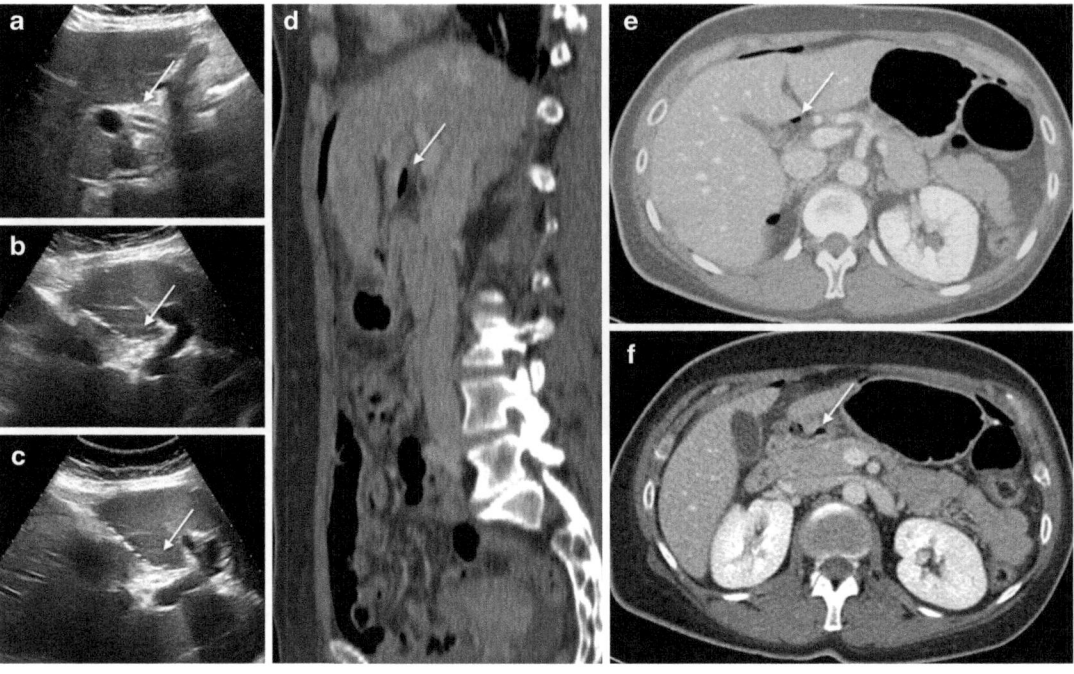

Fig. 17.15 Female, 46 years old, presenting with acute pain in the upper abdominal quadrants. US shows free air bubbles in the lesser sac (**a**, **b**, **c**, arrows). Contrast-enhanced CT confirms free air in the lesser sac and above the right liver (**d**, **e**, **f**, arrows), due to a defect of the ventral wall of the duodenal bulb (Video 17.12)

much less prominent after slight pressure with the probe on the abdominal wall, with patient in supine position, due to displacement of the free intraperitoneal air in other sites of the peritoneal cavity. When the pressure on the probe decreases, the free gas returns to the region anterior to the liver, and the reverberation artifact becomes more prominent.

This is the "scissors maneuver" because on real time, the repetition of this maneuver appears like the opening and closing of scissors on US images [75, 83].

- Enhanced peritoneal stripe allows to differentiate free intraperitoneal air from intraluminal bowel gas.

US indirect signs of pneumoperitoneum are:

- Presence of intraperitoneal free fluid
- Decreased bowel motility in GI perforation due to peritonitis leading to paralytic ileus with gas-fluid stasis and resulting in reduction of intestinal peristalsis [20]

In patients with suspected GI perforation and localized pain, US may help in identifying the site of the perforation. "Inflamed fat" next to a GI tract is one of the hallmarks of bowel perforation because it represents the defense mechanism of the omentum and mesentery to stop the bowel perforation; it appears as an hyperechoic area surrounding the affected site of perforation. However, this finding may be present in a lot of inflammatory conditions of alimentary tract, and so it is high sensitive but low specific for bowel perforation (Fig. 17.1).

An expert radiologist should focalize his attention on specific anatomical sites if there is high suspicion for perforation; for example, in case of gastroduodenal perforation, it is possible to identify little bubbles of air in the lesser omentum (Fig. 17.15). Moreover US can evaluate the bowel movements and can detect the presence of intraperitoneal free fluid.

In GI perforation due to foreign bodies, US may be a useful modality for the identification of cause and site; foreign bodies appear as a linear echogenic structure with or without posterior acoustic shadow, embedded in a large reactive inflammatory mass [75].

17.2.3 Computed Tomography

CT is considered the most valuable imaging technique for detecting the presence, site, and cause of alimentary tract perforations [32, 84].

CT sensitivity and specificity is high for gastrointestinal perforation, ranging between 80 and 100 % [85].

It usually constitutes the second-line imaging approach, following plain radiograph and abdominal US, because of its costs, availability, and ionizing exposure [86], except for patients presenting to the emergency department with acute abdomen for whom CT constitutes the best imaging modality approach [48].

CT protocol is the same as adopted and described for bowel obstruction, and MPR images are helpful to individuate the affected bowel segment and the distribution of air bubbles and free air.

CT diagnosis of gastrointestinal perforation is based on direct CT findings, as presence of extraluminal air and discontinuity of the bowel wall, and on indirect CT findings, as bowel wall thickening, abnormal bowel wall enhancement, abscesses, and inflammatory mass or free fluid collection in the surrounding soft tissues adjacent to the bowel [87].

CT is highly sensitive for detection of extraluminal free air such as small free air bubbles, pneumoperitoneum, and/or pneumoretroperitoneum, in contrast to the low sensitivity of plain radiograph [32, 88]. Different width of HU window can be used: soft tissue to identify the discontinuity of the bowel wall and lung window to detect free air [62, 89].

In open perforation, distribution of free air obviously depends on patient position with free air bubbles located in antideclive position, generally in the anterosuperior part of the involved peritoneal recess, such as in the subphrenic spaces, around the liver, along the mesenteric folds, and in the peritoneal recesses of the pelvic cavity.

When there is a small amount of air, the presence of concentrated free air bubbles in close proximity to the bowel wall can correctly suggest the site of perforation with high sensitivity and specificity (Fig. 17.15, Video 17.12), also without a clear CT depiction of focal discontinuity of bowel wall [90].

The distribution of extraluminal free air depends on the site of perforation if intraperitoneal or retroperitoneal; therefore a good knowledge of the anatomy, particularly of the peritoneum folds, may help the radiologist to hypothesize the site of perforation, focusing the attention on a specific GI segment to find bowel wall discontinuity. In the perforation of the posterior wall of the stomach or of the duodenum, free air is located in the lesser sac (Fig. 17.15, Video 17.12); when perforation is in the duodenal bulb or stomach, free air is confined in the intrahepatic fissure or in the ligamentum teres.

In the small bowel and colon perforation, free air is generally located in mesenteric folds [75]. The presence of free air along portal vein is the most significant sign to differentiate upper from lower GI tract perforation because of the anatomical relationship between the portal tract and the gastric antrum or duodenal bulb [75]. In case of pneumoretroperitoneum, a perforation of the extraperitoneal gastrointestinal tracts should be suspected, such as descending and horizontal portions of duodenum (right anterior pararenal space), ascending (right anterior pararenal space) and descending colon (left anterior pararenal space), rectum (bilateral pneumoretroperitoneum) [91, 92], or also perforation of the sigmoid diverticula (left anterior-pararenal space) as a lot of these are localized in the extraperitoneal space [91, 92]. In the presence at the same time of intraperitoneal and extraperitoneal air, the perforation site is generally located in extraperitoneal structure [92].

Massive pneumoperitoneum with a large amount of free air in abdomen and pelvis is usually caused by gastroduodenal or colonic perforation. If the free air is present in supramesocolic space, the site of perforation is probably the small bowel, if free air is present only in the pelvis, the colon is the site of perforation [9–13]. However, the air distribution described above loses its power when too much time is elapsed after perforation or in presence of a massive amount of free air [93].

The detection of free air in the abdomen is highly suggestive for hollow viscus perforation, even if this sign is not pathognomonic; there are other causes of pneumoperitoneum and retroperitoneum, such as mechanical ventilation and pulmonary barotraumas, peritoneal lavage performed prior to CT, pneumothorax, chest injury, and entry of air via the female genital tract [94–96]. Bowel wall discontinuity, seen as a low-attenuating cleft that usually runs perpendicular to the bowel wall, is a pathognomonic image finding for bowel perforation because it represents the direct visualization of the perforation site [87, 88] (Fig. 17.16, Video 17.13). Because of the small size of the lesion, this finding is seen in less than 50% of the patients with GI tract perforation [90, 94]. CT with MPR can be helpful in identifying disconti-

nuity of the bowel wall, especially when the axial CT images are indeterminate [55, 97].

A further specific finding of alimentary tract perforations is the extraluminal leakage of oral contrast medium (Fig. 17.14). Oral contrast medium administration (diluted water-soluble iodinated solution) during CT exam is controversial; actually, when an extravasation of ingested contrast material is seen, this is considered diagnostic for bowel perforation with a high specificity in the diagnosis of the perforation site. On the other hand, the sensitivity varies from 19 to 42% [98], due to the rapid sealing of perforation sites, the supine position during the CT exam, and the decreased bowel motility (paralytic or adynamic ileus, with gas-fluid stasis) that interfere with the progression of oral contrast through the entire bowel; so, the absence of visible extravasation does not exclude a perforation. In addition, it is necessary a large quantity of oral contrast to opacify the entire alimentary tract, but patient with suspected perforation may not be able to cooperate

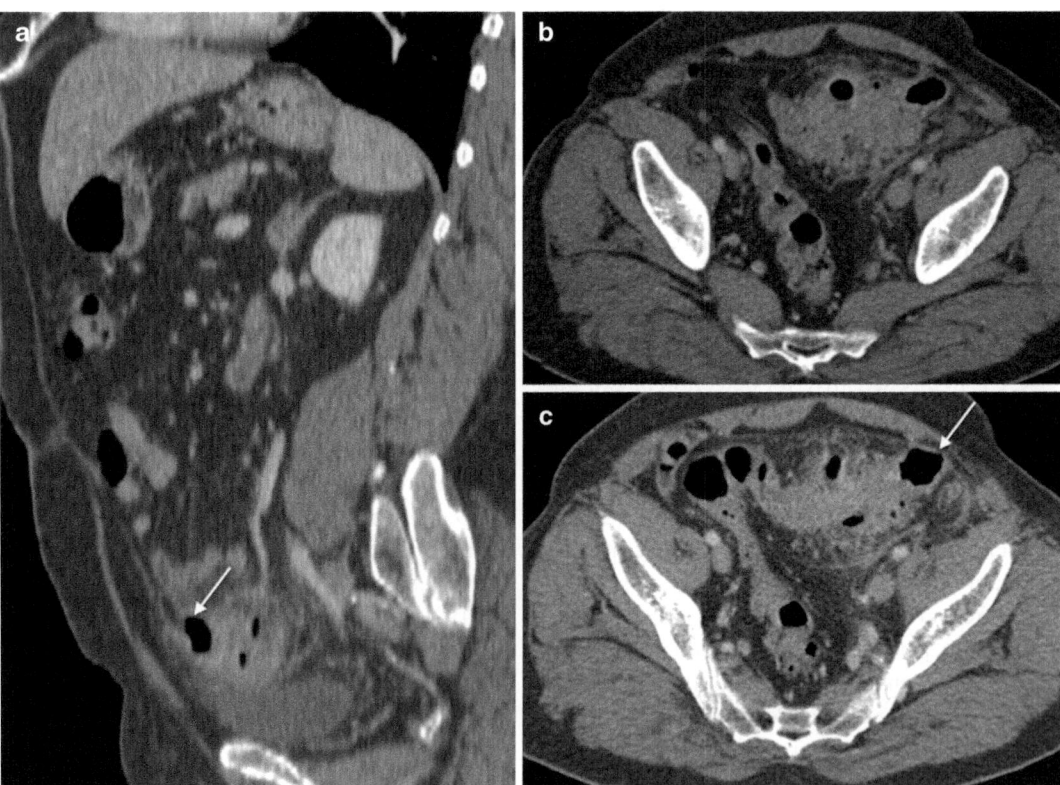

Fig. 17.16 Male, 34 years old, presenting with diffuse abdominal pain and rigid abdomen. Contrast-enhanced CT images in sagittal (**a**) and axial planes (**b, c**) show dif-fuse sigmoid diverticulitis with perivisceral free bubbles. Moreover wall discontinuity (**a, c** arrows) and perivisceral reaction are present

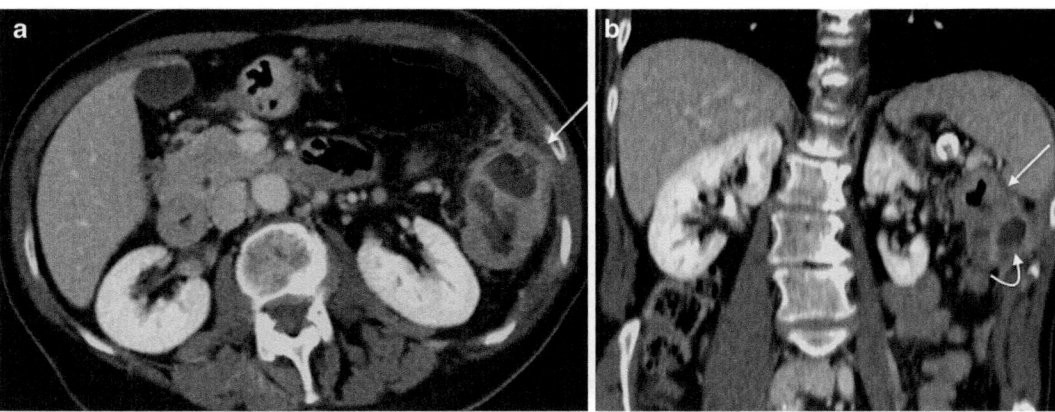

Fig. 17.17 Female, 68 years old, presenting with weight loss and fever. Contrast-enhanced CT images show a large colonic mass at the splenic flexure (**a**, **b**, straight arrows) with some peripheral low fluid hypodensities consistent with abscesses (**b**, curved arrow). These findings are keeping with a complicated colonic neoplasm

if they complain for pain, nausea, and/or vomiting [35, 84]. In our experience, oral contrast medium may be administered after the execution of CT exam with intravenous injection of contrast media (iodine) to confirm the clinical/radiological suspicion of gastroduodenal perforation in cases in which a previous CT examination resulted inconclusive.

CT allows to depict the so-called "covered perforations," consisting in little and self-limiting conditions characterized by minute air bubbles grouped contiguous to a bowel wall, usually associated with a limited amount of free peritoneal fluid. These findings can be associated with bowel wall alterations (bowel wall thickening, abnormal bowel wall enhancement) and perivisceral fat modifications (increased peripheral density of the infiltrated or inflamed surrounding fat tissue) (Fig. 17.17, Video 17.14) and may heal with conservative treatment or may evolve in abscess collections, demonstrated by a low-density unilocular or multilocular collection with air-fluid level or air bubbles, and in retro- or intraperitoneal free perforation (Fig. 17.18, Video 17.15 and Fig. 17.19, Video 17.16) [75].

Bowel wall thickening, abnormal bowel wall enhancement, abscess, and an inflammatory mass adjacent to the bowel are indirect CT findings of GI perforation and can be observed in open perforation or covered perforation, providing a correct diagnosis of perforation and its site of origin [55] (Fig. 17.20, Video 17.17). Fat tissue adjacent to the perforation site usually shows a focal or

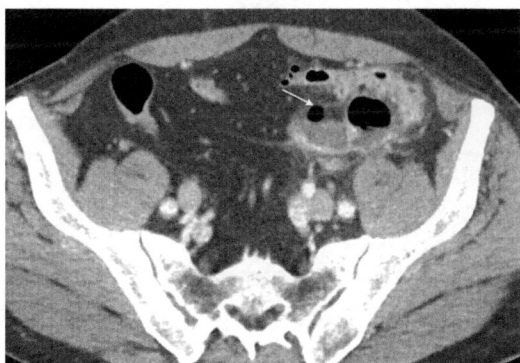

Fig. 17.18 Male, 71 years old, presenting with acute abdominal pain, fever, and diarrhea. Contrast-enhanced CT images show the presence of multiple diverticula connected to an abscess collection, referable to covered perforation (arrow). After few days, free air in the retroperitoneal space was detected (Video 17.15)

diffuse increase of attenuation called "dirty fat sign"; in colonic perforation it is possible to see a focal collection of extraluminal fecal matter containing small air bubbles, called "dirty mass," which is a specific finding of colonic perforation [99, 100] (Fig. 17.19, Video 17.16). Dirty mass is associated with fecal peritonitis (diffuse or localized dirty mass) and high risk of morbidity and mortality [101].

CT offers many advantages, as the possibility to study the whole gastrointestinal tract and to detect the site of perforation following carefully the described signs. In the last decades, CT has gained a pivotal role in the diagnosis of conditions

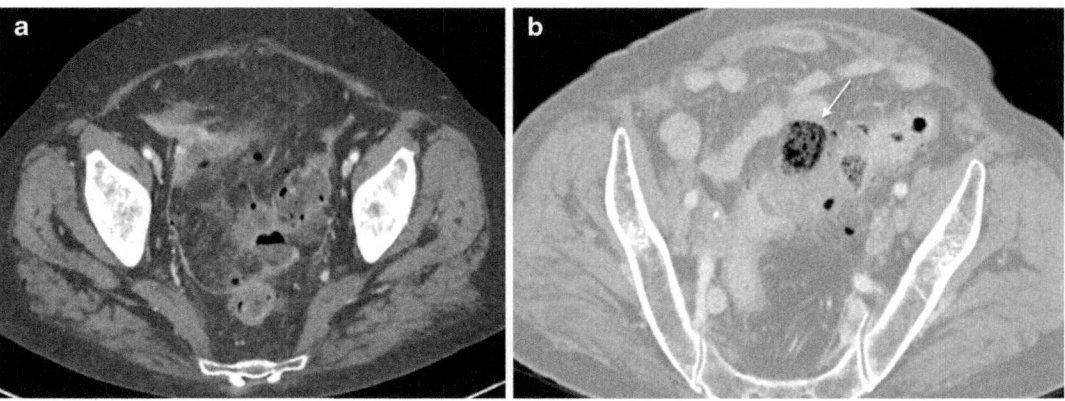

Fig. 17.19 Female, 86 years old, presenting with acute abdominal pain in the epigastrium and fever. Contrast-enhanced CT shows submucosal sigmoid thickening and multiple diverticula (**a**). Note the wall discontinuity with associated extraluminal dirty mass (**b**, arrow)

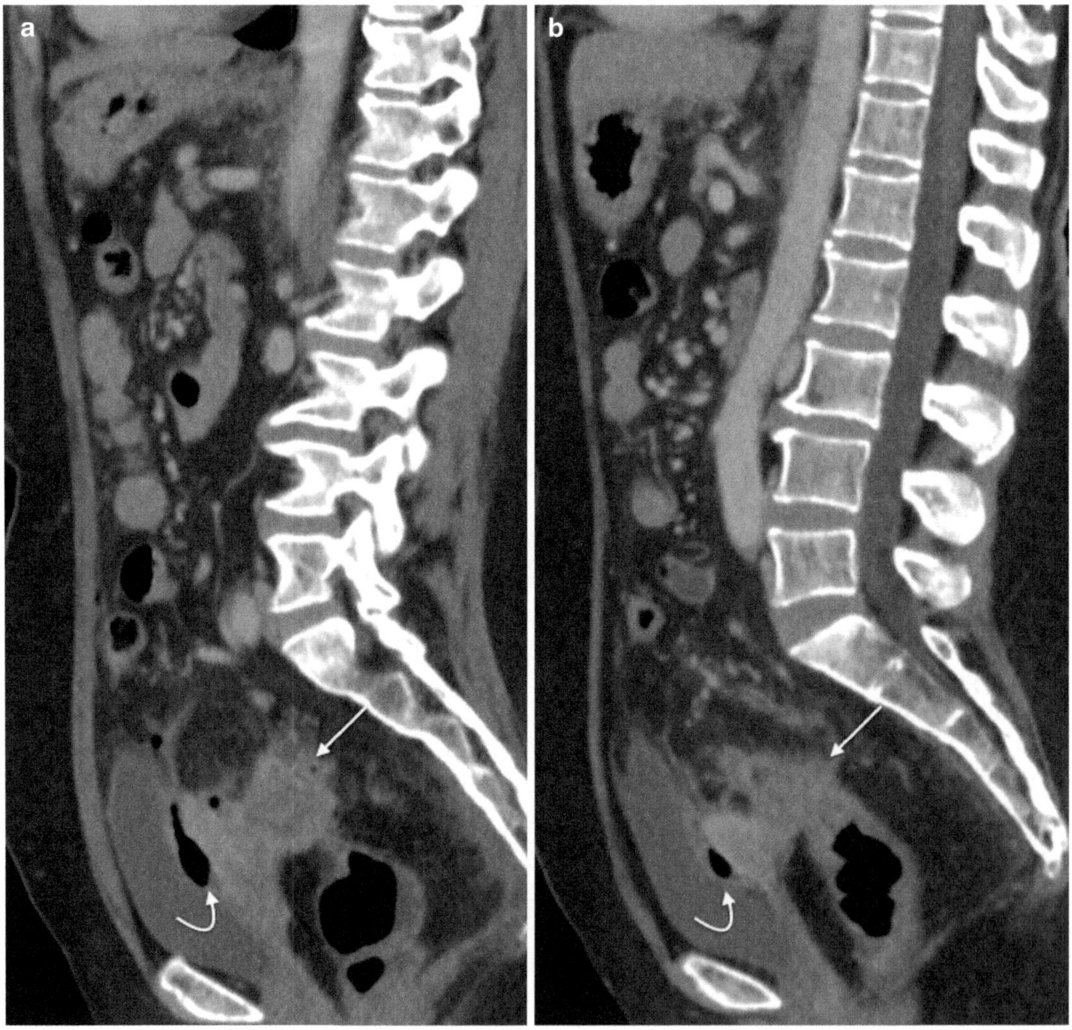

Fig. 17.20 Female, 74 years old, presenting with diffuse abdominal pain. Contrast-enhanced CT images show a large sigmoid mass (**a**, **b**, straight arrows) with an adjacent perivisceral inflammation. Note also the presence of free air (**a**, **b**, curved arrows)

associated with acute abdomen, and in such cases of covered perforation, it can also guide a conservative management [77].

17.3 Conclusion

Bowel obstruction and bowel perforation are common etiology for patient presenting at the emergency department with acute abdominal pain. In these patients, the diagnostic assessment begins with abdominal radiograph and abdominal US, both allowing in most cases to validate the clinical suspicion and to estimate its severity. These are followed by CT with intravenous cm, to delineate the etiology, to make a differential diagnosis, and to establish the surgical urgency in relationship with the vascular involvement. In case of clinical presentation of acute abdomen, the diagnostic approach is first-line CT due to its high diagnostic potential.

References

1. Scaglione M, Linsenmaier U, Schueller G. Emergency radiology of the Abdomen. Diagnostic imaging. Berlin: Springer; 2012.
2. Loo JT, Duddalwar V, Chen FK, Tejura T, Lekht I, Gulati M. Abdominal radiograph pearls and pitfalls for the emergency department radiologist: a pictorial review. Abdom Radiol. 2017;42(4):987–1019.
3. Scrima A. Value of MDCT and clinical and laboratory data for predicting the need for surgical intervention in suspected small-bowel obstruction. AJR Am J Roentgenol. 2017;208(4):785–93.
4. Gore RM, Silvers RI, Thakrar KH, Wenzke DR, Mehta UK, Newmark GM, Berlin JW. Bowel obstruction. Radiol Clin North Am. 2015;53(6):1225–40.
5. Di Mizio R, D'Amario F, Di Mizio V, Colasante MA, D'Amico G, Maggi G, Innocenti P, Scaglione M. In: Di Mizio R, Scaglione M, editors. Ileo meccanico del tenue. Springer; 2007.
6. Grassi R, Cappabianca S, Porto A, Sacco M, Montemarano E, Quarantelli M, Di Mizio R, De Rosa R. Ogilvie's syndrome (acute colonic pseudo-obstruction): review of the literature and report of 6 additional cases. Radiol Med. 2005;109(4):370–5. Review. English, Italian.
7. Vilz TO, Stoffels B, Strassburg C, Schild HH, Kalff JC. Ileus in adults. Dtsch Arztebl Int. 2017;114(29–30):508–18.
8. Jaffe T, Thompson WM. Large-bowel obstruction in the adult: classic radiographic and CT findings, etiology, and mimics. Radiology. 2015;275(3):651–63.
9. Di Mizio V, Di Mizio R, Romano L, Pinto A, D'Amario F, Gagliardi N, Scaglione M, Silva M. Ileo Meccanico. In: Di Mizio R, Scaglione M, editors. TCMD del piccolo intestino in elezione ed urgenza. Verduci Editore; 2012.
10. Di Mizio R, Scaglione M, editors. Small-bowel obstruction CT features with plain film and US correlations. Springer; 2007. p. 2012.
11. Paulson EK, Thompson WM. Review of small-bowel obstruction: the diagnosis and when to worry. Radiology. 2015;275(2):332–42.
12. Somma F, Faggian A, Serra N, Gatta G, Iacobellis F, Berritto D, et al. Bowel intussusceptions in adults: the role of imaging. Radiol Med. 2015;120(1):105–17.
13. Rami Reddy SR, Cappell MS. A systematic review of the clinical presentation, diagnosis, and treatment of small bowel obstruction. Curr Gastroenterol Rep. 2017;19(6):28.
14. Federle MP. CT of the acute (emergency) abdomen. Eur Radiol. 2005;15(Suppl 4):D100–4.
15. Dubuisson V, Voïglio EJ, Grenier N, Le Bras Y, Thoma M, Launay-Savary MV. Imaging of non-traumatic abdominal emergencies in adults. J Visc Surg. 2015;152(6):S57–64.
16. Gangadhar K, Kielar A, Dighe MK, O'Malley R, Wang C, Gross JA, Itani M, Lalwani N. Multimodality approach for imaging of non-traumatic acute abdominal emergencies. Abdom Radiol (NY). 2016;41(1):136–48.
17. Nicolaou S, Kai B, Ho S, Su J, Ahamed K. Imaging of acute small-bowel obstruction. AJR Am J Roentgenol. 2005;185(4):1036–44.
18. Di Mizio R, Di Mizio V, Della Marra R, Di Rocco D, Sciarra R, Grassi R. Radiological correlations. Chapter 5. In: Di Mizio R, Scaglione M, editors. Small-bowel obstruction CT features with plain film and US correlations. Springer; 2007. p. 75–111.
19. Burgess LK, Lee JT, DiSantis DJ. The string of pearls sign. Abdom Radiol (NY). 2016;41(7):1435–6.
20. Grassi R, Di Mizio R, Pinto A, Romano L, Rotondo A. Serial plain abdominal film findings in the assessment of acute abdomen: spastic ileus, hypotonic ileus, mechanical ileus and paralytic ileus. Radiol Med. 2004;108(1–2):56–70.
21. Grassi R, Romano S, D'Amario F, Giorgio Rossi A, Romano L, Pinto F, Di Mizio R. The relevance of free fluid between intestinal loops detected by sonography in the clinical assessment of small bowel obstruction in adults. Eur J Radiol. 2004;50(1):5–14.
22. Di Mizio R, Grassi R, Marchese E, Basti M, Di Campli G, Catalano O, Rotondo A, Fanucci A. "Uncompensated" small bowel obstruction in adults. Ultrasonographic findings of free fluid between loops and its prognostic value. Radiol Med. 1995;89(6):787–91.
23. Iacobellis F, Iadevito I, Romano F, Altiero M, Bhattacharjee B, Scaglione M. Perforated appendicitis: assessment with multidetector computed tomography. Semin Ultrasound CT MR. 2016;37(1):31–6.
24. Lassandro F, Giovine S, Pinto A, De Lutio Di Castelguidone E, Sacco M, Scaglione M, Romano

L. Small bowell volvulus - combined radiological findings. Radiol Med. 2001;102(1–2):43–7.

25. Grassi R, Pinto A, Scaglione M, Ragozzino A, Gagliardi N, Pellegrino G, Amitrano M. Volvulus of the splenic flexure of the colon. Report of a case. Radiol Med. 1997;93(6):783–4.

26. Scaglione M, Grassi R, Pinto A, Giovine S, Gagliardi N, Stavolo C, Romano L. Positive predictive value and negative predictive value of spiral CT in the diagnosis of closed loop obstruction complicated by intestinal ischemia. Radiol Med. 2004;107(1–2):69–77.

27. Caracino V, D'Amico G, Di Mizio R, D'Amario F. Rare cases of bowel obstruction: internal hernias. Chir Ital. 2009;61(5–6):617–21.

28. Scaglione M, Romano S, Pinto F, Flagiello F, Farina R, Acampora C, Romano L. Helical CT diagnosis of small bowel obstruction in the acute clinical setting. Eur J Radiol. 2004;50(1):15–22.

29. Iacobellis F, Berritto D, Belfiore MP, Di Lanno I, Maiorino M, Saba L, Grassi R. Meaning of free intraperitoneal fluid in small-bowel obstruction: preliminary results using high-frequency microsonography in a rat model. J Ultrasound Med. 2014;33(5):887–93.

30. Wongwaisayawan S, Kaewlai R, Dattwyler M, Abujudeh HH, Singh AK. Magnetic resonance of pelvic and gastrointestinal emergencies. Magn Reson Imaging Clin N Am. 2016;24(2):419–31.

31. Del Gaizo AJ, Lall C, Allen BC, Leyendecker JR. From esophagus to rectum: a comprehensive review of alimentary tract perforations at computed tomography. Abdom Imaging. 2014;39(4):802–23.

32. Furukawa A, Sakoda M, Yamasaki M, Kono N, Tanaka T, Nitta N, et al. Gastrointestinal tract perforation: CT diagnosis of presence, site, and cause. Abdom Imaging. 2005;30(5):524–34.

33. Faggian A, Berritto D, Iacobellis F, Reginelli A, Cappabianca S, Grassi R. Imaging patients with alimentary tract perforation: literature review. Semin Ultrasound CT MR. 2016;37(1):66–9.

34. Stoker J, van Randen A, Laméris W, Boermeester MA. Imaging patients with acute abdominal pain. Radiology. 2009;253(1):31–46.

35. Scaglione M, Linsenmaier U, Schueller G. Emergency radiology of the abdomen imaging features and differential diagnosis for a timely management approach. Milan/New York: Springer; 2012.

36. Brown CVR. Small bowel and colon perforation. Surg Clin North Am. 2014;94:471–5.

37. Grassi R, Pinto A, Rossi G, Rotondo A. Conventional plain-film radiology, ultrasonography and CT in jejuno-ileal perforation. Acta Radiol. 1998;39(1):52–6.

38. Pinto A, Grassi R, Rossi G, Romano L, Scaglione M, Pinto F. Computerized tomography in the study of jejuno-ileal perforations. Personal case load. Radiol Med. 1998;96(6):602–6.

39. Romano F, Iacobellis F, Guida F, Laccetti E, Sorbo A, Grassi R, Scaglione M. Traumatic injuries: mechanisms of lesions. In: Miele V., Trinci M, editors. Diagnostic imaging in Polytrauma patients. Springer; 2018.

40. Pinto A, Magliocca M, Grassi R, Scaglione M, Romano L, Angelelli G. Role of computerized tomography in the diagnosis of peritoneo-intestinal lesions resulting from closed trauma. Experience at 2 emergency departments. Radiol Med. 2001;101(3):177–82.

41. Pinto A, Muzj C, Stavolo C, Pepe M, Cinque T, Romano L. Pictorial essay: foreign body of the gastrointestinal tract in emergency radiology. Radiol Med. 2004;107(3):145–52.

42. Pinto A, Reginelli A, Pinto F, Sica G, Scaglione M, Berger FH, et al. Radiological and practical aspects of body packing. Br J Radiol. 2014;7(1036):20130500.

43. Rossi G, Grassi R, Pinto A, Ragozzino A, Romano L. New computerized tomography sign of intestinal infarction: isolated pneumoretroperitoneum or associated with pneumoperitoneum or late findings of intestinal infarction. Radiol Med. 1998;95(5):474–80.

44. Grassi R, Pinto A, Rossi G. Isolated pneumoretroperitoneum secondary to acute bowel infarction. Clin Radiol. 2000;55(4):321–3.

45. Scaglione M, de Lutio di Castelguidone E, Scialpi M, Merola S, Diettrich AI, Lombardo P, et al. Blunt trauma to the gastrointestinal tract and mesentery: is there a role for helical CT in the decision-making process? Eur J Radiol. 2004;50(1):67–73.

46. Espinoza R, Rodriguez A. Traumatic and non traumatic perforation of hollow viscera. Surg Clin North Am. 1997;77(6):1291–13042.

47. Pinto A, Miele V, Schillirò ML, Nasuto M, Chiaese V, Romano L, Guglielmi G. Spectrum of signs of pneumoperitoneum. Semin Ultrasound CT MR. 2016;37(1):3–9.

48. ACR appropriateness criteria, 2006. American College of Radiology Web site. http://www.acr.org/SecondaryMainMenuCategories/quality_safety/app_criteria/pdf/ExpertPanelonGastrointestinalImagingAcuteAbdominalPainandFeverorSuspectedAbdominalAbscessDoc1.aspx.

49. Grassi R, Romano S, Pinto A, Romano L. Gastroduodenal perforations: conventional plain film, US and CT findings in 166 consecutive patients. Eur J Radiol. 2004;50(1):30–6.

50. Smith JE, Hall EJ. The use of plain abdominal x rays in the emergency department. Emerg Med J. 2009;26(3):160–3.

51. Reginelli A, Mandato Y, Solazzo A, Berritto D, Iacobellis F, Grassi R. Errors in the radiological evaluation of the alimentary tract: part II. Semin Ultrasound CT MR. 2012;33(4):308–17.

52. Chen SC, Yen ZS, Wang HP, Lin FY, Hsu CY, Chen WJ. Ultrasonography is superior to plain radiography in the diagnosis of pneumoperitoneum. Br J Surg. 2002;89:351–4.

53. Hefny AF, Abu-Zidan FM. Sonographic diagnosis of intraperitoneal free air. J Emerg Trauma Shock. 2011;4(4):511–3.
54. Miller RE, Nelson SW. The roentgenologic demonstration of tiny amounts of free intraperitoneal gas: experimental and clinical studies. AJR Am J Roentgenol. 1971;112:574–85.
55. Singh JP, Steward MJ, Booth TC, Mukhtar H, Murray D. Evolution of imaging for abdominal perforation. Ann R Coll Surg Engl. 2010;92:182–8.
56. Pendergrass EP, Kirk E. Significance of gas under right dome of diaphragm with discussion of hepatoptosis. Am J Roentgenol. 1995;22:238–46.
57. Woodring JH, Heiser MJ. Detection of pneumoperitoneum on chest radiographs: comparison of upright lateral and posteroanterior projections. AJR Am J Roentgenol. 1995;165(1):45–7.
58. Baker SR. Plain film radiology of the perito- neal and retroperitoneal spaces. In: Baker SR, editor. The abdominal plain film. Norwalk/San Mateo: Appleton & Lange; 1990. p. 71–125.
59. Grassi R, Pinto F, Rotondo A, Smaltino F. Pneumoperitoneo. Napoli: Guido Gnocchi; 1996.
60. Weiner CI, Diaconis JN, Dennis JM. The inverted V: a new sign of pneumoperitoneum. Radiology. 1973;107:47–8.
61. Riegler LG. Spontaneous pneumoperitoneum: a roentgenologic sign found in the supine position. Radiology. 1941;37:604–7.
62. Cho KC, Baker SR. Extraluminal air diagnosis and significance. Radiol Clin North Am. 1994;32:829–44.
63. Cho KC, Baker SR. Air in the fissure for the ligamentum teres: new sign of intraperitoneal air on plain radiographs. Radiology. 1991;178:489–92.
64. Radin R, Van Allan RJ, Rosen RS. The visible gallbladder: a plain film sign of pneumoperitoneum. AJR Am J Roentgenol. 1996;167:69–70.
65. Brill PW, Olson SR, Winchester P. Neonatal necrotizing enterocolitis: air in Morison pouch. Radiology. 1990;174:469–71.
66. Menuck L, Siemers PT. Pneumoperitoneum: importance of right upper quadrant features. AJR Am J Roentgenol. 1976;127:753–6.
67. Cho KC, Baker SR. Depiction of diaphragmatic muscle slips on supine plain radiographs: a sign of pneumoperitoneum. Radiology. 1997;203:431–3.
68. Han SY. Variations in falciform ligament with pneumoperitoneum. Can Assoc Radiol J. 1880;31:171–3.
69. Cho KC, Baker SR. Visualization of the extra- hepatic segment of the ligamentum teres: a sign of free air on plain radiographs. Radiology. 1997;202:651–4.
70. Jelaso DV, Schultz EH. The urachus – an aid to the diagnosis of pneumoperitoneum. Radiology. 1969;92:295–6.
71. Grassi R, Catalano O, Pinto A, Fanucci A, Rotondo A, Di Mizio R. Case report: identification of the transverse mesocolon and root of small bowel mesentery; a new sign of pneumoperitoneum. Br J Radiol. 1996;69:774–6.
72. Miller RE. Perforated viscus in infants: a new roentgen sign. Radiology. 1960;74:65–7.
73. Rampton JW. The football sign. Radiology. 2004;231:81–2.
74. Mindelzun RE, McCort JJ. The cupola sign of pneumoperitoneum in the supine patient. Gastrointest Radiol. 1986;11:283–5.
75. Romano L, Pinto A, editors. Imaging of alimentary tract perforation. Cham: Springer; 2015.
76. Merchea A, Cullinane DC, Sawyer MD, Iqbal CW, Baron TH, Wigle D, Sarr MG, Zielinski MD. Esophagogastroduodenoscopy-associated gastrointestinal perforations: a single-center experience. Surgery. 2010;148:876–80.
77. Solis CV, Chang Y, De Moya MA, Velmahos GC, Fagenholz PJ. Free air on plainfilm: do we need a computed tomography too? J Emerg Trauma Shock. 2014;7(1):3–8.
78. Grassi R, Di Mizio R, Pinto A, Cioffi A, Romano L, Rotondo A. Sixty-one consecutive patients with gastrointestinal perforation: comparison of conventional radiology, ultrasonography, and computerized tomography, in terms of the timing of the study. Radiol Med. 1996;91(6):747–55.
79. Puylaert J, van der Zant F, Rijke A. Sonography and the acute abdomen: practical considerations. AJR Am J Roentgenol. 1997;168:179–86.
80. Lee DH, Lim JH, Ko YT, Yoon Y. Sonographic detection of pneumoperitoneum in patients with acute abdomen. AJR Am J Roentgenol. 1990;154:107–9.
81. Coppolino F, Gatta G, Di Grezia G, Reginelli A, Iacobellis F, Vallone G, et al. Gastrointestinal perforation: ultrasonographic diagnosis. Crit Ultrasound J. 2013;5(Suppl 1):S4.
82. Ghaffar A, Siddiqui TS, Haider H, Khatri H. Postsurgical pneumoperitoneum – comparison of abdominal ultrasound findings with plain radiography. J Coll Phys Surg Pak. 2008;18:477–80.
83. Karahan O, Kurt A, Yikilmaz A, Kahriman G. New method for the detection of Intraperitoneal free air by sonography: scissors maneuver. J Clin Ultrasound. 2004;32:381–5.
84. Maniatis V, Chryssikopoulos H, Roussakis A, Kalamara C, Papadopoulos A, Andreou J, Stringaris K. Perforation of the alimentary tract: evaluation with com- puted tomography. Abdom Imaging. 2000;25:373–9.
85. Cadenas Rodríguez L, Martí de Gracia M, Saturio Galán N, Pérez Dueñas V, Salvatierra Arrieta L, Garzón Moll G. Use of multidetector computed tomography for locating the site of gastrointestinal tract perforations. Cir Esp. 2013;91:316–23.
86. Kunin JR, Korobkin M, Ellis JH, Francis IR, Kane NM, Siegel SE. Duodenal injuries caused by blunt abdominal trauma: value of CT in differentiating perforation from hematoma. AJR Am J Roentgenol. 1993;160:1221–3.
87. Kim SH, Shin SS, Jeong YY, Heo SH, Kim JW, Kang HK. Gastrointestinal tract perforation: MDCT findings according to the perforation sites. Korean J Radiol. 2009;10(1)

88. Imuta M, Awai K, Nakayama Y, Murata Y, Asao C, Matsukawa T, Yamashita Y. Multidetector CT findings suggesting a perforation site in the gastrointestinal tract: analysis in surgically confirmed 155 patients. Radiat Med. 2007;25:113–8.

89. Gerhardt RT, Nelson BK, Keenan S, Kernan L, MacKersie A, Lane MS. Derivation of a clinical guideline for the assessment of nonspecific abdominal pain: the guideline for abdominal pain in the ED setting (GAPEDS) phase 1 study. Am J Emerg Med. 2005;23:709–17.

90. Hainaux B, Agneessens E, Bertinotti R, De Maertelaer V, Rubesova E, Capelluto E, Moschopoulos C. Accuracy of MDCT in predicting site of gastrointestinal tract perforation. AJR Am J Roentgenol. 2006;187:1179–83.

91. Shaffer HA. Perforation and obstruction of the gastrointestinal tract. Assessment by conventional radiology. Radiol Clin North Am. 1992;30:405–26.

92. Meyers MA. The extraperitoneal space: normal and pathologic anatomy. In: Meyers MA, editor. Dynamic radiology of the abdomen. New York: Springer; 2000. p. 333–492.

93. Badgwell BD, Camp ER, Feig B, Wolff RA, Eng C, Ellis LM, Cormier JN. Management of bevacizumab associated bowel perforation: a case series and review of the literature. Ann Oncol. 2008;19:577–82.

94. Brofman N, Atri M, Hanson JM, Grinblat L, Chughtai T, Brenneman F. Evaluation of bowel and mesenteric blunt trauma with multidetector CT. Radiographics. 2006;26:1119–31.

95. Scaglione M, Romano L, Gagliardi N, Palumbo P, Diettrich AI, Vicenzo L. Pneumoperitoneum secondary to blunt trauma of the thorax: report of a case of clinical and radiologic significance. Radiol Med. 1997;93(1–2):136–8.

96. Romano L, Rossi G, Pinto A, Grassi R, Violini M. A case of tracheal rupture caused by blunt trauma associated with pneumoretroperitoneum and intraspinal gas. Radiol Med. 1996;92(5):642–4.

97. Sung HK, Sang SS, Jeong YY, et al. Gastrointestinal tract perforation: MDCT findings according to the perforation sites. Korean. J Radiol. 2009;10: 63–70.

98. Haianaux B, Agneessens E, Bertinotti R, De Maertelaer V, Rubesova E, Capelluto E, Moschopoulos C. Accuracy of MDCT in predicting site of gastrointestinal tract perforation. AJR Am J Roentgenol. 2006;187(5):1179–83.

99. Biondo S, Kreisler E, Millan M, Fraccalvieri D, Golda T, Martí Ragué J, Salazar R. Differences in patient postoperative and long-term outcomes between obstructive and perforated colonic cancer. Am J Surg. 2008;195:427–32.

100. Liguori P, Reginelli A, Sparano A, Ruggiero G, Pinto A. Pneumoretroperitoneum associated with "Dirty Mass": an unusual case of rectal perforation. Radiol Case Rep. 2016;2(1):22–3.

101. Rubesin SE, Levine MS. Radiologic diagnosis of gastrointestinal perforation. Radiol Clin North Am. 2003;41:1095–115.

Chronic Inflammatory Bowel Disease

Emilio Quaia

18.1 Introduction

Chronic inflammatory disease includes Crohn's disease (CD) and ulcerative colitis. CD is a chronic lifelong condition, manifesting both in adults and children, and characterized by transmural inflammation of the bowel wall and progressive bowel damage with tissue remodeling and fibrosis. Based on the epidemiological, genetic, and immunological data, CD is considered to be a heterogeneous disorder with multifactorial etiology in which genetics and environment interact to manifest the disease. CD is associated with a significantly elevated malignancy risk of up to 0.5–1.0% per year after 10 years of disease.

Although CD may affect any part of the gastrointestinal tract from the mouth to perianal area, the most common areas affected by CD are the terminal ileum and proximal colon, followed by the ano-rectum and distal colon. In terms of distribution of the disease, 25% of the patients have colitis only, 25% have ileitis only, and 50%

Electronic Supplementary Material The online version of this chapter (https://doi.org/10.1007/978-3-319-99822-0_18) contains supplementary material, which is available to authorized users.

E. Quaia (✉)
Department of Radiology, University of Padova
Via Giustiniani 2, Padova, Italy
e-mail: emilio.quaia@unipd.it

have ileocolitis. Perianal disease varies between 14 and 76% and represents the most common presenting symptom in pediatric patients, while involvement of the upper gastrointestinal tract is uncommon.

The transmural inflammation, involving discontinuous intestinal segments separated by uninvolved "skip areas," spreads into the layers of affected bowel tract, often involving extraintestinal soft tissues and adjacent mesentery fat and causing significant pain. Mural wall inflammatory infiltrate consists in macrophages (also called epithelioid cells), lymphocytes, usually CD4+ T cells, noncaseating granulomas consisting in a collection of monocyte/macrophage cells and other inflammatory cells with or without giant cells, and microgranulomas consisting in clusters of histiocytes and lymphocytes. Transmural inflammation can be complicated by the development of fibrotic strictures, perforation, abscess formation, and fistulization.

Abdominal pain remains the dominant symptom in patients with CD, and it represents an essential parameter in grading the disease inflammatory activity. Continuous chronic pain due to chronic bowel inflammation can be debilitating and often may lead to life-threatening complications. The cumulative rates of complications—including bowel obstruction or fistulization with abscesses and phlegmons or even perforation—in patients with CD range from 48 to 52% at 5 years and between 69 and 70% at 10 years after diagnosis, with approximately half of the patients

M. A. Cova, F. Stacul (eds.), *Pain Imaging*, https://doi.org/10.1007/978-3-319-99822-0_18

developing a stricture [1]. Postoperative recurrence of stenosis at the ileocolic or ileoileal anastomosis commonly occurs [2].

Chronology of pharmacologic treatment should reduce disease activity followed by maintenance therapy of adequate response or remission. The medications which are highly effective in inducing remission include steroids and antitumor necrosis factor (TNF), while medications used to maintain pain remission include 5-aminosalicyclic acid products, immunomodulators, (azathioprine, 6-mercaptopurine, methotrexate), and anti-TNF biologic drugs (infliximab, adalimumab, certolizumab, and golimumab). Surgical interventions like bowel resection, stricturoplasty, or drainage of abscess are required in up to two thirds of CD patients during their lifetime.

Ulcerative colitis (UC) affects only the colon, always with rectal involvement, manifests in young adults (15–40 years of age), and is more prevalent in males [3]. UC manifests with hemorrhagic diarrhea, urgency of defecation, and tenesmus, often associated with fever, pain, and weight loss [3]. Generally, abdominal pain is lower than in CD. Although ulcerative colitis and CD account for the majority of cases, indeterminate colitis, an entity that demonstrates overlapping clinical, imaging, and histologic features, represents up to 6% of cases.

Since the role of imaging is limited in ulcerative colitis, we will concentrate our essay mainly on CD.

18.2 Disease Classification and Correlation to Pain

All CD clinical and endoscopic scores are directly or indirectly related to patient's pain. Patient's pain is essential in grading the disease inflammatory activity in CD being one of the parameters which are included in the Crohn's disease activity index (CDAI) [4, 5]. The grade of daily abdominal pain represents a crucial parameter in CDAI. CDAI represents the most employed clinical score in patients with CD and includes the number of liquid or soft stools, the grade of daily abdominal pain and patient well-being, presence or absence of complications,

evidence of abdominal inflammatory mass, hematocrit, and body weight. Unfortunately, CDAI has low specificity since it is based mainly on subjective symptoms and it is difficult to use the CDAI value as a clinical biomarker to adjust pharmacologic treatment.

Other clinical scores are based on patient's abdominal pain as well, including Harvey-Bradshaw index (HBI), based on patient's well-being, patient's abdominal pain, number of liquid or soft stools, abdominal mass, and complications, and Mayo score, based on stool frequency, rectal bleeding, endoscopic findings, and physician's global assessment.

The Vienna classification [6] considers age of onset, disease location, and disease behavior as the fundamental parameters to classify CD clinical subtypes, namely, inflammatory, stricturing (fibrostenotic), and penetrating (fistulizing) subtypes. According to the Montreal revision of Vienna Classification, patients with CD can be stratified according to the age at diagnosis (<16 years = A1, 17–40 years = A2, >40 years = A3), disease location (terminal ileum = L1, colon = L2, ileocolic = L3, upper gastrointestinal tract = L4), and disease behavior (non-stricturing and non-penetrating = B1 [B1p if perianal], stricturing = B2 [B2p if perianal], penetrating = B3 [B3p if perianal]) [7]. Most patients with CD present with predominantly inflammatory phenotype at diagnosis; however, the majority of them develop disease complications such as strictures and fistulae over time. Finally, Maglinte and colleagues [8] proposed an imaging-based classification of CD into four broad subtypes: active inflammatory, perforating and fistulating, fibrostenotic, and reparative and regenerative subtypes.

Endoscopic scores are considered the reference techniques to measure CD inflammatory activity, and they are used more commonly in the clinical trials to measure the efficacy of various drugs on inducing and maintaining mucosal healing and pain relief. The endoscopy scores, including Crohn's disease activity index of severity (CDEIS) [9], and simple endoscopic score for Crohn's disease (SES-CD) are both based on mucosal ulcers and disease diffusion which are both related to patient's pain.

Fig. 18.1 (a, b) 35-year-old male patient with Crohn's disease and inflammatory ileal stricture. Patient attends the A and E department with abdominal crampy pain on the right lower quadrant of the abdomen. Gray-scale US. Diffuse thickening (calipers) of the terminal ileum with layered appearance of the bowel wall and submucosal layer thickening

At endoscopy, the mucosa may appear normal or may show multiple small (1–2 mm in size) punctiform, rounded nodules or superficial erosions known as aphthoid lesions [10] which progressively become confluent and lead to larger longitudinal ulcers, known as serpiginous ulcers. The combination of longitudinal and transverse ulceration in an edematous mucosa induces the characteristic "cobblestone" aspect [10]. Ulcerations are commonly located on the mesenteric border of the small intestine and can become deeply situated fissuring ulcers reaching the muscularis propria or pass through the muscularis and give rise to abscesses or fistulas between involved segments and adjacent organs or nearby uninvolved loops. The mesenteric fat adjacent to the involved bowel tract becomes hypertrophied and partially surrounds the intestine, extending from the mesenteric attachment anteriorly and posteriorly corresponding to the involved segment. This phenomenon is known as creeping fat.

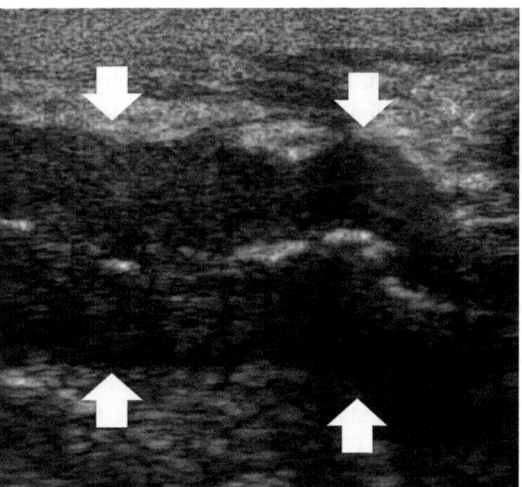

Fig. 18.2 45-year-old woman patient with Crohn's disease and inflammatory ileal stricture. Patient presenting with fever and abdominal pain on the right lower quadrant of the abdomen. Gray-scale US. Diffuse thickening (arrows) of the distal ileum with loss of layered appearance of the bowel wall and evidence of lumen stricture. Lumen corresponds to the thin central hyperechoic layer

18.3 Imaging Findings

The key features for diagnosing CD comprise a combination of imaging, endoscopic, and pathological findings [11]. However, endoscopy does not show the transmural extent of CD, and intubation of the distal ileum can be completed in only 80% of patients with CD. Ultrasound [US], computed tomography [CT], and magnetic resonance [MR] imaging allow to demonstrate the transmural and extraintestinal extent of CD based on mural wall and adjacent mesentery enhancement after contrast injection.

US can be considered the first-line imaging technique to detect CD in patients with abdominal pain based on mural thickening (>3 mm) (Fig. 18.1). The thickened bowel wall with loss of layered pattern is strictly related to active inflammatory disease with diffuse inflammatory edema involving the bowel wall (Fig. 18.2). Active inflammatory disease reveals increased mural vascularity on color Doppler analysis (Fig. 18.3).

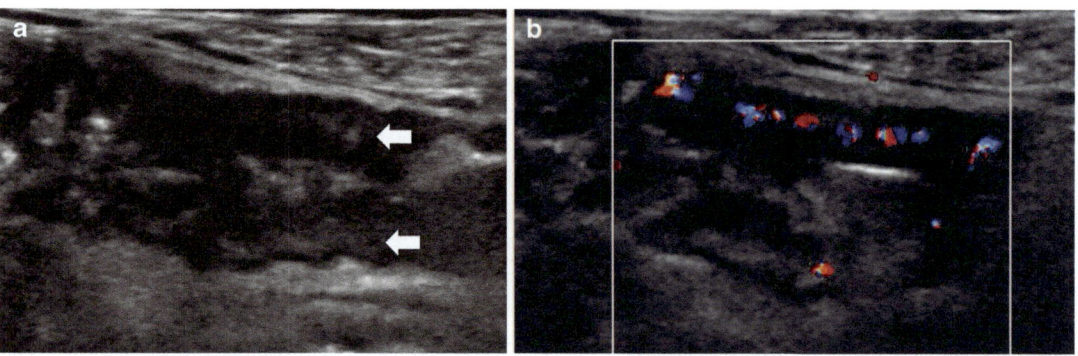

Fig. 18.3 (**a, b**) 22-year-old male patient with Crohn's disease and inflammatory ileal stricture. Patient presenting with diffuse abdominal pain on the right lower quadrant of the abdomen. (**a**) Gray-scale US. (**b**) Color Doppler US. Diffuse thickening (calipers) of the terminal ileum with layered appearance of the bowel wall and evidence of thickened submucosal layer (arrows). Color Doppler reveals increased mural vascularity corresponding to high inflammatory activity

Although CT and MRI enterography still represent the reference imaging techniques to grade CD activity, contrast-enhanced US (CEUS) may represent an alternative imaging modality to assess the grade of inflammatory disease activity [12–15], and, compared to the other modalities, it offers several advantages including low financial cost, portability, availability, lack of restrictions in performing frequent serial examinations at short intervals, and an absence of radiation exposure. In patients with CD and active inflammatory disease, CEUS reveals diffuse transmural enhancement after microbubble contrast agent injection (Figs. 18.4 and 18.5).

Abdominal CT enterography is the most employed imaging technique used in the assessment of patients with CD and presents the advantage of reduced scanning time even though it involves ionizing radiation exposure especially if repeated during a strict follow-up schedule, as in CD patients undergoing surveillance during pharmacologic treatment. CT [16, 17] and MRI [18–20] can demonstrate the transmural and extraintestinal extent of CD, even though they require the administration of large amounts of enteric contrast material. Although MR enterography/enteroclysis presents a higher contrast-to-noise ratio compared to CT, both cross-sectional

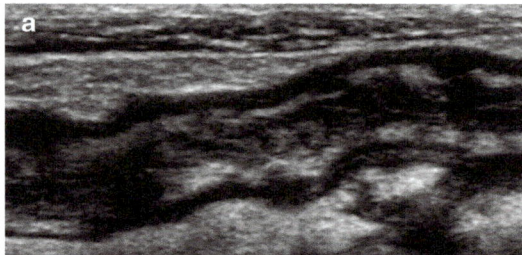

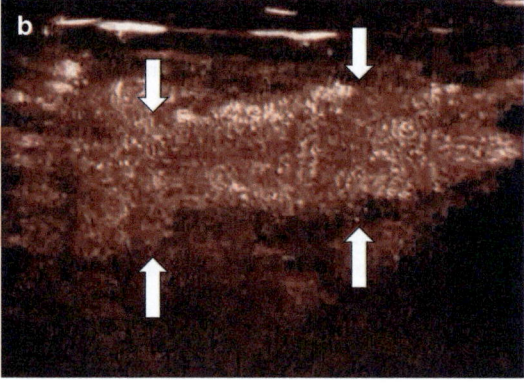

Fig. 18.4 (**a, b**) 24-year-old male patient with Crohn's disease. Patient with diffuse abdominal pain on the right lower quadrant of the abdomen. (**a**) Gray-scale US. (**b**) Contrast-enhanced US. Thickening of distal ileal tract with layered appearance of the bowel wall and evidence of thickened heterogeneous submucosal layer. (**b**) Contrast-enhanced US reveals diffuse transmural contrast enhancement (arrows) corresponding to high inflammatory activity

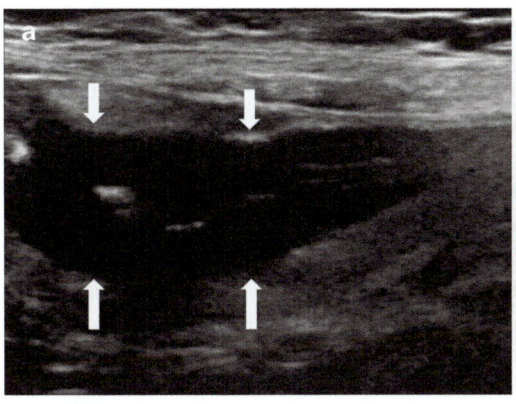 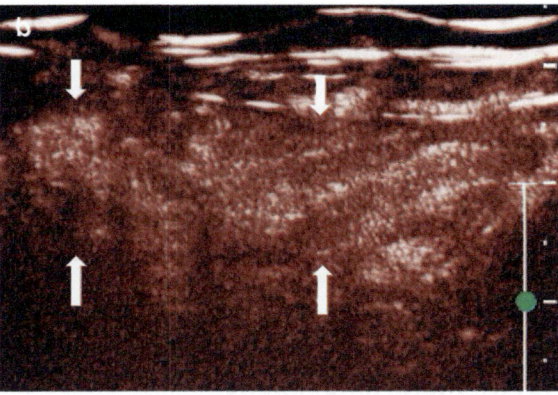

Fig. 18.5 18-year-old woman patient with Crohn's disease with previous total colectomy with ileostomy. Patient presenting with moderate pain close to ileostomy with high disease activity indices. (**a**) Gray-scale US. (**b**) Contrast-enhanced ultrasound. (**a**) Gray-scale US reveals diffuse thickening of the distal ileal tract (arrows) close to ileostomy with loss of layered appearance and extensive hypertrophic adjacent creeping fat in keeping with high disease inflammatory activity. (**b**) Contrast-enhanced ultrasound reveals diffuse transmural contrast enhancement (arrows) corresponding to high disease activity

techniques present a comparable diagnostic accuracy in detecting mural thickening and lumen stricture.

However, MRI is superior to CT in the visualization of ulceration, fistulas, bowel edema, and creeping fat [21] which makes MRI more suitable for patient's long-term follow-up during pharmacologic treatment. The grade of disease activity may be quantified by MR imaging by using the MR index of activity (MARIA) [22] which includes mural wall thickness in mm, mural relative contrast enhancement, and the presence of edema and ulcers, and it is calculated using the following formula:

$$MARIA = \left(1.5 \times \text{wall thickness in mm}\right) + \left(0.02 \times RCE^*\right) + \left(5 \times \text{edema}^\S\right) + \left(10 \times \text{ulceration}\right)$$

*= RCE corresponds to relative contrast enhancement, [(wall SI postgadolinium—wall SI pregadolinium)/(wall SI pregadolinium)] × 100 × (SD noise pregadolinium/SD noise postgadolinium). § = T2-w hyperintensity of the bowel wall relative to the signal of psoas muscle.

MARIA index >11 is related to high inflammatory disease activity with high probability of ulcerative disease.

A further index of disease activity is the Clermont score [23] which corresponds to:

$$\text{Clermont score} = \left(1.646 \times \text{wall mm}\right) - \left(1.321 \times ADC\right) + \left(5.613 \times \text{edema}\right) + \left(8.306 \times \text{ulcers}\right) + 5.039$$

ADC = apparent diffusion coefficient as measured through diffusion-weighted MR imaging sequences with at least two b values.

Clermont score >8 is related to high inflammatory disease activity with high probability of ulcerative disease.

18.4 Clinical Causes of Pain and Imaging Correlation

In patients with CD, several causes of pain can be identified according to the location of disease. The main causes of patient's pain are high grade of mural inflammation, abscesses and phlegmons, ileal strictures leading to bowel obstruction, and fistulas.

18.4.1 Mural Inflammation

Mural inflammation is the most common cause of pain in patients with CD. Inflammatory subtype of CD manifests with inflammation with superficial and deep ulcers, transmural inflammation with granuloma's formation, and mural thickening. CEUS [12–14] CT and MR imaging [22, 24–26] are considered reliable imaging techniques in assessing the inflammatory activity of CD.

Intestinal mucosal ulcers, representing the main cause of abdominal pain in patients with inflammatory CD type, may be identified by imaging techniques. On gray-scale US, intestinal transmural ulcers (sinus tracts) appear as hypoechoic lines perpendicular to the bowel penetrating within the adjacent mesenteric fat (creeping fat) (Fig. 18.6).

Intestinal ulcers, the main cause of abdominal pain in patients with inflammatory CD type, may be identified at CT or MR imaging studies after luminal distension as nidus of high signal surrounded by a rim of moderate signal intensity [21] (Fig. 18.7). Another significant feature of CD, and a further source of patient's pain, is thickening (>3 mm) of the inflamed bowel wall (Figs. 18.8 and 18.9). Active inflammation is also associated with patient's pain and mucosal hyperemia, often with a layered appearance after contrast administration due to submucosal edema. Mural active inflammation is readily visualized on MRI after i.v. gadolinium-based contrast administration as intense enhancement (Figs. 18.8 and 18.9). The peak signal intensity of mucosal enhancement has been shown to have good correlation with Crohn's disease activity index and hence to patient's pain [21]. Enhancing mesenteric vessels supplying an inflamed bowel segment—known as comb sign—represents a further sign of active inflammation and is related to patient's pain [21].

Abdominal pain and bowel wall inflammatory activity may be reduced by anti-inflammatory treatment, particularly anti-TNF biologic drugs. The progressive reduction of mural edema on diffusion-weighted MR imaging sequences is usually related to patient pain relief (Fig. 18.10).

18.4.2 Abscesses and Phlegmons

Abdominal and pelvic abscesses in CD occur spontaneously or as a postoperative complication [27]. Approximately 10–30% of patients with CD will spontaneously develop an abdominal or pelvic abscess during the course of their illness, due to transmural inflammation and microperforation of diseased bowel [28].

Abdominal and pelvic abscesses are hypoechoic on gray-scale US and appear as nonenhancing structures after microbubble contrast agent injection on CEUS (Fig. 18.6).

In the great majority of cases, the terminal ileum, the ileocecal region, or even the site of anastomosis after previous bowel segmental resection are the foci of CD activity and the most frequent sites of abscesses and phlegmons. The majority of abscesses occur on the right side near the diseased bowel and almost always at the site of a prior anastomosis. Abdominal pain, fever, and a palpable mass are the most common findings in patients with abscesses and phlegmons. Most abscesses originate from contained perforations, while free perforations are rare in CD. On the other hand, fistulas arising from the diseased bowel are often associated with the abscess cavity. If the abscess is drainable percutaneously, the next step is to aspirate the collection in order to demonstrate the nature of the fluid which usually is polymicrobial.

Even abdominal phlegmon is an inflammatory mass that can develop in the setting of penetrating CD. Anti-TNF antibody therapy is typically avoided in CD complicated by phlegmon because of concern for peritoneal infection.

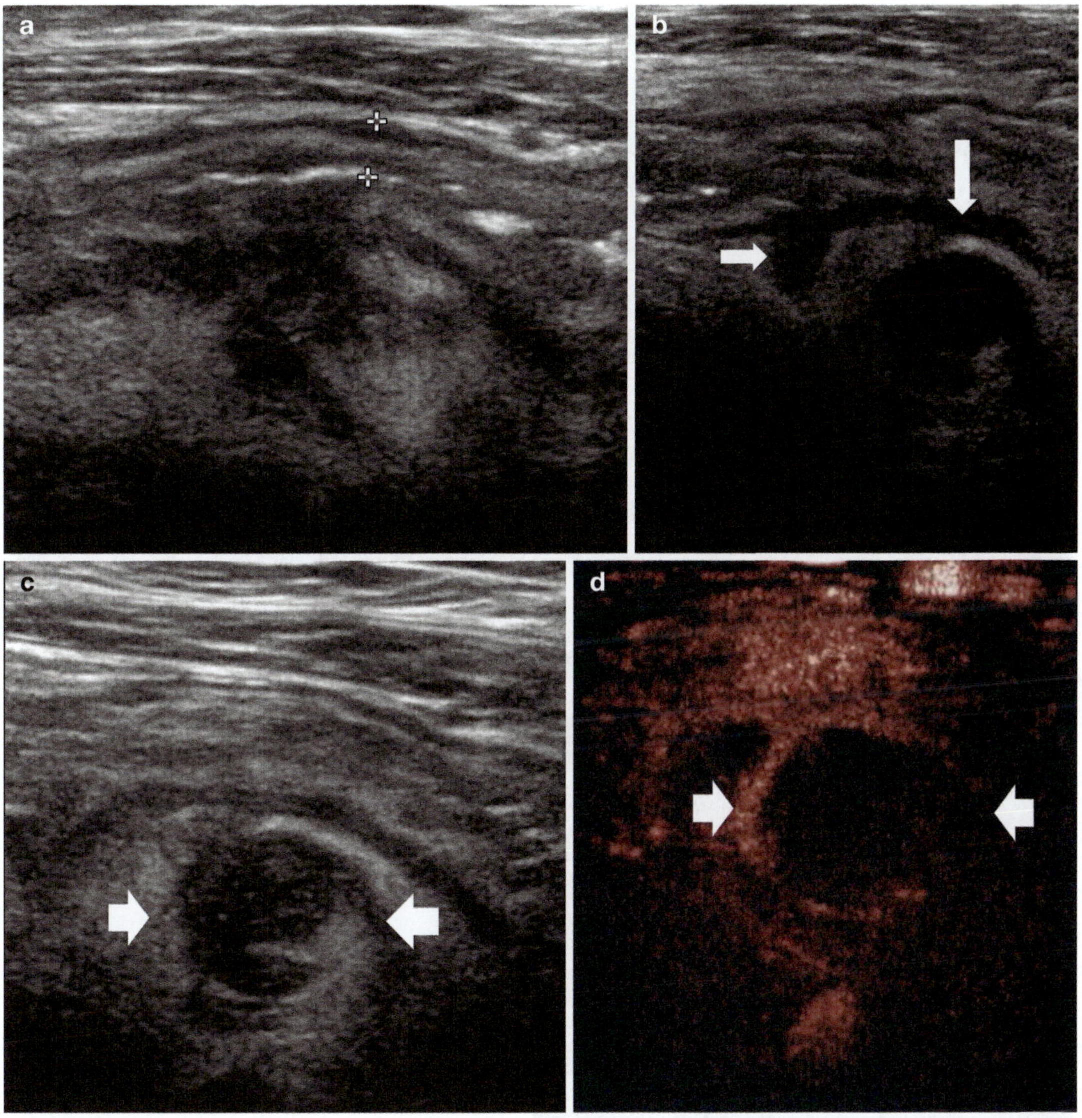

Fig. 18.6 40-year-old woman patient attending the emergency department with acute abdominal pain on the right lower quadrant and increased white blood cell counts (17,000/mm³). Acute appendicitis was suspected. (**a–c**) Gray-scale US. (**d**) Contrast-enhanced ultrasound. (**a–c**). Gray-scale US reveals diffuse thickening of the terminal ileal tract (calipers) with layered appearance, hypertrophic creeping fat, and sinus tract (horizontal line) and abscess (vertical line) adjacent to the mural wall. (**d**) The abscess does not present any enhancement after microbubble injection (arrows)

18.4.3 Bowel Obstruction

Fibrostenotic subtype is characterized by bowel obstruction. The crampy abdominal pain due to ileal stricture represents the most common presenting symptom leading CD patients to the emergency unit. Strictures are characterized by luminal narrowing and bowel wall thickening with or without prestenotic dilatation [10], while ileal mucosa is always ulcerated. CD patients with ileal disease develop clinically apparent strictures—corresponding to a constant luminal narrowing with prestenotic dilatation or obstructive signs/symptoms without presence of

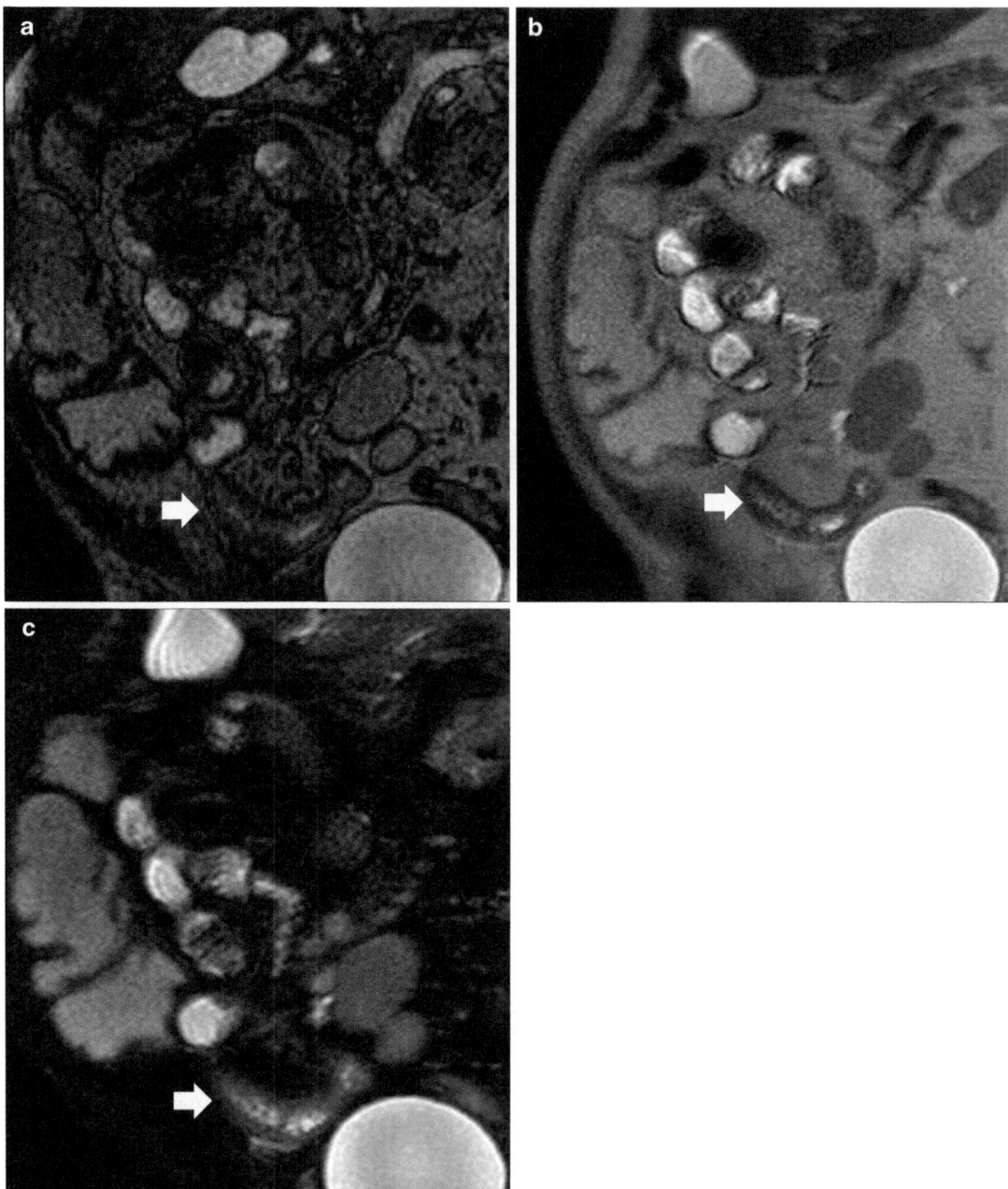

Fig. 18.7 (a–c) 25-year-old male patient with Crohn's disease and inflammatory ileal stricture with mucosal ulcers. Patient presenting with abdominal crampy pain and increased fecal calprotectin and frequent stool. (a) Coronal T1-weighted FFE MR imaging sequence; (b) coronal T2-weighted turbo spin-echo MR imaging sequence; (c) coronal T2-weighted SPAIR MR imaging sequence with fat suppression. One extended ileal stricture (arrows) with wall thickening and mucosal irregularities corresponding to mucosal ulcers

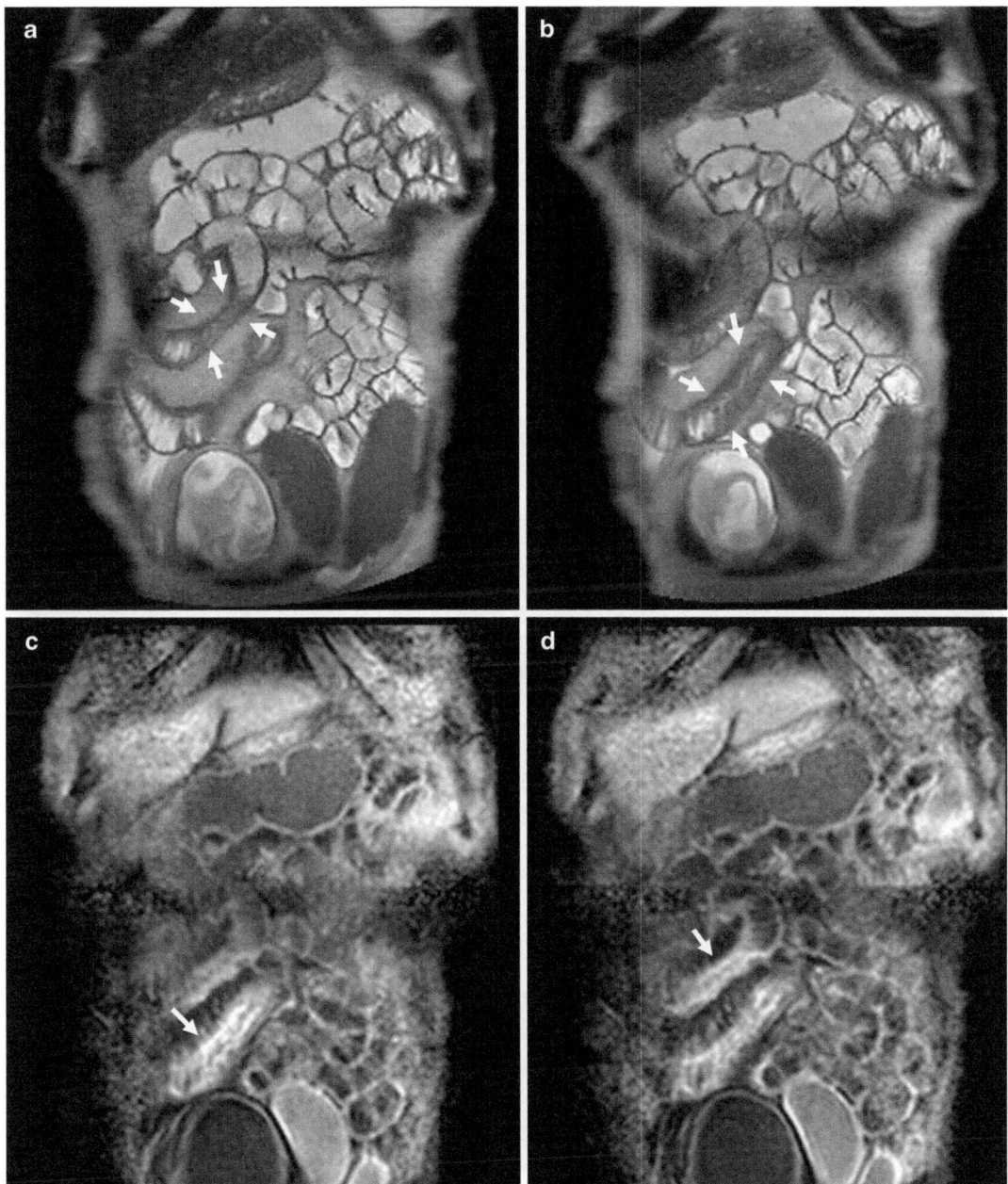

Fig. 18.8 (**a–d**) 35-year-old male patient with Crohn's disease and inflammatory ileal strictures. Patient with normal terminal ileal loop at colonoscopy and presenting with abdominal crampy pain and increased fecal calprotectin. (**a, b**) Coronal T2-weighted turbo spin-echo MR imaging sequences. There are two adjacent ileal strictures (arrows) with wall thickening. (**c, d**) Coronal T1-weighted breath-hold dynamic sequences with fat suppression after gadolinium-based contrast agent injection. Diffuse mural contrast enhancement with adjacent comb sign related to disease active inflammation

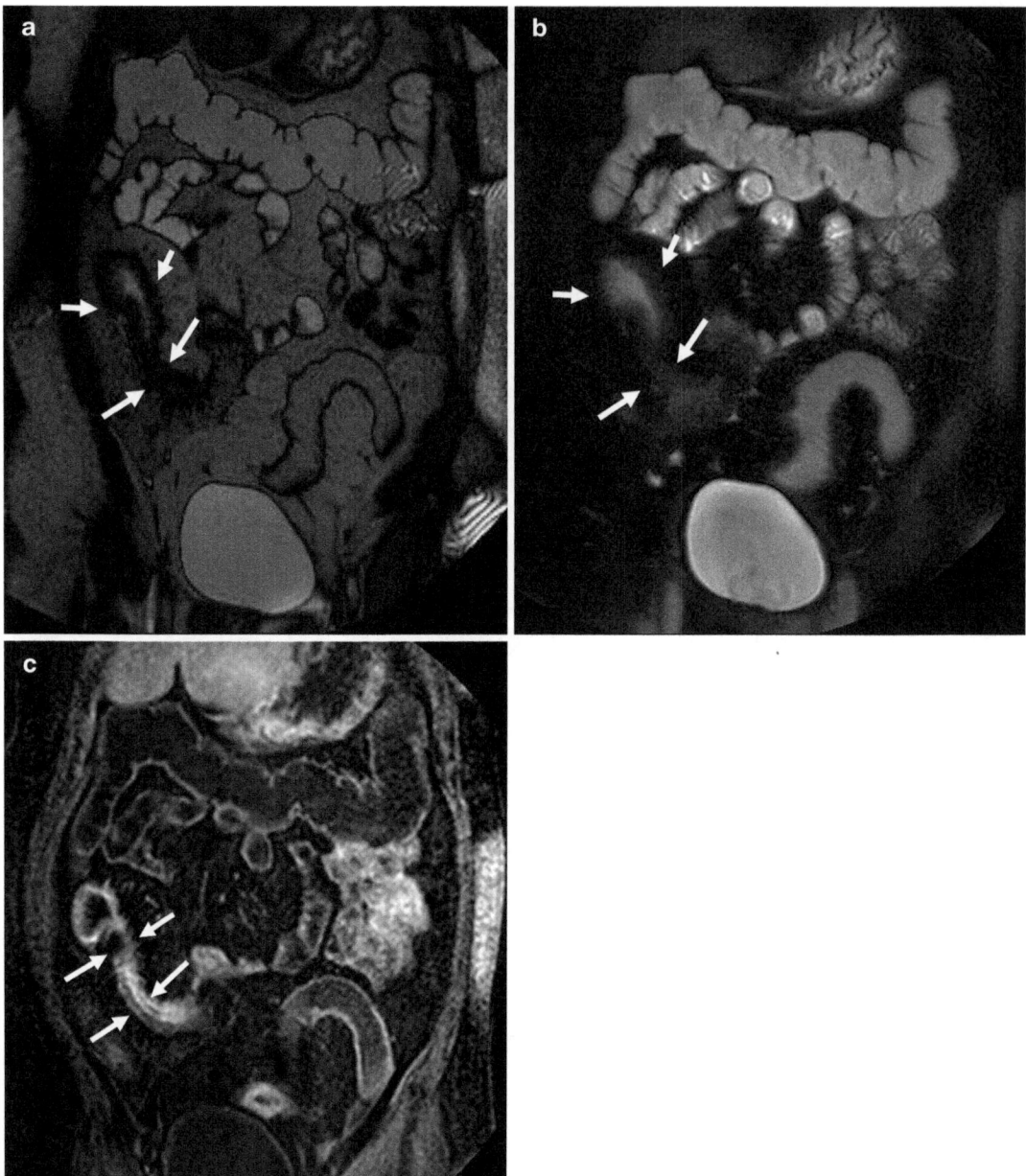

Fig. 18.9 (a–c) 25-year-old female patient with Crohn's disease and inflammatory ileal stricture. Patient presenting with abdominal crampy pain and increased fecal calprotectin. (**a**) Coronal T1-weighted FFE MR imaging sequence. One extended ileal stricture (arrows) with wall thickening; (**b**) coronal T2-weighted SPAIR MR imaging sequence with fat suppression. The thickened bowel wall reveals increased signal intensity related to active inflammatory disease; (**c**) coronal T1-weighted breath-hold dynamic sequence with fat suppression after gadolinium-based contrast agent injection on arterial phase (30 s after contrast injection). Diffuse mural contrast enhancement with adjacent comb sign related to disease active inflammation

penetrating disease—in approximately 40% of cases during the long-term course of the disease, and approximately 60% of patients require surgery within 20 years after diagnosis.

The differentiation of predominantly inflammatory bowel strictures from primarily fibrotic strictures is crucial since pharmacologic anti-inflammatory treatment is indicated in the

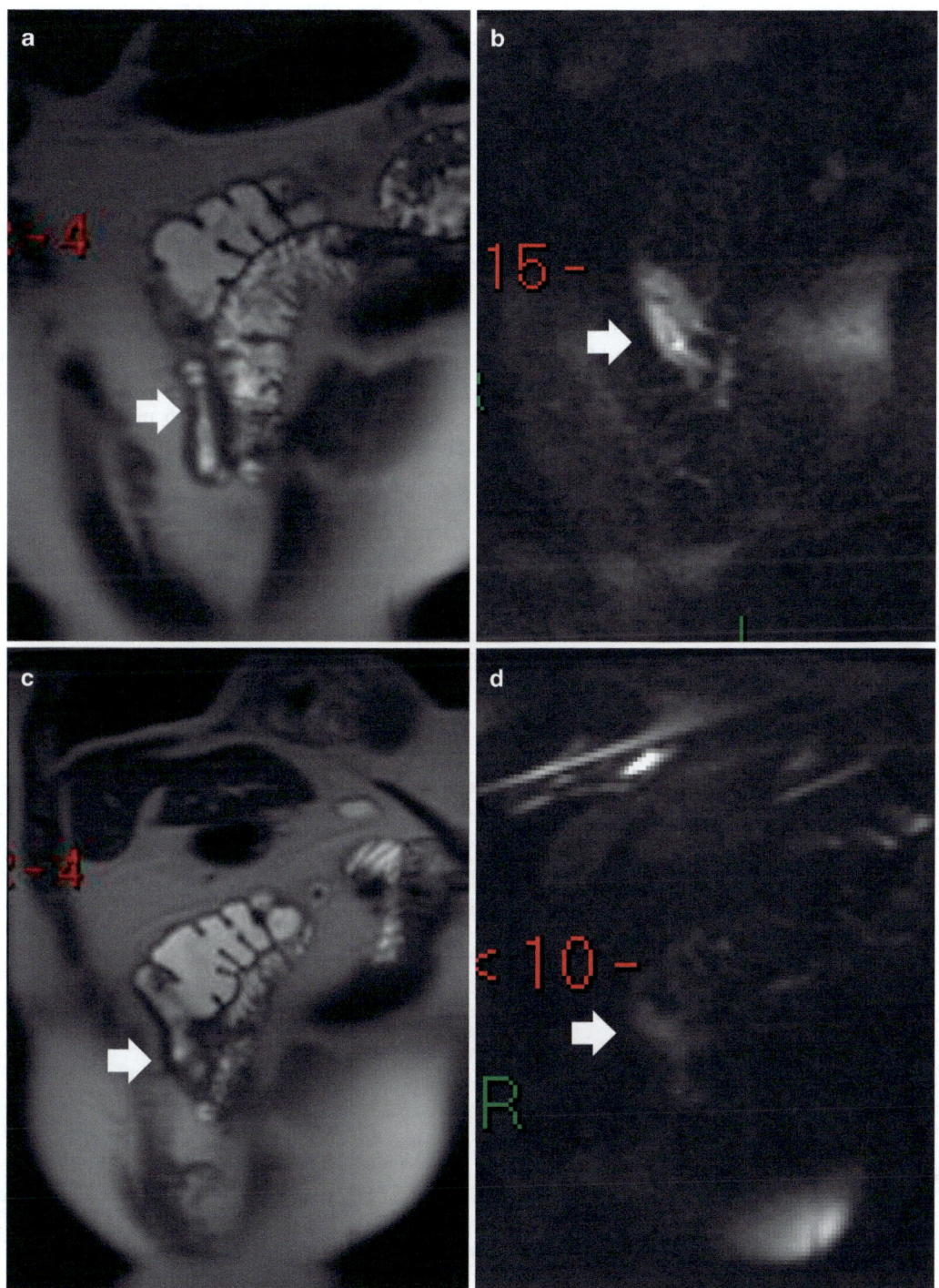

Fig. 18.10 (a–d) 35-year-old female patient with Crohn's disease and inflammatory ileal stricture before (**a, b**) and 3 months after beginning of therapy (**c, d**) with adalimumab. Before therapy patient had intense abdominal crampy pain and increased fecal calprotectin. (**a, c**) Coronal T2-weighted SPAIR MR imaging sequence. (**b, d**) Diffusion-weighted MR imaging sequence, *b* value = 800 s/mm². Before therapy (**a, b**) there was diffuse mural thickening with signal restriction on diffusion-weighted MR imaging sequences. After therapy (**c, d**) there is a clear decrease in ileal wall signal restriction on diffusion-weighted MR imaging sequences in keeping with decreased inflammatory activity and abdominal pain relief

presence of inflammatory changes, whereas endoscopic dilation or surgical resection is required in the presence of fibrosis [29]. All imaging techniques present a limited accuracy to differentiate mural fibrosis from inflammation mainly because both fibrosis and active inflammation coexist within the bowel wall. According to a recent study [30], only a combination of MR enteroclysis and US as well as a combination of 2-deoxy-2-[fluorine-18] fluoro-D-glucose integrated with computed tomography (18F-FDG PET/CT) and US resulted in a 100% detection rate of fibrotic strictures requiring surgery or endoscopic dilation therapy. Even more recently, another study showed that PET/MR enterography may differentiate purely fibrotic strictures from mixed or inflammatory strictures, while no significant differences between inflammation and fibrosis were observed on T2-weighted and diffusion-weighted MR images [31].

Intestinal fibrosis and subsequent stricturing of the intestine in CD result in substantial patient morbidity and mortality and are responsible for a significant proportion of hospitalizations, surgeries, and healthcare costs of CD. MR fluoroscopy may reveal fixity of the affected segment with proximal dilation of the bowel. Chronic fibrotic strictures are typically hypointense on both T1- and T2-weighted MRI sequences, whereas acute inflammatory strictures due to acute inflammatory edema show the target sign with layered enhancement after contrast administration [21]. Fibrotic strictures may show minor, inhomogeneous contrast enhancement on arterial phase (30 s after contrast injection) with progressively increasing contrast enhancement up to the delayed phase (3–5 min after contrast injection) (Figs. 18.11 and 18.12).

18.4.4 Fistulas

Beside mural inflammation and bowel stricture, the third cause of pain in patients with CD is fistulas which represent the distinctive feature of penetrating subtype of disease. This subtype is characterized by severe inflammation with

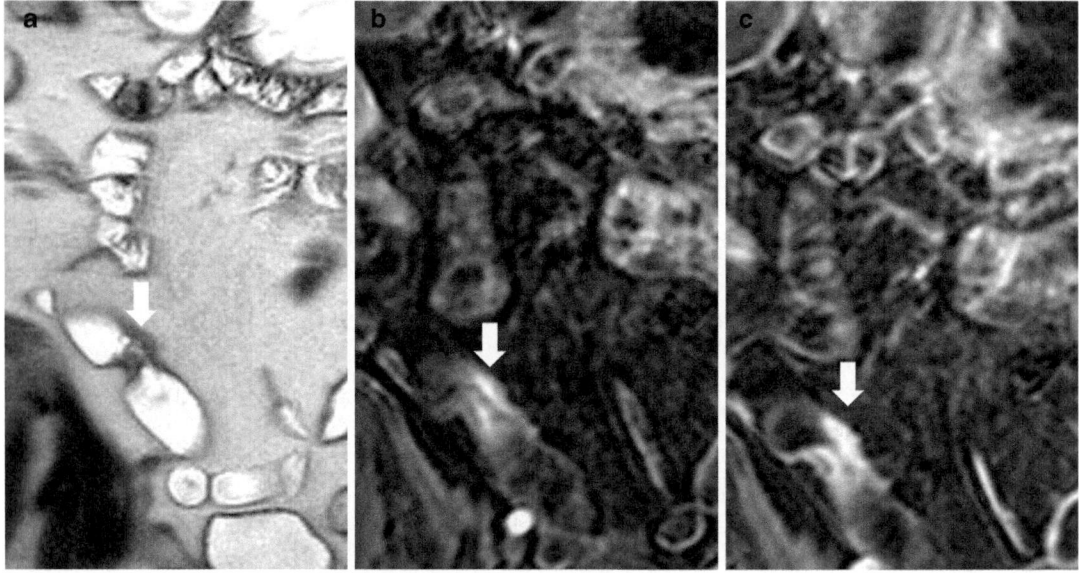

Fig. 18.11 (**a–c**) 40-year-old male patient with Crohn's disease and fibrotic ileal stricture. Patient presenting with abdominal crampy pain and clinical signs of occlusion. (**a**) Coronal T2-weighted turbo spin-echo MR imaging sequence. Focal stricture on the terminal ileum (arrow) is identified; (**b**, **c**) coronal T1-weighted breath-hold dynamic sequences with fat suppression after gadolinium-based contrast agent injection on arterial (**b**) and delayed phase (3 min after contrast injection) (**c**). Progressive increase in mural signal intensity (arrow) from arterial to delayed phase due to progressive gadolinium-based contrast agent leakage within the interstitial fibrotic space

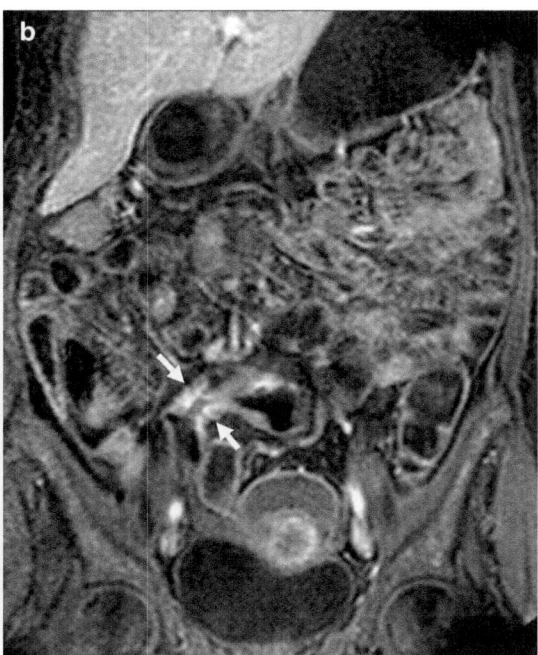

Fig. 18.12 (**a, b**) 45-year-old female patient with Crohn's disease and fibrotic ileal stricture. Patient presenting with abdominal crampy pain and vomiting. (**a**) Coronal T2-weighted turbo spin-echo MR imaging sequence. Extensive irregular strictures with evidence of mucosal ulcerations involving the terminal ileum; (**b**) coronal T1-weighted breath-hold dynamic sequence with fat suppression after gadolinium-based contrast agent injection on delayed phase (3 min after contrast injection). Transmural delayed mural contrast enhancement related to bowel wall fibrosis

progression to transmural ulceration and fistulation. Fistulas—defined as abnormal connections between an organ and another structure—represent a very common complication of CD and are often associated with bowel strictures. Histologically, fistulas are composed of granulation tissue, while lumen is mostly filled up by nuclear debris and inflammatory cells, in particular neutrophils [10]. Granulomas are present in approximately 25% of the perianal fistulas or abscesses [10].

Fistulas occur as a result of deep transmural ulcers or fissures that eventually penetrate the bowel muscle layer and cause inflammation in the adjacent mesenteric tissue leading to formation of small abscesses and blind-ending sinus tracts. Classification of fistulas in CD is based on the origin and terminus of the fistulous tract. The most common types of fistulas found in patients with CD correspond to enteroenteric or enterocolic, anal or perianal, enterocutaneous, enterovesical or colovesical, and enterovaginal. Perianal fistulas may arise from inflamed or infected anal glands (fistula-in-ano) and/or penetration of fissures or ulcers of the rectum or anal canal and lead to anal pain, discharge and incontinence, and impairing patients' social life [32].

Fistulas occur in up to one third of patients with CD at some time during the course of the disease and can be easily detected by MR imaging due to the concomitant inflammatory reaction. The reported sensitivity value for the detection of internal fistulas ranges between 83.3 and 84.4% and the specificity is 100% [21]. Enteroenteric fistulas [33] manifest as multiple ileal loops radiating from a central region on CT and MR imaging sequences (Fig. 18.13) and usually manifest with abdominal pain. Enterocutaneous fistulas (Fig. 18.14) manifest with cutaneous discharge and pain if fistula becomes infected.

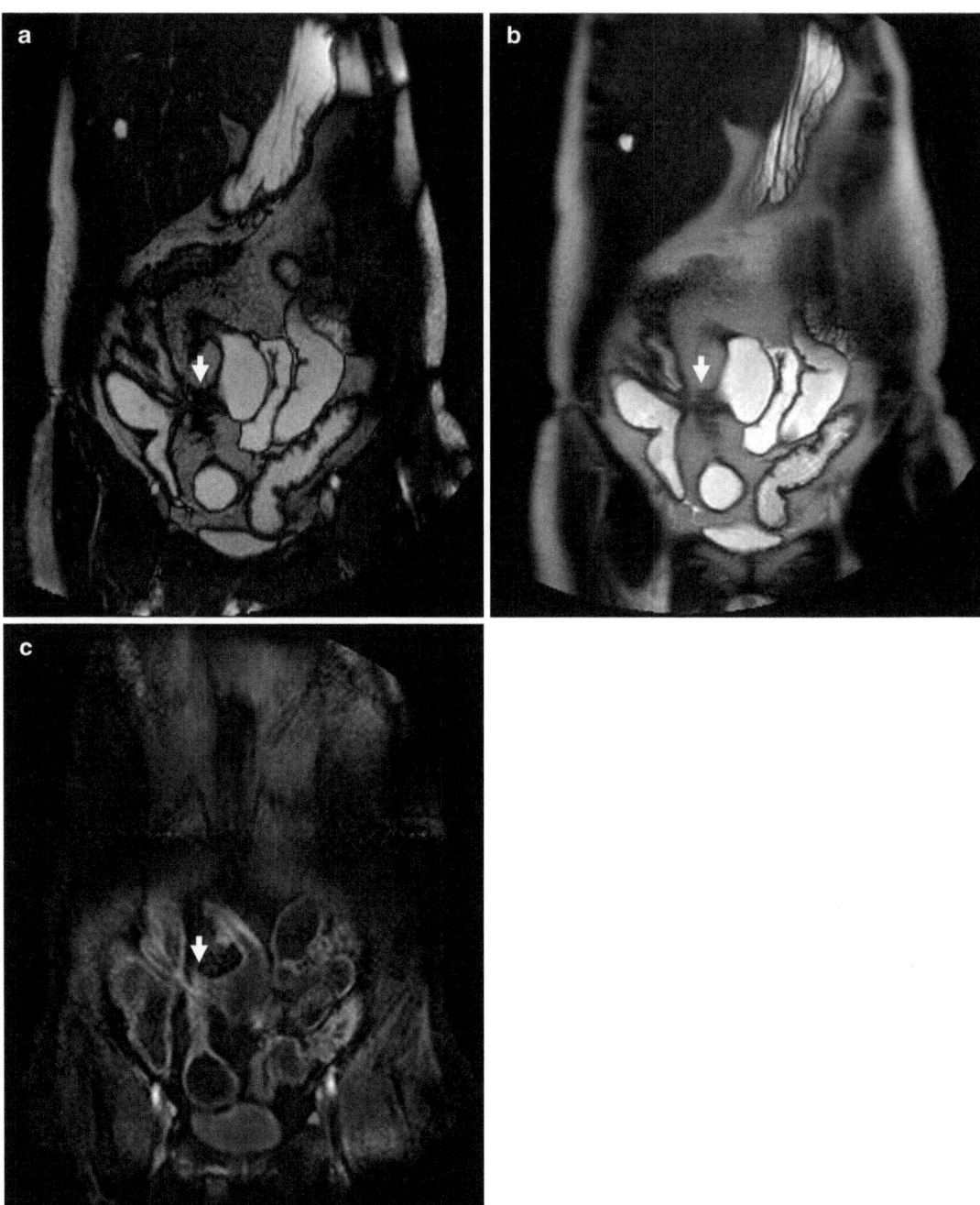

Fig. 18.13 (a–c) 22-year-old female patient with Crohn's disease and ileoileal enteroenteric fistula. Patient presenting with abdominal crampy pain and vomiting. (a) Coronal T1-weighted FFE MR imaging sequence; (b) coronal T2-weighted turbo spin-echo MR imaging sequence; (c) coronal T1-weighted breath-hold dynamic sequence with fat suppression after gadolinium-based contrast agent injection on arterial phase (30 s after contrast injection). All MR imaging sequences show stricture and distortion of distal ileum with adjacent luminal dilatation proximal to the stricture with evidence of converging point (arrow) of enteroenteric fistula from where bowel loops radiate

18.5   Ulcerative Colitis

UC is generally a superficial inflammatory process that affects the colonic mucosa [3], and the role of imaging technique is limited, while colonoscopy represents the reference technique for diagnosis. Button-shaped ulcers represent the most typical pattern at barium studies, while remaining islands of mucosa provide it a pseudopolyp appearance. Damage to the

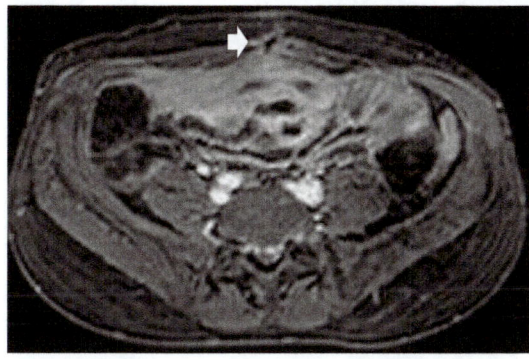

Fig. 18.14 40-year-old female patient with Crohn's disease and enterocutaneous fistula. Patient presenting with abdominal crampy pain and cutaneous mucous discharge. Transverse T1-weighted breath-hold dynamic sequence with fat suppression after gadolinium-based contrast agent injection on portal venous phase (60 s after contrast injection). Evidence of enterocutaneous fistula (arrow)

muscularis propria results in colonic dilation and loss of haustra. Toxic megacolon, a potentially fatal complication, is seen in less than 5% of patients and is characterized by both nonobstructive dilation of the colon to at least 6 cm and evidence of systemic toxicity, electrolyte disturbance, fluid loss, hemorrhage, and perforation.

CD and UC differentiation could be challenging, but UC does not involve the ileum with the exception of backwash reactive ileitis which, differently from CD, presents a patulous ileocecal valve and the absence of ileal mucosa ulceration [3].

Bowel wall thickening, even though less evident than in CD, represents the source of pain and can be easily identified by imaging techniques (Figs. 18.15 and 18.16) manifesting by mural enhancement after contrast administration.

18.6   Conclusion

Pain represents an extremely characteristic symptom of CD and may be due to transmural inflammation, fistulas, abscesses, phlegmons, and bowel strictures. Clinical assessment is essential in diagnosis and monitoring of CD although imaging represents a more effective tool in the objective assessment of CD inflammatory activity and correlation to patient pain.

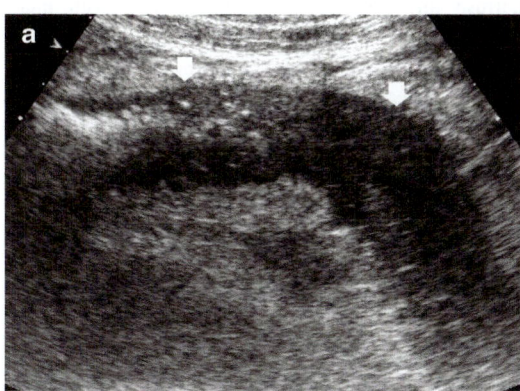
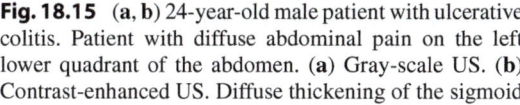
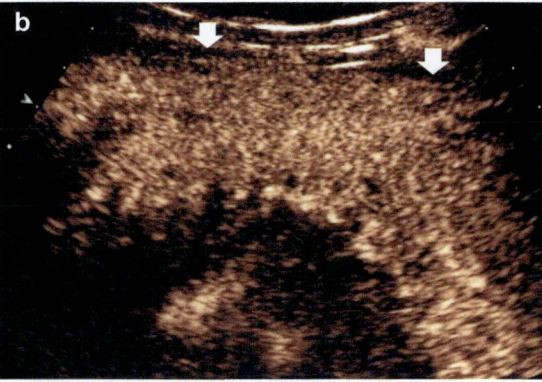

Fig. 18.15 (**a**, **b**) 24-year-old male patient with ulcerative colitis. Patient with diffuse abdominal pain on the left lower quadrant of the abdomen. (**a**) Gray-scale US. (**b**) Contrast-enhanced US. Diffuse thickening of the sigmoid colon (arrows) with adjacent creeping fat. (**b**) Contrast-enhanced US reveals diffuse contrast enhancement (arrows) corresponding to high inflammatory activity

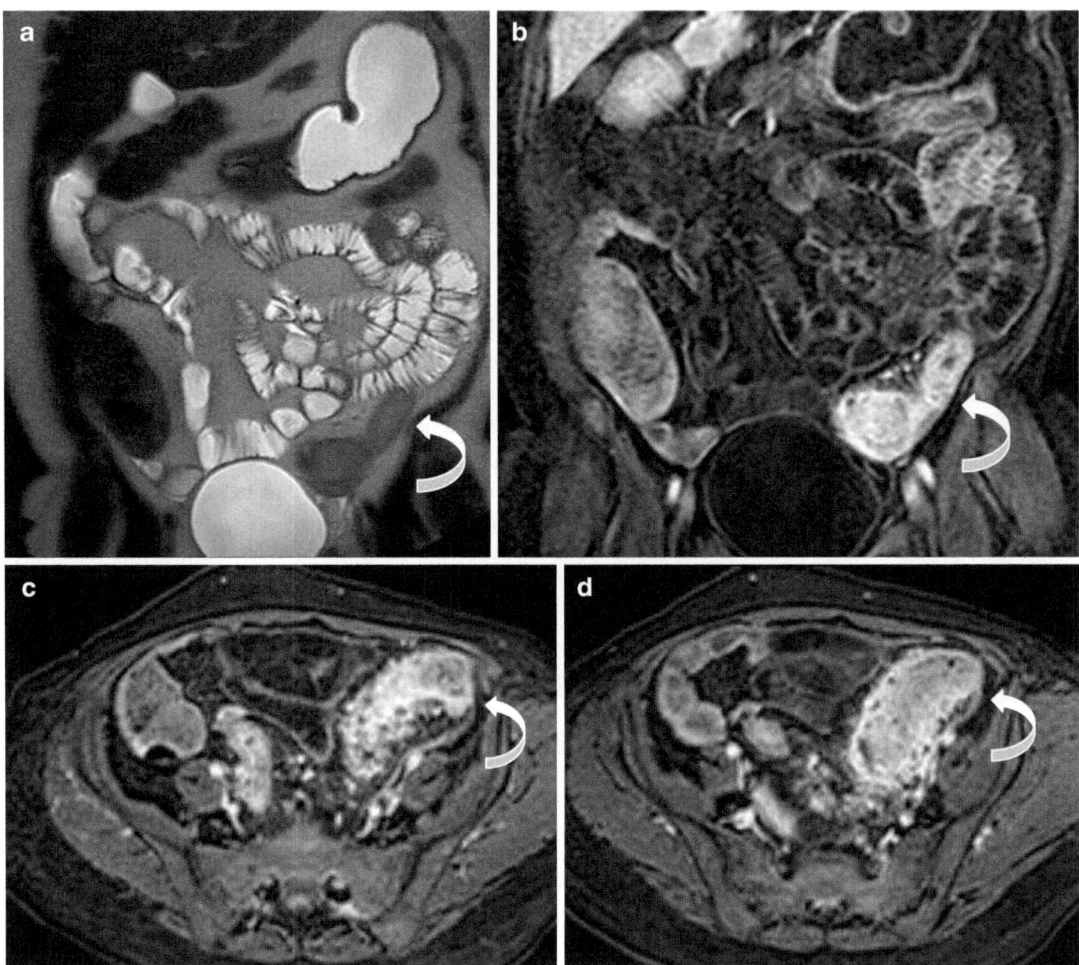

Fig. 18.16 33-year-old male patient with ulcerative colitis. Patient presenting with moderate abdominal pain, hemorrhagic diarrhea, urgency of defecation, and fever. (**a**) Coronal T2-weighted turbo spin-echo MR imaging sequence; (**b–d**) coronal (**b**) and transverse (**c, d**)

T1-weighted breath-hold dynamic sequence with fat suppression after gadolinium-based contrast agent injection on arterial phase (30 s after contrast injection). Diffuse thickening of the sigmoid tract with mural enhancement after contrast administration related to inflammation

References

1. Rieder F, Zimmermann EM, Remzi FH, et al. Crohn's disease complicated by strictures: a systematic review. Gut. 2013;62:1072–84.
2. Scarpa M, Angriman I, Barollo M, Polese L, Ruffolo C, Bertin M, Pagano D, D'Amico DF. Risk factors for recurrence of stenosis in Crohn's disease. Acta Biomed. 2003;74(Suppl 2):80–3.
3. Roggeveen MJ, Tismenetsky M, Shapiro R. Best cases from the AFIP: ulcerative colitis. Radiographics. 2006;26:947–51.
4. Best WR, Becktel JM, Singleton JW, Kern F. Development of a Crohn's disease activity index. Gastroenterology. 1976;70:439–44.
5. Onali S, Calabrese E, Pallone F. Measuring disease activity in Crohn's disease. Abdom Imaging. 2012;37:927–32.
6. Gasche C, Scholmerich J, Brynskov J, et al. A simple classification of Crohn's disease: report of the working party for the world congresses of gastroenterology, Vienna 1998. Inflamm Bowel Dis. 2000;6:8–15.
7. Ahmad T, Armuzzi A, Bunce M, et al. The molecular classification of the clinical manifestations of Crohn's disease. Gastroenterology. 2002;122:854–66.

8. Maglinte DD, Gourtsoyiannis N, Rex D, Howard TJ, Kelvin FM. Classification of small bowel Crohn's subtypes based on multimodality imaging. Radiol Clin North Am. 2003;41:285–303.

9. Mary JY, Modigliani R. Development and validation of an endoscopic index of the severity for Crohn's disease: a prospective multicentre study. Gut. 1989;30:983–9.

10. Geboes K. Histopathology of Crohn's disease and ulcerative colitis. In: Satsangi J, Sutherland L, editors. Inflammatory bowel disease. 4th ed. London: Harcourt; 2003. p. 255–76.

11. Gajendran M, Loganathan P, Catinella AP, Hashash JG. A comprehensive review and update on Crohn's disease. Dis Mon. 2018;64(2):20–57. https://doi.org/10.1016/j.disamonth.2017.07.001.

12. Ripollés T, Martínez-Pérez MJ, Blanc E, et al. Contrast-enhanced ultrasound (CEUS) in Crohn's disease: technique, image interpretation and clinical applications. Insights Imaging. 2011;2:639–52.

13. De Franco A, Marzo M, Felice C, et al. Ileal Crohn's disease: CEUS determination of activity. Abdom Imaging. 2012;37:359–68.

14. Quaia E, De Paoli L, Stocca T, Cabibbo B, Casagrande F, Cova MA. The value of small bowel wall contrast enhancement after sulphur hexaflu-oride-filled micro-bubble injection to differentiate inflammatory from fibrotic strictures in patients with Crohn's disease. Ultrasound Med Biol. 2012;38:1324–32.

15. Quaia E. Contrast-enhanced ultrasound of the small bowel in Crohn's disease. Abdom Imaging. 2013;38:1005–13.

16. Bodily KD, Fletcher JG, Solem CA, et al. Crohn's disease: mural attenuation and thickness at contrast-enhanced CT enterography—correlation with endoscopic and histologic findings of inflammation. Radiology. 2006;238:505–16.

17. Paulsen SR, Huprich JE, Fletcher JG, et al. CT enterography as a diagnostic tool in evaluating small bowel disorders: review of clinical experience with over 700 cases. Radiographics. 2006;26:641–57.

18. Gourtsoyiannis N, Papanikolaou N, Grammatikakis J, Papamastorakis G, Prassopoulos P, Roussomoustakaki M. Assessment of Crohn's disease activity in the small bowel with MR and conventional enteroclysis: preliminary results. Eur Radiol. 2004;14:1017–24.

19. Sempere GAJ, Martinez Sanjuan V, Medina Chulia E, et al. MRI evaluation of inflammatory activity in Crohn's disease. Am J Roentgenol. 2005;184:1829–35.

20. Tolan DJ, Greenhalgh R, Zealley IA, Halligan S, Taylor SA. MR enterographic manifestations of small bowel Crohn's disease. Radiographics. 2010;30:367–84.

21. Sinha R, Verma R, Verma S, Rajesh A. MR enterography of Crohn disease: Part 2, imaging and pathologic findings. Am J Roentgenol. 2011;197:80–5.

22. Rimola J, Rodríguez S, García-Bosch O, et al. Magnetic resonance for assessment of disease activity and severity in ileocolonic Crohn's disease. Gut. 2009;58:1113–20.

23. Buisson A, Hordonneau C, Goutte M, et al. Diffusion-weighted magnetic resonance enterocolonography in predicting remission after anti-TNF induction therapy in Crohn's disease. Dig Liver Dis. 2016;48:260–6.

24. Panes J, Bouzas R, Chaparro M, et al. Systematic review: the use of ultrasonography, computed tomography and magnetic resonance imaging for the diagnosis, assessment of activity and abdominal complications of Crohn's disease. Aliment Pharmacol Ther. 2011;34:125–45.

25. Panes J, Bouhnik Y, Reinisch W, et al. Imaging techniques for assessment of inflammatory bowel disease: joint ECCO and ESGAR evidence-based consensus guidelines. J Crohns Colitis. 2013;7:556–85.

26. Rimola J, Ordás I, Rodriguez S, et al. Magnetic resonance imaging for evaluation of Crohn's disease: validation of parameters of severity and quantitative index of activity. Inflamm Bowel Dis. 2011;17:1759–68.

27. Richards RJ. Management of abdominal and pelvic abscess in Crohn's disease. World J Gastrointest Endosc. 2011;3(11):209–12.

28. Yamaguchi A, Matsui T, Sakurai T, Ueki T, Nakabayashi S, Yao T, Futami K, Arima S, Ono H. The clinical characteristics and outcome of intraabdominal abscess in Crohn's disease. J Gastroenterol. 2004;39:441–8.

29. Bettenworth D, Nowacki TM, Cordes F, Buerke B, Lenze F. Assessment of stricturing Crohn's disease: current clinical practice and future avenues. World J Gastroenterol. 2016;22:1008–16.

30. Lenze F, Wessling J, Bremer J, Ullerich H, Spieker T, Weckesser M, Gonschorrek S, Kannengiesser K, Rijcken E, Heidemann J, Luegering A, Schober O, Domschke W, Kucharzik T, Maaser C. Detection and differentiation of inflammatory versus fibromatous Crohn's disease strictures: prospective comparison of 18F-FDG-PET/CT, MR enteroclysis, and transabdominal ultrasound versus endoscopic/histologic evaluation. Inflamm Bowel Dis. 2012;18:2252–60.

31. Catalano OA, Gee MS, Nicolai E, Selvaggi F, Pellino G, Cuocolo A, Luongo A, Catalano M, Rosen BR, Gervais D, Vangel MG, Soricelli A, Salvatore M. Evaluation of quantitative PET/MR enterography biomarkers for discrimination of inflammatory strictures from fibrotic strictures in Crohn disease. Radiology. 2016;278:792–800.

32. Lo Re G, Tudisca C, Vernuccio F, et al. MR imaging of perianal fistulas in Crohn's disease: sensitivity and specificity of STIR sequences. Radiol Med. 2016;121:243–51.

33. Erden A, Ünal S, Eser Akkaya E, et al. MR enterography in Crohn's disease complicated with enteroenteric fistula. Eur J Radiol. 2017;94:101–6.

Imaging of Vascular Abdominal Pain

Fabio Pozzi Mucelli and Roberta Pozzi Mucelli

19.1 Introduction

Abdominal pain is one of the top five causes for presentation to the emergency department and accounts for 18% of hospital admissions. It has one of the broadest differential diagnosis the hospitalist will confront, and therefore a methodological approach is paramount.

In order to promptly identify the underlying etiology of abdominal pain, the physician must identify the specific characteristics of the symptoms. Factors such as history of trauma, constitutional symptoms, surgical history, relation to food intake, and appetite must be considered. In addition, a careful history must be taken, considering the patient's previous diagnosis, dietary habits, travel history, medication, substance, and environmental exposures.

As with symptoms of other systems and organs, one must first consider basic features to get an idea of the acuity and character of the

abdominal pain, by asking questions pertaining to frequency, associated symptoms, radiation, characteristic, onset, location, duration, exacerbating factors, and relieving factors. A useful acronym to remember all these points is: FAR COLDER.

The differential diagnosis for generalized abdominal pain is vast. In order to remember the various entities that cause abdominal pain, it is helpful to consider broader categories first, such as inflammation, vascular causes, obstruction, cardiac causes, superficial entities, and systemic etiologies.

Focusing on vascular causes, these include either aneurysmatic and occlusive diseases of large vessels (aorta) or main vessels arising from the aorta (celiac trunk, hepatic, splenic, mesenteric, and renal arteries) and smaller vessels (gastroduodenal artery, pancreaticoduodenal arcade, Riolano's arcade). Also abdominal veins can be responsible of abdominal pain, although less frequently.

It must be underlined that abdominal pain of vascular origin generally reflects severe intestinal involvement and lesions that are rapidly irreversible. Diagnosis is difficult, and treatment is often delayed. Such involvement should be considered systematically when confronted with any atypical abdominal pain, especially if it is intense and appears abruptly, in any patient with vascular disease or having cardiac rhythm disorder. At an early stage, the contrast between the severity of pain and the lack of general and physical signs

Electronic Supplementary Material The online version of this chapter (https://doi.org/10.1007/978-3-319-99822-0_19) contains supplementary material, which is available to authorized users.

F. Pozzi Mucelli (✉)
SC (UCO) Radiologia Diagnostica e Interventistica, Azienda Sanitaria Universitaria Integrata di Trieste (ASUITS), Trieste, Italy
e-mail: fabio.pozzimucelli@asuits.sanita.fvg.it

R. Pozzi Mucelli
University of Trieste, Department of Radiology, Cattinara Hospital, Trieste, Italy

should suggest emergency CT scan followed by GI arteriography for diagnosis and deciding treatment. If such measures are impossible, laparotomy should be performed. At the stage of infarct, the presence of an unstable hemodynamic condition and peritoneal signs requires emergency laparotomy without paraclinical examinations. The severity of prognosis depends on the causes, the extent of lesions, patient background, and the rapidity with which treatment is initiated.

19.2 Abdominal Aortic Aneurysm

Abdominal aortic aneurysms (AAAs) are focal dilatations of the abdominal aorta that are 50% greater than the proximal normal segment or >3 cm in maximum diameter. The prevalence of AAAs increases with age, and approximately 10% of individuals older than 65 have an AAA. Males are much more commonly affected than females, with a ratio of 4:1. History of hypertension and smoking are predisposing factors [1]. They are the tenth most common cause of death in the Western world. Most AAAs are asymptomatic unless they leak or rupture and are therefore diagnosed incidentally when the abdomen is imaged for other indications. Unruptured aneurysms may uncommonly cause abdominal or back pain or a pulsatile mass if large.

The most common and feared complication is that of abdominal aortic rupture which presents with severe abdominal or back pain, hypotension and shock, and pulsatile abdominal mass. This classical triad of pain, hypotension, and pulsatile mass however is only seen in 25–50% of patients.

A chronic rupture may escape detection for about weeks to months and is known as sealed aneurysmal rupture or spontaneously healed aneurysmal rupture or abdominal aortic aneurysmal leak.

Unusual presentations of ruptured abdominal aortic aneurysm are transient lower limb paralysis, right upper quadrant pain, groin pain, testicular pain, testicular ecchymosis (blue scrotum sign of Bryant), and iliofemoral venous thrombosis. Flank ecchymosis (appearance of a bruise) is a sign of retroperitoneal bleeding and is also called Grey Turner's sign.

The mortality rate from a ruptured AAA is high (59–83% of patients die before they make it to a hospital or undergo surgery). The operative mortality rate for those who make it to surgery tends to be around 40%. Elective surgery mortality is much lower (4–6%).

Other reported complications include the development of a pseudoaneurysm from chronic contained leak/rupture or of aortic fistulas (aortocaval fistula, aortoenteric fistula). Other reported complications are distal thromboembolism or thrombotic occlusion of a branch vessel and infection/mycotic aneurysm.

The aneurysmal rupture is thought to occur when the mechanical stress is in excess of the wall strength. Thus, the aortic aneurysmal wall tension and the aneurysmal diameter are a significant predictor of impending rupture.

The commonest sites of rupture and their relative incidences are intraperitoneal rupture (20%), retroperitoneal rupture (80%), aortocaval fistula (3–4%), and primary aortoenteric fistula (<1%).

Precise prediction of rupture in patients with AAA continues to be a problem. In routine clinical practice, the maximum aortic diameter is the criterion most often used for AAA repair. The European Society of Vascular Surgery guidelines report an exponentially increasing annual rupture risk for patients exceeding diameters of 5.0–5.5 cm [2], but this sole parameter does not necessarily reflect the true risk of rupture in each patient. The potential for several additional parameters, including the geometrical AAA shape [3], female gender, arterial hypertension, smoking history, familial AAA predisposition [4, 5], and large amount of intraluminal thrombus formation, to elevate the individual rupture risk has been discussed, but these are rarely included in clinical decision-making regarding AAA repair. Recently, Erhart et al. evaluated the contribution of biomechanical parameters such as peak wall rupture risk index, peak wall stress, and rupture risk equivalent diameter in three subgroups of patients with AAA (asymptomatic, symptomatic, and ruptured AAA) and found that PWRI parameter distinguishes most precisely between asymptomatic and symptomatic AAAs. If elevated, this value may represent a negative prognostic factor for asymptomatic AAAs [6].

Imaging Findings Ultrasound is quite sensitive and specific because it is able to identify direct and undirect signs of a ruptured AAA. These signs are focal dilatation of the aorta (aneurysm), periaortic fluid, free intraperitoneal fluid, and retroperitoneal fluid, representing retroperitoneal hemorrhage.

In the acute clinical setting, obtaining unenhanced CT through the abdomen and pelvis may be helpful to detect impending rupture in AAA and also retroperitoneal or intraperitoneal rupture. Thereafter, thin section slices after contrast material administration will be obtained. The most common finding in the case of AAA rupture is retroperitoneal hemorrhage adjacent to the aneurysm. The periaortic blood may be seen to extend into perirenal or pararenal spaces or the psoas muscles. Intraperitoneal extension of the hemorrhage may be seen as an immediate or a delayed finding. On post-contrast studies or CT angiography, active extravasation of contrast material can be seen (Fig. 19.1a,b). The role of angiography is crucial in guiding endovascular repair of not ruptured but also ruptured AAA (Fig. 19.1c,d).

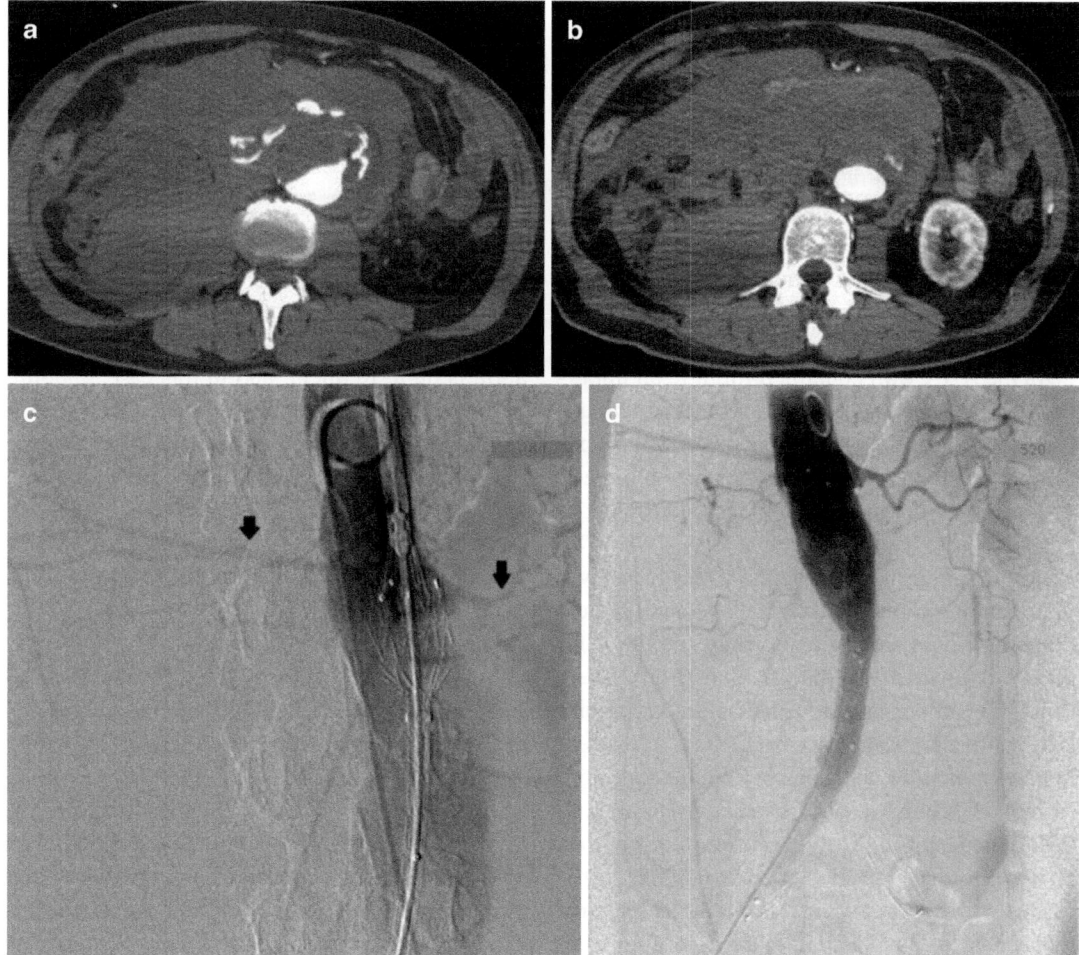

Fig. 19.1 Ruptured abdominal aortic aneurysm. Male, 60 years old. Sudden onset of acute abdominal pain, pulsatile abdominal mass, and shock. (**a**, **b**) CT angiography shows active extravasation from the aorta. A large hematoma is seen anteriorly and posteriorly in the right retroperitoneal space. (**c, d**) Emergent endovascular repair was performed: the stent graft was advanced till the level of renal arteries (arrows), and an aorto-uniliac stent graft was deployed

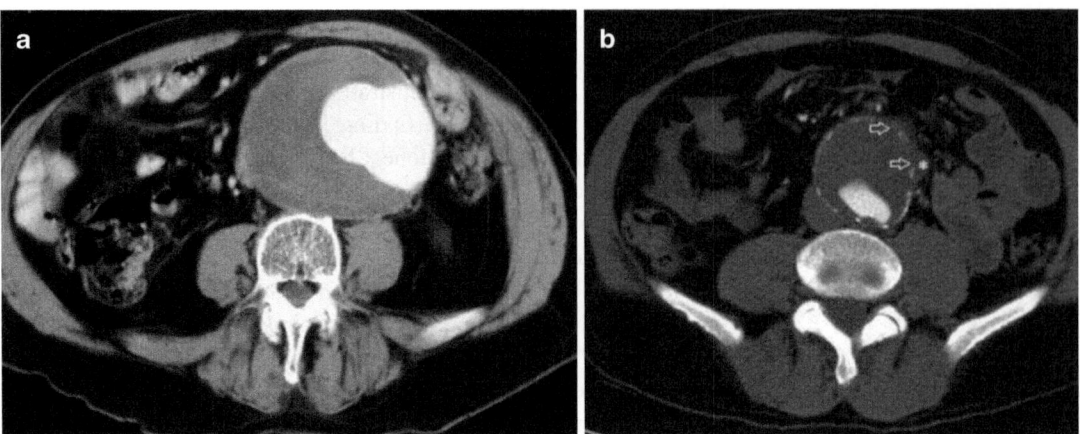

Fig. 19.2 Impending signs of AAA rupture. (**a**) Large AAA with nonhomogeneous thrombus (crescent sign). (**b**) 6.8 cm diameter AAA with focal interruption of aortic wall (arrows) and initial periaortic extension (*)

In hemodynamically stable patients with imaging features of contained aneurysmal rupture, providing preoperative management and avoidance of urgent repair are essential to prevent substantial morbidity and mortality. Previous rupture into a confined anatomic compartment should be suspected in patients with known history of AAA, previous episodes of abdominal pain, and stable hemodynamic status.

In the AAA with contained rupture, an important feature seen is the draped aorta sign, which is present when the posterior part of AAA drapes over the adjacent vertebrae and/or when there is no distinct border between the posterior aspect of AAA and its adjacent structures [7].

Another helpful radiological finding, in favor of impending rupture, is a hyperattenuating crescent sign which reflects hemorrhage in the mural thrombus or in the aneurysm wall (Fig. 19.2a). This sign, if present, appears as an intramural area with attenuation of more than the patent luminal region on unenhanced computed tomography or more than that of psoas muscle on contrast-enhanced CT [8]. Extravasation of contrast media into the mural thrombus of AAA, in the absence of frank retro- or intraperitoneal hemorrhage, is also considered another sign of impending rupture and represents the dissection of the blood from the patent lumen into the luminal thrombus which has not disrupted the aneurysm wall yet. Another sign is the focal interruption of the aortic wall (Fig. 19.2b).

19.3 Aortic Dissection

Aortic dissection is generally a pathology of the thoracic aorta, but involvement of abdominal aorta is quite frequent, and in this case, abdominal symptoms are important and depend on the extension of the dissection to the aorta and on the occlusion of the splanchnic branches which may lead to organ ischemia. The incidence of aortic dissection has been reported to be 2000 new cases per year in the United States and 3000 in Europe [9, 10, 11, 12].

Dissection is the result of a spontaneous longitudinal separation of the aortic intima and adventitia caused by the circulating blood gaining access to and splitting the media of the aortic wall [13].

The intimal tear allows the blood to enter the media from the vessel lumen. The blood-filled space within the medial layer becomes the false lumen. This results in two lumina, a true lumen and a false lumen, with the false lumen having pressures greater than or equal to those in the true lumen [14].

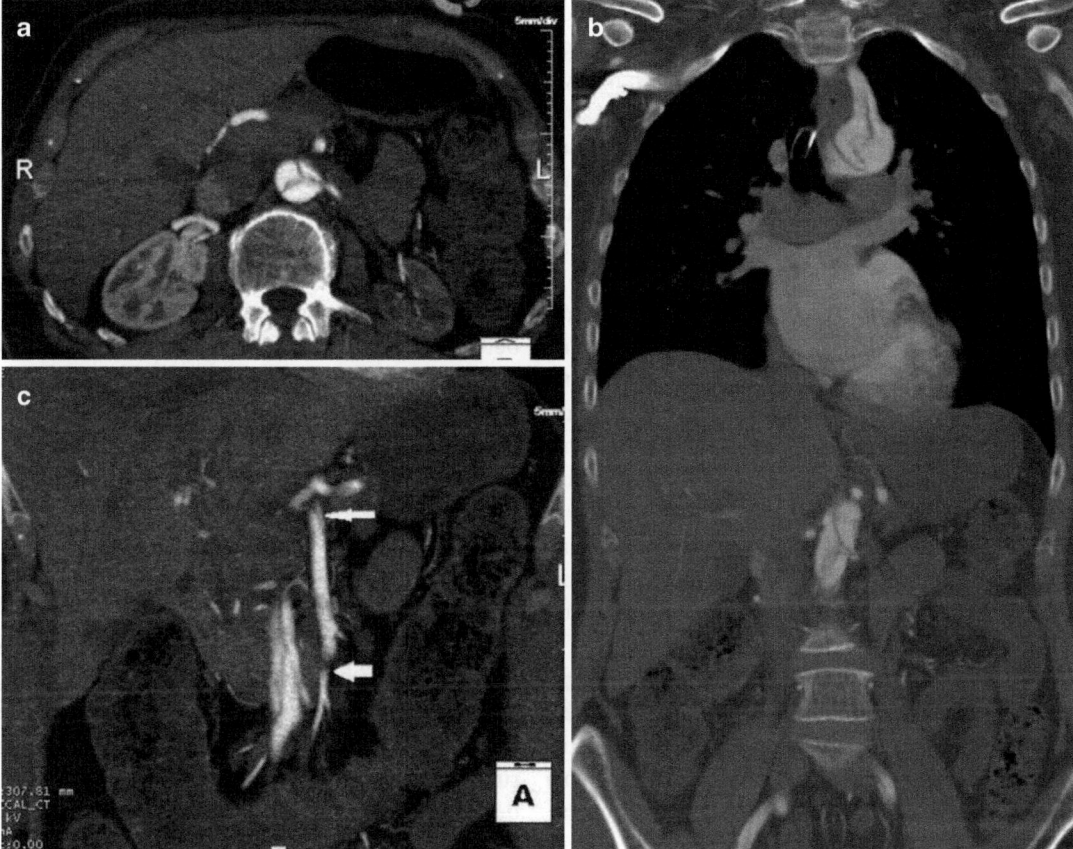

Fig. 19.3 Acute aortic dissection (Stanford A): Female, 71 years old. Sudden thoracic pain, faint brachial pulse on the left arm, and abdominal pain on the left side. (**a, b**) CT angiography: the abdominal aorta shows a complex inti- mal flap involving the ostium of the left renal artery. The left kidney appears hypoperfused. (**c**) An intimal flap (arrow) and a distal short occlusion (fat arrow) are visible also in the superior mesenteric artery

Imaging Findings Main abdominal arterial branch involvement has been reported in 27% of cases [15]; the celiac trunk, superior and inferior mesenteric arteries, and renal arteries can all be involved (Fig. 19.3). Occlusion of the celiac trunk may lead to splenic or hepatic infarction with pain and abnormal liver blood test results. Involvement of the mesenteric branches can lead to mesenteric ischemia with nausea, vomiting, nasogastric aspirates, abdominal pain, bloody diarrhea, recurrent sepsis, and abnormal hepatic and pancreatic enzymes [16]. Compromise of the renal arteries can lead to ischemia with oliguria, anuria, and abnormal renal blood parameters (Fig. 19.3a,b). Renal arteries supplied by the false lumen are rarely compromised [16].

19.4 Visceral Artery Aneurysms and Pseudoaneurysms

The term visceral artery aneurysm (VAA) has been used to refer to any intra-abdominal aneurysm excluding those of the aortoiliac axis. VAA is a rare entity and includes true aneurysms and pseudoaneurysms. True aneurysms are often asymptomatic and are discovered on cross-sectional imaging performed for unrelated clinical indications. The main etiology for VAA is degenerative atherosclerosis, sometimes with the aspect of a post-stenotic aneurysm. Visceral artery pseudoaneurysms are potentially severe vascular lesions that arise from splanchnic circulation, as a result of various causes including inflammation, infection, trauma, and neoplasm [17, 18]. Unlike true aneurysms that have all three arterial wall layers, pseudoaneurysms develop from the disruption of intimal and medial layers of the arterial wall and do not contain any epithelized wall. They are outlined by thin fibrous tissue and are usually surrounded by periarterial hematoma.

The incidence of rupture of pseudoaneurysms varies from 2 to 80% depending on the location, with untreated mortality rates reaching up to 100% [19–21]. Pseudoaneurysms have various etiologies such as inflammation (pancreatitis and cholecystitis), infection (abscess), vasculitis, trauma (iatrogenic or penetrating injury), collagen vascular disease, segmental arterial mediolysis, and malignancy [21, 22]. The distinction between true or false aneurysm is not always possible.

The more frequent location of visceral aneurysm is the splenic artery (60%), followed by the coeliac trunk, the renal artery, the hepatic artery, the superior mesenteric artery (SMA) and its branches, the gastroduodenal artery, the pancreaticoduodenal artery, the gastric artery, and a combination of these.

As previously said, visceral artery aneurysms are often asymptomatic. In fact, a recent paper [23] describing 233 patients with 255 aneurysms, only 62/233 patients (26.6%) had symptoms, and of these, only 11 presented with abdominal pain. Presentation of pseudoaneurysms may vary from the absence of symptoms to life-threatening hemorrhage and death [24]. The most common symptom (50–63% cases) is hemorrhage, which can present as gastrointestinal bleeding due to rupture of a pseudoaneurysm arising from celiac, SMA, and inferior mesenteric arteries (IMA) or hematuria, from renal artery pseudoaneurysm or intra-abdominal hematoma [19, 25, 26].

Patients with severe hemorrhage may present with hypotension and shock. Pain is the next common presentation, seen in one third of patients [25]. Uncommonly, a hematoma can cause mass effect and present with symptoms like jaundice secondary to common bile duct compression [27]. The incidental detection of visceral pseudoaneurysms is reported in one third of patients [25].

Sizes of VAA at the moment of diagnosis are quite variable, going from 15 mm to 9–10 cm. In the analysis of Pitton et al. no correlation was found between diameter and risk of rupture, and the mean transverse diameter of non-ruptured and ruptured cases was nearly equal (15.9 ± 7.4 mm vs. 14.3 ± 7.5 mm, respectively). Moreover, there was no significant difference between the mean diameters of false aneurysms compared to true aneurysms (15.6 ± 7.6 mm vs. 16.3 ± 10.3 mm, respectively).

19.4.1 Splenic Artery Aneurysms (SAAs)

SAAs are four times more common in women than in men. Most aneurysms are small (2–4 cm), asymptomatic, solitary, saccular, and located in the middle to distal splenic artery. Impending rupture of an SAA can produce left upper quadrant pain radiating to the subscapular region. Rupture is a catastrophic event, manifesting with pain and hypotension. SAA has strong associations with female gender, pregnancy [28], and portal hypertension [29]. Most of SAAs are degenerative, with fragmentation of the elastic fibers and loss of smooth muscle in the media [30]. Pseudoaneurysms associated with pancreatitis and pancreatic pseudocysts are another frequent cause of SAA [31] (Fig. 19.4).

There is a strong association of SAA with female gender, pregnancy, and parity that is likely related to the hormonal effects of estrogen and progesterone, both with receptor sites in the arterial wall [32]. Relaxin, a hormone seen late in pregnancy and responsible for the elasticity of the symphysis pubis, may also alter the elasticity of the arterial wall [33]. The high-flow state associated with pregnancy further contributes to the deleterious effects on the arterial wall. Rupture of a SAA during pregnancy, most often in the third trimester, is a catastrophic event, with reported maternal and fetal mortality rates of 70 and 90%, respectively [34].

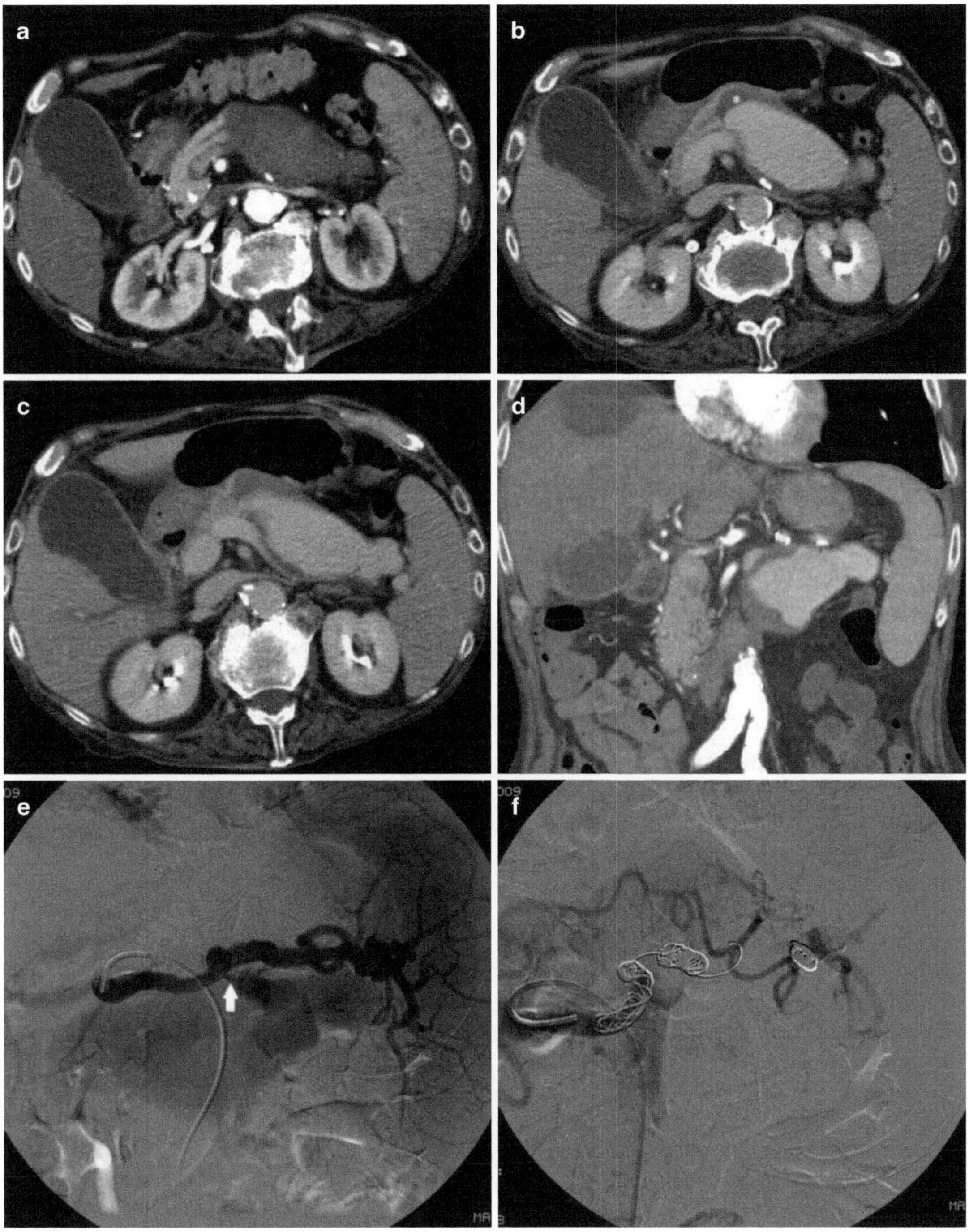

Fig. 19.4 Splenic artery pseudoaneurysm. Male, 82 years old, abdominal pain, known as splenic pseudoaneurysm significantly increased in size at follow-up. (a) CT angiography: in the arterial phase, a hypodense oval mass is visible anteriorly to the splenic vessels. (b–d) This mass shows a huge enhancement in the portal phase suggesting the vascular nature. A thin parietal thrombus is visible peripherally (*). (e) Selective angiography of the splenic artery confirms the presence of a focal active bleeding (arrow). (f) Endovascular treatment: the bleeding was stopped by deploying coils in the splenic artery distally and proximally to the hole

Imaging Findings Although ultrasonography (US) can be used to identify SAA, this technique has some limitations due to the retrogastric position of the aneurysm, the presence of wall calcifications, and the size of the aneurysm. Multidetector CT, on the contrary, does not have any limitation and is considered the modality of choice for the detection and planning of treatment of this pathology. Plain CT may detect linear calcification on the wall of the SAA, suggesting a true aneurysm, while the arterial phase can differentiate the real lumen of the sac from the wall thrombus (Fig. 19.4b). Furthermore, the arterial phase may give information concerning the morphology of the aneurysm, in particular, the size of the neck and the afferent and efferent vessels. All these informations are useful for the therapeutic approach. Angiography has a fundamental role for endovascular treatment of such aneurysms and pseudoaneurysms which can be excluded with different modalities such as proximal and distal occlusion of the splenic artery (Fig. 19.4) or filling of the sac with coils.

19.4.2 Hepatic Artery Aneurysms

Hepatic artery aneurysm is the second most common VAA and unlike SAAs demonstrates a male predilection of 2:1 [35]. Most hepatic artery aneurysms are solitary and involve the hepatic artery outside the liver (66% of cases) [36]. Aneurysm location often helps identify both cause and treatment strategy. Intrahepatic branch aneurysms/pseudoaneurysms are most frequently the result of trauma, iatrogenic injury from biopsy or intervention, infection, or vasculitis (Fig. 19.5). In contrast, extrahepatic aneurysms are most often degenerative or dysplastic [37], and less frequently pancreatitis may be responsible of pseudoaneurysm located in the common or proper hepatic artery. [38].

Although hepatic artery aneurysms may be discovered incidentally, many are symptomatic. These aneurysms may manifest with rupture into the peritoneal cavity or with gastrointestinal hemorrhage. The triad of epigastric pain, hemobilia, and obstructive jaundice (Quincke's

triad) is seen in one third of symptomatic patients [39]. Risk factors associated with rupture are poorly defined, and the prevalence of rupture is difficult to assess. Rupture has been reported in 20–80% of cases [40], with mortality rates ranging from 21 to 35% [41].

Imaging Findings Color Doppler US is quite sensitive and specific in identifying hepatic artery aneurysms or pseudoaneurysms especially when these are located at the liver hilum. MDCT is superior in the detection also of those aneurysm located in the hepatic artery before the liver. Angiography plays an important role as a first therapeutic option by means of embolization procedure (Fig. 19.5c,d).

19.4.3 Renal Artery Aneurysms

Although RAAs have traditionally not been included in reviews of VAA, they are in fact the second or third most common VAA (15–22% of cases) [42]. RAAs are discovered at 0.3–0.7% of autopsies and up to 1% of renal arteriographic procedures [43]. These aneurysms have a female predilection. Most are saccular and noncalcified and tend to occur at the bifurcation of the MRA. Fibromuscular dysplasia is a common cause of RAAs, with degenerative aneurysms, vasculitis, and trauma accounting for most of the others [44].

Another unusual cause of renal aneurysms are angiomyolipomas (AMLs) which are common benign tumors of the kidney composed of varying amounts of fat, smooth muscle, and abnormal thick-walled blood vessels. AMLs may occur as isolated lesions or are associated with tuberous sclerosis (TS). Isolated or sporadic AMLs account for 80–90% of reported cases and commonly occur in women aged 40–70. The lesions in this group are usually unilateral and focal. AMLs associated with TS are usually bilateral and multifocal and can occur at any age and in either sex. Most patients are asymptomatic, and the tumor is often incidentally detected during US or CT [45, 46]. When symptoms do occur, common presenting symptoms are flank or

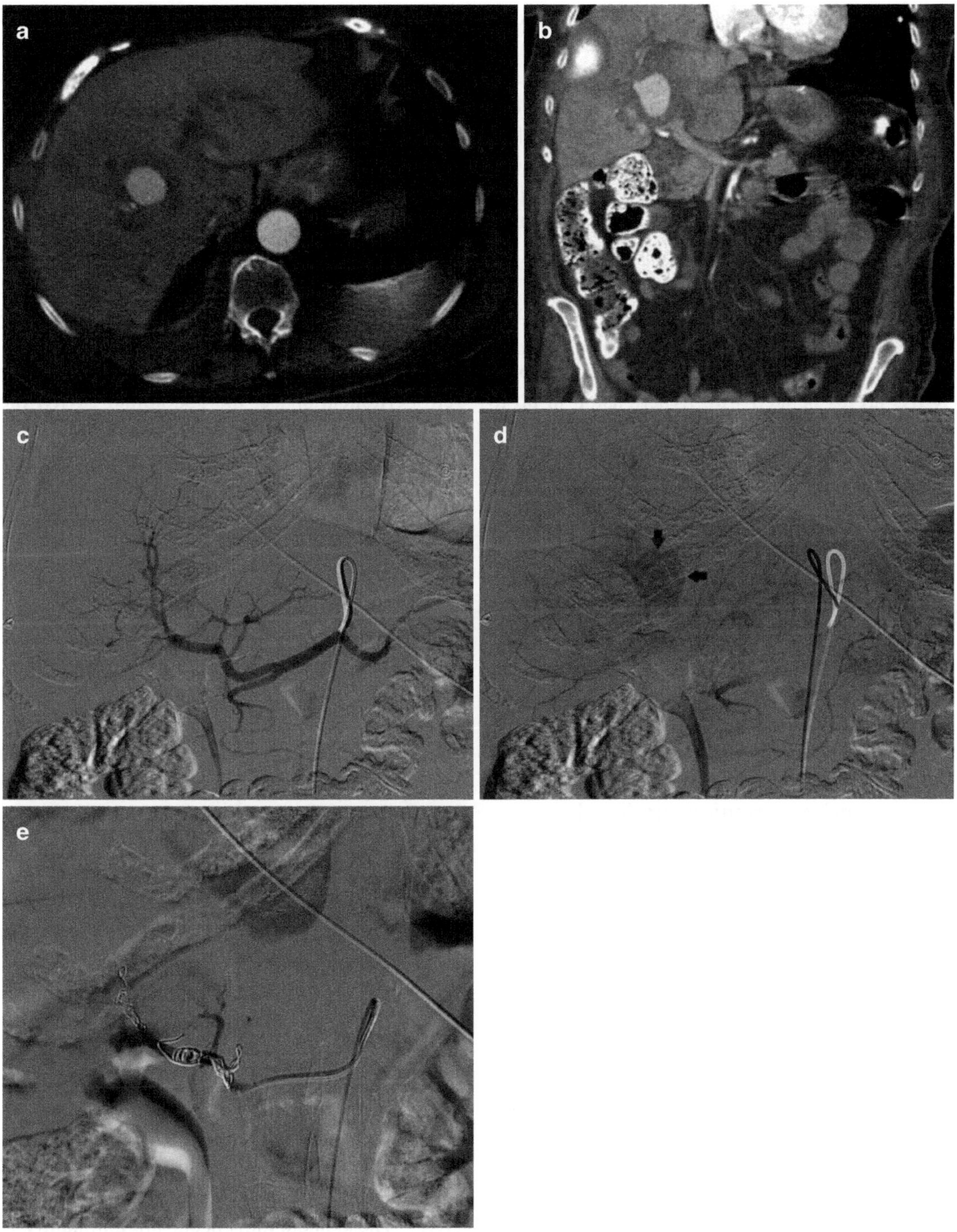

Fig. 19.5 Hepatic artery pseudoaneurysm. Female, 77 years old, 1 month before a biliary drainage was deployed for an obstructive jaundice. Sudden onset of right flank pain, drop of hemoglobin values, and hemobilia. (**a, b**) CT angiography reveals a pseudoaneurysm of an intrahepatic segmental artery at the level of the hilum. In the meantime, the biliary drainage was removed (the subcapsular hyperdense lesion visible in the upper right lobe is expression of contrast media extravasation during biliary drainage removal). (**c, d**) Angiography confirms the pseudoaneurysm (arrows). Embolization was performed deploying some coils in a right segmental arterial branch but also at the level of main bifurcation of proper hepatic artery

abdominal pain, palpable mass, and hematuria related to spontaneous intramural or extramural hemorrhage. The main complication of AMLs is hemorrhage, which is related to the tumor size, increased vascularity, and abnormal thick-walled vessels that are predisposed to the formation of micro-/macroaneurysms which can rupture spontaneously or after minor trauma (Fig. 19.6). AMLs larger than 4 cm in diameter increase the risk for hemorrhage [47].

Most RAAs are asymptomatic, but symptoms may develop from rupture, embolization of the peripheral vascular bed, or arterial thrombosis. RAAs are associated with hypertension in up to 73% of cases [44]. Hypothesis regarding the pathophysiologic basis of hypertension includes coexisting renal artery stenosis, microembolization from the aneurysm, compression or kinking of the renal artery or its branches, and turbulent flow. Improvement in hypertension following treatment has been reported [44], and hematuria has been reported in 30% of RAAs [42].

19.4.4 Aneurysms and Pseudoaneurysms of the Gastroduodenal and Pancreaticoduodenal Arteries

Gastroduodenal artery (GDA) aneurysms are often complications of acute and chronic pancreatitis and pancreatic surgery. GDA aneurysm is among the rarest VAAs, accounting only for 1.5% of the total, second in its rarity only to inferior mesenteric artery aneurysm. Despite its rarity, it represents an important subcategory of VAAs on account of having up to 75% risk of rupture [48], with gastrointestinal bleeding being the presenting feature in up to 52% of cases. They may also be dysplastic or degenerative in otherwise healthy patients [28].

GDA aneurysms, as the other VAAs, may be classified into false or true aneurysms, with the former being more common. Pancreatitis and atherosclerosis are the most common etiological factors associated with GDA aneurysm formation. Leakage of proteolytic enzymes in the setting of

pancreatitis can result in destruction of the vessel wall with subsequent false aneurysm formation. Weakening of the arterial wall secondary to atherosclerosis is the usual pathogenetic event for true aneurysms. However, some authors proposed that atherosclerotic celiac trunk stenosis may cause retrograde flow of the blood through the superior mesenteric and then pancreaticoduodenal arteries with consequent building of pressure in the GDA and aneurysm formation.

Pancreaticoduodenal artery (PDA) aneurysms are rare but a clinically important form of vascular disease that can cause death by bleeding into the retroperitoneal space, the abdominal cavity, the gastrointestinal tract, or a combination of them. Most of the publications about PDA aneurysms are case reports [49]. Aneurysms of the PDA can be divided into "true" and "false." False aneurysms are caused by a local factor, such as pancreatitis, tumor, abdominal trauma, surgery, or septic emboli. True aneurysms are variously caused by atherosclerosis, fibromuscular dysplasia, stenosis/occlusion of the celiac artery, and connective tissue disorders. A small proportion of PDA aneurysms are indirectly caused by compression by the median arcuate ligament (MAL), as a result of a high-flow state in the pancreatic arterial arcade (due to stenosis of the celiac artery) (Fig. 19.7a–c). Technical progress has made it possible to diagnose PDA using contrast-enhanced computed tomography (CT). Angiography is used mainly for selective embolization (Fig. 19.7d–f).

19.4.5 Superior Mesenteric Artery Aneurysm

SMA aneurysms account for 5.5% of all VAAs. SMA aneurysms can be saccular or fusiform and are commonly found in the proximal 5 cm of the artery. These aneurysms occur predominantly in men and are most often diagnosed in the fifth decade of life. Although the number of reported mycotic aneurysms has declined in recent years, such aneurysms still commonly affect the SMA (33–66% of cases) [50, 51]. Recent reports suggest an increase in the prevalence of both true

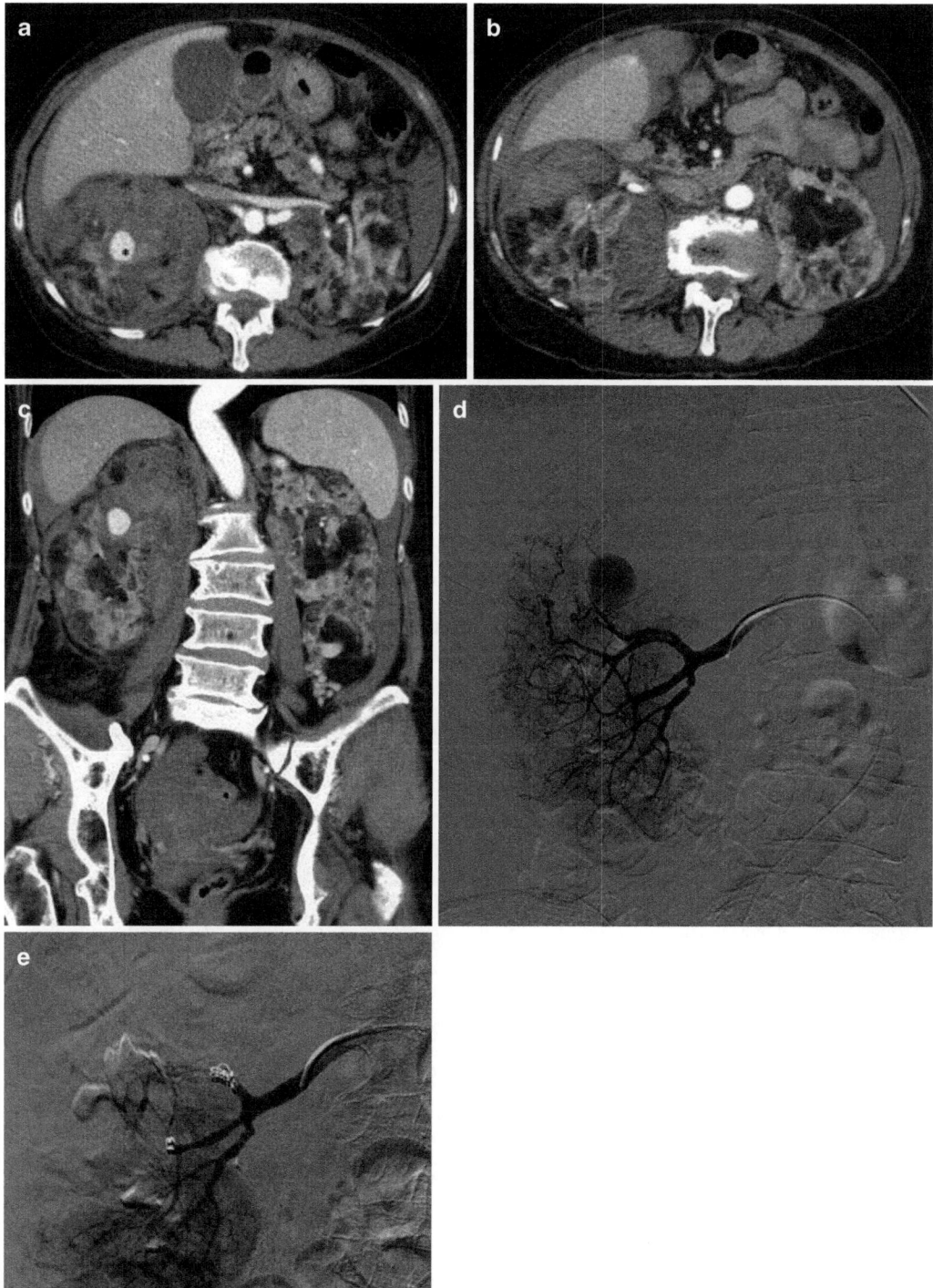

Fig. 19.6 Bleeding angiomyolipoma. Female, 75 years old. Right flank pain, severe anemia, and hematuria. (**a–c**) CT angiography shows multiple fat containing masses in both kidneys with a typical aspect of tuberous sclerosis. On the right kidney, a hyperattenuating mass (*) suggestive for pseudoaneurysm is clearly visible and also a fluid collection in the perirenal space and in the intraperitoneal spaces around the liver and spleen. (**c, d**) The lady underwent an emergent endovascular procedure of embolization with coils of the feeding arteries with complete resolution of symptoms

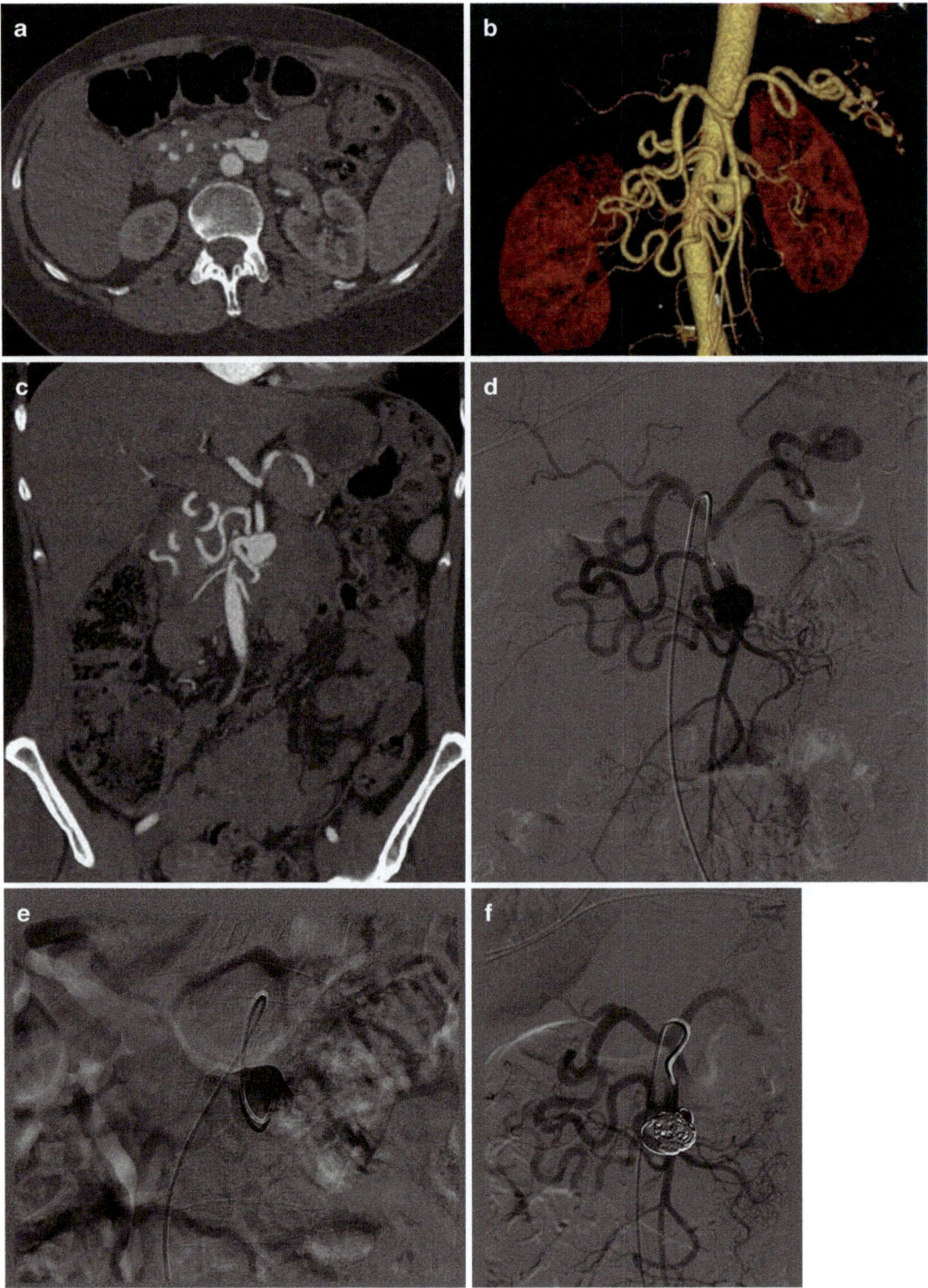

Fig. 19.7 Pancreatic-duodenal artery aneurysm in a female with Dunbar's syndrome. Female, 52 years old, history of postprandial pain. (**a–c**) CT angiography (axial view, VR and MIP coronal view) shows a 4.5 cm aneurysm arising close to the SMA from one of two pancreatic-duodenal arteries which appear hypertrophic and, in a retrograde way, feed the gastroduodenal, hepatic, and splenic artery. The celiac trunk is occluded at the origin. (**d**) Catheter angiography confirms CT finding. After selective catheterization of the aneurysmatic sac (**e**), embolization was performed with pushable coils with a satisfactory result (**f**)

and false aneurysms of the SMA [52, 53]. Other causes of SMA aneurysm include inflammation, vasculitis, trauma, arterial dissection, and dysplastic and degenerative aneurysms [28]. SMA aneurysms are often symptomatic, manifesting with acute and colicky upper abdominal pain, nausea, or vomiting. Symptoms may arise from aneurysm embolization of the peripheral vascular bed to narrowing of the arterial lumen. A palpable mass has been reported in up to 50% of patients [28].

Imaging Findings The diffuse use of CT, US, and MR has increased the detection of VAAs either when they are asymptomatic or when they became symptomatic. Plain abdominal film does not have a significant role and may detect only large calcifications with a laminar aspect which can be seen quite frequently in splenic artery aneurysm. US, with the use of color Doppler imaging, has the ability to detect aneurysm also if it is limited by the location of the lesion frequently hidden by the bowel or gastric gas or the position, as in the case of splenic artery aneurysm, located posteriorly to the stomach. Also calcification in the wall of the aneurysm may obscure detection of visceral aneurysm in US.

CT does not have significant limitations: at plain CT, VAA appears as a low attenuation round lesion, without homogeneous content in case of thrombus inside the aneurysm and sometimes laminar peripheral calcifications. After intravenous contrast injection, VAA shows a marked enhancement with Hounsfield values similar to that of contiguous arteries. The margins of the lesions are well defined if the wall of the aneurysm or pseudoaneurysm is unbroken. In the case of wall rupture, a fluid collection is visible surrounding the aneurysm with attenuation values lower than those of the aneurysm. At plain CT, high value inside this collection can be found suggesting the presence of fresh blood. With fast CT acquisition during contrast media injection, active bleeding outside the aneurysm or pseudoaneurysm can be detected.

19.4.6 Mesenteric Ischemia

Mesenteric ischemia accounts for approximately 1% of acute abdomen hospitalizations and occurs in 0.1% patients presenting to emergency department [54]. Despite growing recognition of this entity and interest in preventing irreversible ischemia, early diagnosis is challenging because symptoms are non-specific [55]. Despite major diagnostic and treatment advances in the last decades, low clinical suspicion leads to persistently high mortality rates of 40–70% for acute mesenteric ischemia (AMI) [56]. Early diagnosis is necessary to start the appropriate treatment, whereas diagnostic delay contributes to poor patient outcomes. A 24-h delay decreases survival rates by 20% [57].

In 70–80% of cases, intestinal ischemia is caused by an arterial embolus or thrombosis within the superior mesenteric artery. Embolic occlusions are more dangerous due to the absence of a well-developed collateral circulation; they cause earlier ischemia and transmural necrosis compared to other causes of mesenteric ischemia. Less common causes are venous thrombosis and non-thrombotic mechanical causes such as strangulated hernia [58]. Patients with a history of arterial emboli, vasculitis, deep venous thrombosis, hypercoagulable state, or chronic postprandial pain are at increased risk [59]. Vasculitis is a common cause of mesenteric ischemia in younger people with autoimmune disease [60]. Finally, case reports implicate vascular anomalies as a cause of mesenteric ischemia [61, 62].

There are a wide variety of clinical presentations for mesenteric ischemia. Classically, AMI is associated with a dramatic onset of severe abdominal pain disproportionate to physical exam findings. Peritonitis and septicemia develop once the ischemia has progressed transmurally. Postprandial pain, nausea, and weight loss often occur in patients with chronic mesenteric ischemia and superior mesenteric artery thrombosis [55]. In chronic mesenteric ischemia, the association of pain with meals leads to fear of eating and subsequent weight loss [59].

Classically, patients with mesenteric ischemia have leukocytosis, metabolic acidosis, an elevated D-dimer, and elevated serum lactate [55].

Imaging Findings Until the introduction of MDCT, mesenteric angiography was considered the gold standard for the diagnosis of mesenteric ischemia [59]. When the clinician was aware of possible AMI, angiography showed good accuracy and increased survival [63]. However, catheter angiography is invasive and time-consuming. Furthermore, the unavailability of this diagnostic modality at most hospitals leads to a critical delay. However over the last two decades, there

has been a major shift toward CT angiography because it is less invasive, less time- and resource-consuming, and more readily available. Today, CT angiography has replaced angiography as the gold standard in diagnosing mesenteric ischemia with a sensitivity and specificity of 96% and 94%, respectively [64, 65]. Typical CT angiography findings are evidence of arterial stenosis (defined as luminal diameter narrowing of more than 50%) or occlusion in the celiac, superior, and inferior mesenteric arteries (Figs. 19.8 and 19.9) and their first-order branches and signs of nonocclusive mesenteric ischemia: diffuse severe narrowing of the main arteries or their branches,

Fig. 19.8 Superior mesenteric artery stenosis responsible of "claudication abdominis." Female 63 years old, postprandial pain and significant weight loss. (**a**) CT angiography reveals a short stenosis at the origin of SMA and an AAA involving the origin of IMA which is occluded. (**b**) Catheter angiography confirms the severe stenosis at the proximal tract of SMA. The stenosis was crossed with a microguidewire, and a balloon-expandable stent was deployed at the origin of the vessel with complete resolution of the stenosis (**c**). The lady had total symptom relief and regained weight

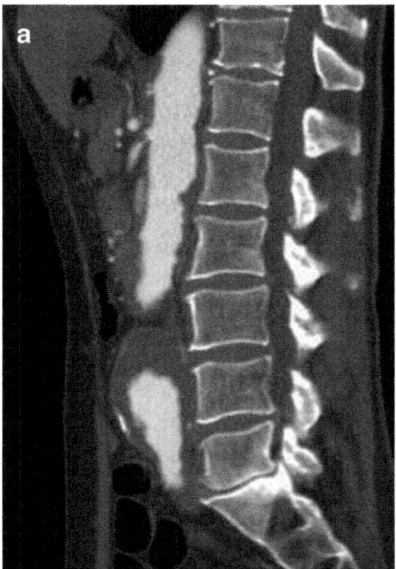
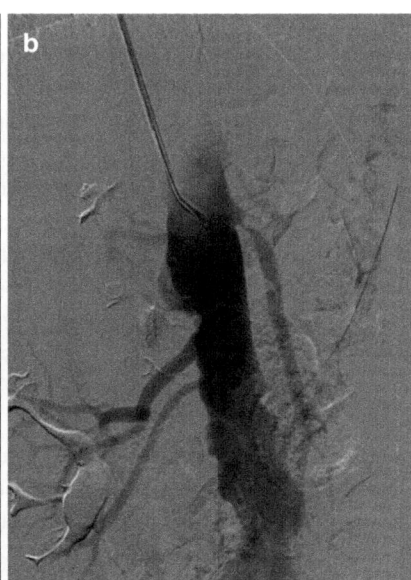
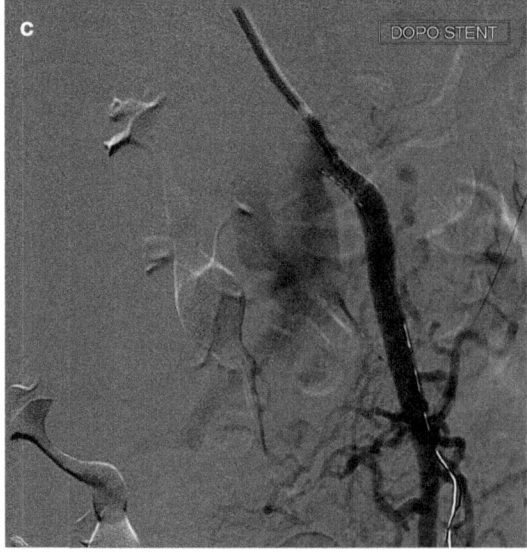

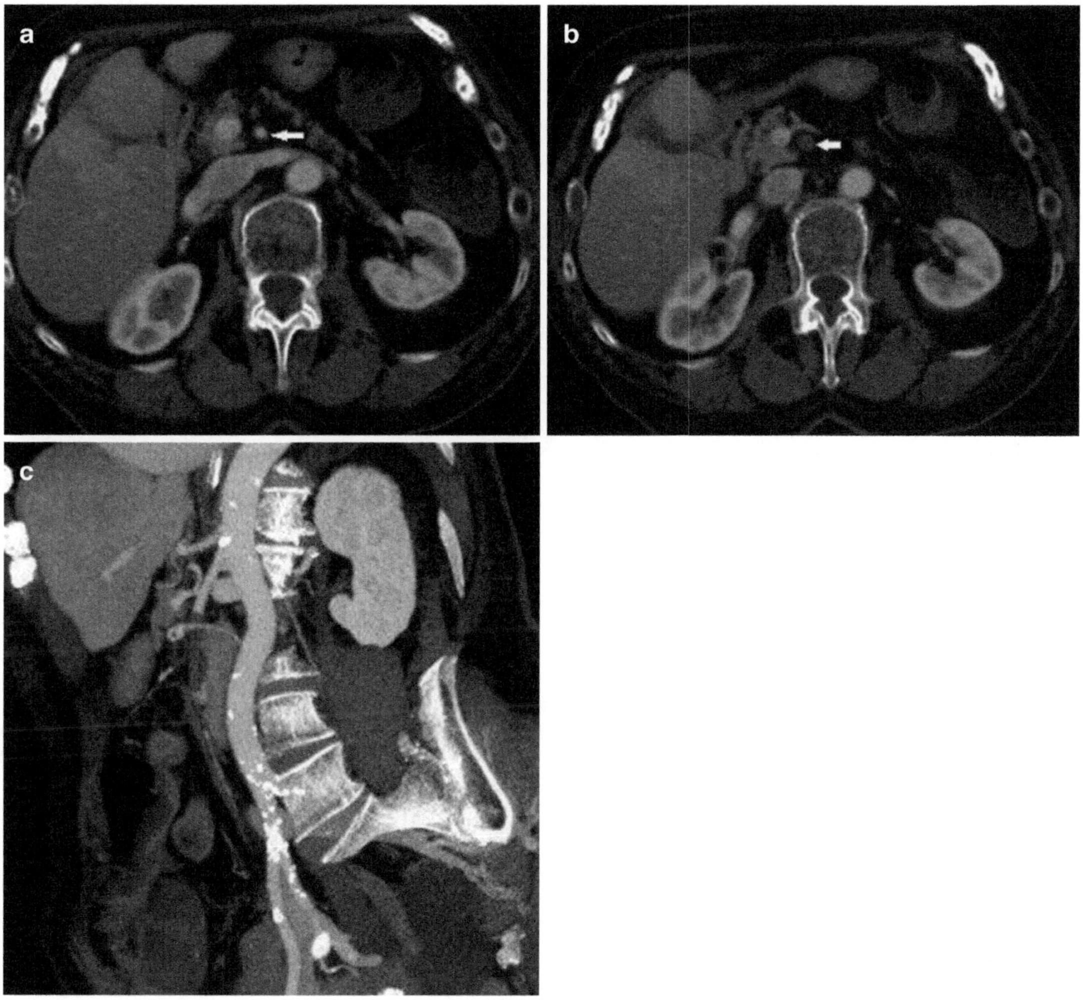

Fig. 19.9 Mesenteric infarction. Female, 96 years old. Acute epigastric pain. (**a, b**) CT angiography: the SMA appears normal in **a** (arrow), while in **b** (5 mm below), it is completely occluded (arrow). (**c**) MIP reconstruction clearly shows the occlusion of the SMA few cm after its origin. Distally, the artery is reperfused with a small caliber

segmental stenosis, and dilations [59]. Atherosclerotic changes were also noted. However, acute mesenteric ischemia can be postulated only in cases of SMA occlusion (embolus or thrombosis) (Fig. 19.9). Other studies [55, 66] relied mostly on indirect signs, such as wall thickening, wall perfusion, abdominal fat stranding, pneumatosis intestinalis, and venous gas, which by definition are a late sequel and reflect end organ damage. These indirect signs have a lower specificity and can result from other abdominal catastrophic events. Although mesenteric angiography has been replaced by noninvasive imaging as MDCT, angiography is still used

for endovascular treatment of stenotic lesion of SMA and IMA (Fig. 19.8 b,c).

A rare cause of abdominal angina is the median arcuate ligament syndrome (MALS) also known as Dunbar's syndrome (Fig. 19.7). This is an unusual condition caused by abnormally low insertion of the median arcuate ligament fibers, resulting in compression and luminal narrowing of the coeliac trunk. These fibers connect the right and left crura of the diaphragm and define the anterior margin of the aortic hiatus. The coeliac trunk supplies blood to digestive splanchnic organs through left gastric, common hepatic, and splenic arteries. Supply to the intestines includes the coeliac trunk, superior mesenteric artery, and inferior mesenteric artery [67]. The coeliac trunk is an essential source of blood because the interconnections with the SMA and IMA are not adequate to sustain sufficient perfusion to splanchnic organs. Typically, the arcuate ligament compresses the coeliac trunk on expiration, thereby eliciting occlusion of the coeliac trunk. Inspiration induces decompression of the ligament with partial release of occlusion of the coeliac trunk. This leads to hypoperfusion of intestinal organs and abdominal angina.

CT angiography generally shows a short-segment stricture at the root of celiac trunk with the pattern of a focal extrinsic compression and a post-stenotic dilatation. Other findings observed are the conspicuous dilation of gastroduodenal artery and pancreaticoduodenal in response to the increased blood flow diverted from pathways with the SMA (Fig. 19.7). Angiography shows the same findings, and it may be able to demonstrate the extrinsic nature of the stenosis at the origin of the celiac trunk if the investigation is performed during inspiration and expiration.

19.5 Renal Infarction

Acute renal infarction is an underreported phenomenon, and it is often misdiagnosed. Characteristic clinical findings in major acute renal infarction include sudden onset of abdominal or flank pain, frequently accompanied by fever and nausea with vomiting. Laboratory findings are those typically seen in acute infarction, which include moderate leukocytosis, albuminuria, microscopic hematuria, elevated serum creatinine (particularly with large embolus or bilateral disease), and rising of LDH levels [68, 69]. These clinical and laboratory findings, although consistent with renal infarction, are non-specific and often suggestive for alternative conditions including acute surgical abdomen or appendicitis with the risk of overlooking the correct diagnosis. It may occur in patients who are at risk of systemic embolization (e.g., patients with atrial fibrillation). However, Bolderman et al.

[70] reported that there are several idiopathic cases where risk factors related to renal infarct are not clear.

Imaging Findings Imaging tools are important to make proper clinical assessment. The first diagnostic work-up of patients with acute abdominal pain includes US, which is widely available and gives a real-time dynamic exploration [71]. Moreover, the use of Doppler technique to evaluate blood flow is an essential component of US study.

Acute renal infarction appears as the absence of perfusion on color and power Doppler examination, complete when the entire kidney is affected or patchy when segmental arteries are involved. The absence of flow may also be directly appreciated in the renal artery or, in rare cases of venous thrombosis causing infarction, the renal vein. After a first hypothesis of renal vascular impairment is made at US, a contrast-enhanced CT scan should be performed to confirm the diagnosis.

Currently, CT has become the gold standard for the diagnosis of renal infarction. Indeed CT angiography allows to identify the occluded vessel while also assessing if there is evidence of ischemia in other organs such as the spleen, liver, or lungs or whether there are indirect signs of cardiac disease responsible for thromboembolism episodes. At contrast-enhanced CT, renal infarction usually appears as wedge-shaped low attenuation area within an otherwise normal-appearing kidney [72] (Figs. 19.10 and 19.11).

Nowadays, with the possibility of detecting renal arterial infarction with US and CT scan, invasive procedures, such as renal arteriography should rarely be performed, and they also help in making a quick differential diagnosis with other more common acute abdominal diseases such as appendicitis [68].

An early identification of the disease allows an appropriate treatment to be started, which is the same for both idiopathic cases and patients with atrial fibrillation-induced embolism and is based on early anticoagulation (low-molecular-weight heparin) with a good prognosis [73].

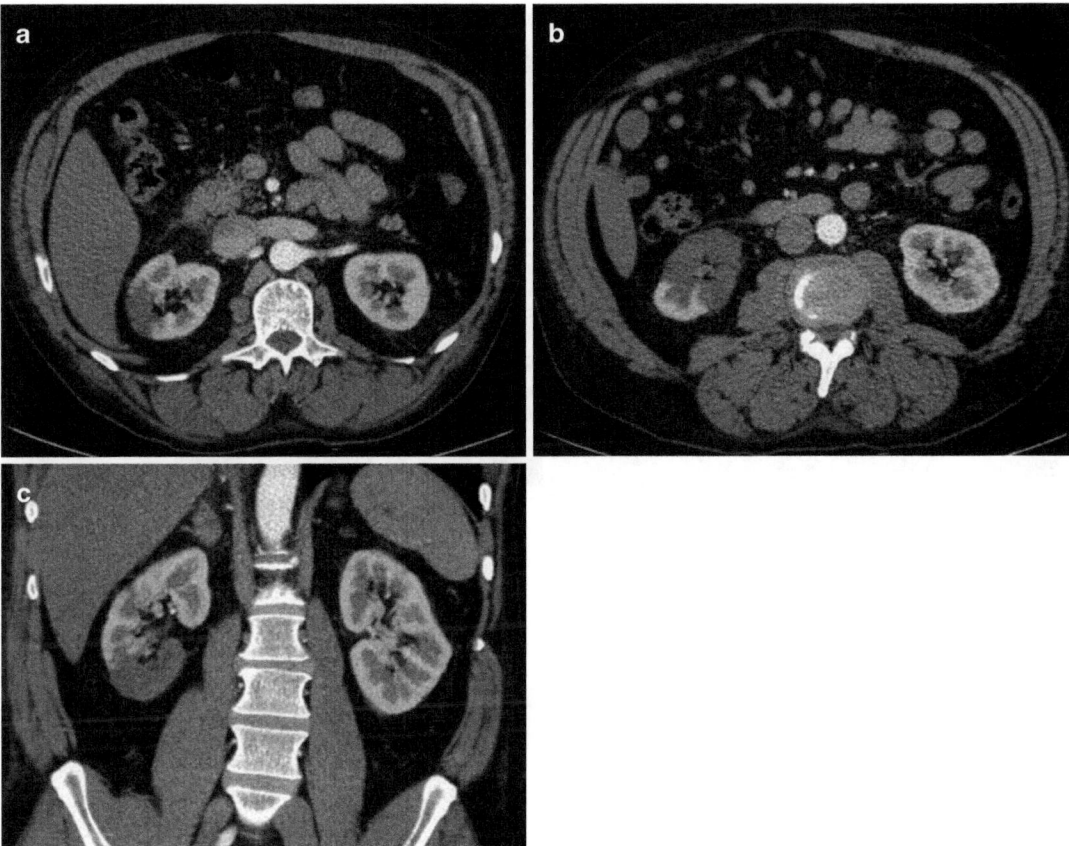

Fig. 19.10 Renal infarction. Male, 47 years old. Sudden cramp-like pain of the lower abdomen. Right lumbar pain (**a–c**). CT angiography clearly shows a hypodense area involving the cortex of the right kidney. The coronal view shows the ischemic involvement of the lower pole

Other possible treatments include endovascular thrombolysis, which is, however, supported by limited data so that its utility is still debated [74]. An alternative approach reported is stent graft deployment in the injured renal artery [75, 76].

19.6 Splenic Infarction

Splenic infarction (SI) occurs when the splenic artery or one or more of its branches become occluded, either by an embolus or by in situ thrombosis. The spleen has a rich vascular supply and receives 5% of the cardiac output making it susceptible to emboli (cardiogenic, aortic, paradoxical) [77]. Furthermore, it is not infre-quently affected by malignant hematological disorders which increase the risk of thrombosis. The current widespread availability and escalating early use of computed tomography (CT) scanning may have changed its etiologic distribution and presenting features [78]. In the retrospective analysis of Schattner et al. [79], the patients' predominant symptom is abdominal pain which is acute in more than 50% of cases but unfrequently intense and severe. Pain location is most often in the left upper quadrant of the abdomen or epigastrium. Sometimes, no abdominal pain is referred. From an etiologic point of view, cardiogenic emboli are by far the major etiologic mechanism, followed by autoimmune disease and infection-associated SI.

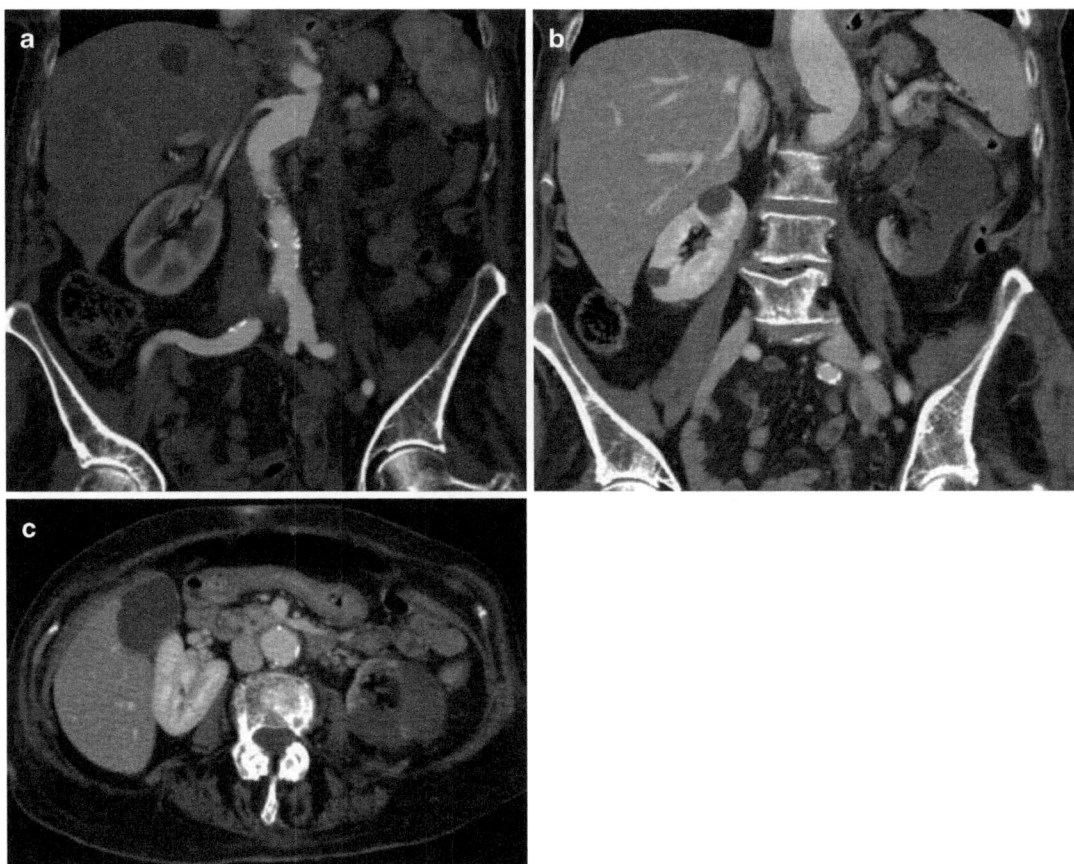

Fig. 19.11 Renal infarction. Female, 84 years old. Sudden onset of left flank and lumbar pain. Acute bowel obstruction was suspected. (**a**–**c**) Occlusion of the left renal artery at the origin (**a**) while the right renal artery is regular. (**b, c**) The left kidney appears almost completely not perfused except that in the medial aspect of the lower pole

Imaging Findings On US, splenic infarcts appear as hypoechoic areas compared to the rest of the spleen with wedge or round or irregular shape. During contrast-enhanced ultrasound, the infarcted area remains hypo-intense throughout all phases of the study.

CT is considered the imaging investigation of choice, ideally performed during the portal venous phase, to avoid confusing heterogeneous enhancement normally seen during arterial phase. Imaging features may vary with the stage of the infarct. In the hyperacute phase, CT may show areas of mottled increased attenuation, representing areas of hemorrhagic infarction. There are various classical patterns of established splenic infarcts on CT: the most typical is the pattern of a peripheral, wedge-shaped hypo-enhancing region (Fig. 19.12); less frequently, the pattern is characterized by multiple, heterogeneous areas of patchy enhancement; in the most severe cases of global splenic infarction, the entire spleen is hypo-enhancing (e.g., in splenic torsion).

19.7 Gastrointestinal Bleedings

GI bleeding can be distinguished in those originating from the upper gastrointestinal tract and those originating from the lower intestinal tract.

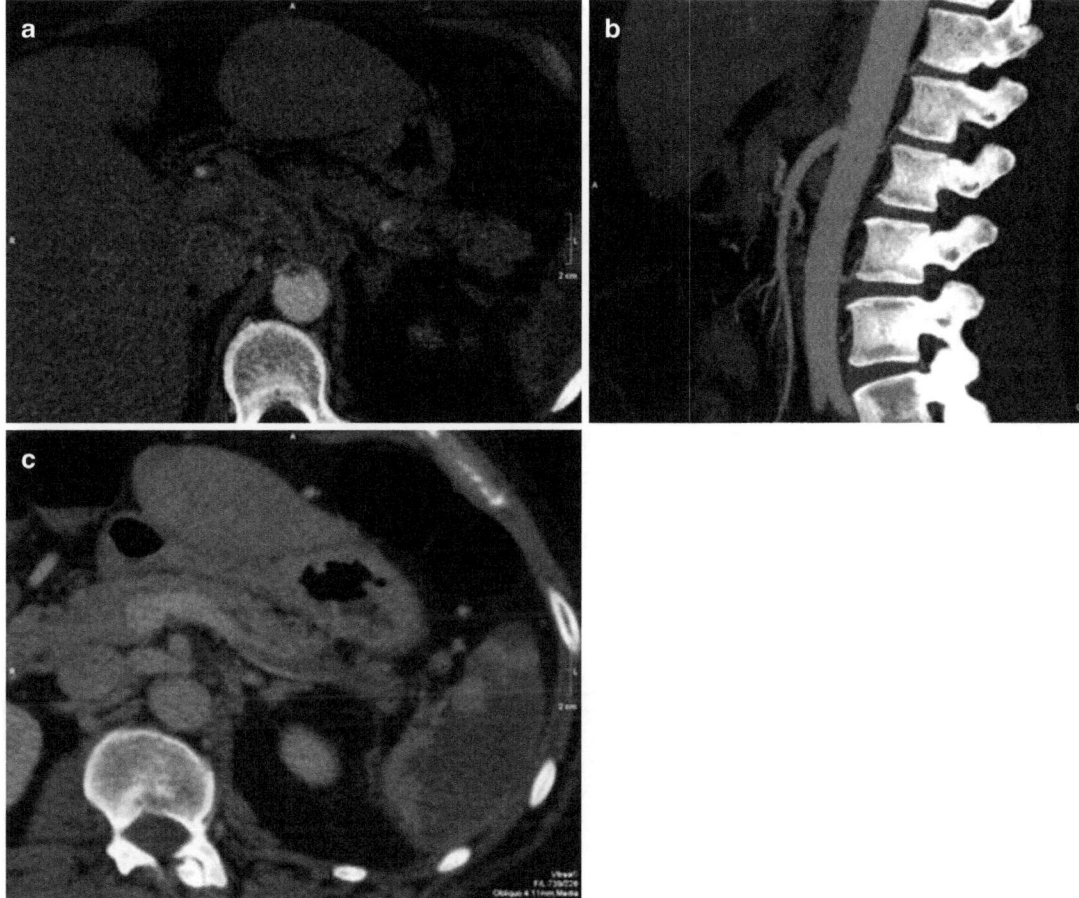

Fig. 19.12 Splenic infarction. Female, 50 years old. Sudden onset of diffuse cramp abdominal pain, mainly on the left flank. (**a, b**) CT angiography shows a filling defect inside the celiac trunk protruding in the aorta. (**c**) The spleen appears diffusely hypodense. A thrombus is visible inside the splenic vein

Upper Gastrointestinal Bleedings Upper gastrointestinal bleeding includes hemorrhage originating from the esophagus to the ligament of Treitz. Peptic ulcer bleeding causes more than 60% of cases of upper gastrointestinal bleeding, whereas esophageal varices cause approximately 6%. Other etiologies include arteriovenous malformations, Mallory-Weiss tear, gastritis, duodenitis, and malignancy.

Patients with history of peptic ulcer report abdominal pain together with coffee-ground-like emesis, dysphagia, black tarry stools, bright red blood per rectum, hematemesis, and chest pain.

Early upper endoscopy (within 24 h of presentation) is recommended in most patients with upper gastrointestinal bleeding because it confirms the diagnosis and allows for targeted endoscopic treatment, resulting in reduced morbidity, hospital stays, risk of recurrent bleeding, and need for surgery. Rebleeding after successful endoscopic therapy occurs in 10–20% of patients.

Imaging Findings Diagnostic imaging is an alternative to be used if endoscopic therapy fails. Multidetector CT has expanded the applications of CT angiography for evaluating patients with vascular diseases, including acute upper and lower GI bleeding. Temporally resolved CT angiography allows the identification of active extravasation of contrast material and the accurate identification of the source of hemorrhage [80]. CT angiography can be used to evaluate the wall of the entire gastrointestinal tract and other digestive structures that may occasionally be the source of bleeding, such as the pancreas and biliary tract. Intraluminal extravasation of contrast material is the main criterion used to define the location of the bleeding point [81, 82] (Fig. 19.13). Identification of this finding requires that active bleeding be present during the period of time that the injected contrast material circulates through the vascular system; CT angiography typically detects active bleeding with a rate that exceeds 0.3–0.5 mL/min, a rate that is slightly higher than the threshold assigned to catheter angiography (0.5 mL/min) and is lower than that of scintigraphy with 99mTc-labeled red blood cells, which can be used to detect active bleeding at a rate higher than 0.1 mL/min [80, 82]. Therefore, severe bleeding episodes, such as those manifesting with hemodynamic instability, increase the pretest probability of a positive result for active bleeding at CT angiography [81, 83, 84]. Intermittent bleeding can cause false-negative findings at CT angiography [80, 83]. The usual appearance of active bleeding is that of an intraluminal blush of contrast-enhanced blood in the arterial phase or a hyperattenuating focus of variable attenuation and morphology in the portal venous phase. The changing morphology of the focus of contrast media extravasation with time (from the arterial phase to the portal venous phase) unequivocally confirms the presence of bleeding (Fig. 19.14a,b), especially when the unenhanced image shows no hyperattenuating intraluminal material.

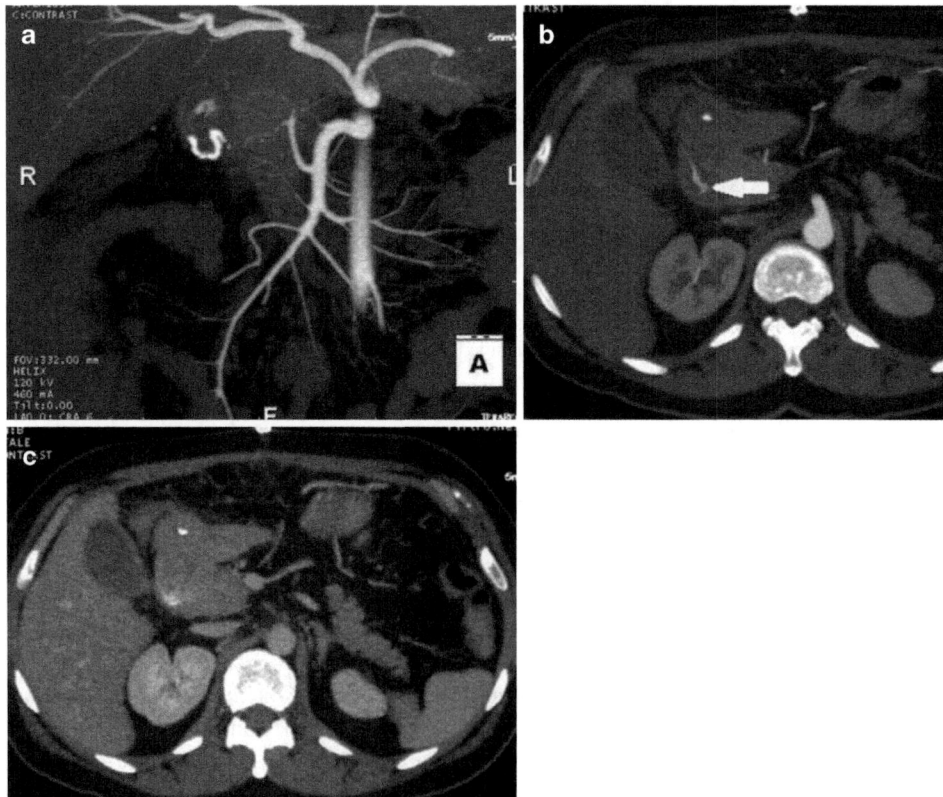

Fig. 19.13 Gastrointestinal bleeding. Male, 70 years old, recent gastric surgery for a duodenal bleeding ulcer. Sudden onset of pain and significant decrease of hemoglobin values. (**a**, **b**) CT angiography (arterial phase): a focal hyperdense irregular-shaped area (arrow) typical for intraluminal arterial bleeding is visible at the level of duodenum. In the delayed phase (**c**), the active bleeding typically modifies its shape

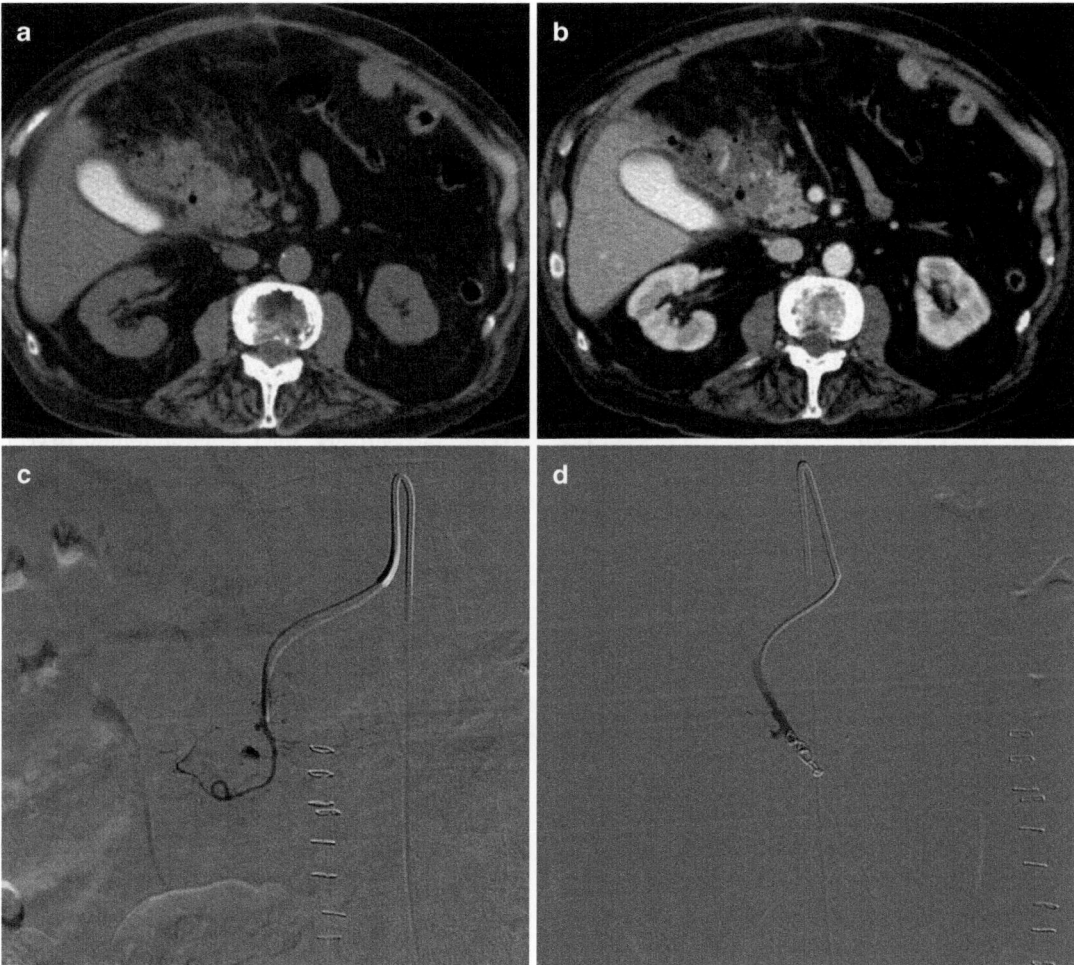

Fig. 19.14 Gastrointestinal bleeding. Male, 39 years old. Recent surgery for a duodenal GIST. Sudden onset of pain and fall of hemoglobin values. (**a**) Plain CT shows a not homogeneous fluid content in the duodenum. After contrast enhancement (**b**), hyperdense striations appear at the level of the duodenum suggesting an active bleeding. (**c**, **d**) Catheter angiography confirms the active bleeding of a collateral branch of the gastroduodenal artery which was stopped by selective embolization (**d**)

Arteriography with embolization usually precedes surgical therapy because both are equally effective in treating patients with persistent bleeding (Fig. 19.14c,d). Surgical therapy is usually recommended if endoscopy and arteriography with embolization have failed to control the bleeding or if interventional radiology expertise is not available after a failed endoscopic attempt.

Lower Gastrointestinal Bleedings Acute colonic bleeding (or lower GI bleeding), defined as that occurring from the colon, rectum, or anus, and presenting as either hematochezia (bright red blood, clots, or burgundy stools) or melena, has an annual incidence of about half of that for upper GI bleeding. The rate of hospitalization is even higher in the elderly [85]. The source of lower gastrointestinal tract bleeding is colorectal in approximately 90% of cases. In the remaining 10%, the bleeding site is situated in the small bowel. Among colorectal lesions, colonic diverticula, angiodysplasia, inflammatory lesions, and malignancies are the most common causes of bleeding [86].

Most cases of acute colonic bleeding will stop spontaneously, thereby allowing nonurgent evaluation. However, for patients with severe hematochezia (continued bleeding within the first 24 h of hospitalization, drop in the hemoglobin of at least 2 g/dL, transfusion requirement), urgent diagnosis and intervention are required to control the bleeding. Clinical factors predictive of severe colonic bleeding include aspirin use, at least two comorbid illnesses, pulse greater than 100/minute, and systolic blood pressure <115 mmHg [87]. The overall mortality rate from colonic bleeding is 2.4–3.9% [85, 88]. Typical clinical findings include abdominal pain and weight loss which is non-specific but may suggest inflammatory bowel disease, ischemia, and/or malignancy, medication use (non-steroidal anti-inflammatory drugs—NSAIDS—and other medications that can cause ulcers or intestinal ischemia), recent colonoscopy with polypectomy (postpolypectomy bleed), prior abdominal/pelvic radiation (radiation proctitis/colitis), prior operations (possible anastomotic ulcers), or a history of abdominal aortic aneurysm with or without surgical repair (possible aortoenteric fistula). A history of alcoholism or chronic liver disease raises the suspicion for bleeding due to portal hypertension, such as varices. The manner in which the patient with bleeding presents can also suggest potential etiologies. Bright red blood is more often seen from anorectal and distal colonic sources, but brisk upper GI bleeding can also manifest this way. Painless severe bleeding with clots is more common with diverticular hemorrhage. Bloody diarrhea often occurs with ischemic and inflammatory colitis.

Colonoscopy generally should be the initial modality used for evaluating acute colonic bleeding or severe hematochezia requiring hospitalization. Because most bleeding stops spontaneously, colonoscopy often is performed semi-electively, 24 h or more after initial hospitalization, to allow the patient to receive blood transfusions and the bowel preparation on the first day of hospitalization. However, the optimal time for performing urgent bowel preparation and colonoscopy is controversial.

Imaging Findings The accuracy of CT angiography for determining the specific cause of lower gastrointestinal bleeding ranges from 80 to 85% in most series [83, 89–91]. CT angiography can be used to easily diagnose bleeding from colonic diverticula, the leading cause of lower gastrointestinal tract bleeding [92]. Colonic angiodysplasia is the second most common cause of lower gastrointestinal tract bleeding, accounting for as many as 40% of cases in patients older than 60 years [82]. Junquera et al. have reported values for the sensitivity, specificity, and positive predictive value of 70%, 100%, and 100%, respectively, for CT angiography [93]. It is important to try to distinguish between bleeding from a diverticulum and angiodysplasia because the probability of rebleeding is as high as 85% in cases of angiodysplasia and is only 25% in cases of diverticular bleeding [81]. In addition, CT angiography can be used to accurately diagnose neoplasms and colitis, which are the third and fourth most common causes of lower gastrointestinal tract bleeding, respectively [81, 86, 89], and CT angiography is also helpful for the diagnosis of benign anorectal lesions. Postoperative bleeding can occur at an anastomotic site or a more distant location.

The ability to visualize active extravasation of contrast material is influenced by many factors related to the nature of the bleeding (severity, intermittence), the patient (hemodynamic status, body mass index, preexistent intestinal contents), the CT technique (examination protocol, scanner generation, iodine concentration of the contrast material used), and the experience of the radiologist [89]. In the studies for the detection of active bleeding with CT angiography, false-negative results are most often due to intermittent or low-intensity bleeding, below the threshold of CT angiographic detection [82, 84]. Dilution of extravasated contrast material in fluid-filled dilated bowel loops is another cause of non-depiction of active bleeding with CT angiography [94]. Inadequate bowel distention precludes detection of subtle tumors or inflammatory lesions that may be better seen at CT enterography.

Mucosal enhancement of collapsed bowel loops can simulate extravasated contrast material [81, 83]. Errors of perception and interpretation (such as satisfaction of search), which are usually related to the inexperience of the radiologist, are other causes of false-negative results.

The main advantage of mesenteric angiography, compared to radionuclide imaging, is its interventional capability. However, the bleeding rate must be at least 0.5 mL/min to detect extravasation into the gut, which is significantly higher than radionuclide imaging. The other disadvantages of radionuclide imaging, the inability to detect non-active bleeding stigmata or to make an etiologic diagnosis, also occur with angiography. Additionally, certain patient factors (such as contrast dye allergy and acute/chronic kidney disease) are potential contraindications to angiography. The diagnostic yield of angiography depends on patient selection, the timing of the procedure, and the skill of the angiographer, with positive results in 10–70% of cases. Previously, angiographic intervention involved injection of vasoconstrictors to control bleeding in preparation for surgery. However, thanks to technological advances, super-selective embolization of distal arterial branches is now possible. A review of several studies using angiographic embolization for colonic bleeding found that immediate hemostasis was achieved in 96%, with 22% experiencing early rebleeding, 26% experiencing minor complications that did not require surgery, and 17% experiencing major complications that required surgery or resulted in death [95].

19.8 Spontaneous Abdominal Muscle Hematoma

Spontaneous abdominal muscle hematomas are an uncommon cause of acute abdominal pain and are often misdiagnosed. They result from bleedings which mainly occur in three anatomical regions:

- Anterior muscles of the abdominal wall: there are four muscles on each side (the rectus, the external oblique, the internal oblique, and the transverse muscle). Vascularization of this muscle group is mainly provided by the deep inferior epigastric arteries, the superior epigastric arteries, and the deep circumflex iliac arteries.
- Posterior muscles of the abdominal wall: there are three muscles per side (the iliac, the psoas, and the erector spinae muscles). These muscles are vascularized by the lumbar arteries and the iliolumbar arteries.
- Buttock muscles: there are three gluteal muscles, the piriformis, and the internal obturators. This muscle group is vascularized by the superior and inferior gluteal arteries, which are the terminal branches of the posterior trunk of the internal iliac artery.

Spontaneous muscle hematomas may occur because of trauma, physical exercise, recent surgery, or injection procedures. They may also occur because of increased intra-abdominal pressure from coughing, sneezing, vomiting, or straining during urination, defecation, and labor [96–100]. Other predisposing factors include increased age, arterial hypertension, atherosclerosis, and systemic anticoagulant therapy. Most abdominal wall hematomas occur in the rectus sheath (Fig. 19.15), while hematoma within the oblique muscles is very rare (Fig. 19.16). Hematomas of the iliopsoas muscles are less frequent than rectus sheath; however, they have a high mortality rate, mostly related to anticoagulation therapy and usually affecting the elderly and fragile patients.

From a clinical point of view, most common presenting signs and symptoms of these hematomas are acute abdominal pain and firm, palpable abdominal wall masses. Because of their rarity, abdominal wall hematomas can be mistaken for several common acute abdominal conditions such as appendicitis, sigmoid diverticulitis, perforated ulcers, ovarian cyst torsion, tumors, or incarcerated inguinal hernias [101]. The most important diagnostic finding suggesting a hematoma of the abdominal wall is the presence of an abdominal wall mass with ecchymosis.

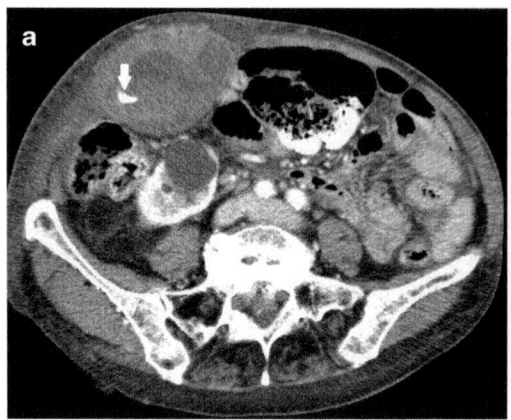 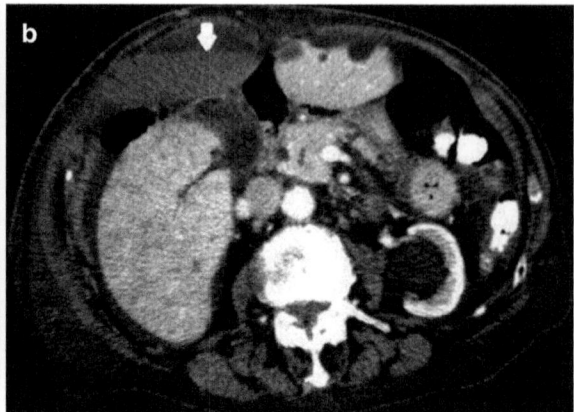

Fig. 19.15 Hematoma of the abdominal wall. Male, 78 years old. Sudden onset of pain, palpable mass, and decrease of hemoglobin values in a man in anticoagulant therapy for atrial fibrillation. (**a**) CT angiography shows a huge mass in the context of the right rectum muscle with an active bleeding (arrow). Another typical finding is the fluid-fluid level (arrow-**b**)

However, abdominal wall ecchymosis is a late sign, and the average time between its presentation and its onset takes about 4 days, as reported in the literature [102].

As previously mentioned, many risk factors have been reported for abdominal wall hematomas. Of these, aging and anticoagulant therapy play an important role. In a review of 126 cases of rectus sheath hematoma, published in 2006, it is reported that most patients (69%) were on some forms of anticoagulation therapy, and the mean age was 67.9 years [99].

Imaging Findings The diagnosis of an oblique muscle hematoma is made by combining medical history, laboratory examination findings, and US and/or radiological findings. US and CT scans can provide useful information for differential diagnosis to avoid unnecessary surgery [100]. US can be useful as a first-line investigation because it is widely available and portable [103]. In addition to US, contrast-enhanced CT can detect and evaluate active bleeding from the rupture site [98] (Figs. 19.15 and 19.16). Another typical CT finding is a fluid-fluid level inside the hematoma due to superior Hounsfield values of fresh blood (Figs. 19.15 and 19.16).

Even in a patient without contrast extravasation at the bleeding site as observed on CT, selective digital subtraction angiography could be a useful imaging technique to identify an active bleeding point [104], and it is the modality of choice for therapeutic treatment of an active bleeding by means of an embolization procedure (Fig. 19.16).

The following grading system has been established for a rectus sheath hematoma on the basis of CT findings. Grade I is an intramuscular hematoma with an observable increase in muscle size.

Grade II is also an intramuscular hematoma but with blood between the muscle and transversalis fascia. Grade III hematoma may or may not affect the muscle, and the blood is seen between the transversalis fascia and muscle in the peritoneum and prevesical space that results in a drop in hemoglobin [105]. Grade I hematoma may resolve rapidly within approximately 30 days, whereas Grade II hematomas require 2–4 months, and Grade III hematomas require more than 3 months to resolve [105]. Hence, a classification based on CT findings could help a physician in predicting a patient's outcome.

Conservative treatment including bed rest and analgesics is appropriate in most patients with abdominal wall hematomas. Although most are self-limiting because the bleeding usually stops without intervention, some patients show significant morbidity, and the overall mortality rate is reported to be 4%. Surgical intervention or transcatheter arterial embolization is recommended when conservative management fails [96, 98].

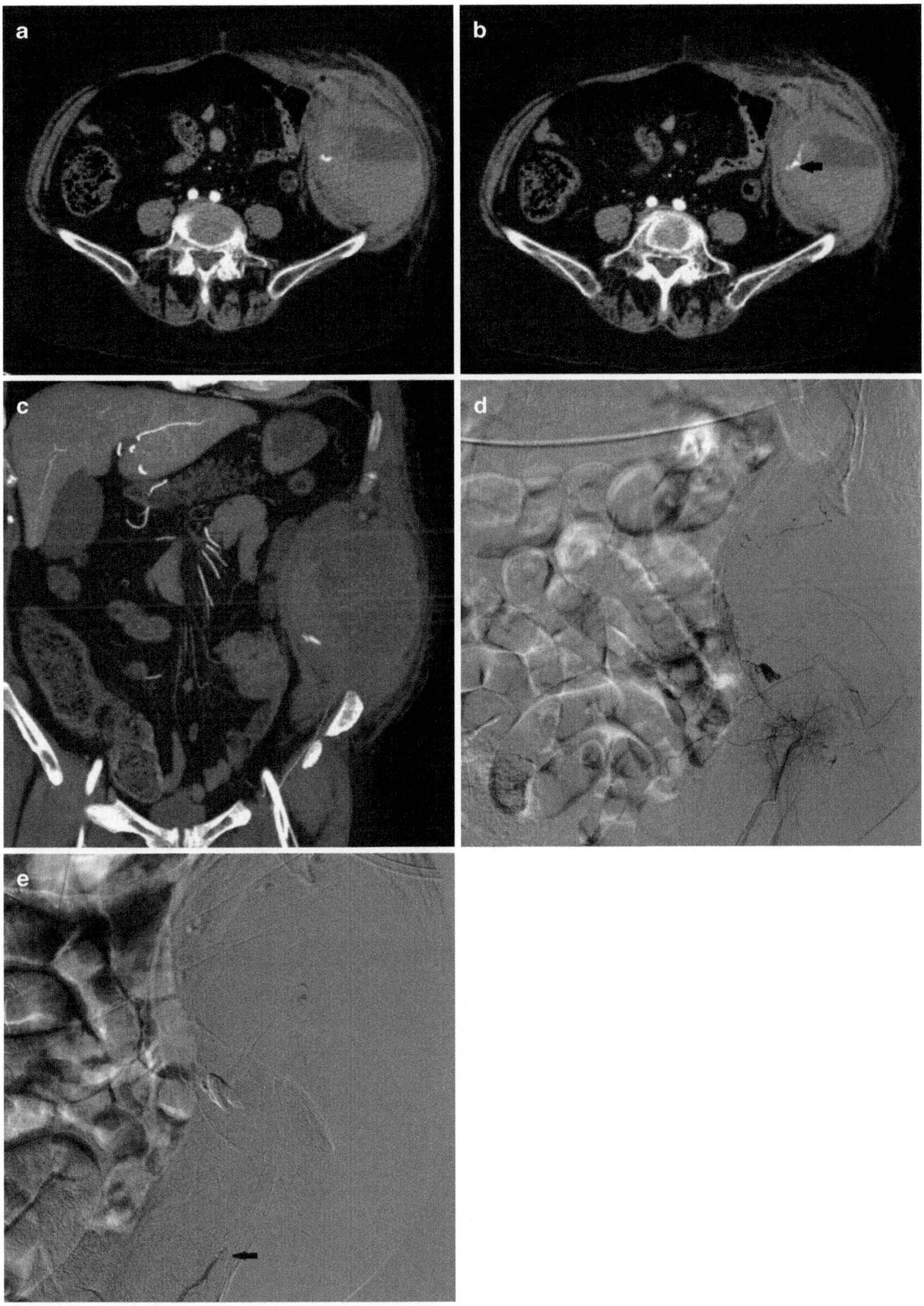

Fig. 19.16 Abdominal wall hematoma. Female, 69 years old, sudden onset of left flank pain, palpable mass, anticoagulant therapy. (**a**, **b**) CT angiography shows a huge hematoma in the contest of the left oblique muscle with an active bleeding (arrow) and a fluid-fluid level. (**c**, **d**) Catheter angiography confirmed the active bleeding which was stopped by means of an embolization procedure with embolizing particles and a coil (arrow) (**e**)

19.9   Nutcracker Syndrome (NCS)

The nutcracker phenomenon refers to compression of the left renal vein most commonly between the abdominal aorta and superior mesenteric artery. The exact prevalence and incidence of NCS are unknown, likely because of the variable presenting features; however it is rare, with a slight female predominance and symptomatic incidence in the second to fourth decade. It often goes undiagnosed, especially in patients who are asymptomatic [106].

Most typical nutcracker morphologic features imply the compression of the left renal vein between the aorta and the SMA, thus known as anterior nutcracker. Less often the retroaortic left renal vein may be compressed between the aorta and the vertebral body, so being called posterior nutcracker or pseudonutcracker [107].

The severity of this phenomenon is variable, and affected patients may be completely asymptomatic or in extreme cases they may present severe pelvic congestion. However the most common clinical manifestation is micro- or macroscopic hematuria. Other symptoms or complications that may occur include left flank pain, pelvic discomfort, varicocele or ovarian vein syndrome in women [108].

Imaging Findings Diagnosis is done through careful history evaluation and a variety of diagnostic tests; in fact imaging studies are not sufficient to confirm the diagnosis.

From an imaging point of view, Doppler ultrasonography (DUS), CT, and venography are the most important. DUS is the first imaging modality, with a sensitivity and specificity that range, respectively, between 69–90% and 89–100%, and is capable of evaluating the velocity of the blood flow within the LRV. Nutcracker syndrome DUS criteria are based on both the ratio of the peak velocity in the narrowed and dilated portions of the LRV and the ratio of the AP diameter of the LRV in the dilated and narrowed portions. The peak velocity ratio cutoff for NCS ranges from 4.1 to 5.0 (narrowed/dilated), and the AP diameter ratio cutoff ranges from 4.0 to 5.0 (dilated/narrowed) [106]. However, despite convenience and affordability, DUS methods are limited by technical difficulties, e.g., very small sample areas and are highly variable depending on the position of the patient [107].

Advanced CT or MRI, with multiplanar images, is able to depict the "beak sign," an abrupt narrowing or compression of the left renal vein between the aorta and SMA, with dilation of left gonadal vein, or pelvic varices and left renal vein variations such as retroaortic type (in the posterior nutcracker syndrome) [109] (Fig. 19.17). This sign has a sensitivity of 91.7% and specificity of 88.9% in the diagnosis of this

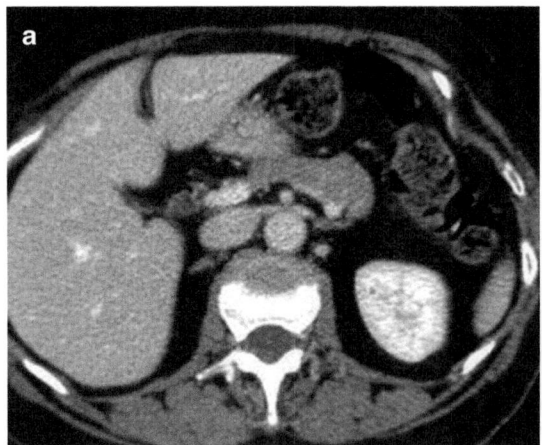
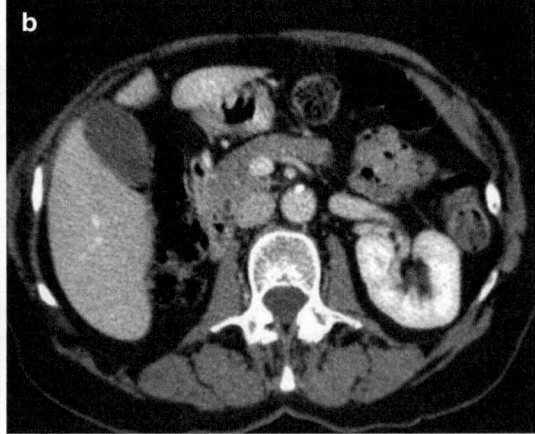

Fig. 19.17 Nutcracker syndrome. Female, 72 years old, pelvic pain, atypical varicose veins. (**a, b**) CT (axial images) shows the compression of the left renal vein between the aorta and SMA; the left renal vein is dilated (**b**), and also the left gonadal vein appears significantly larger than normal (**c, d**)

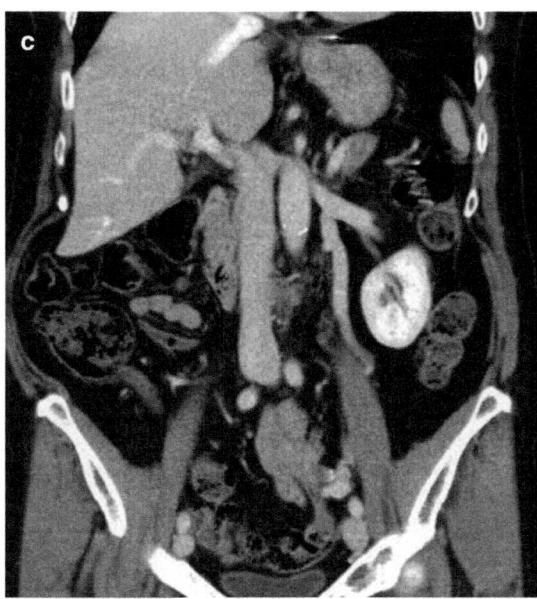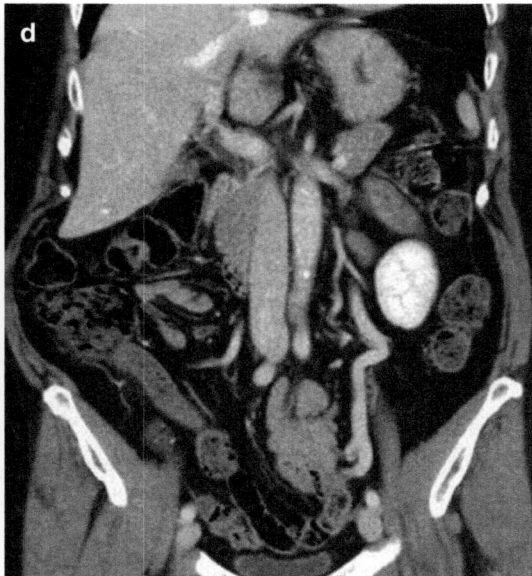

Fig. 19.17 (continued)

syndrome [108]. Therefore, the demonstration of left renal vein compression at imaging in the absence of clinical symptoms and varices should be termed nutcracker phenomenon, and not nutcracker syndrome. CT also plays the key role to differentiate the various causes of left renal vein compression such as retroperitoneal tumors, retroperitoneal fibrosis, or lymphadenopathy.

There is no definite guideline about which clinical manifestations are sufficiently enough to warrant appropriate management. Gross hematuria, severe pain, and renal failure may be the indications for surgical treatment [107], ranging from a left renal vein bypass to the more conventional approach of nephrectomy. Recently, endovascular stent placement in the left renal vein as modality of treatment has been reported with encouraging outcomes [110].

References

1. LaRoy LL, Cormier PJ, Matalon TA, Patel SK, Turner DA, Silver B. Imaging of abdominal aortic aneurysms. AJR Am J Roentgenol. 1989;152(4):785–92.
2. Moll FL, Powell JT, Fraedrich G, Verzini F, Haulon S, Waltham M, et al. Management of abdominal aortic aneurysms clinical practice guidelines of the European society for vascular surgery. Eur J Vasc Endovasc Surg. 2011;41(Suppl. 1):S1–S58.
3. Vorp DA, Raghavan ML, Webster MW. Mechanical wall stress in abdominal aortic aneurysm: Influence of diameter and asymmetry. J Vasc Surg. 1998;27(4):632–9.
4. Powell JT, Worrel P, MacSweeney S, Franks P, Greenhalgh R. Smoking as a risk factor for abdominal aortic aneurysm. Ann N Y Acad Sci. 1996;800:246–8.
5. Larsson E, Granath F, Swedenborg J, Hultgren R. A population-based case-control study of the familial risk of abdominal aortic aneurysm. J Vasc Surg. 2009;49(1):47–51.
6. Erhart P, Hyhlik-Dürr A, Geisbüsch P, Kotelis D, Müller-Eschner M, Gasser TC, et al. Finite element analysis in asymptomatic, symptomatic, and ruptured abdominal aortic aneurysms: In search of new rupture risk predictors. Eur J Vasc Endovasc Surg. 2015;49(3):239–45.
7. Schwartz SA, Taljanovic MS, Smyth S, O'Brien MJ, Rogers LF. CT findings of rupture, impending rupture, and contained rupture of abdominal aortic aneurysms. AJR Am J Roentgenol. 2007;188:W57–62.
8. Rakita D, Newatia A, Hines JJ, Siegel DN, Friedman B. Spectrum of CT findings in rupture and impending rupture of abdominal aortic aneurysms. Radiographics. 2007;27(2):497–507.
9. Mehta RH, Suzuki T, Hagan PG, Bossone E, Gilon D, Llovet A, et al. Predicting death in patients with acute type A aortic dissection. Circulation. 2002;105(2):200–6.
10. Hagan PG, Isselbacher EM, et al. NCA. The international registry of acute aortic dissection

(irad): new insights into an old disease. JAMA. 2000;283(7):897–903.

11. Wheat MW. Acute dissecting aneurysms of the aorta: diagnosis and treatment-1979. Am Heart J. 1980;99(3):373–87.

12. Nienaber CA, Fattori R, Mehta RH, Richartz BM, Evangelista A, Petzsch M, et al. Gender-related differences in acute aortic dissection. Circulation. 2004;109(24):3014–21.

13. Dahnert W. Radiology review manual. 5th ed. Philadelphia: Lippincott Williams & Wilkins; 2003. p. 394–6.

14. Williams DM, Lee DY, Hamilton BH, Marx MV, Narasimham DL, Kazanjian SN, et al. The dissected aorta: part III. Anatomy and radiologic diagnosis of branch-vessel compromise. Radiology. 1997;203:37–44.

15. Cambria RP, Brewster DC, Gertler J, Moncure AC, Gusberg R, Tilson MD, et al. Vascular complications associated with spontaneous aortic dissection. J Vasc Surg. 1988;7(2):199–209.

16. Castañer E, Andreu M, Gallardo X, Mata JM, Cabezuelo MÁ, Pallardó Y. CT in nontraumatic acute thoracic aortic disease: typical and atypical features and complications. Radiographics. 2003;23(Suppl 1):S93–110.

17. Belli AM, Markose G, Morgan R. The role of interventional radiology in the management of abdominal visceral artery aneurysms. Cardiovasc Interv Radiol. 2012;35:234–43.

18. Gabelmann A, Gorich J, Merkle EM. Endovascular treatment of visceral artery aneurysms. J Endovasc Ther [Internet]. 2002;9(1):38–47.

19. Lu M, Weiss C, Fishman E, Johnson P, Verde F. Review of visceral aneurysms and pseudoaneurysms. J Comput Assist Tomogr. 2015;39(1):1–6.

20. Guillon R, Garcier JM, Abergel A, Mofid R, Garcia V, Chahid T, et al. Management of splenic artery aneurysms and false aneurysms with endovascular treatment in 12 patients. Cardiovasc Intervent Radiol. 2003;26(3):256–60.

21. Cordova AC, Sumpio BE. Visceral artery aneurysms and pseudoaneurysms—should they all be managed by endovascular techniques? Ann Vasc Dis. 2013;6(4):687–93.

22. Nosher JL, Chung J, Brevetti LS, Graham AM, Siegel RL. Visceral and renal artery aneurysms: a pictorial essay on endovascular therapy. Radiographics. 2006;26:1687–704. quiz 1687.

23. Pitton MB, Dappa E, Jungmann F, Kloeckner R, Schotten S, Wirth GM, et al. Visceral artery aneurysms: Incidence, management, and outcome analysis in a tertiary care center over one decade. Eur Radiol. 2015;25(7):2004–14.

24. Saad NE, Saad WE, Davies MG, Waldman DL, Fultz PJ, Rubens DJ. Pseudoaneurysms and the role of minimally invasive techniques in their management. Radiographics. 2005;25(Suppl 1):S173–89.

25. Loffroy R, Rao P, Ota S, De Lin M, Kwak BK, Krause D, et al. Packing technique for endovascular coil embolisation of peripheral arterial pseudoaneurysms with preservation of the parent artery: safety, efficacy and outcomes. Eur J Vasc Endovasc Surg. 2010;40(2):209–15.

26. Fankhauser GT, Stone WM, Naidu SG, Oderich GS, Ricotta JJ, Bjarnason H, et al. The minimally invasive management of visceral artery aneurysms and pseudoaneurysms. J Vasc Surg. 2011;53(4):966–70.

27. Julianov A, Georgiev Y. Hepatic artery aneurysm causing obstructive jaundice. Quant Imaging Med Surg. 2014;4(4):294–5.

28. Messina LM, Shanley CJ. Visceral artery aneurysms. Surg Clin North Am. 1997;77(2):425–42.

29. Lee PC, Rhee RY, Gordon RY, Fung JJ, Webster MW. Management of splenic artery aneurysms: the significance of portal and essential hypertension. J Am Coll Surg. 1999;189(5):483–90.

30. Mattar SG, Lumsden AB. The management of splenic artery aneurysms: experience with 23 cases. Am J Surg. 1995;169(6):580–4.

31. Stanley JC, Fry WJ. Pathogenesis and clinical significance of splenic artery aneurysms. Surgery. 1974;76(6):898–909.

32. Trastek VF, Pairolero PC, Joyce JW, Hollier LH, Bernatz PE. Splenic artery aneurysms. Surgery. 1982;91(6):694–9.

33. Hallett JW Jr. Splenic artery aneurysms. Semin Vasc Surg. 1995;8(4):321–6.

34. Holdsworth R, Gunn A. Ruptured splenic artery aneurysm in pregnancy. Br J Obs Gynaecol. 1992;99(7):595–7.

35. Shanley CJ, Shah NL, Messina LM. Uncommon splanchnic artery aneurysms: pancreaticoduodenal, gastroduodenal, superior mesenteric, inferior mesenteric, and colic. Ann Vasc Surg. 1996;10:506–15.

36. Baggio E, Migliara B, Lipari G, Landoni L. Treatment of six hepatic artery aneurysms. Ann Vasc Surg. 2004;18(1):93–9.

37. Shanley CJ, Shah NL, Messina LM. Common splanchnic artery aneurysms: splenic, hepatic, and celiac. Ann Vasc Surg. 1996;10(3):315–22.

38. Sethi H, Peddu P, Prachalias A, Kane P, Karani J, Rela M, et al. Selective embolization for bleeding visceral artery pseudoaneurysms in patients with pancreatitis. Hepatobiliary Pancreat Dis Int. 2010;9(6):634–8.

39. Harlaftis NN, Akin JT. Hemobilia from ruptured hepatic artery aneurysm. Report of a case and review of the literature. Am J Surg. 1977;133(2):229–32.

40. Abbas MA, Stone WM, Fowl RJ, Gloviczki P, Oldenburg WA, Pairolero PC, et al. Splenic artery aneurysms: two decades experience at Mayo Clinic. Ann Vasc Surg. 2002;16(4):442–9.

41. O'Driscoll D, Olliff SP, Olliff JF. Hepatic artery aneurysm. Br J Radiol. 1999;72(862):1018–25.

42. Klein GE, Szolar DH, Breinl E, Raith J, Schreyer HH. Endovascular treatment of renal artery

aneurysms with conventional non-detachable microcoils and Guglielmi detachable coils. Br J Urol. 1997;79(6):852–60.

43. Tham G, Ekelund L, Herrlin K, Lindstedt EL, Olin T, Bergentz SE. Renal artery aneurysms. Natural history and prognosis. Ann Surg. 1983;197(3):348–52.

44. Henke PK, Cardneau JD, Welling TH, Upchurch GR, Wakefield TW, Jacobs LA, et al. Renal artery aneurysms: a 35-year clinical experience with 252 aneurysms in 168 patients. Ann Surg. 2001;234(4):454-62-3.

45. Arenson AM, Graham RT, Shaw P, Srigley J, Herschorn S. Angiomyolipoma of the kidney extending into the inferior vena cava: sonographic and CT findings. Am J Roentgenol. 1988;151(6):1159–61.

46. Carter T, Angtuaco TL, Shah H. US case of the day. Large, bilateral angiomyolipomas of the kidneys with tuberous sclerosis. Radiographics. 1999;19(2):555–8.

47. Steiner MS, Goldman SM, Fishman EK, Marshall FF. The natural history of renal angiomyolipoma. J Urol. 1993;150(6):1782–6.

48. Harris K. Gastroduodenal artery aneurysm rupture in hospitalized patients: an overlooked diagnosis. World J Gastrointest Surg. 2010;2(9):291.

49. Chivot C, Rebibo L, Robert B, Regimbeau J. Ruptured pancreaticoduodenal artery aneurysms associated with celiac stenosis caused by the median arcuate ligament: a poorly known etiology of acute abdominal pain. Eur J Vasc Endovasc Surg. 2016;51(2):295–301.

50. Stone WM, Abbas M, Cherry KJ, Fowl RJ, Gloviczki P. Superior mesenteric artery aneurysms: is presence an indication for intervention? J Vasc Surg. 2002;36(2):234–7.

51. Komori K, Mori E, Yamaoka T, Ohta S, Takeuchi K, Matsumoto T, et al. Successful resection of superior mesenteric artery aneurysm. A case report and review of the literature. J Cardiovasc Surg (Torino). 2000;41(3):475–8.

52. Ogino H, Banno T, Sato Y, Hara M, Shibamoto Y. Superior mesenteric artery stent-graft placement in a patient with pseudoaneurysm developing from a pancreatic pseudocyst. Cardiovasc Intervent Radiol. 2004;27(1):68–70.

53. Lorelli DR, Cambria RA, Seabrook GR, Towne JB. Diagnosis and management of aneurysms involving the superior mesenteric artery and its branches--a report of four cases. Vasc Endovascular Surg. 2003;37(1):59–66.

54. Menke J. Diagnostic accuracy of multidetector CT in acute mesenteric ischemia: systematic review and meta-analysis. Radiology. 2010;256(1):93–101.

55. Oldenburg WA, Lau LL, Rodenberg TJ, Edmonds HJ, Burger CD. Acute mesenteric ischemia: a clinical review. Arch Intern Med. 2004;164(10):1054–62.

56. Kassahun WT, Schulz T, Richter O, Hauss J. Unchanged high mortality rates from acute occlusive intestinal ischemia: six year review. Langenbeck's Arch Surg. 2008;393:163–71.

57. Boley SJ, Feinstein FR, Sammartano R, Brandt LJ, Sprayregen S. New concepts in the management of emboli of the superior mesenteric artery. Surg Gynecol Obstet. 1981;153(4):561–9.

58. Sabiston D, Lyerly H. Textbook of surgery: the biological basis of modern surgical practice. 15th ed. Pennsylvania: WB Saunders Company; 1997. p. 1752–6.

59. Brandt LJ, Boley SJ. AGA technical review on intestinal ischemia. American Gastrointestinal Association. Gastroenterology. 2000;118(5):954–68.

60. Hokama A, Kishimoto K, Ihama Y, Kobashigawa C, Nakamoto M, Hirata T, et al. Endoscopic and radiographic features of gastrointestinal involvement in vasculitis. World J Gastrointest Endosc. 2012;4(3):50–6.

61. Dutta U, Bapuraj R, Yadav TD, Lal A, Singh K. Mesenteric ischemia and portal hypertension caused by splenic arteriovenous fistula. Indian J Gastroenterol. 2004;23(5):184–5.

62. Kayacetin E, Karak S, Karabacakoglu A, Emlik D. Mesenteric ischemia: an unusual presentation of fistula between superior mesenteric artery and common hepatic artery. World J Gastroenterol. 2004;10(17):2605–6.

63. Clark RA, Gallant TE. Acute mesenteric ischemia: angiographic spectrum. Am J Roentgenol. 1984;142(3):555–62.

64. Kirkpatrick IDC, Kroeker M, Greenberg HM. Biphasic CT with mesenteric CT angiography in the evaluation of acute mesenteric ischemia: initial experience. Radiology. 2003;229(1):91–8.

65. Wyers MC. Acute mesenteric ischemia: diagnostic approach and surgical treatment. Semin Vasc Surg. 2010;23(1):9–20.

66. Block T, Nilsson TK, Björck M, Acosta S. Diagnostic accuracy of plasma biomarkers for intestinal ischaemia. Scand J Clin Lab Invest. 2008;68(3):242–8.

67. Carboni GP, Visconti S, Battisti S, Zobel BB. A rare cause of abdominal angina. BMJ Case Rep. 2011;2011:8–10.

68. Di Serafino M, Severino R, Gullotto C, Lisanti F, Scarano E. Idiopathic Renal Infarction Mimicking Appendicitis. Case Rep Emerg Med. 2017; 2017:8087315.

69. Saeed K. Renal infarction. Int J Nephrol Renovasc Dis. 2012;5:119–23.

70. Bolderman R, Oyen R, Verrijcken A, Knockaert D, Vanderschueren S. Idiopathic renal infarction. Am J Med. 2006;119(4):356.e9-12.

71. Stoker J, Van Randen A, Laméris W, Boermeester MA. Imaging patients with acute abdominal pain. Radiology. 2009;253(1):31–46.

72. Antopolsky M, Simanovsky N, Stalnikowicz R, Salameh S, Hiller N. Renal infarction in the ED: 10-year experience and review of the literature. Am J Emerg Med. 2012;30(7):1055–60.

73. Huang CC, Lo HC, Huang HH, Kao WF, Yen DHT, Wang LM, et al. ED presentations of acute renal infarction. Am J Emerg Med. 2007;25(2):164–9.

74. Decoste R, Himmelman JG, Grantmyre J. Acute renal infarct without apparent cause: a case report and review of the literature. J Can Urol Assoc. 2015;9(3–4):E237–9.

75. Vidal E, Marrone G, Gasparini D, Pecile P. Radiological treatment of renal artery occlusion after blunt abdominal trauma in a pediatric patient: is it never too late? Urology. 2011;77(5):1220–2.

76. Dowling JM, Lube MW, Smith CP, Andriole J. Traumatic renal artery occlusion in a patient with a solitary kidney: case report of treatment with endovascular stent and review of the literature. Am Surg. 2007;73(4):351–3.

77. Wilkins BS. The spleen. Br J Haematol. 2002;117(2):265–74.

78. Kocher KE, Meurer WJ, Fazel R, Scott PA, Krumholz HM, Nallamothu BK. National trends in use of computed tomography in the emergency department. Ann Emerg Med. 2011;58(5):452-62. e3.

79. Schattner A, Adi M, Kitroser E, Klepfish A. Acute Splenic infarction at an academic general hospital over 10 years. Medicine (Baltimore). 2015;94(36):e1363.

80. Kerr SF, Puppala S. Acute gastrointestinal haemorrhage: the role of the radiologist. Postgrad Med J. 2011;87:362–8.

81. Laing CJ, Tobias T, Rosenblum DI, Banker WL, Tseng L, Tamarkin SW. Acute gastrointestinal bleeding: emerging role of multidetector CT angiography and review of current imaging techniques. Radiographics. 2007;27(4):1055–70.

82. Yoon W, Jeong YY, Kim JK. Acute gastrointestinal bleeding: contrast-enhanced MDCT. Abdominal Imaging. 2006;31:1–8.

83. Scheffel H, Pfammatter T, Wildi S, Bauerfeind P, Marincek B, Alkadhi H. Acute gastrointestinal bleeding: detection of source and etiology with multi-detector-row CT. Eur Radiol. 2007;17(6):1555–65.

84. Geffroy Y, Rodallec MH, Boulay-Coletta I, Julles M-C, Fulles M-C, Ridereau-Zins C, et al. Multidetector CT angiography in acute gastrointestinal bleeding: why, when, and how. Radiographics. 2011;31(3):E35–46.

85. Laine L, Yang H, Chang SC, Datto C. Trends for incidence of hospitalization and death due to GI complications in the United States from 2001 to 2009. Am J Gastroenterol. 2012;107(8):1190–5.

86. Friebe B, Wieners G. Radiographic techniques for the localization and treatment of gastrointestinal bleeding of obscure origin. Eur J Trauma Emerg Surg. 2011;37(4):353–63.

87. Strate LL, Orav EJ, Syngal S. Early predictors of severity in acute lower intestinal tract bleeding. Arch Intern Med. 2003;163(7):838.

88. Strate LL, Ayanian JZ, Kotler G, Syngal S. Risk factors for mortality in lower intestinal bleeding. Clin Gastroenterol Hepatol. 2008;6(9):1004–10.

89. Martí M, Artigas JM, Garzón G, Álvarez-Sala R, Soto JA. Acute lower intestinal bleeding: feasibility

90. Ernst O, Bulois P, Saint-Drenant S, Leroy C, Paris J-C, Sergent G. Helical CT in acute lower gastrointestinal bleeding. Eur Radiol. 2003;13(1):114–7.

91. Sabharwal R, Vladica P, Chou R, Law WP. Helical CT in the diagnosis of acute lower gastrointestinal haemorrhage. Eur J Radiol. 2006;58(2):273–9.

92. Barnert J, Messmann H. Diagnosis and management of lower gastrointestinal bleeding. Nat Rev Gastroenterol Hepatol. 2009;6:637–46.

93. Junquera F, Quiroga S, Saperas E, Perez-Lafuente M, Videla S, Alvarez-Castells A, et al. Accuracy of helical computed tomographic angiography for the diagnosis of colonic angiodysplasia. Gastroenterology. 2000;119(2):293–9.

94. Stuber T, Hoffmann MHK, Stuber G, Klass O, Feuerlein S, Aschoff AJ. Pitfalls in detection of acute gastrointestinal bleeding with multi-detector row helical CT. Abdom Imaging. 2009;34(4):476–82.

95. Strate LL, Naumann CR. The role of colonoscopy and radiological procedures in the management of acute lower intestinal bleeding. Clin Gastroenterol Hepatol. 2010;8(4):333–43.

96. Shimizu T, Hanasawa K, Yoshioka T, Mori T, Kajinami T, Yokoyama K, et al. Spontaneous hematoma of the lateral abdominal wall caused by a rupture of a deep circumflex iliac artery: report of two cases. Surg Today. 2003;33(6):475–8.

97. Linhares MM, Lopes Filho GJ, Bruna PC, Ricca AB, Sato NY, Sacalabrini M. Spontaneous hematoma of the rectus abdominis sheath: a review of 177 cases with report of 7 personal cases. Int Surg. 1999;84(3):251–7.

98. Nakayama T, Ishibashi T, Eguchi D, Yamada K, Tsurumaru D, Sakamoto K, et al. Spontaneous internal oblique hematoma successfully treated by transcatheter arterial embolization. Radiat Med. 2008;26(7):446–9.

99. Cherry WB, Mueller PS. Rectus sheath hematoma: review of 126 cases at a single institution. Medicine (Baltimore). 2006;85(2):105–10.

100. Moreno Gallego A, Aguayo JL, Flores B, Soria T, Hernández Q, Ortiz S, et al. Ultrasonography and computed tomography reduce unnecessary surgery in abdominal rectus sheath haematoma. Br J Surg. 1997;84(9):1295–7.

101. Luhmann A, Williams EV. Rectus sheath hematoma: a series of unfortunate events. World J Surg. 2006;30(11):2050–5.

102. Zainea GG, Jordan F. Rectus sheath hematomas: their pathogenesis, diagnosis, and management. Am Surg. 1988;54(10):630–3.

103. Klingler PJ, Wetscher G, Glaser K, Tschmelitsch J, Schmid T, Hinder RA. The use of ultrasound to differentiate rectus sheath hematoma from other acute abdominal disorders. Surg Endosc. 1999;13(11):1129–34.

104. Rimola J, Perendreu J, Falcó J, Fortuño JR, Massuet A, Branera J. Percutaneous arterial embolization in

the management of rectus sheath hematoma. AJR Am J Roentgenol. 2007;188(6):W497–502.

105. Berná JD, Garcia-Medina V, Guirao J, Garcia-Medina J. Rectus sheath hematoma: diagnostic classification by CT. Abdom Imaging. 1996;21(1):62–4.

106. Wilson Denham SL, Hester FA, Weber TM. Abdominal pain of vascular origin: nutcracker syndrome. Ultrasound Q. 2013;29(3):263–5.

107. Kurklinsky AK, Rooke TW. Nutcracker phenomenon and nutcracker syndrome. Mayo Clin Proc. 2010;85(6):552–9.

108. Fong JKK, Poh ACC, Tan AGS, Taneja R. Imaging findings and clinical features of abdominal vascular compression syndromes. Am J Roentgenol. 2014;203:29–36.

109. Srisajjakul S, Prapaisilp P, Bangchokdee S. Imaging features of vascular compression in abdomen: Fantasy, phenomenon, or true syndrome. Indian J Radiol Imaging. 2017;27:216–24.

110. Policha A, Lamparello P, Sadek M, Berland T, Maldonado T. Endovascular treatment of nutcracker syndrome. Ann Vasc Surg. 2016;36:295.e1–7.

Pelvic Pain: Clinical Features

20

Giuseppe Ricci, Giovanni Di Lorenzo,
Gabriella Zito, Simona Franzò,
and Federico Romano

20.1 Introduction and Epidemiology

There is no consensus on the definition of chronic pelvic pain (CPP). Various definitions of CPP have been proposed by scientific societies. Diagnosis is purely clinical, based on the presence of a noncyclic pain perceived in the pelvic area that persists continuously or episodically for 3–6 months or longer and is unrelated to pregnancy [1, 2]. Chronic pelvic pain (CPP) is typically severe enough to cause functional disability or require treatment; it is often cause of absence from work, multiple medical consultations, and it affects quality of life and mood [3–5]. Most of the classifications do not include perineal or vulvar pain [6].

Chronic pelvic pain (CPP) can be an expression of a great number of conditions, and it is often due to multiple components. The causes are not well understood, hardly definable, and usually multifactorial. The correct assessment should aim to examine all the contributory factors, to treat reversible specific ones and approach central chronic situations.

The estimated prevalence of CPP ranges from 4 to 16 percent among fertile women, but numbers are distorted because of epidemiology, lack of concordance on the definition, and referral patterns, as most women tend not to discuss it with their doctor [4, 7–9]. CPP prevalence is definitely higher in women than in men, often leading to a great number of invasive diagnostic and therapeutic procedures [10–12].

Efforts have been made to find organic causes such as endometriosis and adhesions syndrome, which were considered directly related to CPP. Besides, there is a growing interest in the role of the central nervous system (CNS) as a key point in the production of such symptom, which could be the expression of a nonorganic neurologic damage, referred to as central sensitization [1, 13, 14]. This hypothesis is firstly based on the gate control theory proposed by Melzack and Wall in 1965 [15]. This theory suggests that the perception of pain depends on a complex interplay of the central nervous system and the peripheral nervous system as they process each pain stimulus in their own way.

Later Melzack's neuromatrix theory introduced the pivotal concept of neuroplasticity [16]. Plasticity related to pain consists in persistent functional changes in the nervous system due to previous injuries or other nonorganic patho-

G. Ricci (✉)
Department of Medicine, Surgery and Health Sciences, University of Trieste, Trieste, Italy

Institute for Maternal and Child Health, IRCCS Burlo Garofolo, Trieste, Italy
e-mail: giuseppe.ricci@burlo.trieste.it

G. Di Lorenzo · G. Zito · F. Romano
Institute for Maternal and Child Health, IRCCS Burlo Garofolo, Trieste, Italy

S. Franzò
Department of Medicine, Surgery and Health Sciences, University of Trieste, Trieste, Italy

© Springer Nature Switzerland AG 2019
M. A. Cova, F. Stacul (eds.), *Pain Imaging*, https://doi.org/10.1007/978-3-319-99822-0_20

logical events. Psychological factors are no more considered as pure reactions to pain. They are now seen as an integral part of pain processing that may change the following response to painful stimuli. Furthermore, inflammatory or specific painful conditions (such as painful bladder syndrome, endometriosis, and irritable bowel syndrome) may affect the whole organism, causing an enhancement in pain sensitivity [17]. This finding is relevant to understand how pain can be provoked by a non-painful stimulus (allodynia) or sensitivity to pain can be increased (hyperalgesia) [18]. Central sensitization to pain reveals genetic and environmental contributors, whose identification will provide additional options to manage this condition [19, 20].

In conclusion, in women affected from a non-cyclic pain localized in the pelvic area or radiating to the abdomen lasting over 6 months, causes of CPP must be suspected and assessed, including both organic and functional factors. Diagnostic pathway can be defined thanks to a cohort of associated symptoms such as urinary or gastrointestinal symptoms and psychiatric symptoms.

20.2 Evaluation of Patients with Chronic Pelvic Pain

For a correct evaluation of causes and, consequently, appropriate management of diagnosis and therapy, a targeted evaluation of the syndrome is needed. Overlapping syndromes including CPP, other chronic pain conditions, or psychiatric conditions are often found [21].

20.2.1 Detailed History

A careful analysis of patient's history is critical [22]. Several standardized forms are available to assess helpful factors in the evaluation of patient's clinical features, including characteristics of the pain; medical and surgical history, with specific reference to gynecological and obstetric history (past pregnancies and deliveries, intrapartum and postpartum complications, history of sexual impairment or dissatisfaction, assault, and vio-

lence); and urinary, gastrointestinal, musculoskeletal symptoms [21].

Assessing psychosocial state and quality of life using a validated questionnaire, such as the Quality of Life Scale, and creating a patient-doctor relationship of trust is of great relevance in this context, due to the frequent association between CPP and previous negative experiences [5, 23]. Moreover, satisfaction in relationship with the doctor has shown to improve compliance and recovery rate [2].

History collection guides the investigator through the most common etiologies of CPP [24]:

1. Endometriosis/adenomyosis, leiomyoma
2. Pelvic floor disorders
3. Interstitial cystitis/painful bladder syndrome
4. Irritable bowel syndrome
5. Peripheral neuropathy

However, given the lack of specificity and the uncertainty on the mechanisms that cause the pain, the possibility of a non-frequent pathology should always be considered. The multifactorial nature of CPP should always be discussed with the patient, who is looking for a diagnosis and a treatment, and management should be agreed with her from the beginning.

After the evaluation of location and pattern of the pain, its characteristics should be evaluated [24]. It should be taken into account the provocative and the palliative factors, the radiation of pain, the setting and timing of pain occurrence, trigger events, and the associated symptoms.

The identification of the factors that provoke or alleviate the pain, such as posture or movement, association with sexual activity, urination and defecation, and response to painkillers, is necessary to perform differential diagnosis.

Asking patients to describe with some words their painful sensation, noting their emotional load, and to quantify the intensity on a numeric rating scale is important, particularly for nonmenstrual pelvic pain dysmenorrhea, dyschezia, dyspareunia, and dysuria. Though, it is important to note that these categories have considerable overlapping with other etiologies. Some recent studies have identified two pain pattern phenotypes in patients with urological CPP: patients with pelvic pain only and those with pelvic pain and beyond, which had more severe non-pelvic symptoms, higher risk of psychiatric diseases, worse quality of life, and poorer outcome with need of a longer medical therapy. Further investigations are needed to validate the usefulness of this or other kinds of classifications [22, 25].

Both visceral and musculoskeletal etiologies may cause radiation of pain, sometimes in specific areas, which can be easily pointed by the patient. This is useful to define a pattern and origin. Differential diagnosis can be carried out with the help of nerve blocks that improves a purely peripheral process [26].

All women should be interrogated on the relation of pain with menses, sexual intercourses, bowel movements, and posture. Assessing possible association with prior events and the pattern of evolution of the symptoms (constant, episodic, or cyclic) can suggest specific diagnosis. A pain diary can help the patient in keeping trace of peculiar situations and concomitances, such as a pelvic or abdominal procedure or trauma, a prior visceral dysfunction, and a cyclical exacerbation related to the menses.

The presence of any red flag symptoms, such as rectal bleeding, new bowel symptoms, new pain after the menopause, presence of a pelvic mass, suicidal ideation, excessive weight loss, irregular vaginal bleeding over 40 years of age, and postcoital bleeding, could help to identify the magnitude of organ system involvement and should suggest further investigations. If the pain wakes the patient from sleep, a certain concern should be raised both on physical and psychic intensity, and treatment efforts should be carried out in both ways.

20.2.2 Psychosocial Evaluation

Assessment for mental health issues and social disability should be conducted by a health psychologist or psychiatrist. In fact, in the population of women with CPP, higher prevalence of primary psychiatric comorbidity was found. Suspecting and investigating mood disturbances

is critical to describe a thorough frame of the patient's condition.

Coexisting factors such as depression, anxiety, sleep impairment, substance abuse, and somatization, as well as sexual abuse, can be associated to CPP. It is unclear if a causal relationship exists or association is casual, although biological and psychological factors seem to interact and the sum of the two to worsen the overall clinical outcome [24, 27–29].

However, it is important not to confuse psychological factors with psychiatric illnesses. In fact, secondary psychological problems are developed by some patients as a consequence of their pain. Since psychological processes have been recognized to have an impact on nociceptive pathways, symptomatology can get worse and assume an affective connotation triggering a vicious circle [30].

Moreover, opioid analgesics have been found to be less effective in CPP patients, requiring higher doses of medication for adequate analgesia, which adds possible side effects and addiction/tolerance. Appropriate psychosocial interventions aim to alleviate the psychological and behavioral sequelae of chronic pain through lifestyle modification and alterations in pain coping style.

Patients with such issues should be referred to a psychologist and physician specialized in pain management for cognitive behavioral therapy and alternative treatment regimen, which have been found to enhance outcomes.

20.2.3 Physical Examination

Evaluation of pelvic pain should always be supported by an accurate physical examination, including complete abdominal and pelvic examinations [30]. During the visit particular attention should be paid to the patient's history to assess the most likely causes in each specific situation.

Vital parameters should be taken and posture and behavior observed preliminarily.

Pain and stress caused by the examination can be limited using a systematic approach and interacting with the patient through eye contact and correct explanation of maneuvers. As patients with CPP are particularly vulnerable, a trust relationship with the doctor is critical and increases patient compliance to the visit and treatment.

These should be conducted slowly and gently, palpating the less painful areas first; looking for tender areas that have to be exactly identified, formations, and other abnormalities; and always asking if they reproduce the pain for which the patient comes to consultation [31].

The main aim of physical examination is to pinpoint the localization and identify the organs from which the pain takes origin. The patient should be aware that findings can be nonspecific and thus inconclusive.

A complete assessment of the back, abdomen, extremities, and pelvis should be carried out [24].

General Examination

General inspection of the patient is the first step to identify the source and some characteristics of the pain, paying attention to movements, agility, ease of changing position and walking, spinal curvature, or asymmetries of hips.

This is followed by back examination that begins with the patient seated. Pain at the palpation of the lower back, sacroiliac joints, paraspinal muscles, and coccyx, as well as referral or radiation to the back and/or abdominal wall, may indicate a musculoskeletal origin of pain.

Proceeding with the abdominal examination is the next step. The abdomen should be palpated with the patient lying supine. Cutaneous allodynia and hyperalgesia can be identified applying a cotton swab to the abdominal skin, suggesting the presence of a neuropathy of abdominal wall. Pattern, severity, and association of pain with quotidian symptoms of the patient should be assessed. Carnett's test should be performed to distinguish between visceral and abdominal wall pain. The examiner palpates the painful site of the abdomen while the patient raises both legs off the table. This maneuver potentially increases musculoskeletal pain, whereas pain lowers if the cause is visceral. Some somatic structures such as pelvic floor, iliopsoas muscle, or abdominal wall are usually underestimated but are often causes of pain. Muscular and nervous pain in the abdomen cause pain at the superficial palpation of the abdominal wall, and it might be diffuse or focal, in which case the examiner should distinguish between trigger points and pain derived from direct muscle damage.

Inguinal area should be examined for hernia; prior surgery on the pelvis should raise attention on iatrogenic nerve damage, and pubic symphysis should be palpated to determine conditions such as symphysis pubis dysfunction (pelvic girdle pain) and osteitis pubis. Pelvic organs should not be abdominally palpable, so every abdominal mass needs further evaluation.

If musculoskeletal involvement is suspected, a more deep analysis of orthopedic problems (legs and hips) should be considered, testing passive and active joint functionality (including hip flexion, extension, internal and external rotation, abduction, and adduction) and muscle strength.

Pelvic Examination

The lithotomy position is the most used for pelvic examination, which is carried out systematically [24].

External Genitalia Evaluation

The external genitalia can present signs of infection, inflammatory dermatologic conditions, vulvar malignancy, scars, and neurogenic disorders. The cotton swab test, consisting of a gentle touch of vulvar skin in all the quadrants (at the 1-, 4-, 6-, 8-, and 11-o'clock locations), is particularly used for women with vulvar pain or superficial dyspareunia [24]. Focal pain at slight touch of the vulva is pathognomonic for vulvodynia (Fig. 20.1).

Speculum Examination

A speculum examination should always be performed before digital examination, especially if an infection is suspected, as in cases of cervicitis, vaginitis, or PID, to be able to collect a proper sample for vaginal and cervical cultures. To reduce discomfort, the smallest speculum should be used that allows an adequate visualization of the cervix and posterior vaginal fornix [24]. This is particularly relevant if symptoms of endometriosis are present, as it can occasionally present transmural deep infiltrative lesions.

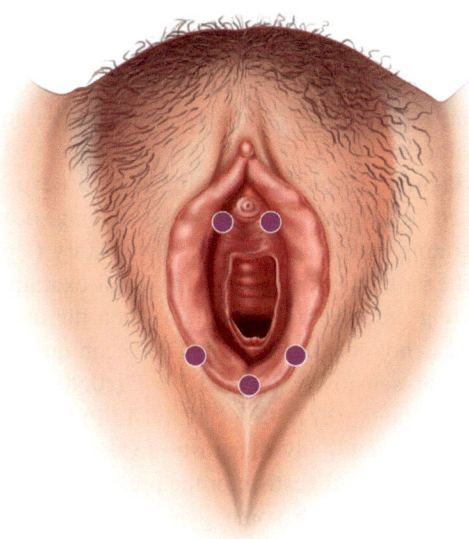

Fig. 20.1 Cotton swab test. Spots indicate the evaluation points on the vestibule

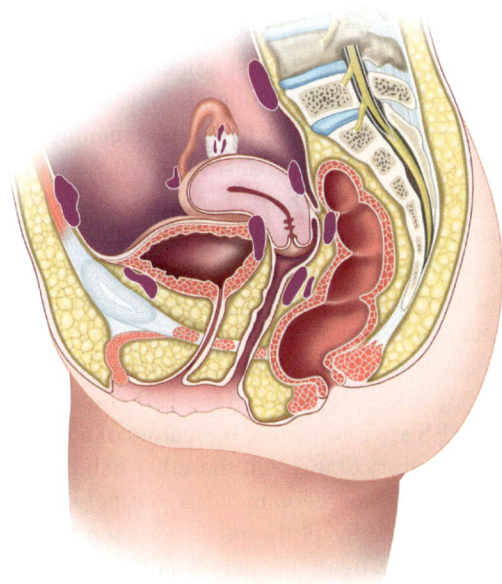

Fig. 20.2 Sagittal section of pelvis with most frequent endometriosis' nodule localization indicated in purple

Single Digit Vaginal Exam

Starting pelvic examination with a single finger allows to clean nociceptive interfering signals from the abdominal wall. Evaluation of the pelvic floor muscles systematically, vagina, cervix, and uterus with a single finger is important to assess for muscular pain and trigger points. To reduce the discomfort of the insertion and to assess the patient's awareness and control over pelvic muscle, the operator asks her to contract and relax perineal muscles. Pelvic floor tension myalgia or vaginismus is a quite common condition that can present both consequently to some other pathologies or as a primitive problem, implicating a dense network of physical and psychological factors. Most frequently, the kind of pain elicited at the visit is similar to the one usually experienced by the woman. The most painful areas should be left at the end to be examined, to avoid distortion of sensibility, and to allow a proper examination of the other sectors. Low urinary tract (bladder and urethra) and rectum anterior wall are also explored. A scoring system to rate relative tenderness in pelvic floor muscle hyperalgesia was proposed; further investigations may be helpful to recognize its value and improve precision [32].

Bimanual Exam

Finally, the abdominal hand is added to investigate volume, tenderness, mobility, and regularity of pelvic organs. Applying a gentle pressure alternatively with the abdominal hand and the vaginal finger, deep pain can be differentiated from wall pain. For example, when palpation of the urethra and the bladder evokes pain, a diagnosis of painful bladder syndrome can be suspected [24]. For deep pelvic pain presentations, rectovaginal examination should be considered, to assess nodularity or tenderness in the rectovaginal septum or uterosacral ligaments, as happens in deep infiltrating endometriosis (Fig. 20.2).

20.3 Diagnostic Strategies

As CPP has a great number of potential etiologies and it is often due to multiple components, differential diagnosis includes a wide range of pathologies that involve a number of organs and functions [24]. For this reason, diagnostic strategy should be tailored on the specific patient, consistently with findings of the history and physical examination, to avoid over testing the patient without any benefit and with increase of costs. Tests choice should be targeted on symptoms, epidemiology, and physical examination. Some first-line screening tests for the most frequent causes of CPP are widely recommended, such as urinalysis, to exclude urinary tract infection if symptoms suggest bladder involvement, a pregnancy test, and microbiologic tests for sexually transmitted infections (gonorrhea, chlamydia, and trichomonas) for active women and victims of abuse [5, 33]. Elevated white blood cell count, PCR, and VES are nonspecific indicators of a general inflammatory status. On the other hand, imaging tests are not recommended routinely. Pelvic ultrasonography is the most common method used to investigate the pelvis and highlight the main organ-specific pathologies that can cause a chronic pelvic pain, such as endometriosis, adenomyosis, or pelvic and adnexal masses [5, 33]. Thanks to its low cost, availability, absence of ionizing radiation, and the detailed anatomic information provided, it is considered a perfect first-line imaging test for abdomen and pelvis. Besides, when ultrasonography results inconclusive, if an organic pathology is suspected, the study can be completed where appropriate by magnetic resonance imaging, computed tomography, or diagnostic laparoscopy [34]. While evaluation of symptoms, physical examination, and ultrasonography are likely to correctly classify ovarian endometriosis, in absence of endometrioma, normal imaging cannot exclude endometriosis of the peritoneal surface [35].

However, the developments in ultrasound have given a new tool in diagnosing deep infiltrating endometriosis (DIE). Indeed, DIE can be recognized by a routine transvaginal scan. Dynamic ultrasound allows examination of the adhesion between pelvic structures, such as rectum and uterus or adnexa and parietal peritoneum, by the absence of sliding among them. This "negative sliding sign" has a sensitivity of 85% and specificity of 96% for DIE [31]. This type of evalua-

tion is likely operator dependent, and the choice between magnetic resonance imaging (MRI) and transvaginal ultrasound should be made based on the experiences of the local gynecologist and radiologist.

Magnetic resonance imaging should be performed in women suspected of having deep infiltrating endometriosis either by history (e.g., dyschezia or dyspareunia) or physical examination (e.g., rectovaginal nodules) when the ultrasound is not conclusive [36]. This technique has excellent sensitivity (0.94, 95% CI 0.90–0.97) and specificity (0.77, 95% CI 0.44–1.00) for DIE, even if not definitely diagnostic [35, 37]. It can also be highly suggestive for the presence of adenomyosis, although some gynecologists prefer ultrasound imaging. A CT scan can be performed when an unclear abdominal acute process is present or when acute enteritis or colitis is suspected; in case of pelvic venous congestion evidence, pelvic venography can be suggested if performed by skilled operators.

Stimulation of the involved organs could be a way to identify the source of pain when visceral hypersensitivity is considered a risk factor for CPP, although these tests are now available only in research protocols [38, 39]. For example, anal manometry has a role in the suspicion of irritable bowel syndrome, and urodynamic testing could be used in women with bladder pain.

20.3.1 Targeted Evaluation

In order to target patient's evaluation on one or few of the possible diagnoses, it is important to note all signs and symptoms collected, and it is as much essential to pay attention to patient history. The aim of targeting the diagnostic pathway is to reach a correct diagnosis and subsequent therapy in the shorter time possible.

A systematic description of the causes as shown in Table 20.1 is proposed, starting from the most frequent, i.e., gynecological pathology.

Table 20.1 Common causes of chronic pelvic pain

Gynecologic
Adhesions
Adenomyosis
Adnexal mass
Dysmenorrhea
Endometritis
Endometriosis
Leiomyomatosis
Ovarian cancer
Ovarian remnant
Pelvic congestion syndrome
Pelvic floor dysfunction
PID
Vestibulitis
Vaginal apex pain
Urologic
Chronic urethral syndrome
Interstitial cystitis/painful bladder syndrome
Neoplasia
Urethral diverticulum
Urinary tract infection
Urolithiasis
Gastrointestinal
Celiac disease
Colon cancer
Constipation
Diverticular colitis
Inflammatory bowel disease
Irritable bowel syndrome
Musculoskeletal
Coccydynia
Fibromyalgia
Piriformis/levator ani syndrome
Myofascial pelvic pain syndrome
Neurologic
Herpes zoster
Nerve entrapment
Psychosocial disorders
Depression
Physical and sexual abuse
Sleep disorders
Somatization

20.4 Gynecological Pathology

The most frequent cause of prolonged pelvic pain is dysmenorrhea, characterized by cyclic symptoms and therefore not properly considered among causes of CPP. Gynecological causes must be investigated in women with pelvic symptoms who do not complain urologic or gastrointestinal problems. A possible role of recurring episodes of severe dysmenorrhea in sensitization of the pelvic nervous system and thus development of CPP seems to be found [40, 41].

20.4.1 Endometriosis

Endometriosis, defined as the presence of ectopic endometrial tissue outside of the endometrial cavity, is the most common diagnosis made in a patient with CPP undergoing laparoscopy, being found in almost one third of these women. This finding reflects the high prevalence of the disease in the selected population of women with pelvic pain, which is estimated to reach 70% [36].

When endometriosis is concerned, it is worth noting that the spread of the disease does not show a linear relation to the severity of symptoms [42, 43]; endometriosis is often found as an incidental discovery during surgery for other reasons, and the position of the symptoms seems to be independent from the localization of the implants. In fact, it is known that endometriosis symptoms are not pathognomonic [44]. Factors explaining the relation between endometriosis and CPP were studied, and many mechanisms have been proposed to explain the origin of the pain associated with endometriosis, inflammatory, nociceptive, and neuropathic ones being the most established [45]. Endometriotic nodules were found to be abundantly innervated by unmyelinated sensory C, myelinated sensory Ad, cholinergic, and adrenergic nerve fibers. The inflammatory milieu, which is critical to the maintenance of endometriosis, also causes overexpression of neurotrophins which may contribute to pain and hypersensitivity [46].

Deeply infiltrating endometriosis differs from ovarian endometriomas from a biologic and clinical point of view. It is characterized by fibrotic, vascular, desmoplastic tissue destruction, adhesions formation, and visceral nerves infiltration; the examination and imaging findings often refer to specific symptoms, showing higher incidence of dyspareunia if rectal-vaginal nodularity is present or dyschezia with intrinsic rectal involvement [47–49].

Treatment of endometriosis is always recommended when identified in symptomatic women; however, it is important to investigate all other possible sources of pain (such as inflammatory bowel disease), as symptoms are not specific and different conditions can coexist.

The medical management, with hormonal suppression and nonsteroidal anti-inflammatory drugs (NSAIDs), can be proposed as first approach to women who do not desire pregnancy at the moment and in which no adnexal masses suspicious for endometrioma were found [50, 51]. On the other hand, laparoscopy for diagnosis and excision of endometriosis lesions is indicated "tout court" in women who cannot use hormonal therapy for medical or personal reasons, in unresponsive patients, and in patients in reproductive age with dysmenorrhea and/or dyspareunia, or an ovarian mass, to avoid delay in diagnosis [52–54]. Moreover, laparoscopic complete surgical excision of deep endometriosis lesions has shown a role in improving fertility issues in women with DIE without involvement of the bowel, despite the lack of definitive data [55].

A future achievement to reach about endometriosis management is the reduction of surgical procedures performed, aiming to provide the optimal surgical intensity of treatment; simultaneously, a comparison in the long-term efficacy of medical therapy versus excisional treatment should be made.

20.4.2 Adhesions and Pelvic Inflammatory Disease

CPP is commonly caused by previous pelvic inflammatory disease. Thirty percent of women with acute pelvic inflammatory disease (PID) will develop CPP. This is more likely to happen in settings where sexually transmitted infections prevalence is higher and after multiple episodes of PID, especially in patients who had severe adhesive disease and tubal damage, long-lasting tenderness after treatment, and social and psychological issues [56]. The Fitz-Hugh-Curtis syndrome, or perihepatitis, is a complication in approximately 10% of cases of PID caused by *Chlamydia trachomatis*. Even though it usually causes right upper quadrant pain in young women, lower abdominal and pelvic pain may precede, follow, or occur simultaneously with upper abdominal pain.

Adhesions' role as a cause of CPP is not well-defined, as they are often asymptomatic; though stretch of the organs or limited organ mobility might be some mechanism, most patients with symptomatic adhesions present a history of surgery or intraabdominal or pelvic inflammatory process [57]. Laparoscopic lysis of adhesions is not always a useful or durable therapy, and it can increase the morbidity [24]. No differences in the overall outcome have been shown between women treated and those who underwent diagnostic laparoscopy alone [58]. Therefore, there is little evidence to support routine use of adhesiolysis in treatment for chronic pain [59]. However, some studies suggest that lysis of dense vascular adhesions might produce a significant pain relief [60], and some patients may benefit from selective removal of hydrosalpinges, distorted tubes, or ovaries. In some cases hysterectomy as a final option could be curative for some patients. Physicians should carefully explain to patients asking for adhesiolysis its scarce likelihood to be beneficial for pain reduction and should focus attention on the central factors amplifying pain with the possible need for medical treatment and physical therapy [24].

A personalized treatment should be offered to patients who develop CPP as a consequence of PID, if no other causes of CPP can be identified. The therapy, which consists neuromodulators, including antidepressants and anticonvulsants, should be mainly oriented to the management of neuropathic pain [24].

20.4.3 Pelvic Congestion Syndrome

Pelvic congestion syndrome refers to a condition in which the valvular incompetence in the ovarian veins results in flux insufficiency, leading to reflux and chronic dilation. It can provoke a chronic pelvic pain that exacerbates especially during the day after standing for a long time, premenstrual phase, and after an intercourse, all situations that increase pelvic veins congestion [61]. It is a common situation and is considered cause of one third of CPP cases, even if its pathophysiology is still unclear and pain is not a hallmark [62]. The stretch and stasis of the engorged ovarian and pelvic veins may be the trigger to activate pain receptors within the venous walls causing a diffuse sensitization [63].

The ideal diagnostic test has not been definitively established yet [24]. Ultrasound scan is widely used but also MRI and venography are valid options. Treatment through hormonal suppression, percutaneous embolization, surgical venous occlusion, hysterectomy, salpingectomy, and ovariectomy seems to solve this problem, although just few of the various study protocols available involving these interventions are controlled trials and more evidence is needed [64].

20.4.4 Adenomyosis

Adenomyosis is the abnormal presence of endometrial tissue within the myometrium. Abnormal uterine bleeding and dysmenorrhea are the major symptoms of adenomyosis. Therefore, their presence associated to CPP could suggest adenomyosis. Bleeding and swelling of endometrial islands in the uterine wall seem to be part of the pain originating factors. Symptoms typically develop between the ages of 40 and 50 years. Increased expression of VEGF in the tissues has been considered as one of the most important pathogenetic mechanisms causing pain in patients with adenomyosis. Angiogenesis and neurogenesis are stimulated by VEGF, which is intensely expressed in eutopic and ectopic endometrium of women with adenomyosis [65].

Finding of an enlarged uterus on examination in a patient with typical symptoms is suggestive of adenomyosis. The imaging study includes ultrasound and MRI, which is often performed and is usually useful showing the uterine profile alterations and the presence of endometrial tissue within the myometrium [36]. Moreover, MRI

allows measuring the exact extension of the adenomyosis areas.

Hormonal treatments such as contraceptive pills (estro-progestin or only progestin) or the levonorgestrel-releasing IUDs or subcutaneous progestin device are the first-line therapy. Hysterectomy remains the final solution in nonresponder patients, even if it does not always resolve pelvic pain. Unfortunately, in 25% of women with CPP due to adenomyosis, pelvic pain persists postoperatively [66]. When a single adenomyoma is identified, hysterectomy can sometimes be avoided and fertility-sparing surgery can be performed by skilled hands, counseling the patient in regard to the augmented risk of uterine rupture in pregnancy [67].

20.4.5 Ovarian Cancer

Despite being usually silent, ovarian cancer may cause nonspecific symptoms that rarely alert the patient, such as lower abdominal and back mild pain, discomfort, pressure, bloating, constipation, fatigue, lack of appetite, nausea, indigestion, irregular menstrual cycles, abnormal vaginal bleeding, dyspareunia, and urinary frequency [24]. Pelvic exam and ultrasound are generally sufficient to rule out malignancy.

20.4.6 Ovarian Remnant

This situation can present if bilateral oophorectomy is performed inadequately and ovarian tissue removal is not complete [22]. In this situation, ovarian tissue left keeps responding to FSH and secreting sexual hormones and becoming enlarged and hypertrophic. In case of DIE or intervention in a woman with extensive pelvic adhesions, the risk of missing part of the ovary is increased. Moreover, in a frame of fibrotic adhesions, the enlarged ovary can determine CPP and dyspareunia [22]. The absence of menopausal symptoms and unilateral cyclic pelvic pain should raise physician's attention on this possibility. If symptoms lead to the suspicion of an ovarian remnant, a pelvic examination with a ultrasound scan should be performed, along with blood exams, which will likely show premenopausal levels of FSH and E2, even if menopausal values, especially in older women, do not exclude the diagnosis [24]. Surgery is needed to remove the ovarian remnant, which should be done after stimulation with clomiphene citrate to make the mass more visible. Unfortunately, there is always the possibility of recurrences, together with the risk of side effects of repeating surgery, such as ureteral obstruction [68].

20.4.7 Residual Ovary Syndrome

After hysterectomy without oophorectomy, ovarian tissue left behind can cause symptoms related to ovulatory function, provoking CPP in a small percentage of women [69]. This can be related to the presence of adhesions of the ovary to the colon or the vaginal dome and rupture or leakage of a cyst prompting [22].

20.4.8 Leiomyoma

Uterine leiomyomas are unlikely to cause chronic pain; when it happens, it is most probably related to pressure- and mass-related symptoms, such as urinary retention, urinary frequency, or constipation [24]. Usually patients with leiomyoma present heavy or irregular vaginal bleeding, whereas acute pain can be related to degeneration, torsion, or expulsion through the cervix [7]. Leiomyoma can be suspected by physical examination if it is big, but most frequently it is diagnosed by imaging study. There are not diagnostic criteria to prove that a leiomyoma is the cause of pelvic pain especially when the diameter is less than 3 cm [24]. The management is personalized, guided by patient's age, symptoms, family planning, and wills. It is possible to start from hormonal suppression, if the woman is young and does not desire pregnancy, or myomectomy for small subserosal myomas in women who desire to preserve fertility. On the other hand, symptomatic women who have completed their family, with big myomas, may benefit of surgical removal of the uterus.

20.4.9 Pelvic Floor Dysfunction

Pelvic organ prolapse (POP) is a condition interesting woman from the menopausal period, which makes them a poor cause for CPP, whose peak of incidence is in the third or fourth decade of life. It usually presents with heaviness, pressure, dropping sensations, or aching related to pelvic relaxation [22]. These symptoms are also related to the tense of levator plate due to patient's attempt to hold in prolapsing organs [22].

Some authors relate the retroverted uterus to CPP, especially in case of deep dyspareunia. Usually retroversion is a common anatomic variation but sometimes is related with dysmenorrhea and dyspareunia and consequently with CPP. In the past corrective surgery is used to reduce pain in these women changing the position of the uterus to an axial or anteverted position, with relief of symptoms in uncontrolled clinical series [70–73].

20.4.10 Vaginal Apex Pain

After hysterectomy, vaginal vault pain may occur, often localized to a fornix. The physical examination can produce pain mostly in the lateral fornix despite the cuff appearing perfectly healed [22]. It is important not to confuse the apical pain with others, for example, bowel adhesions, pelvic scarring, or from the remaining ovary. It is possible to distinguish them with the aid of a cotton applicator to touch gently only the vaginal cuff and fornices or with injection of a local anesthetic that does not eliminate the internal pain but only the apex pain [22].

This kind of pain is defined as neuropathic, and it is treated with lidocaine, oral nortriptyline, amitriptyline, or gabapentin. Laparoscopic revision can reduce symptoms but tends to recur in 2–3 years but at less intense level [74].

20.4.11 Other

CPP is often associated with vulvar pain and dyspareunia and postsurgical neuropathy, such as pudendal nerve (and other regional nerve) entrapment.

20.5 Urologic Pathology

CPP can relate to some urologic pathologies as interstitial cystitis/painful bladder syndrome, renal stones, bladder foreign bodies, or urethral diverticulum (Table 20.1). The associated symptoms are pain with voiding, urinary urgency and/or frequency, nocturia, dyspareunia, urethral mass, urinary incontinence, and hematuria [24]. Physical examination, ultrasound, cystourethroscopy, and urodynamic testing are the most commonly utilized diagnostic methods. The prevalent features are slow urine stream, sensation of incomplete emptying, and difficulty voiding, but acute causes can present with suprapubic pelvic and/or genital area pain, such as in case of compressing mass or urethral lesion [24].

20.5.1 Interstitial Cystitis/Painful Bladder Syndrome

Interstitial cystitis/painful bladder syndrome is a complex condition often associated with vulvodynia, endometriosis, and pelvic floor dysfunctions, and it may be a common cause of CPP [75]. Often it mimics urinary tract infection, but urine cultures are negative. It is a chronic inflammatory condition of the bladder with voiding dysfunction (exaggerated urge to void and urinary frequency), pelvic pain, dyspareunia, nocturia, vulvar discomfort, and, rarely, incontinence [76]. Bladder pain syndrome seems to be associated with endometriosis in 48% of cases. Treatment tools include behavioral changes; physical therapy; medications such as amitriptyline, which is the first-line oral drug; and invasive treatments such as bladder hydrodistention or intravesical instillation of glycosaminoglycans [76].

20.5.2 Other

Urinary tract infection is the most common urinary tract disease causing acute pain, but in some cases the recurrence of it can cause CPP, and it is characterized by chronic suprapubic pain, with frequency, urgency, and/or hematuria [76].

Urethral diverticulum should be considered if a suburethral mass, fullness, or tenderness is detected. Symptoms of interstitial cystitis can mask bladder neoplasia or chronic urethral syndrome [76]. The first presents in women with hematuria, a history of smoking, or who are over 60 years of age; the second, which appears as an interstitial cystitis, represents a distinct pathology from this.

20.6 Gastrointestinal Tract Pathology

CPP can find a cause in irritable bowel syndrome, inflammatory bowel disease, diverticular colitis, celiac disease, chronic constipation, and cancer (Table 20.1). In these cases, CPP may be associated with diarrhea, constipation, rectal bleeding, urgency, and tenesmus [24]. Chronic pelvic pain is reported in literature to be present in one third of the irritable bowel syndrome patients, twice as much as in the inflammatory bowel disease [77]. Distinction between gastroenterological and gynecological causes should be assessed, although sometimes different etiologies give similar symptoms, such as dyschezia that was reported in 44% of patients with endometriosis and in 24% of women without pelvic findings, undergoing laparoscopy [78]. Another confounding symptom of endometriosis is hematochezia; in this case colonoscopy is mandatory.

20.6.1 Irritable Bowel Syndrome

Irritable bowel syndrome (IBS) is a gastrointestinal functional pain syndrome in which abdominal pain is chronic and has an intermittent trend. This is a frequent condition that affects 10% of the general population, having an incidence that is double in women than in men [79–81]. Besides, children and adolescents with CPP are frequently affected from IBS, even if this condition is under-diagnosed and undertreated [82]. Irritable bowel syndrome diagnosis is based on patient's history; on the contrary, physical examination is generally unremarkable. CPP is more frequently associated with IBS in patients with history of dysthymic disorder, panic disorder, somatization disorder, childhood sexual abuse, and hysterectomy [76, 83]. It is mainly a diagnosis of exclusion [77].

Specific functional abdominal pain disorders include functional dyspepsia, abdominal migraine, and functional abdominal pain syndrome.

20.6.2 Inflammatory Bowel Disease

Crohn's disease presents with fatigue, diarrhea with crampy abdominal pain, weight loss, and fever, with or without gross bleeding [84]. Ulcerative colitis has a similar presentation, but rectal bleeding is more common with ulcerative colitis than with Crohn's disease [84].

20.6.3 Celiac Disease

Celiac disease (or sprue) can present variously also as chronic pelvic pain, often associated with diarrhea and weight loss, due to a mucosal immune reaction to gluten. It is characterized by impaired absorption and digestion of nutrients by the small bowel [77].

20.6.4 Diverticular Colitis

Diverticular colitis develops in the frame of diverticular disease [85]. Its pathogenic mechanism is not well understood, it seems to be due to chronic mucosal inflammation that usually involves the sigmoid colon, resulting in variable endoscopic and histological features. Its cause may be multifactorial, related to mucosal prolapse, fecal stasis, or localized ischemia.

20.6.5 Colon Cancer

Most patients with colorectal cancer have abdominal pain, accompanied by other findings such as hematochezia or melena, abdominal pain, and changes in bowel habits.

20.6.6 Other

Chronic intestinal pseudo-obstruction and chronic constipation are both common in women, the first usually presenting with acute pelvic pain, whereas CPP is most frequent in the second.

20.7 Musculoskeletal Problems

The main musculoskeletal processes that can cause CPP include myofascial pelvic pain syndrome and fibromyalgia (Table 20.1). Musculoskeletal changes could be cause or consequence of CPP [22]. Damages or spasms of the abdominal wall or pelvic floor muscles or nerves may be a source of pain, which can be misdiagnosed as visceral pain. It associates with movements, posture, surgery, or trauma. Recent studies indicate significant clinical improvement of physiotherapy for CPP and female sexual dysfunction [86].

20.7.1 Myofascial Pelvic Pain Syndrome

Myofascial pelvic pain syndrome is often associated with visceral pain in organs in continuity with pelvic floor, such as vagina, vulva, rectum, or bladder, or in distant areas such as the thighs, buttocks, hips, or lower abdomen. Sometimes, the patients complain of visceral symptoms like heaviness, bladder urgency or frequency, and tenesmus [24]. The physical examination is the preferred diagnostic method. The identification of tender pelvic muscles and trigger points is the sign that defines the pathology [87, 88]. Possible treatments available are physical therapy and physiatry. Myofascial pain often is associated with the other pain syndromes seen in CPP [24].

20.7.2   Fibromyalgia

Fibromyalgia is present in as much as 2–8% of the population; is characterized by widespread pain; is a clinical diagnosis characterized by widespread pain, typically in the muscles and joints and multiple tender points on examination; and is often accompanied by fatigue, memory problems, and sleep disturbances [24, 89]. This disorder is characterized by pain of uncertain origin, felt in all four quadrants of the body and especially at physical pressure in at least 11 trigger points out of 18 (e.g., knees, shoulders, elbows, neck), including the pelvis [90]. Other clinical syndromes of unknown origin overlap with fibromyalgia such as systemic exertion intolerance disease, also known as chronic fatigue syndrome, and IBS; moreover, patients are more likely to suffer from depression and have somatization symptoms [81]. It is characterized by failure of the diffuse noxious inhibitory control (DNIC) system. The pain from a trigger point may then become self-perpetuating, and sometimes visceral pain can lead to muscular tension and pain. This sensitization constitutes a pain amplifying factor that must be considered regardless of whether it is the consequence or the underlying cause of chronic pain. Clear evidence regarding diagnostic tests and therapeutic options is lacking.

20.7.3   Other

Coccydynia, piriformis/levator ani syndrome, pelvic floor tension myalgia, or pelvic myofascial pain is caused by involuntary spasm of the pelvic floor muscles [91, 92]. In particular, the levator ani muscle group can undergo pain processes after hypertonus, myalgia, overuse, and fatigue, caused by inflammatory disorder, childbirth, pelvic surgery, and trauma. It is increased by sitting for prolonged periods and relieved by heat and lying down with the hips flexed. The pelvic floor tension myalgia may sometimes be a direct consequence of endometriosis or painful bladder syndrome/interstitial cystitis [93]. Faulty posture can cause muscle imbalance in different muscular groups giving local or referred pain.

Osteitis pubis is a noninfectious inflammation of the pubic symphysis causing abdominal and pelvic pain as complication of surgery or most frequently related to pregnancy/childbirth, athletic activities, trauma, or rheumatological disorders [94]. Common feature is pain aggravated by movements, and the pubis symphysis is tender to palpation.

Chronic abdominal wall pain may be related to muscular injury or strain or nerve injury. It is frequently unrecognized or confused with visceral pain. Chronic abdominal wall pain occurs in 7–9% of women after a Pfannenstiel incision [95].

Abdominal wall hernias can also cause CPP.

20.8   Psychosocial Disorders

Disturbances such as depression, anxiety, and somatization can be part of CPP and require specific multidisciplinary and targeted treatments [22]. It is more likely to find a story of sexual abuse in patients who experience chronic pelvic pain. Migraine, temporomandibular joint, and fibromyalgia provoke a central sensitization that can have repercussions on the whole body.

Women with CPP are characterized by pain-catastrophizing thinking associated to greater anxiety, somatization, and depression [84, 85, 96–99].

20.8.1   Depression

Depression frequently occurs in women with CPP [99]. The modulation of nociceptive pathways by psychological processes probably plays an important role in amplifying pain symptomatology [30].

It is unclear if a causal relationship exists or association is casual, although biological and psychological factors seem to interact. Some authors believe that in some cases CPP takes part of a specific syndrome, the pain-prone disorder, which has been considered as a variant of depression [100]. Moreover, a strict relation between childhood sexual abuse, CPP, and depression has been found [76, 101]. It is important to distinguish patients with a story of primary psychiatric comorbidity from patients who are developing secondary psychological problems in reaction to their pain. A possible therapy should be aimed to reduce this hypervigilant response, through cognitive behavioral therapy methods used to treat other chronic pain conditions [89].

20.8.2 Physical and Sexual Abuse

Previous physical or sexual abuse is related to chronic pain, mostly with CPP. Studies report a prevalence of a history of physical and/or sexual abuse in more than 47% of women with CPP [91, 92, 102]. Traumatic experiences may alter both the modulation of pain signals and pituitary-adrenal/autonomic responses to stress. According to studies on trauma populations, the hypervigilance and autonomic response to peripheral stimuli should be reduced by cognitive behavioral therapy (i.e., mind-body methods) [94].

20.8.3 Sleep Disorders

Sleep disorders are very frequent in women with chronic pain and are related to CPP in a two-way relationship. CPP could be the cause of sleep disorder as well as a consequence of it, with negative effect on depressive symptoms, starting a vicious cycle [103]. Stopping this strong bond referring the patients to his physician for a sleep evaluation is critical.

20.8.4 Somatization

Somatization is a syndrome of nonspecific physical symptoms (such as fatigue, widespread pain, and/or sleep disturbance) that cannot be fully explained by a known medical condition after appropriate investigation. Some study describes patients with somatic syndrome as individuals more prone to experiencing pain-related distress and not as a condition that they develop [104, 105]. This explanation can help provide an etiology and could find a therapy in mind-body methods to reduce threat hypervigilance and reduce autonomic response to peripheral stimuli [24].

20.8.5 Opiate Dependency

The use of opioids must be cautious in patients with CPP for two reasons; (1) the risk of addiction disorder 3–26% [106–108] and (2) patients with chronic pain are less responsive to opioid analgesics [22]. For these motivations the use of opioid should be considered only after a careful evaluation, in case of other treatment modalities and counseling of risks.

Moreover, there are other two considerations about opioid analgesic in long-term therapy for chronic pain: (1) there are no significant benefits using opioid monotherapy and (2) in nonresponder patients, worsening of symptoms at increasing opioid doses should be considered opioid-induced hyperalgesia [109]. In these cases, it should be considered to refer the patients to a psychologist for a cognitive behavioral therapy and potential elimination of opioids [31].

References

1. Fall M, Baranowski AP, Elneil S, Engeler D, Hughes J, Messelink EJ, et al. EAU guidelines on chronic pelvic pain. Eur Urol. 2010;57(1):35–48.
2. RCOG. The initial management of chronic pelvic pain. RCOG Green-top Guideline No 41. 2012.
3. Zondervan KT, Yudkin PL, Vessey MP, Jenkinson CP, Dawes MG, Barlow DH, et al. The community prevalence of chronic pelvic pain in women and associated illness behaviour. Br J Gen Pract. 2001;51(468):541–7.
4. Mathias SD, Kuppermann M, Liberman RF, Lipschutz RC, Steege JF. Chronic pelvic pain: prevalence, health-related quality of life, and economic correlates. Obstet Gynecol. 1996;87(3):321–7.
5. Howard FM. Chronic pelvic pain. Obstet Gynecol. 2003;101(3):594–611.
6. Merskey H, Bogduk N. Visceral and other syndromes of the trunk apart from spinal and radicular pain. In: IASP Press S, editor. Classification of chronic pain: descriptions of chronic pain syndromes and definitions of pain terms. 2nd ed. Seattle, WA: IASP Press; 2002. p. 1–37.
7. Lippman SA, Warner M, Samuels S, Olive D, Vercellini P, Eskenazi B. Uterine fibroids and

gynecologic pain symptoms in a population-based study. Fertil Steril. 2003;80(6):1488–94.

8. Zondervan KT, Yudkin PL, Vessey MP, Dawes MG, Barlow DH, Kennedy SH. Prevalence and incidence of chronic pelvic pain in primary care: evidence from a national general practice database. Br J Obstet Gynaecol. 1999;106(11):1149–55.

9. Grace VM, Zondervan KT. Chronic pelvic pain in New Zealand: prevalence, pain severity, diagnoses and use of the health services. Aust N Z J Public Health. 2004;28(4):369–75.

10. Tu FF, Beaumont JL. Outpatient laparoscopy for abdominal and pelvic pain in the United States 1994 through 1996. Am J Obstet Gynecol. 2006;194(3):699–703.

11. Farquhar CM, Steiner CA. Hysterectomy rates in the United States 1990–1997. Obstet Gynecol. 2002;99(2):229–34.

12. Howard FM. The role of laparoscopy in chronic pelvic pain: promise and pitfalls. Obstet Gynecol Surv. 1993;48(6):357–87.

13. Suter MR. Microglial role in the development of chronic pain. Curr Opin Anaesthesiol. 2016;29(5):584–9.

14. Bagarinao E, Johnson KA, Martucci KT, Ichesco E, Farmer MA, Labus J, et al. Preliminary structural MRI based brain classification of chronic pelvic pain: A MAPP network study. Pain. 2014;155(12):2502–9.

15. Melzack R, Wall PD. Pain mechanisms: a new theory. Science. 1965;150(3699):971–9.

16. Melzack R. Pain and the neuromatrix in the brain. J Dent Educ. 2001;65(12):1378–82.

17. Giamberardino MA, Costantini R, Affaitati G, Fabrizio A, Lapenna D, Tafuri E, et al. Viscero-visceral hyperalgesia: characterization in different clinical models. Pain. 2010;151(2):307–22.

18. Hellman KM, Patanwala IY, Pozolo KE, Tu FF. Multimodal nociceptive mechanisms underlying chronic pelvic pain. Am J Obstet Gynecol. 2015;213(6):827.e1–9.

19. Phillips K, Clauw DJ. Central pain mechanisms in chronic pain states--maybe it is all in their head. Best Pract Res Clin Rheumatol. 2011;25(2):141–54.

20. Phillips ML, Gregory LJ, Cullen S, Coen S, Ng V, Andrew C, et al. The effect of negative emotional context on neural and behavioural responses to oesophageal stimulation. Brain. 2003;126(Pt 3):669–84.

21. Engeler D (Chair) APB, Borovicka J, Cottrell AM, Dinis-Oliveira P, Elneil S, Hughes J, Messelink EJ (Vice-chair), de C Williams AC, Guidelines Associates: B. Parsons SG. The 2017 EAU guidelines on chronic pelvic pain 2017.

22. Griffith JW, Stephens-Shields AJ, Hou X, Naliboff BD, Pontari M, Edwards TC, et al. Pain and urinary symptoms should not be combined into a single score: psychometric findings from the MAPP research network. J Urol. 2016;195(4):949–54.

23. Jamieson DJ, Steege JF. The association of sexual abuse with pelvic pain complaints in a primary care population. Am J Obstet Gynecol. 1997;177(6):1408–12.

24. Su N, Lobbezoo F, van Wijk A, van der Heijden GJ, Visscher CM. Associations of pain intensity and pain-related disability with psychological and socio-demographic factors in patients with temporomandibular disorders: a cross-sectional study at a specialised dental clinic. J Oral Rehabil. 2017;44(3):187–96.

25. Fenton BW, Grey SF, Tossone K, McCarroll M, Von Gruenigen VE. Classifying patients with chronic pelvic pain into levels of biopsychosocial dysfunction using latent class modeling of patient reported outcome measures. Pain Res Treat. 2015;2015:940675.

26. Randy Jinkins J. The anatomic and physiologic basis of local, referred and radiating lumbosacral pain syndromes related to disease of the spine. J Neuroradiol. 2004;31(3):163–80.

27. Di Tella M, Ghiggia A, Tesio V, Romeo A, Colonna F, Fusaro E, et al. Pain experience in fibromyalgia syndrome: the role of alexithymia and psychological distress. J Affect Disord. 2017;208:87–93.

28. Bharucha AE, Lee TH. Anorectal and pelvic pain. Mayo Clin Proc. 2016;91(10):1471–86.

29. Richter HE, Holley RL, Chandraiah S, Varner RE. Laparoscopic and psychologic evaluation of women with chronic pelvic pain. Int J Psychiatry Med. 1998;28(2):243–53.

30. Eisendrath SJ. Psychiatric aspects of chronic pain. Neurology. 1995;45(12 Suppl 9):S26–34; discussion S5–6.

31. Hudelist G, English J, Thomas AE, Tinelli A, Singer CF, Keckstein J. Diagnostic accuracy of transvaginal ultrasound for non-invasive diagnosis of bowel endometriosis: systematic review and meta-analysis. Ultrasound Obstet Gynecol. 2011;37(3):257–63.

32. Bhide AA, Puccini F, Bray R, Khullar V, Digesu GA. The pelvic floor muscle hyperalgesia (PFMH) scoring system: a new classification tool to assess women with chronic pelvic pain: multicentre pilot study of validity and reliability. Eur J Obstet Gynecol Reprod Biol. 2015;193:111–3.

33. Gambone JC, Mittman BS, Munro MG, Scialli AR, Winkel CA, Group CPPEW. Consensus statement for the management of chronic pelvic pain and endometriosis: proceedings of an expert-panel consensus process. Fertil Steril. 2002;78(5):961–72.

34. Ganeshan A, Upponi S, Hon LQ, Uthappa MC, Warakaulle DR, Uberoi R. Chronic pelvic pain due to pelvic congestion syndrome: the role of diagnostic and interventional radiology. Cardiovasc Intervent Radiol. 2007;30(6):1105–11.

35. Nisenblat V, Bossuyt PM, Farquhar C, Johnson N, Hull ML. Imaging modalities for the non-invasive diagnosis of endometriosis. Cochrane Database Syst Rev. 2016;2:CD009591.

36. Howard FM. The role of laparoscopy in the evaluation of chronic pelvic pain: pitfalls with a negative laparoscopy. J Am Assoc Gynecol Laparosc. 1996;4(1):85–94.

37. Tirlapur SA, Daniels JP, Khan KS, collaboration Mt. Chronic pelvic pain: how does noninvasive imaging compare with diagnostic laparoscopy? Curr Opin Obstet Gynecol. 2015;27(6):445–8.

38. Hanno P. Potassium sensitivity test for painful bladder syndrome/interstitial cystitis: con. J Urol. 2009;182(2):431–2. 4

39. Whitehead WE, Palsson OS. Is rectal pain sensitivity a biological marker for irritable bowel syndrome: psychological influences on pain perception. Gastroenterology. 1998;115(5):1263–71.

40. Iacovides S, Baker FC, Avidon I, Bentley A. Women with dysmenorrhea are hypersensitive to experimental deep muscle pain across the menstrual cycle. J Pain. 2013;14(10):1066–76.

41. Jarrell J, Arendt-Nielsen L. Evolutionary considerations in the development of chronic pelvic pain. Am J Obstet Gynecol. 2016;215(2):201.e1–4.

42. Porpora MG, Koninckx PR, Piazze J, Natili M, Colagrande S, Cosmi EV. Correlation between endometriosis and pelvic pain. J Am Assoc Gynecol Laparosc. 1999;6(4):429–34.

43. Milingos S, Protopapas A, Kallipolitis G, Drakakis P, Loutradis D, Liapi A, et al. Endometriosis in patients with chronic pelvic pain: is staging predictive of the efficacy of laparoscopic surgery in pain relief? Gynecol Obstet Invest. 2006;62(1):48–54.

44. Hsu AL, Sinaii N, Segars J, Nieman LK, Stratton P. Relating pelvic pain location to surgical findings of endometriosis. Obstet Gynecol. 2011;118(2 Pt 1):223–30.

45. Howard FM. Endometriosis and mechanisms of pelvic pain. J Minim Invasive Gynecol. 2009;16(5):540–50.

46. Kobayashi H, Yamada Y, Morioka S, Niiro E, Shigemitsu A, Ito F. Mechanism of pain generation for endometriosis-associated pelvic pain. Arch Gynecol Obstet. 2014;289(1):13–21.

47. Vercellini P, Fedele L, Aimi G, Pietropaolo G, Consonni D, Crosignani PG. Association between endometriosis stage, lesion type, patient characteristics and severity of pelvic pain symptoms: a multivariate analysis of over 1000 patients. Hum Reprod. 2007;22(1):266–71.

48. Fauconnier A, Chapron C, Dubuisson JB, Vieira M, Dousset B, Bréart G. Relation between pain symptoms and the anatomic location of deep infiltrating endometriosis. Fertil Steril. 2002;78(4):719–26.

49. dell'Endometriosi GIplS. Relationship between stage, site and morphological characteristics of pelvic endometriosis and pain. Hum Reprod. 2001;16(12):2668–71.

50. Medicine PCotASfR. Treatment of pelvic pain associated with endometriosis: a committee opinion. Fertil Steril. 2014;101(4):927–35.

51. Dunselman GA, Vermeulen N, Becker C, Calhaz-Jorge C, D'Hooghe T, De Bie B, et al. ESHRE guideline: management of women with endometriosis. Hum Reprod. 2014;29(3):400–12.

52. Sinaii N, Plumb K, Cotton L, Lambert A, Kennedy S, Zondervan K, et al. Differences in characteristics among 1,000 women with endometriosis based on extent of disease. Fertil Steril. 2008;89(3):538–45.

53. Hickey M, Ballard K, Farquhar C. Endometriosis. BMJ. 2014;348:g1752.

54. Facchin F, Barbara G, Saita E, Mosconi P, Roberto A, Fedele L, et al. Impact of endometriosis on quality of life and mental health: pelvic pain makes the difference. J Psychosom Obstet Gynaecol. 2015;36(4):135–41.

55. Angioni S, Cela V, Sedda F, Stochino Loi E, Cofelice V, Pontis A, et al. Focusing on surgery results in infertile patients with deep endometriosis. Gynecol Endocrinol. 2015;31(8):595–8.

56. Trautmann GM, Kip KE, Richter HE, Soper DE, Peipert JF, Nelson DB, et al. Do short-term markers of treatment efficacy predict long-term sequelae of pelvic inflammatory disease? Am J Obstet Gynecol. 2008;198(1):30.e1–7.

57. Surgeons PCoASfRMicwSoR. Pathogenesis, consequences, and control of peritoneal adhesions in gynecologic surgery. Fertil Steril. 2008;90(5 Suppl):S144–9.

58. Molegraaf MJ, Torensma B, Lange CP, Lange JF, Jeekel J, Swank DJ. Twelve-year outcomes of laparoscopic adhesiolysis in patients with chronic abdominal pain: a randomized clinical trial. Surgery. 2017;161(2):415–21.

59. van den Beukel BA, de Ree R, van Leuven S, Bakkum EA, Strik C, van Goor H, et al. Surgical treatment of adhesion-related chronic abdominal and pelvic pain after gynaecological and general surgery: a systematic review and meta-analysis. Hum Reprod Update. 2017;23(3):276–88.

60. Swank DJ, Swank-Bordewijk SC, Hop WC, van Erp WF, Janssen IM, Bonjer HJ, et al. Laparoscopic adhesiolysis in patients with chronic abdominal pain: a blinded randomised controlled multi-centre trial. Lancet. 2003;361(9365):1247–51.

61. Beard RW, Reginald PW, Wadsworth J. Clinical features of women with chronic lower abdominal pain and pelvic congestion. Br J Obstet Gynaecol. 1988;95(2):153–61.

62. Rozenblit AM, Ricci ZJ, Tuvia J, Amis ES. Incompetent and dilated ovarian veins: a common CT finding in asymptomatic parous women. AJR Am J Roentgenol. 2001;176(1):119–22.

63. Phillips D, Deipolyi AR, Hesketh RL, Midia M, Oklu R. Pelvic congestion syndrome: etiology of pain, diagnosis, and clinical management. J Vasc Interv Radiol. 2014;25(5):725–33.

64. Tu FF, Hahn D, Steege JF. Pelvic congestion syndrome-associated pelvic pain: a systematic review of diagnosis and management. Obstet Gynecol Surv. 2010;65(5):332–40.

65. Orazov MR, Nosenko EN, Radzinsky VE, Khamoshina MB, Lebedeva MG, Sounov MA. Proangiogenic features in chronic pelvic pain caused by adenomyosis. Gynecol Endocrinol. 2016;32(sup2):7–10.

66. Stovall TG, Ling FW, Crawford DA. Hysterectomy for chronic pelvic pain of presumed uterine etiology. Obstet Gynecol. 1990;75(4):676–9.

67. Osada H, Silber S, Kakinuma T, Nagaishi M, Kato K, Kato O. Surgical procedure to conserve the uterus for future pregnancy in patients suffering from massive adenomyosis. Reprod Biomed Online. 2011;22(1):94–9.

68. Vilos GA, Marks-Adams JL, Vilos AG, Oraif A, Abu-Rafea B, Casper RF. Medical treatment of ureteral obstruction associated with ovarian remnants and/or endometriosis: report of three cases and review of the literature. J Minim Invasive Gynecol. 2015;22(3):462–8.

69. Bukovsky I, Liftshitz Y, Langer R, Weinraub Z, Sadovsky G, Caspi E. Ovarian residual syndrome. Surg Gynecol Obstet. 1988;167(2):132–4.

70. Halperin R, Padoa A, Schneider D, Bukovsky I, Pansky M. Long-term follow-up (5–20 years) after uterine ventrosuspension for chronic pelvic pain and deep dyspareunia. Gynecol Obstet Invest. 2003;55(4):216–9.

71. Batioglu S, Zeyneloglu HB. Laparoscopic plication and suspension of the round ligament for chronic pelvic pain and dyspareunia. J Am Assoc Gynecol Laparosc. 2000;7(4):547–51.

72. Carter JE. Carter-Thomason uterine suspension and positioning by ligament investment, fixation and truncation. J Reprod Med. 1999;44(5):417–22.

73. Masters WH, Johnson VE. Human Sexual Response. Boston: Little Brown; 1966.

74. Lamvu G, Robinson B, Zolnoun D, Steege JF. Vaginal apex resection: a treatment option for vaginal apex pain. Obstet Gynecol. 2004;104(6):1340–6.

75. Stanford EJ, Dell JR, Parsons CL. The emerging presence of interstitial cystitis in gynecologic patients with chronic pelvic pain. Urology. 2007;69(4 Suppl):53–9.

76. Walker E, Katon W, Harrop-Griffiths J, Holm L, Russo J, Hickok LR. Relationship of chronic pelvic pain to psychiatric diagnoses and childhood sexual abuse. Am J Psychiatry. 1988;145(1):75–80.

77. Pain AAoPSoCA. Chronic abdominal pain in children. Pediatrics. 2005;115(3):812–5.

78. Schliep KC, Mumford SL, Peterson CM, Chen Z, Johnstone EB, Sharp HT, et al. Pain typology and incident endometriosis. Hum Reprod. 2015;30(10):2427–38.

79. Parsons CL. Diagnosing chronic pelvic pain of bladder origin. J Reprod Med. 2004;49(3 Suppl):235–42.

80. O'Leary MP, Sant GR, Fowler FJ, Whitmore KE, Spolarich-Kroll J. The interstitial cystitis symptom index and problem index. Urology. 1997;49(5A Suppl):58–63.

81. Lane TJ, Manu P, Matthews DA. Depression and somatization in the chronic fatigue syndrome. Am J Med. 1991;91(4):335–44.

82. Williams RE, Hartmann KE, Sandler RS, Miller WC, Savitz LA, Steege JF. Recognition and treatment of irritable bowel syndrome among women with chronic pelvic pain. Am J Obstet Gynecol. 2005;192(3):761–7.

83. Walker EA, Gelfand AN, Gelfand MD, Green C, Katon WJ. Chronic pelvic pain and gynecological symptoms in women with irritable bowel syndrome. J Psychosom Obstet Gynaecol. 1996;17(1):39–46.

84. Heddini U, Bohm-Starke N, Nilsson KW, Johannesson U. Provoked vestibulodynia--medical factors and comorbidity associated with treatment outcome. J Sex Med. 2012;9(5):1400–6.

85. Nickel JC, Tripp DA, Pontari M, Moldwin R, Mayer R, Carr LK, et al. Psychosocial phenotyping in women with interstitial cystitis/painful bladder syndrome: a case control study. J Urol. 2010;183(1):167–72.

86. Berghmans B. Physiotherapy for pelvic pain and female sexual dysfunction: an untapped resource. Int Urogynecol J. 2018;29(5):631–8.

87. Simons DG, Travel JG, Simons PT. Upper half of body. In: Williams & Wilkins B, editor. Travell and Simons' myofascial pain and dysfunction: the trigger point manual. 2nd ed. Baltimore: Williams & Wilkins; 1999.

88. Lavelle ED, Lavelle W, Smith HS. Myofascial trigger points. Anesthesiol Clin. 2007;25(4):841–51. vii-iii.

89. Center CPFR. MiBetterBack symptom management program for low back pain. University of Michigan Health System; 2017.

90. Wolfe F, Smythe HA, Yunus MB, Bennett RM, Bombardier C, Goldenberg DL, Tugwell P, Campbell SM, Abeles M, Clark P. The American College of Rheumatology 1990 criteria for the classification of fibromyalgia. Report of the multicenter criteria committee. Arthritis Rheum. 1990;33(2):160.

91. Walling MK, Reiter RC, O'Hara MW, Milburn AK, Lilly G, Vincent SD. Abuse history and chronic pain in women: I. Prevalences of sexual abuse and physical abuse. Obstet Gynecol. 1994;84(2):193–9.

92. Meltzer-Brody S, Leserman J, Zolnoun D, Steege J, Green E, Teich A. Trauma and posttraumatic stress disorder in women with chronic pelvic pain. Obstet Gynecol. 2007;109(4):902–8.

93. Tu FF, Fitzgerald CM, Kuiken T, Farrell T, Harden RN, Norman HR. Comparative measurement of pelvic floor pain sensitivity in chronic pelvic pain. Obstet Gynecol. 2007;110(6):1244–8.

94. Deblinger E, Pollio E, Runyon MK, Steer RA. Improvements in personal resiliency among youth who have completed trauma-focused cognitive behavioral therapy: A preliminary examination. Child Abuse Negl. 2017;65:132–9.

95. Loos MJ, Scheltinga MR, Mulders LG, Roumen RM. The Pfannenstiel incision as a source of chronic pain. Obstet Gynecol. 2008;111(4):839–46.

96. Clemens JQ, Brown SO, Calhoun EA. Mental health diagnoses in patients with interstitial cystitis/painful bladder syndrome and chronic prostatitis/chronic pelvic pain syndrome: a case/control study. J Urol. 2008;180(4):1378–82.

97. Granot M, Lavee Y. Psychological factors associated with perception of experimental pain in vulvar vestibulitis syndrome. J Sex Marital Ther. 2005;31(4):285–302.

98. Lowenstein L, Kenton K, Mueller ER, Brubaker L, Heneghan M, Senka J, et al. Patients with painful bladder syndrome have altered response to thermal stimuli and catastrophic reaction to painful experiences. Neurourol Urodyn. 2009;28(5):400–4.

99. Lorençatto C, Petta CA, Navarro MJ, Bahamondes L, Matos A. Depression in women with endometriosis with and without chronic pelvic pain. Acta Obstet Gynecol Scand. 2006;85(1):88–92.

100. Blumer D, Zorick F, Heilbronn M, Roth T. Biological markers for depression in chronic pain. J Nerv Ment Dis. 1982;170(7):425–8.

101. Randolph ME, Reddy DM. Sexual functioning in women with chronic pelvic pain: the impact of depression, support, and abuse. J Sex Res. 2006;43(1):38–45.

102. Rapkin AJ, Kames LD, Darke LL, Stampler FM, Naliboff BD. History of physical and sexual abuse in women with chronic pelvic pain. Obstet Gynecol. 1990;76(1):92–6.

103. Nolan TE, Metheny WP, Smith RP. Unrecognized association of sleep disorders and depression with chronic pelvic pain. South Med J. 1992;85(12):1181–3.

104. Ablin K, Clauw DJ. From fibrositis to functional somatic syndromes to a bell-shaped curve of pain and sensory sensitivity: evolution of a clinical construct. Rheum Dis Clin North Am. 2009;35(2):233–51.

105. Grinberg K, Granot M, Lowenstein L, Abramov L, Weissman-Fogel I. A common pronociceptive pain modulation profile typifying subgroups of chronic pelvic pain syndromes is interrelated with enhanced clinical pain. Pain. 2017;158(6):1021–9.

106. Fleming MF, Balousek SL, Klessig CL, Mundt MP, Brown DD. Substance use disorders in a primary care sample receiving daily opioid therapy. J Pain. 2007;8(7):573–82.

107. Boscarino JA, Rukstalis M, Hoffman SN, Han JJ, Erlich PM, Gerhard GS, et al. Risk factors for drug dependence among out-patients on opioid therapy in a large US health-care system. Addiction. 2010;105(10):1776–82.

108. Liebschutz JM, Saitz R, Weiss RD, Averbuch T, Schwartz S, Meltzer EC, et al. Clinical factors associated with prescription drug use disorder in urban primary care patients with chronic pain. J Pain. 2010;11(11):1047–55.

109. Dowell D, Haegerich TM. Using the CDC guideline and tools for opioid prescribing in patients with chronic pain. Am Fam Physician. 2016;93(12):970–2.

Imaging of Uterine Disease-Related Pain

21

Maria Milagros Otero-García, Patricia Blanco-Lobato, and Maria Cristina Prado-Monzo

Abbreviations

2D	Two-dimensional
3D	Three-dimensional
ACR	The American College of Radiology
ADC	Apparent diffusion coefficient
ALARA	As low as reasonably achievable
ASMR	The American Society of Reproductive Medicine
CT	Computed tomography
DCE	Dynamic contrast enhanced
DWI	Diffusion-weighted imaging
ESHRE/ESGE	The European Society of Human Reproduction and Embryology/European Society of Gynecologic Endoscopy
ESS	Endometrial stroma sarcoma
ESUR	The European Society of Urogenital Radiology
FIGO	The International Federation of Gynecology and Obstetrics
FOV	Field of view
Gd	Gadolinium
GRE	Gradient echo
HPV	Human papillomavirus
HSG	Hysterosalpingography
ICM	Iodinated contrast media
IUD	Intrauterine devices
LDH	Lactate dehydrogenase
LMS	Leiomyosarcomas
MDA	Müllerian ducts anomalies
MRI	Magnetic resonance imaging
PET	Positron emission tomography
PID	Pelvic inflammatory disease
T1WI	T1-weighted imaging
T2WI	T2-weighted imaging
TOF	Time-of flight
TAPS	Traumatic abruptio placental scale
UAE	Uterine artery embolization
UES	Undifferentiated endometrial sarcoma
US	Ultrasound
VCUAM	Vagina, cervix, uterus, adnexa, and associated malformations
β-hCG	Beta-human chorionic gonadotropin

Electronic supplementary material The online version of this chapter (https://doi.org/10.1007/978-3-319-99822-0_21) contains supplementary material, which is available to authorized users.

M. M. Otero-García (✉) · P. Blanco-Lobato
M. C. Prado-Monzo
Complejo Hospitalario Universitario de Vigo (CHUVI), Hospital Álvaro Cunqueiro, Vigo, Pontevedra, Spain
e-mail: milagros.otero.garcia@sergas.es; patricia.blanco.lobato@sergas.es; maria.cristina.prado.monzo@sergas.es

21.1 Introduction

Several uterine disorders can cause pelvic pain in both pregnant and nonpregnant women. This pain may or may not be associated with menstruation (dysmenorrhea). It can be chronic and often disabling or acute, warranting in the latter case, a differential diagnosis with other gynecological or non-gynecological entities in the emergency room.

The purpose of this chapter is to review the most common uterine diseases manifesting clinically with pain in both pregnant and nonpregnant women and the role of diagnostic imaging techniques in their evaluation and management.

21.2 Diagnostic Imaging Techniques

Symptoms and physical examination findings in uterine diseases are often non-specific; hence, diagnostic imaging techniques play an important and useful role in achieving an early and accurate diagnosis, in planning the treatment, and in the follow-up of these entities, enabling better clinical outcomes.

21.2.1 Ultrasound

Ultrasound (US) in both its modalities—transvaginal and transabdominal—is the imaging technique of choice to assess female pelvic pain when a gynecological cause is suspected; especially in pregnant women, because it is easy to perform, cost-effective and widely available, without a risk of radiation, and has an acceptable sensitivity and specificity for diagnosing most pelvic pathological entities [1]. However, it also has disadvantages, such as its relatively small field of view (FOV), the difficulties arising from a poor acoustic window in patients with a large body habitus, or in the presence of extensive bowel gas or calcification [2]. Another important limitation of this technique is its dependence on the operator's experience.

Because of this, the study must often be carried out using additional imaging techniques, such as magnetic resonance imaging (MRI) or computed tomography (CT).

Transabdominal US is best performed with a low-middle frequency transducer (1–5 MHz). It requires an adequate acoustic window, which is obtained by filling the bladder, thus generating a wide FOV of the pelvis, as well as a good view of the uterine fundus, the high positioned adnexa, and the possible presence of intraperitoneal free fluid or hemorrhage. Transvaginal US uses a high-frequency endovaginal probe (>7 MHz) following bladder voiding, allowing an excellent assessment of the endometrium and adnexal structures.

21.2.2 Magnetic Resonance Imaging

MRI is considered an excellent imaging tool for evaluating gynecological pathological entities due to its lack of ionizing radiation, high soft tissue resolution, and multiplanar imaging capabilities; therefore, it is frequently used as a second-choice imaging modality when the US findings are inconclusive [1].

To improve MRI performance, patients must have fasted for 4–6 h, and bladder and rectal voiding is recommended to reduce motion artifacts caused by bowel peristalsis. The intramuscular or intravenous injection of an antiperistaltic agent (hyoscine butylbromide or glucagon) is also advised to further reduce motion artifacts, not only from bowel peristalsis but also from uterine peristalsis, and improve image quality. Patients should be imaged in the supine position, using 1.5 or 3.0 T MRI equipment with a body, pelvic or cardiac phase-array surface coil, and fat saturation bands are applied to eliminate motion artifacts from the anterior abdominal wall [3–8].

MRI protocols should be optimized and tailored to address a specific indication for uterine pathology.

Recommended sequences and their main indications for nonpregnant and pregnant patients are included in Table 21.1.

Table 21.1 MR technique in uterine pathology

Sequence	Anatomical Anomalies	Adenomyosis/other benign entities	Leiomyomas pre/ post UFE	Malignant diseases	Pregnancy[5]
NFST2WI (axial oblique, sagittal coronal)* Or 3DT2WI**	+	+	+	+	± (3D T2WI)
Axial FS/NFS T1WI or Dixon Technique [$]	+	+	±	±	–
2D T2WI—HASTE[%]	+	+	–	+	+
DWI (sagittal, axial) b: 0, 500, 800, 1000,1500 ADC maps[1]	–	±	±	+	+
GRE T1WI In- and out-of-phase	–	±	–	–	+
3D GRE-T1WI +C[2]	–	±	+	+	±
MRA[3]	–	–	+	–	–
(2D) TOF image[4]	–	–	±	–	±

±: optional sequences. *, nonfat saturated (NFS) fast spin-echo (FSE) sequences; **, volumetric acquisition; FS, fat saturated; $, to detect fat and hemorrhage. Thin-section acquisition, useful for characterization of uterus and adnexal processes; %, single-shot FSE (SSFSE)-HASTE with large FOV (36–40 cm), useful in characterizing and detecting genetic anomalies of the kidney and ureter and assessment of para-aortic lymphadenopathy and hydronephrosis, recommended for the evaluation of uterine peristalsis in adenomyosis/endometriosis and for MR urography in pregnant women. 1: Echo planar sequence. 2: Gradient echo (GRE) sequences pre-/post-gadolinium injection. 3: MR arteriography for fibroid/adenomyosis embolization. 4: TOF (time-of flight). Obtained from the renal veins to the symphysis pubis to screen for a venous clot. 5: Pregnant women should be scanned using 1.5 T magnets and large FOV sequences (40 cm)

21.2.2.1 T2-Weighted Imaging

T2-weighted images (T2WI) are the mainstay of pelvic MR imaging. They are best performed without fat suppression due to the inherent contrast between the signal intensity of the uterus and the surrounding fat. Three-dimensional (3D) T2-weighted volumetric sequence is optional and provides submillimeter section thickness along with multiplanar reformatting capability [3, 5–8].

In uterine malignant diseases, thin sections (3–4 mm) and a small FOV (20–24 cm) are recommended. Image acquisition must be optimized for T2WI angled perpendicularly to the endometrium or cervix (Fig. 21.1). Since the uterus can have a variable position and tilted within the pelvis, the realization of real perpendicular images can be difficult. To obtain axial oblique images, a "double oblique image" angled both in the sagittal and coronal planes create a "true oblique" that is exactly orthogonal to the endometrial or endocervical cavities [6, 7].

21.2.2.2 T1-Weighted Imaging

T1-weighted images (T1WI) sequences without and with fat suppression are advisable since they allow the characterization of hemorrhagic or fat content in a specific lesion. The two-dimensional (2D) or 3D Dixon technique, providing four simultaneous different T1WI contrast during the same acquisition and a stronger fat suppression in the female pelvis. It may be used as an alternative to standard T1WI sequence [5]. Axial/coronal T2WI or T1WI from renal hila to pubic bone (36–44 cm) is useful in characterizing and detecting genetic anomalies of kidney and ureter, and in the assessment of para-aortic lymphadenopathies, hydronephrosis, endometriosis extension, and bone metastases [4, 6–8].

21.2.2.3 Functional Imaging

Diffusion-Weighted Imaging

Diffusion-weighted imaging (DWI) is mandatory in malignant suspected uterine diseases because

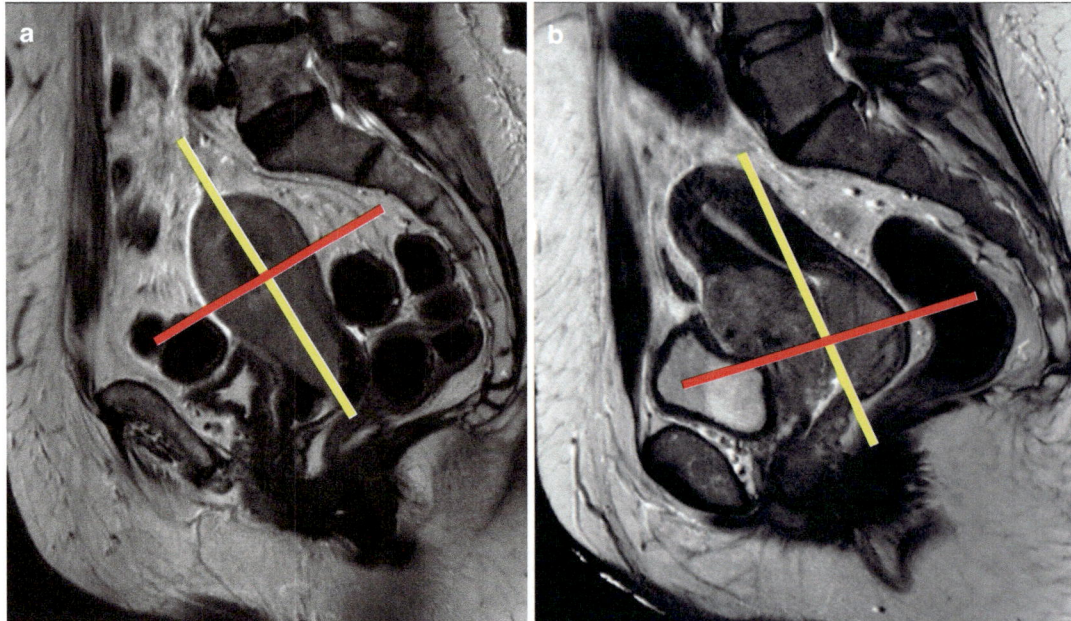

Fig. 21.1 Planning of MRI sequences in endometrial (**a**) and cervical (**b**) cancers. (*Yellow line*) indicates the coronal plane, (*red line*) indicates the axial-oblique plane

it improves the detection and characterization of uterine tumors and the visualization of small implants in peritoneal carcinomatosis. Moreover, the apparent diffusion coefficient (ADC) measurement may be useful for monitoring the therapeutic outcome after chemotherapy and/or radiation therapy [6–13]. DWI images should always be evaluated together with ADC maps and anatomic images to prevent pitfalls.

DWI protocol should include in at least one but preferably in two planes (axial oblique along the uterus with the same orientation as axial oblique T2WI and sagittal), with a minimum of two *b*-values (e.g., b:0, b: 1000). Acquiring T2WI and DWI on the same plane allows image fusion and optimizes anatomic correlation [6–9].

Dynamic Contrast Enhanced
Dynamic contrast-enhanced (DCE) images are obtained with a 3D gradient echo (GRE) T1WI and fat-saturated sequence after the administration of 0.1 mmol/kg of gadolinium (Gd) at a rate of 2 mL/s. Images are traditionally acquired before contrast injection, and then during multiple phases of enhancement in sagittal/axial planes

at 25 s, 1 min, and 2 min after injection. A delayed sequence is acquired on axial oblique 4 min after injection. DCE images should be obtained whenever additional characterization of incidentally seen disease is necessary, and in malignant diseases for adequate staging purposes [6, 7, 14–20].

21.2.3 Computed Tomography

CT provides poor soft tissue contrast of reproductive organs [1]. However, it is often used as a first-line imaging tool in the case of a chief complaint of abdominal acute pain in the emergency room, especially in elderly women, when a non-gynecological entity is suspected, or in the context of trauma injuries.

Regarding CT performance, previous fasting for 4–6 h is recommended. Patients are scanned in the supine position. It is important to administer both oral and intravenous contrast media, except in a context of emergency studies in which oral contrast is not considered essential. Oral contrast media may aid in distinguishing bowel loops from adenopathies and adnexal structures, and intravenous contrast media improves the delimitation of the uterus and adnexa [21].

Our 64-multidetector CT protocol includes the oral administration of 1000–1500 mL of positive iodinated contrast media (ICM) (sodium diatrizoate and meglumine diatrizoate—Gastrografin®) or negative contrast (1000–1500 mL of water) and the intravenous injection of 120 mL of nonionic ICM at a rate of 3 mL/s, obtaining images from the level of the diaphragm domes to the pubic symphysis, with a delay of 70–80 s postinjection (portal-venous phase). The scan parameters usually used are 120 kVp; 250 mAs; acquisition width, 1.25 mm; interval, 0.625 mm; pitch and velocity/rotational, 0.984:1; and iterative reconstructions for diminishing patient radiation dose.

21.2.4 Technique Protocols in Pregnant Women

US and MRI are the imaging techniques of choice because of the lack of ionizing radiation. The American College of Radiology (ACR) stated that MRI is a useful problem-solving tool in the evaluation of pelvic pain in pregnant women. This statement refers to machines in clinical use at 1.5 T or less. Contrast injection should only be administered to a pregnant patient "if the potential benefit justifies the potential risk to the fetus and using the smallest dose of the most stable gadolinium agent" [22–29].

MR study should be focused to solve a particular clinical question and to ensure that the diagnostic information is obtained with the minimum of sequences and/or energy dissipation (Table 21.1). If a patient is uncomfortable or feels faint lying supine within the MR gantry (especially in the third trimester), imaging with the patient in the lateral decubitus position is appropriate (decreasing the pressure on the inferior vena cava) [1, 2, 22, 26–29].

Regarding CT, given its radiation issues, it can only be justified in pregnant women when the study is overwhelmingly in the best health interest of the mother. We must take into account the risk/benefit ratio and always keeping radiation

doses according to the ALARA (as low as reasonably achievable) principle. On the other hand, CT is the primary tool to use when there is a life-threatening situation, and a rapid diagnosis is required (e.g., hypovolemia due to blunt or penetrating trauma or severe sepsis) [1, 2, 22, 26–30].

Pregnant patients should be informed about contrast (Gd and ICM) and MR and CT imaging safety issues, and a written informed consent is also advisable, as recommended in the European Society of Urogenital Radiology (ESUR) and ACR contrast media guidelines. Neonatal screening for hypothyroidism should follow for all neonates whose mothers received ICM during pregnancy [24, 25].

21.3 Pain Related to Uterine Disease

21.3.1 Menstrual-Related Pain (Dysmenorrhea)

Dysmenorrhea is defined as a cramping pain in the lower abdomen occurring just before or during menstruation. It is the first cause of gynecological morbidity in women of childbearing age and can be severe and disabling, thus being a common cause of absenteeism [31].

Dysmenorrhea can be classified into two categories: primary and secondary.

21.3.1.1 Primary or Idiopathic Dysmenorrhea

Primary dysmenorrhea is defined as menstrual pain without an underlying identifiable gynecological pathology. Its initial onset typically occurs during adolescence, once the ovulation cycles have been established. Women with primary dysmenorrhea show increased production of endometrial prostaglandins, which, in turn, results in increased myometrial contractility and causes uterine ischemia and pain [31, 32].

The typical pain begins a few hours before or at the time of onset of the menstruation, peaks with maximum blood flow, and lasts up to 2–3 days. It mainly involves the pelvis but can spread to the lumbar area or the thighs, being acute and intermittent as cramps. It may be associated with nausea and vomiting, diarrhea, fatigue, mild headache, dizziness, and even fever or syncope [31, 32].

The diagnosis is based on the patient's clinical history and standard physical examination findings. A gynecological examination is not usually necessary in patients with typical symptoms, although some authors recommend examining the external genitalia to rule out the existence of hymen anomalies [31, 32].

Nonsteroidal anti-inflammatory drugs alone or combined with oral contraceptives are the mainstay of treatment. If the patient does not respond to these measures, secondary causes of dysmenorrhea must be considered. In this case, the use of diagnostic imaging techniques is recommended, with US being the first choice followed by an MRI, if necessary, to rule out possible causes of secondary menstrual pain [31, 32].

21.3.1.2 Secondary Dysmenorrhea

Secondary dysmenorrhea is defined as menstrual pain associated with underlying gynecological conditions.

Anatomical Abnormalities

Müllerian duct anomalies (MDAs) are a group of congenital uterine disorders resulting from malformations occurring during the embryologic development of the Müllerian ducts. Fusion of the Müllerian ducts normally occurs between the 6th and 11th weeks of gestation to form the uterus, fallopian tubes, cervix, and the proximal two-thirds of the vagina [4, 33].

The prevalence of MDAs in the general population ranges between 4 and 7%. However, in a population of women with recurrent pregnancy loss, this incidence increases to as much as 18% [33].

Concomitant renal abnormalities are reported in 29% of cases of MDA (up to 40% in cases of unicornuate uterus). The spectrum of renal abnormalities includes agenesis, horseshoe kidney, renal dysplasia, ectopic kidney, and duplicated collecting systems [4].

Over the last few decades, several classification systems have been proposed to describe MDAs. Buttram and Gibbons [34] proposed an MDA classification in 1979, which was subsequently modified by the American Society of Reproductive Medicine (ASRM) in 1988 (formerly the American Fertility Society) [35]. Other classifications include the vagina, cervix, uterus, adnexa, and associated malformations (VCUAM) classification [36] and, most recently, The European Society of Human Reproduction and Embryology (ESHRE)/European Society for Gynecologic Endoscopy (ESGE) classification, updated in 2013 [37]. The most widely accepted classification system is the ASRM classification described in Table 21.2.

A septate uterus (ASRM class V) is the most common type of uterine developmental abnormality, accounting for 55% of cases [4]. It may be suspected in patients with a history of midtrimester pregnancy loss.

MDAs are diagnosed while investigating fertility issues, and some can present with pelvic pain (malformations with some type of obstructive component).

Imaging studies play an essential role in the diagnosis and treatment planning of MDAs. Given the high prevalence of associated renal abnormalities, it is important to take cross-section images of the kidneys (US or MRI). The time of onset of symptoms often dictates the initial imaging modality of choice (e.g., primary amenorrhea, pelvic pain, or infertility).

Hysterosalpingography (HSG) can be used to examine the endometrial cavity and can reliably establish tubal patency. Given that the myometrium and external uterine contour are not viewed with this technique, HSG is of limited use in the evaluation of MDAs. Contrarily, (3D) US imaging (transabdominal or endovaginal) does allow for an accurate evaluation of MDAs. Following its acquisition, the data set can be manipulated to generate 3D images of the uterus from virtually any angle. Coronal images reveal essential details of the endometrial cavity and serosal surface of the uterus. MDAs are best evaluated during the secretory phase of the menstrual cycle, when viewing of the endometrial echo complex thickness is optimal [4, 33]. In expert hands, this technique yields a sensitivity of 98.3% and a specificity of 99.4% in detecting MDAs [38].

Table 21.2 The ASRM classification of MDA (adapted from Ref. [35], with permission)

Class I Hypoplasia/agenesis				
(a) Vaginal	(b) Cervical	(c) Fundal	(d) Tubal	(e) Combined

Class II unicornuate				Class III didelphus
(a) Communicating	(b) Noncommunicating	(c) No cavity	(d) No horn	

Class IV bicornuate		Class V septate		Class VI arcuate
(a) Complete	(b) Partial	(a) Complete	(d) Partial	

Class VII DES drug related				

MRI is considered the ideal imaging modality for detecting MDAs, as it provides clear anatomic detail of both the internal uterine cavity and the external contour. T2WI is best performed without fat suppression due to the inherent contrast between the signal intensity of the uterus and the surrounding fat. On the other hand, T1WI can be useful to detect hyperintense blood products in cases of hematocolpos or endometriosis (Table 21.1) [4, 33].

The following obstructive anomalies are the most frequent type of malformation presenting with pelvic pain in premenarchal young women:

Mayer-Rokitansky-Kuster-Hauser Syndrome (ASRM class I): a malformation characterized by hypoplasia of the uterus and upper two-thirds of the vagina. The rudimentary uterus may contain a normal functional endometrium. Its main presenting symptoms are amenorrhea, hematometra, or cyclic pelvic pain in postpubertal patients, secondary to the accumulation of hemorrhagic products within the rudimentary uterus [4, 33, 39].

Unicornuate Uterus (ASRM class II): an abnormality resulting from the failure of one of the Müllerian ducts to elongate, while the other duct develops in a normal fashion. It accounts for approximately 20% of all MDAs. A single uterine horn can be observed in up to 35% of patients. More often, a small rudimentary horn is seen arising from the primary single horn in 65% of cases. This rudimentary horn may contain endometrium in 50% of patients and communicate with the dominant horn in up to 33% of cases. Conversely, there is no communication between the rudimentary and primary horns in 66% of cases. The presence of endometrial tissue in a noncommunicating rudimentary horn may manifest clinically with pelvic pain, owing to the increased prevalence of endometriosis secondary to the retrograde flow of menses through the obstructed horn. Furthermore, the presence of endometrium in a rudimentary horn carries an increased risk of miscarriage, ectopic pregnancy, preterm labor, and uterine rupture during pregnancy [4, 33].

A unicornuate uterus is diagnosed by the presence of a solitary, deviated, and often atrophic horn. The solitary horn is typically fusiform or banana-shaped; the endometrium is narrow and described as bullet-shaped, tapering toward the apex. MR imaging is the most sensitive imaging modality for detecting a rudimentary horn. Additionally, when the rudimentary horn contains endometrium, the zonal anatomy generally shows up well on T2WI.

Herlyn-Werner-Wunderlich Syndrome (variant of ASRM class III): a very rare congenital malformation of the urogenital tract characterized by a triad of didelphys uterus, obstructed hemivagina, and ipsilateral renal anomalies. After menarche, menstrual blood accumulates gradually within the vagina (hematocolpos), uterus (hematometra), and the ipsilateral fallopian tube (hematosalpinx). Instillation of an endovaginal gel before conducting an MRI scan better reveals the existence of a duplicated vagina. The presence of a unilateral hemivaginal septum obstructing one of the uterine horns will cause that horn to be markedly distended due to the accumulation of hemorrhagic products, showing a hyperintense signal on T1WI (Fig. 21.2) [4, 33, 40].

Imperforate Hymen: a common associated obstructive disorder of the female reproductive system, with a reported incidence of 0.014–0.024%. Its most common symptoms are the presence of a bulging bluish-black membrane in the vulva, cyclic abdominal pain, a pelvic mass, and primary amenorrhea [41].

Adenomyosis

Adenomyosis is a common benign gynecological disease characterized by the presence of ectopic endometrial glands and stroma within the myometrium, as well as hypertrophy and hyperplasia of the myometrial smooth muscle [42, 43]. It usually affects multiparous, premenopausal women over the age of 30, being rare and with no typical characteristics in adolescents [42].

Up to one-third of patients with adenomyosis are asymptomatic. Clinical symptoms include menorrhagia (50%), dysmenorrhea (30%), metrorrhagia (20%), and, occasionally, dyspareunia. These symptoms are non-specific being also common in myomatous uterus, that can coexist with adenomyosis in up to 50% of cases or in endometriosis (defined by the presence of ectopic endometrium outside the uterus). Both endometriosis and adenomyosis coexist in up to 11% of cases. For these reasons, clinical diagnosis is often difficult [21, 42–45].

Transvaginal US and MRI findings in this entity include an enlarged, globular uterus with small cystic areas corresponding to diffuse dilated endometrial glands.

MR is the best imaging tool for diagnosing adenomyosis (sensitivity of 70–86%, specificity of 86–93%, and mean accuracy of 87.5%). MRI findings may be stratified into direct and indirect signs [42–44]:

Direct signs are related to the presence of endometrial glands within the myometrium:

- *Submucosal microcysts* (size, 2–7 mm) are detected in 50% of cases as hypointense foci on T1WI and a hyperintense signal on T2WI and, if they contain hemorrhagic products, on T1WI.
- *Adenomyoma* is a solid, mass-like, localized form of adenomyosis. Differentiating it from leiomyoma may be challenging; however, adenomyomas usually show a hypointense signal on T2WI but may contain disperse foci of high intensity on T1WI (Fig. 21.3). Unlike leiomyomas, adenomyomas have ill-defined margins; minimal mass effect on the endometrium as

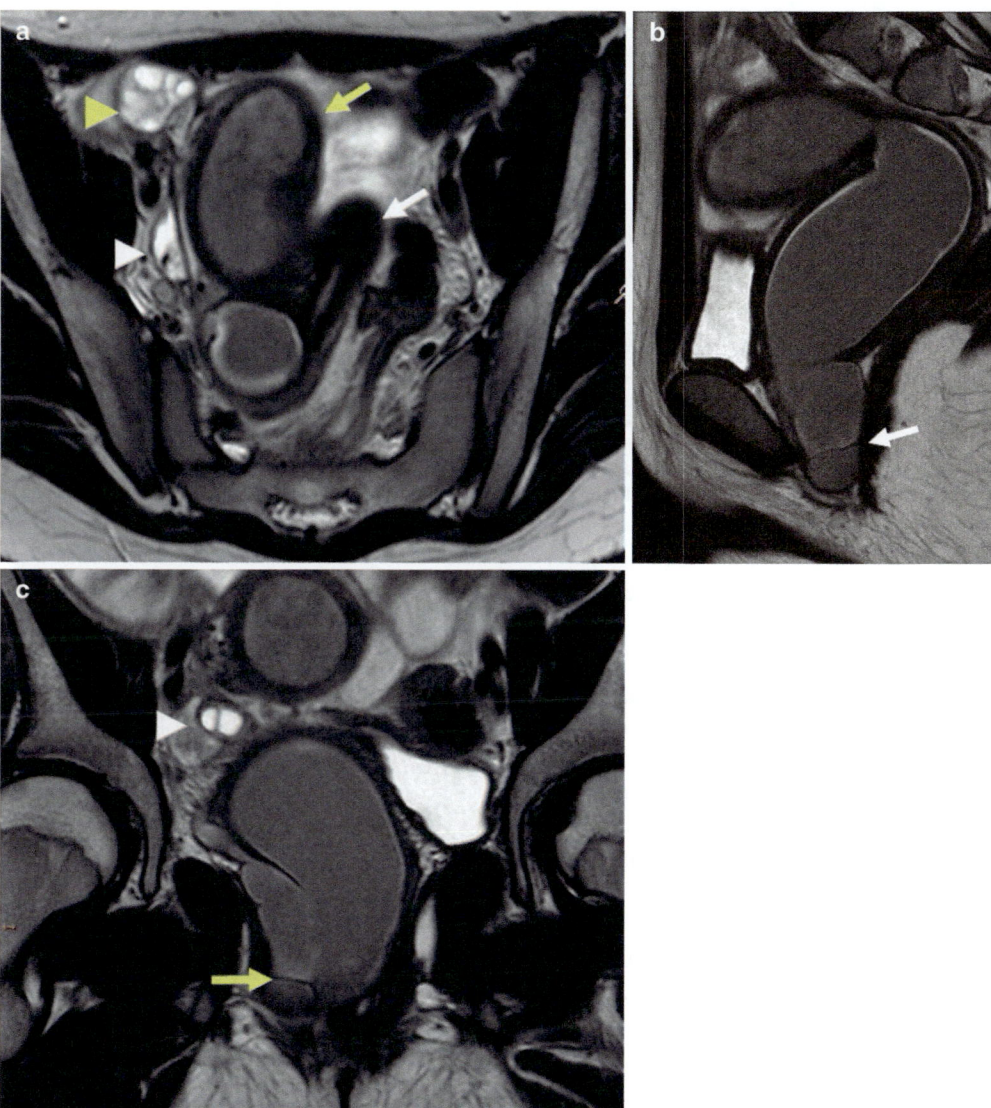

Fig. 21.2 12 year-old girl with chronic pelvic pain that worsened in the previous month. (**a**) MR (Axial oblique T2WI): right dysplastic and ectopic kidney (*yellow arrowhead*), right ovary (*white arrowhead*) and two uterine cavities (*arrows*), one of them distended by hypointense fluid content (hyperintense in T1WI- not shown), with a peripheral hyperintense rim, suggesting accumulation of hemorrhagic products (*yellow arrow*). (**b**) Sagittal T2WI: distended uterine and vaginal cavities with a thin obstructing hypointense band (white arrow). (**c**) Coronal T2WI: dilated right ureter leading to right hemivagina. A thin hypointense band obstructing the ureter is shown (*arrow*), right ovary (*arrowhead*). Diagnosis: **Herlyn-Werner-Wunderlich Syndrome:** Uterus didelphys + pelvic multi-cystic dysplastic right kidney and ectopic ureter + septated right hemivagina (associated hematometra and hematocolpos). Left hemivagina was collapsed at gynecological examination

compared to a leiomyoma of similar size; an elliptical, rather than round shape; may display linear striations radiating from the endometrium; and their margins do not contain dilated vessels [42, 43]. Identifying this entity is important for patient management, as myomectomy may be curative for leiomyomas but ineffective for adenomyomas.

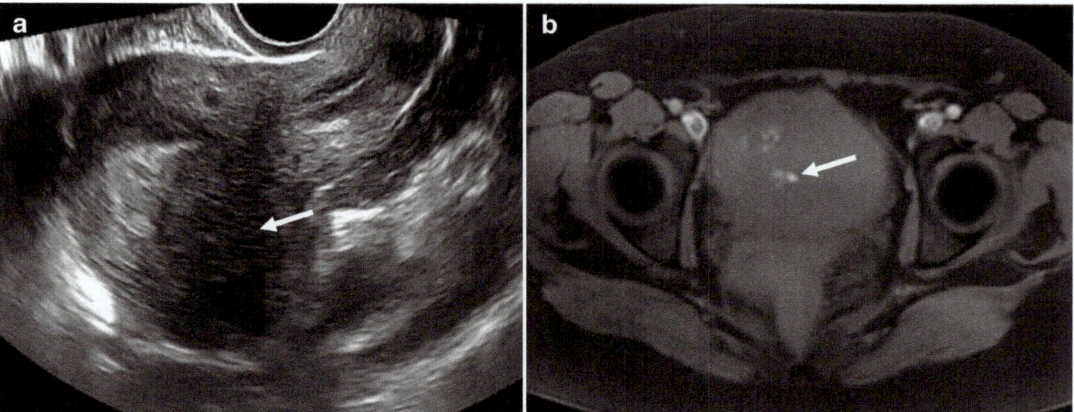

Fig. 21.3 40-year-old woman with pelvic complaints. (**a**) Transvaginal US: a globular uterus is shown with an ill-defined hypoechoic area in the posterior fundus (*arrow*), which contain small cystic areas. (**b**) Fat Sat T1WI: these cystic areas are hyperintense because of the blood content (*arrow*)

Indirect signs are the result of reactive changes in the myometrium:

- *Thickening of the junctional zone (JZ) -12 mm*; either focal or diffuse, resulting from smooth muscle hypertrophy, is caused by the presence of ectopic endometrial glands within the myometrium. This sign is highly sensitive, specific, and accurate in diagnosing adenomyosis (63%, 96%, and 85%, respectively) [46].
- *The JZ differential sign* is a difference >5 mm between the maximal and minimal thickness of the anterior and posterior uterine JZ. This sign is more reliable than a JZ thickness >12 mm (Fig. 21.4) [47].

Furthermore, there are two unusual forms of adenomyosis:

- *Cystic adenomyoma* is a single nodular myometrial lesion with a central cavity filled with blood products due to profuse menstrual bleeding in the ectopic endometrium. It appears with high-intensity signal on T1WI and with low intensity signal on T2WI. Cystic adenomyoma is more common in adolescents and young women and usually causes intense dysmenorrhea.
- *Swiss cheese appearance* is characterized by large cysts, which represents dilated endometrial glands and nodules within the myometrium, associated to other more typical signs such as thickening and poor definition of the JZ [42].

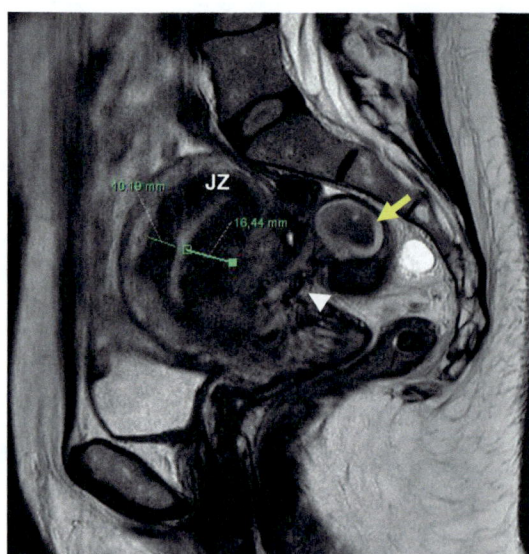

Fig. 21.4 Sagittal T2 WI. Endometriosis and adenomyosis: thickening of the junctional zone (JZ) and JZ differential sign (>5 mm thicker the posterior JZ). Deep fibrotic endometriosis (*arrowhead*) and ovarian endometriosis (yellow *arrow*)

Benign Uterine Neoplasms: Leiomyomas

Leiomyomas, the most common type of uterine neoplasm in women of childbearing age, may cause menstrual disorders such as menorrhagia and, consequently, dysmenorrhea, especially in cases of severe hypermenorrhea associated with passing of large blood clots.

The exact pathophysiological mechanism of this entity is unknown; however, it is probably related to an increased endometrial surface area associated with elongation and even inflammation and/or ulceration of the endometrium overlying the leiomyomas; increased uterine vascularity, probably secondary to dysregulation of the leiomyoma growth factors, which impacts vascular function and angiogenesis; interference of intramural leiomyomas with the normal symmetric uterine contractions; and venous myometrial and endometrial congestion resulting from venous compression caused by the leiomyoma [48–50].

In the following section, we will describe the characteristic imaging findings and other aspects of leiomyomas.

21.3.2 Pain Unrelated to the Menstrual Cycle

21.3.2.1 Pelvic Infection

Pelvic infection may be divided into two important categories according to the source of the infection: gynecological and non-gynecological causes (Table 21.3).

Pelvic Inflammatory Disease

Pelvic inflammatory disease (PID) is typically an infection of the upper genital tract resulting from spreading of a vaginal infection to the cervix, fallopian tubes, ovaries, and, finally, to the peritoneal cavity. Hematogenous spread of an infection originating in adjacent organs is a less frequent cause of PID [51].

PID is considered a sexually transmitted disease caused by microorganisms such as *Chlamydia trachomatis*, *Neisseria gonorrhoeae*, *Mycoplasma genitalium*, and gram-negative bacteria. Polymicrobial infections account for 30–40% of reported cases of PID. Infections by *Mycobacterium tuberculosis* and *Actinomyces sp.* are less common. Risk factors for this condition include a history of multiple sexual partners, young age, a prior uterine procedure, intrauterine devices, vaginal douching, and a low socioeconomic status [51, 52].

The most frequent form of PID is inflammation of the fallopian tube, also known as salpingitis. Involvement of the uterine cervix (cervicitis) or endometrium (endometritis) usually goes

Table 21.3 Causes of pelvic infections

Gynecological causes	Non-Gynecological causes
Pelvic inflammatory disease (PID)	*Intestinal:* appendicitis, diverticulitis, Crohn
Cervicitis	
Salpingitis	
Tubo-ovarian abscess	
Peritonitis (Fitz-Hugh-Curtis Syndrome)	
Puerperal infections	Fistulae (intestinal, urinary, postradiotherapy)
Cesarean section	
Vaginal delivery	
Postoperative gynecological surgery	*Chronic infections*
Pelvic abscess	Tuberculosis
Post leiomyomas embolization infection	Actinomycosis
Fistulae	
Abortion-associated infections	
Endometritis	
Incomplete septic abortion	

unnoticed and takes place at the beginning of the infection.

Regarding its clinical presentation, up to 60% of women are asymptomatic, 36% experience moderate symptoms, and 4% have severe symptoms, with the most common symptoms being pelvic pain, fever, vaginal discharge, and dyspareunia with coexisting leukocytosis [51, 53].

The diagnosis of PID is based on the patient's clinical history, physical examination, and US findings. Given the presence of non-specific symptoms, CT is usually the first imaging modality of choice for its assessment. It is very useful in assessing the extent of peritoneal disease, detecting disease complications, and excluding other potential differential diagnoses. MRI is also useful in delimiting the uterine and adnexal structures and differentiating PID from other pathologic processes (e.g., diverticulitis or appendicitis) (Fig. 21.5).

PID is generally treated conservatively with a short course of oral antibiotic therapy. Patients with complicated PID must usually be hospitalized and treated with intravenous antibiotics, as well as with percutaneous or surgical drainage of any pelvic abscess, if present (Fig. 21.6).

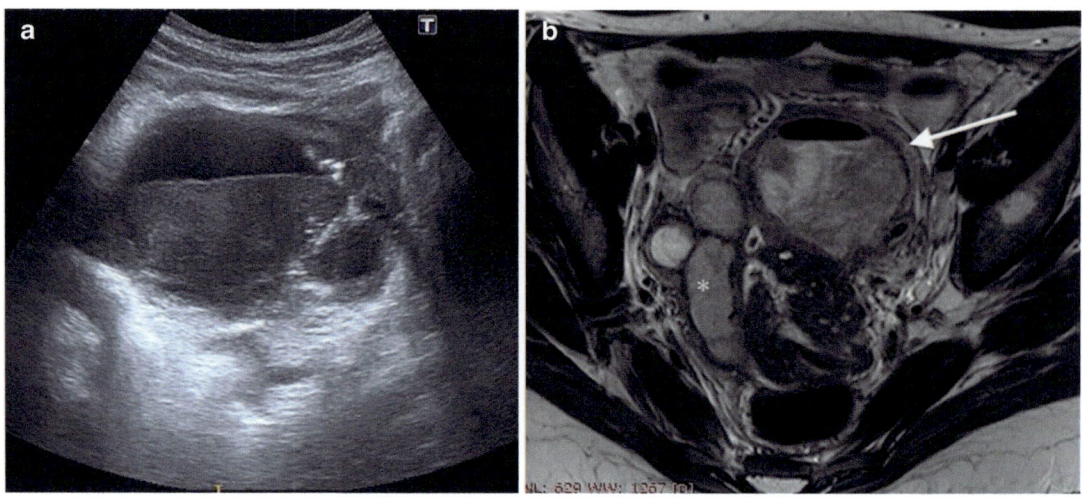

Fig. 21.5 Woman with intense pelvic pain, fever, and leukocytosis. (**a**) Abdominal ultrasound of the pelvic region: large collection in the left adnexal region with fluid-fluid level. (**b**) MRI- axial T2WI: collection with heterogeneous content and hydro-aerial level (*arrow*), in addition, a right hydrosalpinx (*) is identified

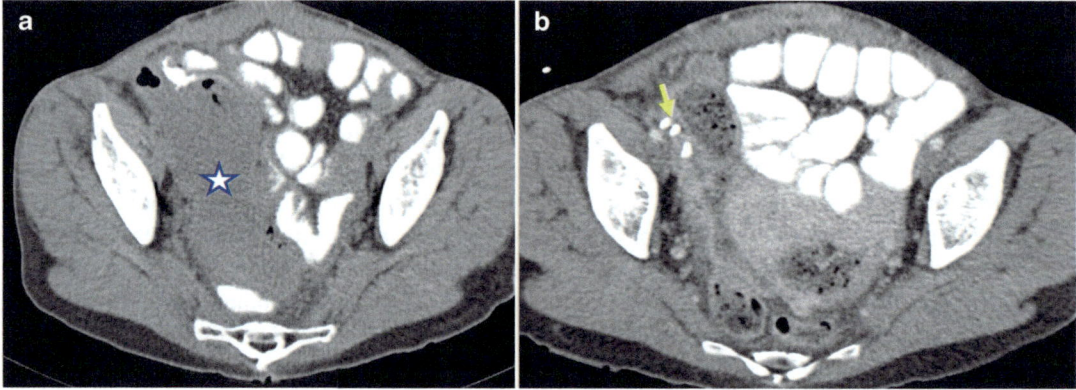

Fig. 21.6 Axial reformatted CT. Complicated PID with pelvic abscess (*) before (**a**) and after drainage (**b**), drainage catheter (*arrow*)

Approximately 25% of women with a single episode of PID will experience sequelae, including ectopic pregnancy, infertility, or chronic pelvic pain.

Cervicitis

Cervicitis is an inflammation of the uterine cervix. It may be acute (frequently caused by infection) or chronic (pelvic radiation, chemical irritation, etc.).

Symptoms of acute cervicitis are a jelly-like, yellow or turbid vaginal discharge, bleeding with intercourse, and a feeling of pelvic pressure or discomfort.

In patients with acute cervicitis, US often shows a cervical mucosa and stroma with a diffusely heterogeneous echotexture. Given that the key finding of this condition is a markedly increased vascularity, the conduct of a color Doppler US is recommended. US, CT, and MR imaging may also reveal an enlarged uterine cervix, abnormal contrast enhancing or hyperemic endocervical canal, and parametrial fat stranding [54, 55].

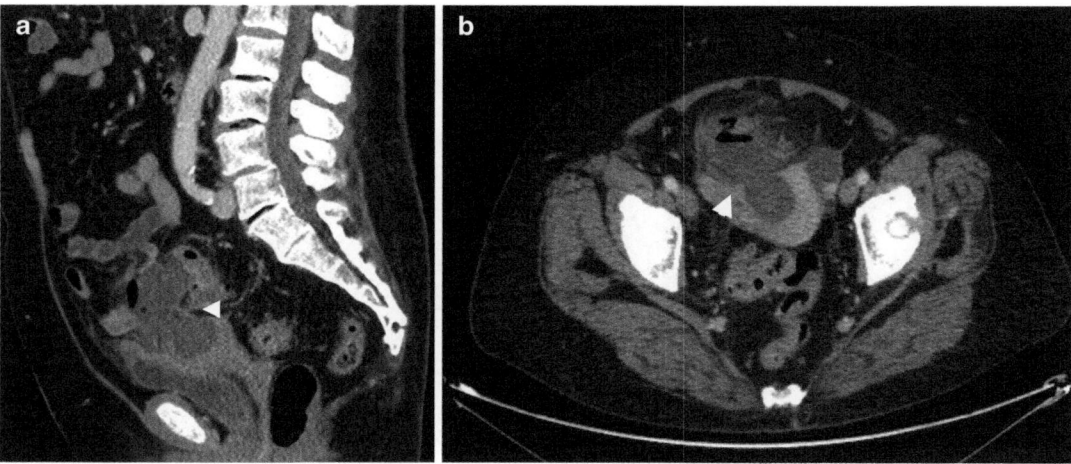

Fig. 21.7 Sagittal and axial reformatted CT image (portal phase) (**a, b**) Sigmoid diverticulitis perforated to the uterine fundus (*arrowhead*)

Endometritis

Endometritis is an inflammatory condition of the uterine lining. It is often seen during pregnancy or the postpartum period. In non-obstetric women, PID and invasive gynecological procedures are the most frequent causes of acute endometritis.

US, CT, or MR imaging findings of endometritis include an enlarged uterus, accumulation of fluid within the endometrial cavity, and an abnormal endometrium secondary to increased vascularity. Loss of the clear separation of the uterus from the adnexal and parametrial fat can also be observed [51].

Pyometra

Pyometra is a form of infectious endometritis characterized by the accumulation of pus within the uterine cavity, usually secondary to the blockage or stenosis of the cervix. It has an incidence of 0.01–0.5% among gynecological infections and mainly affects postmenopausal women, with a prevalence as high as 13.6% in this group. Fifty percent of patients are asymptomatic. Symptomatic patients usually complain of pelvic pain, fever, and a purulent vaginal discharge. Imaging findings of this condition include accumulation of a complex fluid within the uterine cavity, inflammatory changes in the surrounding parametrial fat, and the

presence of free fluid in the posterior cul-de-sac. Gas bubbles or an air-fluid level may also be seen within the endometrial canal [51, 52].

Secondary Uterine Infection

Although the uterus provides a protective barrier against an inflammatory or malignant metastatic disease, a colouterine fistula may develop due to the spontaneous rupture of a gravid uterus, obstetric trauma such as curettage, uterine or sigmoid colon cancer, or radiation therapy. Furthermore, inflammatory processes such as a periappendiceal abscess or diverticulitis may also cause a colouterine fistula. Inflammatory adhesion of the colon and uterus can occur during an episode of diverticulitis, resulting in necrosis and the subsequent formation of a fistula (Fig. 21.7) [56].

Actinomycosis

Actinomycosis is a chronic disease caused by *Actinomyces israelii*. Female genital involvement has been associated with IUDs. The disease is characterized by disemination through the soft tissue planes and the formation of granulation tissue and fibrosis (Fig. 21.8). The ability to release proteolytic enzymes explains its invasive nature, resulting in the formation of abscesses, fistulas, and sinus tracts. Infection by *A. israelii* involves

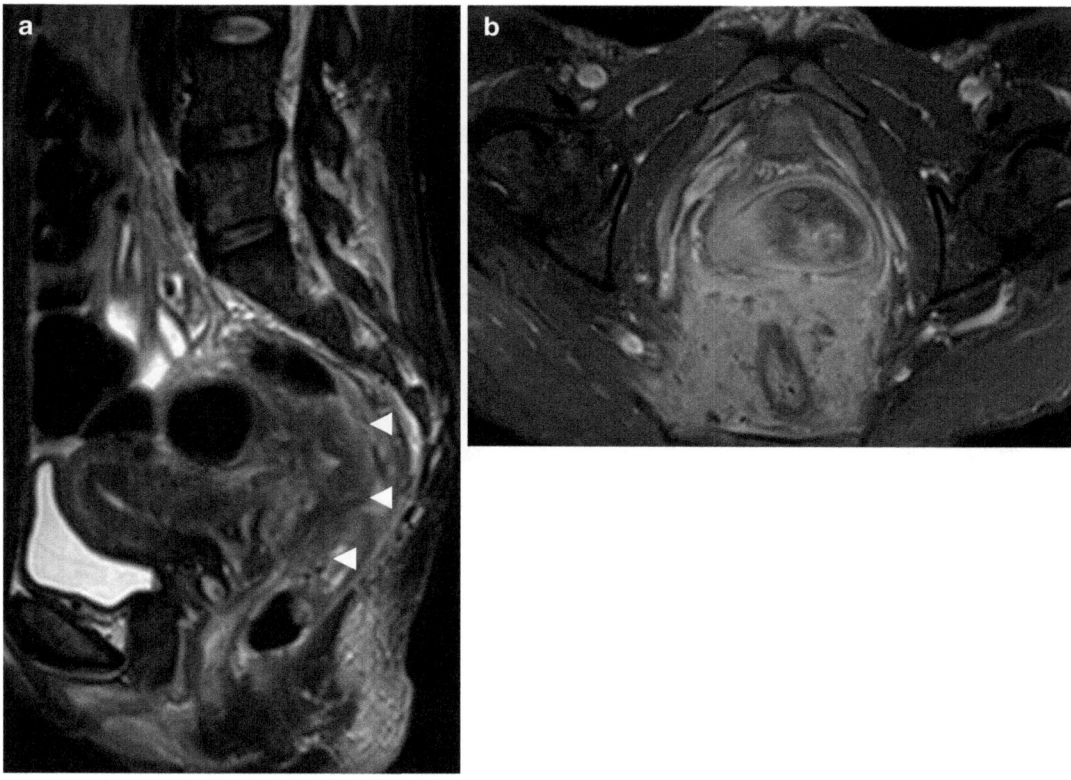

Fig. 21.8 Pelvic actinomycosis. (**a**) T2WI sagittal: infiltrative mass in T2WI that extends through rectouterine and rectovaginal spaces, surrounds the rectum and perirectal space (*arrowheads*). (**b**) Axial Fat Sat T1WI +Gd: a homogeneous and retarded uptake is shown due to the fibrotic characteristics of the mass. There were no abscesses in this case

both fallopian tubes in 50% of cases; however, the infection can spread and form fistulas along the pelvic and abdominal structures. CT imaging in this disease demonstrates enhancement of the solid components of the adnexal and soft tissue masses, along with small rim-enhancing hypoattenuating foci representing small abscesses. In MRI, the solid components of the adnexal mass show up as hypointense foci on T2WI and areas of contrast enhancement after intravenous administration of a Gd-based contrast material, whereas the small abscesses are viewed as hyperintense areas with peripheral rim enhancement [57].

21.3.2.2 Uterine Neoplasms

Benign Uterine Neoplasms: Leiomyomas

Uterine leiomyomas, also known as myomas or fibroids, are benign monoclonal smooth muscle tumors of myometrial origin. They are the most common pelvic masses in women of childbearing age, affecting up to 80% of women throughout their lifetime [1, 44, 48, 50, 58].

Leiomyomas are hormone-dependent tumors, with estrogen being their main growth factor. They tend to grow during pregnancy and with the intake of oral hormonal contraceptives and regress after the menopause [1, 48, 58, 59].

FIGO classified uterine leiomyomas based on their location (i.e., submucosal, intramural, subserosal, and hybrid) (Table 21.4). This classification is clinically significant, since both their symptoms and treatment depend on the leiomyoma subtype [44, 48, 50, 60].

Leiomyomas are usually asymptomatic but between 20 and 50% can cause abnormal uterine bleeding (both cyclic and noncyclic) as the most common symptom. Other manifestations include acute or chronic pelvic pain, symptoms resulting

Table 21.4 FIGO Leiomyomas sub-classification system

Type	Subtype	Location	Scheme
SM (Submucosal)	0	Pedunculated intracavitary	
	1	Submucosal and <50% intramural	
	2	Submucosal and ≥50% intramural	
O (Others: intramural and subserosal)	3	100% intramural and contact endometrium	
	4	100% intramural and don't contact endometrium	
	5	Subserosal and ≥50% intramural	
	6	Subserosal and <50% intramural	
	7	Pedunculated subserosal	
Hibrid leiomyomas (Impact both endometrium and serosa)	Two numbers separated by a hyphen (First number refers to the relationship with the endometrium and the second one to the relationship with the serosa)	Combination types	
	8	Others (parasitic, cervical…)	

from the pressure caused on adjacent organs, a palpable abdominal mass, and reproductive or sexual dysfunction. These symptoms have a significant negative impact on women's quality of life [44, 48–50, 58]. Pain is usually the result of degeneration, but it may also occur secondary to the presence of a mass effect, severe hemorrhage, torsion and necrosis of a pedunculated leiomyoma, or prolapse of a pedunculated submucosal leiomyoma [1, 21, 48].

US is the first-line imaging modality used to evaluate leiomyomas; however, MRI is the most accurate technique at depicting the number and location of the lesions, as well as the internal tissue characteristics, with sensitivity, specificity, and positive predictive values of 94%, 68.7%, and 95.7%, respectively. CT is rarely used to evaluate leiomyomas but may be performed to rule out complications (e.g., torsion of a pediculated leiomyoma or infection...) [1, 21, 44, 48, 50].

Degeneration

As leiomyomas increase in size, they may outgrow their blood supply, resulting in ischemia and consequently hyaline, cystic, myxoid, or red degeneration. Red degeneration mainly occurs during pregnancy, and it is also associated with the use of oral contraceptives. It is caused by thrombosis and occlusion of the venous outflow, which leads to venous congestion, significant tumor growth, and acute hemorrhagic infarction. Patients with degenerated leiomyomas may present with abdominal pain, low-grade fever, leukocytosis, and physical examination findings that mimic other gynecological or non-gynecological acute pelvic processes, such as acute appendicitis, adnexal torsion, or PID [1, 44, 48, 58, 59, 61].

The appearance of leiomyomas varies depending on the degree and type of degeneration. The characteristic findings of degenerating leiomyomas on all the different imaging modalities are their heterogeneity, resulting from cystic, hemorrhagic, or necrotic changes, with poorly or non-enhancing areas following the administration of a contrast agent [1, 44].

On US, non-degenerated leiomyomas appear as well-defined solid masses arising within or attached to the myometrium, with a hypoechoic and discreetly heterogeneous echotexture and,

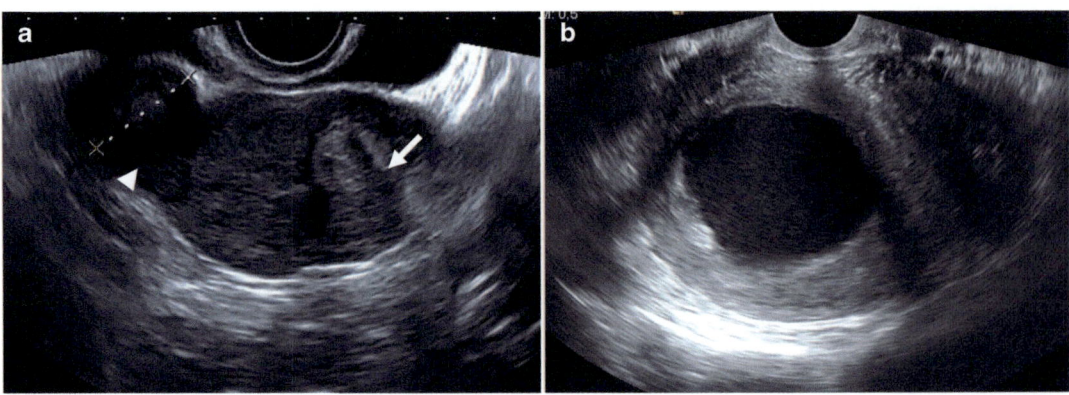

Fig. 21.9 Intramural (*arrow*) and right subserous (*arrowhead*) non-degenerated leiomyomas (**a**) and cystic (degenerated) leiomyoma (**b**) on transvaginal ultrasound

occasionally, acoustic reinforcement or an acoustic shadow. The degeneration leads to the formation of cystic areas (Fig. 21.9). Red degeneration shows a decreased or absent flow in Doppler studies [59, 61].

The most common CT findings are uterine enlargement with associated focal masses that may deform the uterine contour or endometrial cavity. Usually, non-degenerated leiomyomas show homogeneous density and post-contrast enhancement similar to that of the myometrium. In contrast, degenerated leiomyomas may have a cystic appearance, with hypodense areas and poor or absent enhancement, that can be difficult to differentiate from cystic ovarian masses. If one leiomyoma becomes infected (pyomyoma), gas bubbles may be seen within it. Leiomyoma calcification is also a frequent CT finding [21, 44, 58, 61, 62].

On MRI, non-degenerated leiomyomas usually appear as well-defined masses showing homogeneous hypointensity on T2WI and isointensity on T1WI as compared to the myometrium and show the blackout effect in DWI. Post-contrast enhancement is variable depending on the size of the myomas. Cellular leiomyomas are a variant characterized by a matrix with little or no collagen that can show hyperintense signal on T2WI, restricted diffusion in DWI, and they enhance homogeneously on post-contrast images (Fig. 21.10) [1, 15, 44, 48].

An early finding of degeneration in MRI is heterogeneous hyperintensity on T2WI due to the presence of an interstitial edema. Areas of hyaline degeneration or calcification may show up with a very hypointense signal or with a mixed pattern of hyper- and hypointense signal on T2WI, with heterogeneous post-contrast enhancement. Cystic degeneration appears as areas with a hyperintense signal on T2WI, without post-contrast enhancement. Myxoid degeneration is characterized by a very hyperintense signal on T2WI and minimal contrast enhancement. Imaging findings indicating red degeneration may depend on the time of evolution of the hemorrhagic infarction and usually appear as diffuse or peripheral hyperintensity on T1WI, related to either T1 shortening of methemoglobin or the protein content of blood; variable signal intensity on T2WI, with or without a rim of hypointense signal due to the presence of abundant intracellular methemoglobin in the obstructed vessels; and lack of enhancement following the administration of contrast media (Fig. 21.11). Leiomyomas with fatty degeneration are hyperintense on T1WI and hypointense in fat-suppressed T1WI [1, 44, 48, 59, 61].

Torsion of a Subserosal Pedunculated Leiomyoma

This is a rare complication of subserosal pedunculated leiomyomas. The twisted leiomyoma shows up on US as a pelvic mass without vascular flow and on CT or MR, as a pelvic mass without contrast enhancement, attached to the normally-enhanced uterus. Usually, the twisted pedicle is hard to identify. Its differential diagnoses include ovarian torsion, ovarian tumor, leiomyoma with massive necrotic infarction, or uterine torsion (Fig. 21.12) [61].

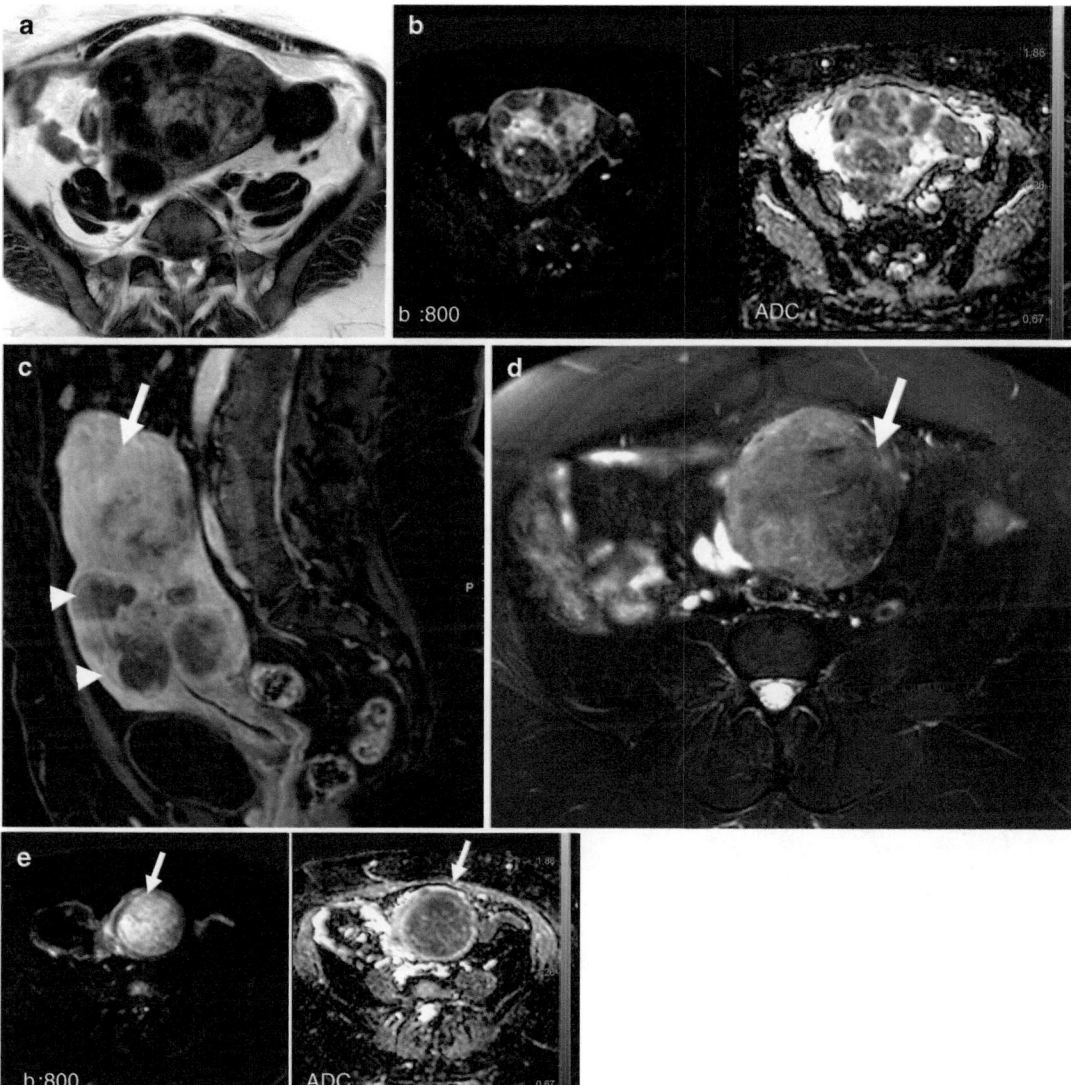

Fig. 21.10 Multiple leiomyomas. (**a**) Axial T2 WI, (**b**) DWI: multiple hypointense leiomyomas with the blackout effect (decrease in signal intensity in the DW image). After contrast injection (**c**), the leiomyomas are hypovascular (*arrowheads*) except one located at the top of the uterus that shows a homogeneous enhancement (*arrow*), is slightly hyperintense in T2WI (**d**), and shows diffusion restriction (arrow) on DWI (**e**) corresponding to a cellular leiomyoma

Prolapse of a Pedunculated Submucosal Leiomyoma

This entity is defined as protrusion of large pedunculated submucosal leiomyomas into the cervix or even into the vagina and perineum, causing vaginal bleeding and pain secondary to the dilation of the cervical canal.

Imaging techniques can be helpful in diagnosing the source of the mass, especially MRI, which allows for identifying the stalk of the mass and its myometrial attachment on sagittal T2WI. The stalk extends from the cervical or vaginal mass, up into the endometrial cavity, and usually has multiple linear structures running through it. The appearance of the stalk and prolapsed leiomyoma has been described as the "*broccoli sign*." Differential diagnosis with a prolapsed endometrial polyp may be difficult, but in MRI, polyps typically show a hyperintense and heterogeneous signal on T2WI,

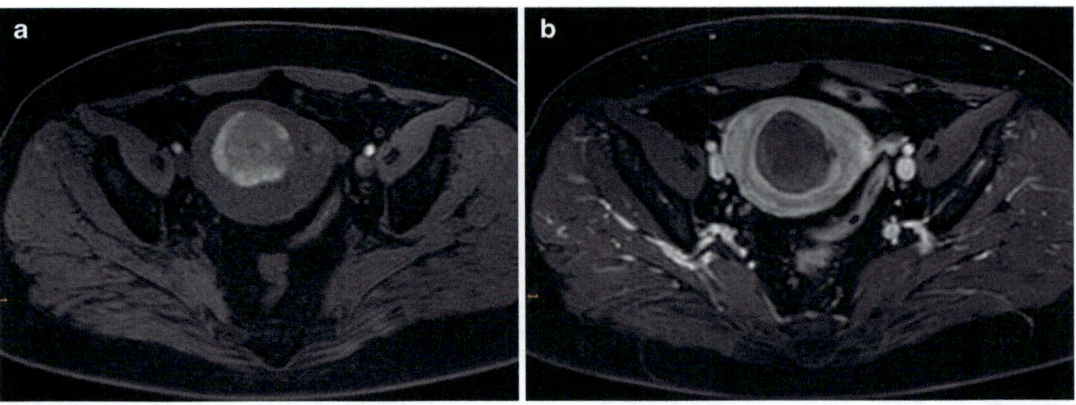

Fig. 21.11 Leiomyoma with hemorrhagic infarction. (**a**, **b**) Uterine fibroid with peripheral hyperintensity and lack of enhancement in 3D-Fat Sat T1 WI (DCE) MRI

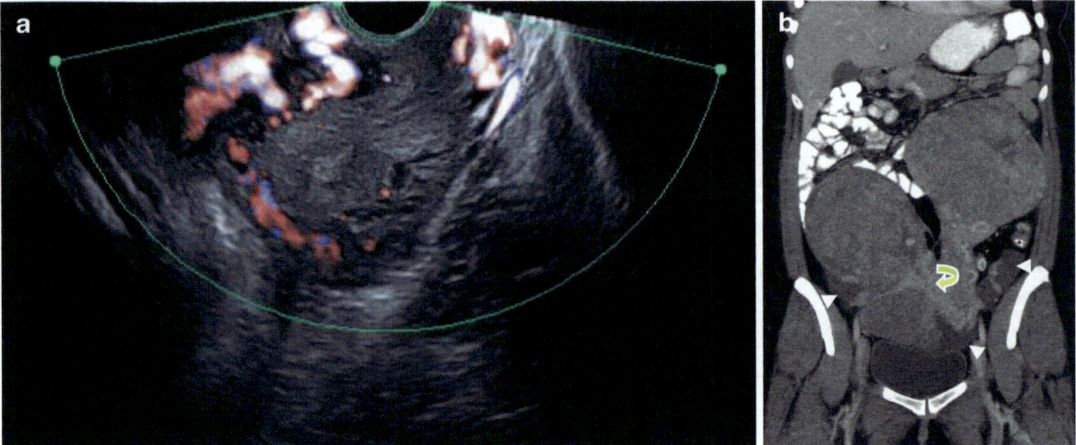

Fig 21.12 36 year-old woman who presented with abdominal and pelvic cramping pain. (**a**) Doppler US: a normal size uterus is seen with an increased vascularization in the fundus and abnormal vessels in the broad uterine ligament. (**b**) Coronal reformatted CT image: pedunculated subserous bilateral leiomyomas that displace intestinal loops and free fluid (*arrowheads*). Surgery was performed; the pedicle of the right leiomyoma was twisted (*curved arrow*)

whereas the T2WI signal of leiomyomas is hypointense, except in cases of torsion and necrosis, which show up with a more heterogeneous signal intensity and no enhancement after the administration of Gd [1, 59].

Uterine Malignant Diseases

At the early stages, uterine cancer in women may be asymptomatic. A symptomatic woman might complain of unusual vaginal bleeding (which is the most common symptom), spotting, or watery vaginal discharge that may be heavy and have a foul odor, difficulty or pain while urinating, dyspareunia, or pelvic pain. Premenopausal women can suffer from menorrhagia and/or intermenstrual uterine bleeding.

At the advanced stages, symptoms are nonspecific and include pelvic or abdominal pain; difficulty eating or reaching early satiety, urinary symptoms such as increased frequency and urgency, pain during urination, and obstructive urinary symptoms. If the tumor has spread toward the rectum or sigmoid colon, the patient may present with chronic constipation, fecal impaction, and abdominal swelling and bloating associated with pain or cramping [63, 64].

In women with a suspected uterine malignancy, screening for the disease begins with an

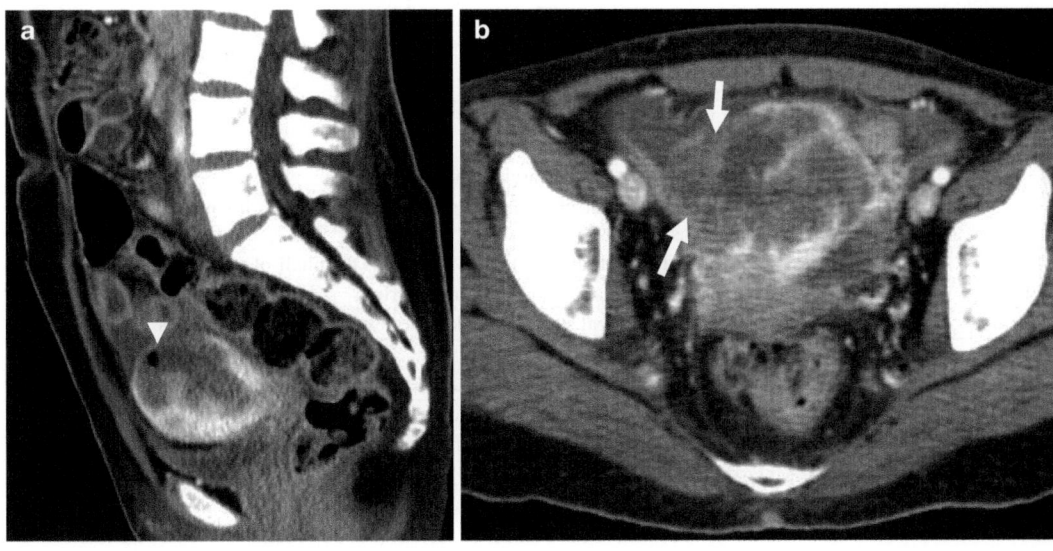

Fig. 21.13 Mentally disabled 45 year-old woman who presented with cramping abdominal pain, and septic shock. A CT (portal phase) was performed to rule out appendicitis. (**a**, **b**) Sagittal and axial reformatted CT: uterine endometrial/myometrial mass with serosal disruption (arrows), a gas bubble (arrowhead) and peri-uterine fluid. Hysterectomy was performed and histo-pathological analysis showed endometrial carcinoma (Endometrioid- type I, grade 3) and endometritis by *Escherichia coli*

evaluation of the patient's medical history and a physical examination, followed with US, a hysteroscopy, an endometrial/cervical biopsy, or dilation and curettage. An MRI is often performed subsequently to reach a final diagnosis and/or staging [3, 6–12, 14].

Endometrial Cancer

Is the most frequent malignant tumor of the female genital tract in Western countries. Its incidence is growing, mainly owing to the population's increased life expectancy and obesity rates. Most cases of endometrial cancer are diagnosed at an early stage, and 75% of cases occur in postmenopausal women [6, 14, 65–67].

There are two histopathological subtypes of endometrial cancer: Type I is the most frequent form (80–85%); it is estrogen-dependent, affects younger patients (premenopausal or perimenopausal women), and is usually diagnosed at an early stage due to an abnormal vaginal bleeding. Histologically, type I endometrial carcinoma is a grade 1 to 2 endometrioid adenocarcinoma with good prognosis (5-year survival of 80%). Conversely, type II endometrial cancer is less frequent (10–15%), affects older women (postmenopause), is diagnosed at an advanced stage (60%), and can develop alongside peritoneal carcinomatosis (such as in ovarian cancer). Histologically, it comprises grade 3 endometrioid adenocarcinomas (Fig. 21.13) and other rare etiologies, such as clear-cell carcinoma, undifferentiated serous carcinoma, and carcinosarcoma. Type II endometrial cancer has an aggressive behavior and a poor prognosis (5-year survival of 40%) [6, 14, 65–67].

Endometrial cancer is staged surgicopathologically according to the FIGO and the TNM systems (Table 21.5) [68–70]. MRI is recommended for endometrial cancer staging and for evaluating patients who would rather avoid surgery in order to preserve their fertility [8]. The combination of T2WI, DWI, and DCE has been accepted as a standard MRI protocol in routine clinical practice (Table 21.1) [6, 66, 67, 71, 72].

A major clinical challenge is the optimal selection of high-risk patients with lymph node metastasis who would benefit from more extensive surgical procedures (lymphadenectomy, pelvic exenteration) while avoiding overtreatment of low-risk patients. Lymphadenectomy is contraindicated in low-risk patients (type I endometrial cancer, grade 1 or 2, without myometrial invasion). The depth of the myometrial invasion

Table 21.5 TNM and FIGO classifications for endometrial cancer

TNM categories	FIGO stages	Definition
Tx		Primary tumor cannot be assessed
T0		No evidence of primary tumor
Tis		Tumor in situ (preinvasive carcinoma)
T1	I	Tumor confined to the corpus uteri (endocervical glandular involvement should be considered as stage I)
T1a	IA	Tumor limited to endometrium or invading less than half of myometrium
T1b	IB	Tumor invades one half or more of myometrium
T2	II	Tumor invades cervical stroma, but does not extend beyond the uterus
T3	III	Local and regional spread
T3a	IIIA	Tumor invades the serosa of the corpus uteri or adnexa (direct extension or metastasis)
T3b	IIIB	Vaginal or parametrial involvement (direct extension or metastasis)
N1, N2	IIIC	Metastasis to pelvic or para-aortic lymph nodes
N1	IIIC1	Metastasis to pelvic lymph nodes
N2	IIIC2	Metastasis to para-aortic lymph nodes, with or without positive pelvic lymph nodes
T4	IVA	Tumor invades mucosa of bladder or rectum (bullous edema is not sufficient to classify a tumor as T4)
Nx		Regional lymph nodes cannot be assessed
N0		No regional lymph node metastasis
N1		Regional lymph node metastasis to pelvic lymph nodes
N2		Regional lymph node metastasis to para-aortic lymph nodes, with or without positive pelvic lymph nodes
M0		No distant metastasis
M1	IVB	Distant metastasis (includes metastasis to inguinal lymph nodes, intraperitoneal disease, or lung, liver, or bone metastases; it excludes metastasis to para-aortic lymph nodes, vagina, pelvic serosa, or adnexa)

(myometrial invasion of less than or $\geq 50\%$) classifies the entity into stages IA and IB, and MRI is known to accurately assess the depth of this parameter [6, 66, 67, 71, 72].

Cervical Cancer

Is the third most common gynecological cancer worldwide, accounting for over 300,000 deaths annually. Nearly 80% of cases of cervical cancer are instanced in developing countries, and most patients are diagnosed with the disease at an advanced stage, thus not being suitable for surgical staging. Most cervical cancers are caused by the sexually transmitted human papillomavirus (HPV), with over 70% of cancers being associated with high-risk subtypes HPV 16 and HPV 18. Increased compliance with screening Pap smears for the detection of precancerous lesions, as well as the approval of HPV prevention vaccines, have drastically decreased the rate of cervical cancer in the United States and other developed regions of the world [65].

Histologically, 85% of cervical carcinomas are of the squamous cell subtype, and the remaining 15% are caused by adenocarcinoma, adenosquamous carcinoma, and undifferentiated carcinoma [65].

Clinical staging of cervical carcinomas is performed by gynecological bimanual and speculum examinations, colposcopy, and cervical biopsy. In developing countries where MRI and positron emission tomography/computed tomography (PET/CT) are not available, additional invasive techniques, including an examination under anesthesia, cystoscopy, intravenous urography, and sigmoidoscopy or barium enema, can be performed to screen for the advanced disease. The revised FIGO staging system recommends the use of MRI together with PET/CT to increase the accuracy of the staging (Table 21.6) [73].

There are significant inaccuracies in the clinical staging system compared to the surgical one, with an error rate of up to 32% in patients with a stage IB disease and of up to 65% in patients with a stage III disease. The greatest difficulties reported in the clinical examination of patients with cervical cancer are the accurate estimation

Table 21.6 TNM and FIGO classifications for cervical cancer

TNM categories	FIGO stages	Definition
Tx		Primary tumor cannot be assessed
T0		No evidence of primary tumor
Tis		Preinvasive carcinoma
T1	I	The carcinoma is strictly confined to the cervix (extension to the uterine corpus should be disregarded)
T1a	IA	Invasive carcinoma that can be diagnosed only microscopy, with maximun depth of invasion <5 mm[a]
T1a1	IA1	Measured stromal invasion <3 mm in depth
T1a2	IA2	Measured stromal invasion ≥3 mm and <5 mm in depth
T1b	IB	Invasive carcinoma with measured deepest invasion ≥5 mm (greater than Stage IA), lesion limited to the cervix uteri[b]
T1b1	IB1	Invasive carcinoma with measured deepest invasion ≥5 mm depth in stromal invasion, and <2 cm in greatest dimension
T1b2	IB2	Invasive carcinoma ≥2 cm and <4 cm in greatest dimension
No TNM equivalent	IB3[d]	Invasive carcinoma >4 cm in greatest dimension
T2	II	The carcinoma invades beyond the uterus, but has not extended onto the lower third of the vagina or to the pelvic wall
T2a	IIA	Involved limited to the upper two-thirds of the vagina without parametrial invasion
T2a1	IIA1	Invasive carcinoma <4 cm in greatest dimension
T2a2	IIA2	Invasive carcinoma ≥4 cm in greatest dimension
T2b	IIB	With parametrial involvement but not up to the pelvic wall
T3	III	The carcinoma involves the lower third of the vagina and/or extends to the pelvic wall and/or causes hydronephrosis or nonfunctioning kidney and/or involves pelvic and/or para-aortic lymph nodes[c]
T3a	IIIA	The carcinoma involves the lower third of the vagina, with no extension to the pelvic wall
T3b	IIIB	Extension to the pelvic wall and/or hydronephrosis or nonfunctioning kidney (unless known to be due to another cause)
Nx		Regional lymph nodes cannot be assessed
N0		No regional lymph nodes metastasis
N[d]	IIIC[d]	Involvement of pelvic and/or para-aortic lymph nodes, irrespective of tumor size and extent (with r and p notations)[c]
No TNM equivalent	IIIC1[d]	Pelvic lymph nodes metastasis only
No TNM equivalent	IIIC2[d]	Para-aortic lymph nodes metastasis
T4	IV	The carcinoma has extended beyond the true pelvis or has involved (biopsy proven) the mucosa of the bladder or rectum. (A bullous edema, as such, does not permit a case to be allotted to Stage IV)
	IVA	Spread to adjacent pelvic organs
M0		No distant metastasis
M1	IVB	Spread to distant organs

When in doubt, the lower staging should be assigned

[a]Imaging and pathology can be used, when available, to supplement clinical findings with respect to tumor size and extent in all stages

[b]The involvement of vascular/lymphatic spaces does not change the staging. The lateral extent of the lesion is no longer considered

[c]The notations of r (imaging) and p (pathology) are added to indicate the findings used to assign a case as Stage IIIC. For example, if imaging indicates pelvic lymph node metastasis, the stage allocation would be Stage IIIC1r, whereas if confirmed by pathologic findings, the stage would be Stage IIIC1p. The type of imaging modality or pathology technique used should always be documented

[d]The revised FIGO classification was recently published (October 2018). TNM (8th Edition) does not include classification for the new FIGO groups IB3, IIIC1, and IIIC2. TNM defines only regional lymph nodes, with N0 (i+) indicating isolated tumor cells in regional lymph node(s) no greater than 0.2 mm, and N1 indicating regional lymph node metastasis

of tumor size, the assessment of parametrial and pelvic sidewall invasion, and the evaluation of lymph node metastases, all of which are very important prognostic factors [14, 73–76].

The ultimate goal of imaging is to appropriately stratify patients into treatment groups, avoid the morbidity and mortality associated with unnecessary surgery, and ensure that all regions of a suspected disease are included in the radiation treatment fields [14, 70, 73–76]. Therefore, imaging is complementary to the clinical assessment, with MRI being the optimal modality to stage cervical carcinoma with a FIGO stage 1B1 or greater. For the detection of nodal metastasis greater than 10 mm, PET/CT is more accurate than CT and MRI, with false-negative results in 4%–15% of cases. PET/CT has a sensitivity of 53%–73% and specificity of 90%–97% for the detection of LN involvement, while in more advanced stages the sensitivity for detecting the involvement of para-aortic nodes increases to 75% with 95% specificity [73]. Regarding treatment, in young patients with small invasive tumors who wish to preserve their fertility, a more conservative surgical procedure (vaginal radical trachelectomy) can be performed. In these cases, MRI staging is mandatory to determine eligibility in terms of tumor size (<2 cm), cervical length (>2.5 cm), and distance between the tumor and the internal cervical os (>1 cm) [8, 75]. Young women with larger tumors (FIGO IB1, IB2) or with a limited vaginal access, are usually selected for abdominal radical trachelectomy or neoadjuvant chemotherapy plus conservative surgery [8, 73].

Patients with an early-stage disease, tumors confined to the uterus, and tumors of less than 4 cm (stage I–IB2) are treated with primary surgical resection and lymphadenectomy. Tumors at stage IB3 or above are treated with concurrent chemoradiotherapy (Fig. 21.14). Moreover, women with an advanced-stage disease (IVB) are offered palliative chemotherapy and symptomatic control [73, 74].

Uterine Sarcomas

Are a heterogeneous group of tumors accounting for 2–3% of all uterine tumors. In studies and systematic reviews of women undergoing hysterectomy or myomectomy for a myometrial mass,

the prevalence of sarcoma was approximately 0.20–0.36%. The black population has a risk factor for uterine sarcoma. Average age at diagnosis is 60 years, thus, most sarcomas develop after menopause [15, 77].

The clinical features of benign leiomyomas and uterine sarcomas are often indistinguishable. They can both present with abnormal uterine bleeding, pelvic pain/pressure, and a pelvic mass. Classically, uterine sarcomas are identified as a rapidly-growing pelvic mass, which may be accompanied by vaginal bleeding and abdominal or pelvic pain in postmenopausal women. Serum markers such as Lactate dehydrogenase (LDH) and LDH isozyme type III can be elevated in leiomyosarcomas (LMS) but also with cellular and degenerated leiomyomas [15].

Uterine sarcomas may originate from the smooth muscle of the myometrium [LMS], the endometrial stroma (endometrial stromal sarcoma [ESS] (Fig. 21.15) and undifferentiated endometrial sarcoma [UES]), or both (adenosarcoma) [15]. LMS is the most commonly instanced histological variant of uterine sarcomas and is considered to be an aggressive tumor associated with poor prognosis and a 5-year survival rate ranging from 18.8 to 68%. ESS is relatively indolent and associated with long-term survival but is characterized by late recurrences (14–60% of women). In contrast, UES has a very aggressive behavior and poor prognosis, with a 5-year survival rate of 25–55%. Adenosarcomas are rare mixed tumors, of both glandular and mesenchymal origin, with a relatively low malignant potential, a slow growth pattern, and a 5-year survival rate of over 80% [15, 65].

Uterine sarcomas are staged with FIGO classification (Table 21.7) [78].

The distinction between different subtypes of uterine sarcomas and other uterine tumors is not made on clinical grounds. Thomassin-Naggara et al. [16] reported that by combining the analysis of T2 signal intensity, b: 1000 images, and ADC map, MRI achieved 92.4% accuracy in distinguishing benign and uncertain or malignant myometrial tumors. More recently, Lackman et al. [79] analyzing qualitative measures to differentiate

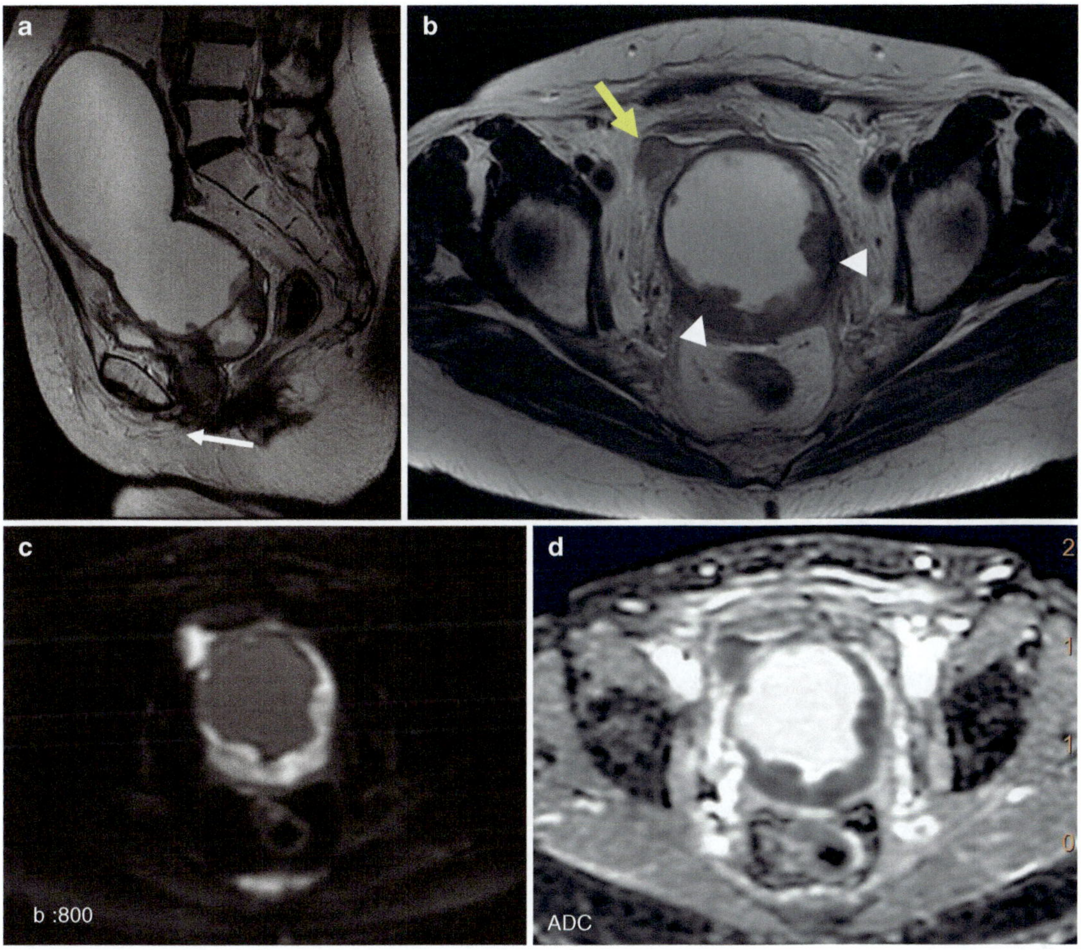

Fig. 21.14 56-year-old woman with abdominal bloating and chronic pelvic pain. (**a, b**) Sagittal and axial oblique T2WI: cervical mass obstructing the endometrial cavity (*white arrow*) which is distended with fluid. There is extrauterine extension (*yellow arrow*) and tumoral vegetations extending into the endometrial cavity. (**c, b**) DWI (b:800, ADC map) shows diffusion restriction. Cervical biopsy and histology: squamous cervical cancer. FIGO: IIB

LMS from atypical leiomyoma showed that the four qualitative MR features most strongly associated with LMS were nodular borders, hemorrhage, "T2 dark" area(s), and central unenhanced area(s). When a lesion had ≥3 of these four features, it was most probably a LMS ($p \leq 0.0001$).

MRI has a developing role in the assessment of these malignancies, being useful in the evaluation of pelvic masses at their onset, in the characterization of the different uterine masses, in an adequate staging (assessment of invasion depth, spread to adjacent organs and lymph nodes), and, consequently, in establishing the appropriate treatment plan [14–16, 79].

Uterine Lymphomas

Primary malignant lymphomas of the uterus or cervix are rare. Most cases of uterine lymphomas are a result of secondary involvement of the disease. Less than 1% of primary malignant lymphomas develop in the female genitalia. Most cases of primary uterine lymphoma are a form of non-Hodgkin lymphoma, mainly diffuse large B-cell lymphoma [80].

The median age at diagnosis of this disease is between 40 and 50 years. Most primary uterine lymphomas arise from the cervix; however, in most cases, both the cervix and uterine body are involved. The most common symptoms of primary uterine lymphoma are abnormal vaginal bleeding

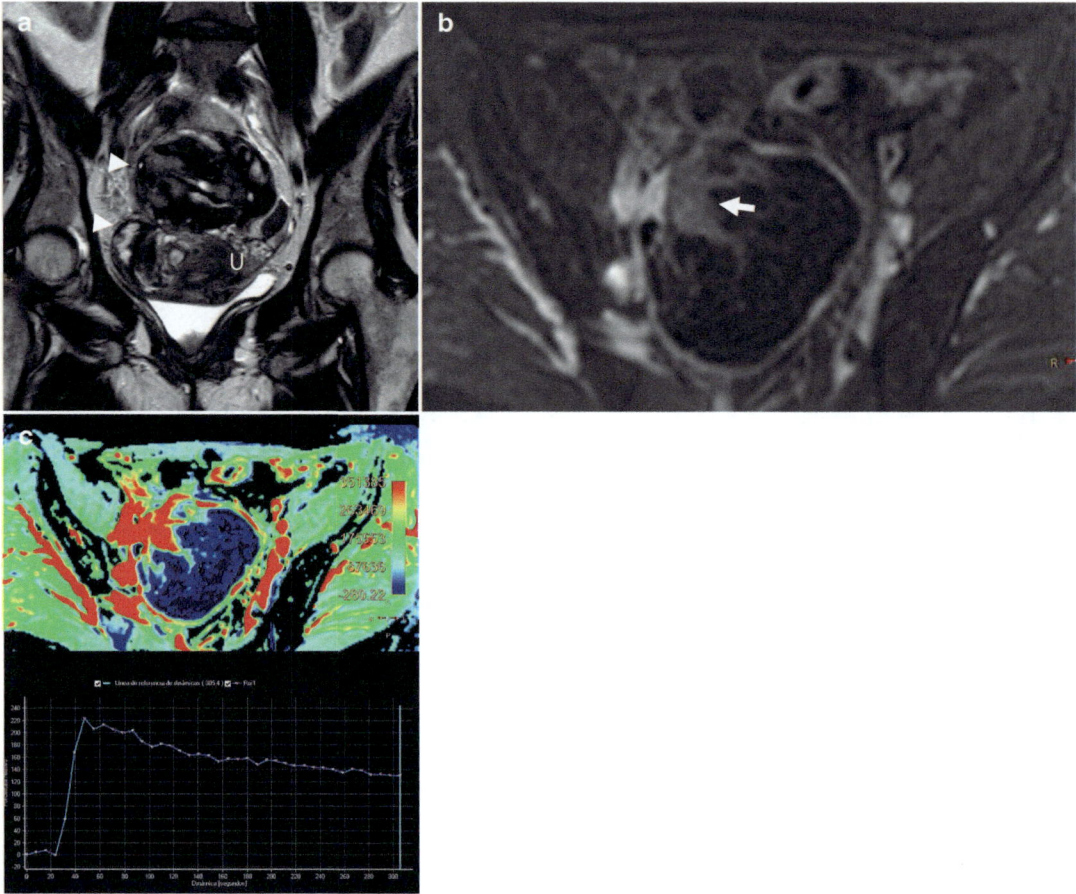

Fig 21.15 60 year-old woman with no complaints. (**a**) Coronal T2WI: pelvic heterogeneous exophytic mass that extends from the right side of the uterine fundus (*U*) with serosa disruption (*arrowheads*), upward to the midline of the pelvis. (**b**, **c**) DCE (*subtraction image*), parametric map and time-intensity curve show a heterogeneous mass with early enhancement in the right aspect (*arrow*) of the mass and early washout-curve type 3. Hysterectomy and histology: undifferentiated endometrial stromal sarcoma, FIGO: IIIB

or discharge, abdominal pain, and mass effect. Pap smear results are usually not abnormal, because primary lymphoma of the cervix or uterus arises from the stroma, and not from the epithelium.

The disease usually presents as diffuse uterine enlargement, but it may appear as a large lobulated mass or as multiple nodules. Significant contrast enhancement with Gd has also been reported, which is a slightly unusual finding compared to lymphoma in solid abdominal organs. Invasion of the bladder and vagina may also be observed. Its possible differential diagnoses include cervical carcinoma, small-cell carcinoma of the uterus, metastases, and sarcoma [81].

Uterine Metastasis

Metastasis to the uterus and cervix from extragenital sites is a rare occurrence. Metastasis of a primary vaginal or ovarian tumor in the female genital tract is more common. Taking into account extragenital tumors, the breast followed by gastrointestinal tumors, are the most common primary source of the metastasis (Fig. 21.16) [82, 83].

Metastatic tumors must be considered in the differential diagnosis of a cervical/uterine mass in women of perimenopausal ages, especially in patients with a prior history of neoplasm presenting with abnormal vaginal bleeding.

Table 21.7 TNM and FIGO classifications for uterine sarcomas (leiomyosarcomas, endometrial stromal sarcomas, adenosarcomas, and carcinosarcomas)

TNM categories	FIGO stage	Surgical-pathologic findings
Leiomyosarcomas and Endometrial Stromal Sarcomas (ESS)		
T1	I	Tumor limited to the uterus
T1a	IA	Tumor ≤5 cm in greatest dimension
T1b	IB	Tumor >5 cm
T2	II	Tumor extends to the pelvis
T2a	IIA	Tumor involves adnexa
T2b	IIB	Tumor extends to extrauterine pelvic tissue
T3	III	Tumor involves abdominal tissues (not just protruding into the abdomen)
T3a	IIIA	One site
T3b	IIIB	>One site
N1	IIIC	Metastasis to pelvic and/or para-aortic lymph nodes
T4	IVA	Tumor invades bladder and/or rectum
M1	IVB	Distant metastases
Adenosarcomas[a]		
T1	I	Tumor limited to the uterus
T1a	IA	Tumor limited to endometrium/endocervix with no myometrial invasión
T1b	IB	Tumor invades to ≤50% of the myometrium
T1c	IC	Tumor invades >50% of the myometrium
T2	II	Tumor extends beyond the uterus, within the pelvis
T2a	IIA	Tumor involves adnexa
T2b	IIB	Tumor involves other pelvic tissue
T3	III	Tumor invades abdominal tissues (not just protruding into the abdomen)
T3a	IIIA	One site
T3b	IIIB	>One site
N1	IIIC	Metastasis to pelvic and/or para-aortic lymph nodes
T4	IVA	Tumor invades bladder and/or rectum
Nx		Regional lymph nodes cannot be assessed
N0		No regional lymph node metastasis
N1		Regional lymph node metastasis
M0		No distant metastasis
M1	IVB	Distant metastases (excluding adnexa, pelvic and abdominal tissues)
Carcinosarcomas		Should be staged as endometrial carcinoma

[a]Simultaneous tumor of the uterine corpus and ovary/pelvis in association with ovarian/pelvic endometriosis should be classified as independent primary tumors

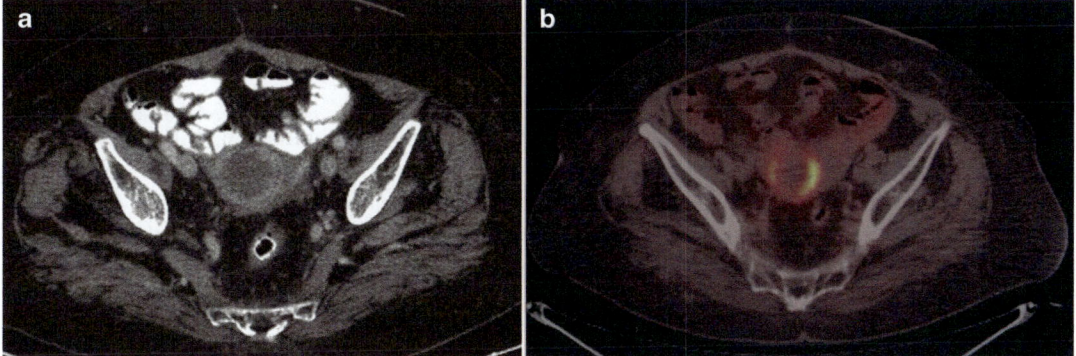

Fig. 21.16 70-year-old woman with history of sigmoid adenocarcinoma treated with Hartmann procedure 5 years before. (**a**) Control CT (portal phase) shows a cystic mass in the uterine fundus with a rim of contrast enhancement. (**b**) FDG-PET/CT: necrotic uterine mass with peripheral rim enhancement (standardized uptake value- SUV:10.6 g/mL). Biopsy and histology: metastasis of colon adenocarcinoma

21.3.2.3 Uterine Torsion

Uterine torsion is a very rare acute disorder entailing a rotation of over 45° of the uterus along its longitudinal axis, usually at the level of the isthmus [61, 84].

Risk factors for this condition include leiomyomas, which are the most common predisposing factor in nonpregnant women, followed by pregnancy, abnormal fetal presentation, external cephalic version, congenital uterine anomalies, adnexal masses, and pelvic adhesions [61, 84–86].

Its most common symptoms are abdominal pain, of mild or acute intensity, associated with shock, vaginal bleeding, and gastrointestinal or urinary discomfort. In pregnant women it can lead to placental abruption [61, 84, 87].

In US, an obvious change can be observed in the location of a known leiomyoma or the placenta of pregnant women (from left to right or vice versa), which may aid in reaching an early diagnosis. Doppler US reveals abnormally positioned ovarian vessels across the uterus, as the bilateral ovaries may be involved in the twisted pedicle, with the broad ligament wrapped around the uterine corpus. CT and T2WI images may reveal a whirlpool sign at the level of the uterine isthmus or either an X-shaped or twisted configuration of the upper vagina on axial images; however, these signs may depend on the extent and level of the torsion [61, 84, 88].

21.3.2.4 Uterine Pain Related to Iatrogenic and Medical Procedures

Intrauterine Contraceptive Devices

Intrauterine devices (IUD) are the most common type of long-term reversible contraceptive method used worldwide. Mispositioning and other complications, such as uterine perforation or PID, may be a cause of pelvic pain in women. In these cases, imaging techniques are useful not only to assess the location of the IUD but also to rule out potential associated complications [89, 90].

US is the first-line imaging modality used to evaluate IUDs; however, other techniques, such as plain radiography or CT, can be helpful if the device cannot be viewed clearly or to further assess complications. In US, a correctly positioned T-shaped IUD (the most common type) shows up as a hyperechogenic device, with or without an acoustic shadow, placed within the endometrial cavity, with the proximal end of the stem being located in the internal cervical os, its distal end in the fundus, and the arms positioned transversally. 3D US allows for a more accurate evaluation of the position of the IUD arms, particularly on coronal views [91, 92].

Mispositioning

A low positioned IUD is less effective as a contraceptive method and may cause pain, especially dyspareunia. US would reveal the misplaced device with its upper tip and crossbar located in the middle or lower uterus and its proximal end positioned within the cervical canal. Some authors defined displacement as a distance >3 mm between the upper tip of the stem and the uterine fundus and associated this condition with a high risk of expulsion, but it has been shown that in many cases, the IUD spontaneously shifts into a correct position within a few months. In women who have had prior uterine surgery, the mispositioning can occur due to the migration of the tip of the IUD to the scar defect [92–94].

Uterine Perforation

Penetration of the arms or stem of device into or through the myometrium at the time of insertion occurs in one to two cases per 1000 insertions. Risk factors for this include insertion by inexperienced operators, the device being placed less than 6 months postpartum, and women with a history of few/no pregnancies or several miscarriages [90, 91].

Clinically, it manifests with pelvic pain, usually moderate, and vaginal bleeding although it can occasionally be asymptomatic. The threads are often not found during the patient's physical examination [91–94].

Penetration may be partial (embedment) or complete (perforation) if the IUD reaches and pierces the serosa, either partially or completely. Secondary migration within the pelvis or even the upper abdomen may occur subsequently, due to chronic inflammation causing erosion of the uterine wall. Migration outside the uterus can lead to additional severe complications such as bowel or bladder perforation [90, 92, 95].

If a known IUD is not found during an US exam, a plain abdominal X-ray may be helpful to ascertain its location, and a CT scan of the abdomen can help determine a more accurate location or assess additional complications for their appropriate management [90, 92, 95].

Uterine Artery Embolization

Uterine artery embolization (UAE) is a percutaneous interventional radiological procedure used in the treatment of clinically selected patients with symptomatic leiomyomas or adenomyosis. It involves the delivery of embolic particles via the uterine arteries to occlude end-arterioles perfusing the leiomyomas, thus resulting in their necrosis [50].

After the procedure, at least 50% of patients suffer a post-embolization syndrome consisting of pelvic pain and cramping, pyrexia, nausea, and vomiting, lasting for up to 48–72 h. Pelvic pain, which is the most common symptom, may last for up to a month. Other complications that may cause severe uterine pain, fever, and recurrent vaginal bleeding are the sloughing of submucosal necrotic fibroids associated or not to their transvaginal delivery, which occurs in 2–5% of cases, endometritis (0.5% of cases), and pyomyoma or uterine infarction (in less than 1% of patients). Other complications, such as tubo-ovarian abscesses, urinary tract infections, urinary retention, or nontarget embolization leading to vaginal or bladder mucosal necrosis, may also cause abdominal pain [50, 58].

After a successful procedure, a follow-up MRI should show a progressive liquefaction of the leiomyoma, with a hyperintense signal on T2WI, until its complete infarction. Complete infarction is characterized by a total lack of enhancement in post-contrast MR images. Occasionally, a hyperintense signal on T1WI and variable signal intensity on T2WI may appear within the leiomyoma, depending on the duration of the hemorrhage, a condition known as hemorrhagic infarction (Fig. 21.17). A small amount of gas showing up as signal voids on T1WI and T2WI may be identified within the necrotic leiomyoma; this finding should not be misdiagnosed as evidence of pyomyoma since gas can arise from the necrotic process itself; therefore, clinical correlation is imperative. Leiomyoma calcification occurs at least 6 months after the procedure and can be observed as a hypointense signal on T1WI and T2WI, along with blooming on GRE images [50].

Complications of Cesarean Delivery: Suture Dehiscence

Dehiscence of cesarean section, and consequent uterine rupture are rare early complications of cesarean delivery. It occurs in about 1 out of every 700–2400 cesarean births, usually in the setting of underlying infection [96].

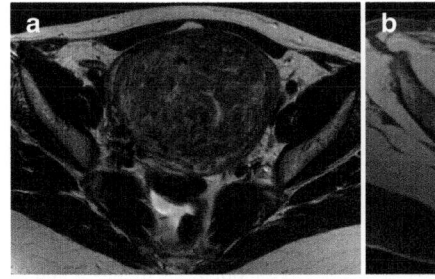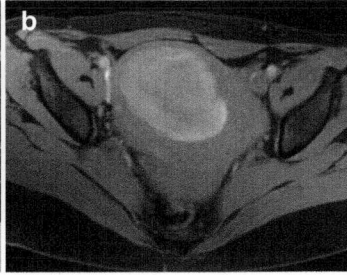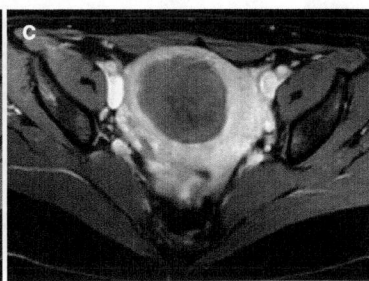

Fig. 21.17 Leiomyoma embolization. (**a**) Axial T2WI (pre-embolization): degenerated leiomyoma. (**b**) Axial Fat Sat T1WI (post-embolization): red (hemorrhagic) leio-myoma. (**c**) Axial Fat Sat T1 +Gd: no enhancement of the leiomyoma (complete infarction)

CT and especially MRI have a higher accuracy than US for the diagnosis of this condition. The parietal gap, located in the anterior lower uterine wall, may be better demonstrated on images in a perpendicular plane to that of the cesarean incision. It is often associated with fluid collections, abscesses, or hematomas. Although a small bladder flap hematoma, in the vesicouterine pouch, is a frequent finding after cesarean delivery, large ≥5 cm hematomas are often associated with infective suture dehiscence (Fig. 21.18) [29, 96].

21.3.3 Painful Pregnancy-Related Conditions

21.3.3.1 Early Miscarriage
Spontaneous miscarriage during the first trimester occurs in approximately 10–12% of known pregnancies. Although it may be asymptomatic, most patients present with pain and vaginal bleeding.

US is the first-line imaging modality of choice when a spontaneous miscarriage is clinically suspected. In 2012, a multispecialty panel convened by the Society of Radiologists in Ultrasound

established new and more conservative US finding criteria for both suspected and definitive diagnoses of early pregnancy failure (Table 21.8) [97, 98]. US suspicious findings must be correlated with the date of the last menstruation and the levels of the beta subunit of human chorionic gonadotropin (β-hCG) and are indication for a new follow-up sonogram in few days.

21.3.3.2 Placental Abruption and Subchorionic Hemorrhage
Placental abruption entails the premature separation of a normally implanted placenta from the myometrium, which affects approximately 1% of all pregnancies and accounts for 10–25% of prenatal deaths [1, 2].

If often occurs between the 24th and 26th weeks of gestation, causing pain and vaginal bleeding, and being the main cause of the latter during the third trimester of pregnancy. Risk factors for placental abruption include chronic hypertension, trauma, and advanced maternal age [1, 99, 100].

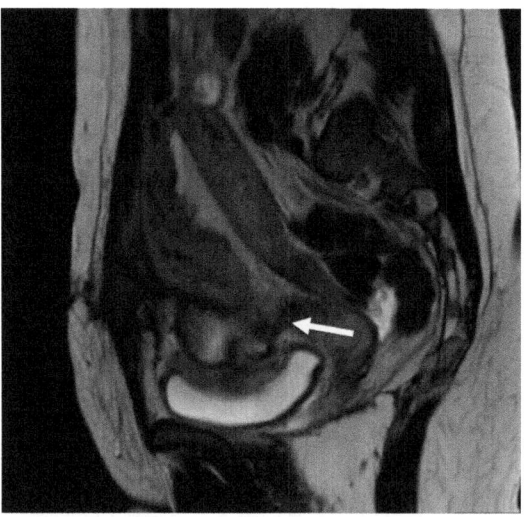

Fig. 21.18 25 year-old woman with a recent C-section due to chorioamnionitis (*Klebsiella and Escherichia coli*), who presented with fever and leukocytosis. MRI. Sagittal oblique T2WI: cesarean scar dehiscence (*arrow*)

Table 21.8 Early miscarriage: diagnostic and suspicious US findings

Diagnosis findings	Suspicious findings
≥7 mm length embryo with no heartbeat	<7 mm length embryo with no heartbeat
≥25 mm gestational sac with no embryo	16–24 mm gestational sac with no embryo
No embryo with heartbeat ≥14 days after prior US showing gestational sac without yolk sac	No embryo with heartbeat 7–13 days after prior US showing gestational sac without yolk sac
No embryo with heartbeat ≥11 days after prior US showing gestational sac with yolk sac	No embryo with heartbeat 7–10 days after prior US showing gestational sac with yolk sac
	No embryo ≥6 weeks after last menses
	Amnion with no visible embryo
	>7 mm length yolk sac
	<5 mm difference between gestational sac diameter and embryo length

The 2012 Society of Radiologists in Ultrasound multispecialty consensus panel criteria (adapted from Ref. [96], with permission)

US is the imaging modality of choice for evaluating the placenta. In US, the normal placenta is discoid, with rounded margins and a thickness of 2–4 cm. It shows homogeneous intermediate echogenicity, with a deep hypoechoic band at the junction between the myometrium and the basal decidual layer, known as the retroplacental hypoechoic space. However, the sensitivity of US for detecting placental abruption is low, approximately 25%, because in most cases of abruptio, the resulting hemorrhage may not be retained within the endometrial cavity [99-100]. A retroplacental hematoma can be suspected in US if the retroplacental hypoechoic zone is thickened to over 2 cm. It may show up as a well-delimited mass with variable echogenicity, that can mimic an abnormally thickened placenta (>4 cm) [2, 100]. Typically, hematomas form between the myometrium and the chorionic membrane (subchorionic), and they are associated with a worse neonatal outcome. [2, 99, 100].

MRI is superior to ultrasound for diagnosing placental abruption due to its greater accuracy at characterizing hemorrhagic products, better soft tissue contrast, and wider FOV [1, 2, 99, 101]. Normal placenta is isointense to the myometrium on T1WI and a hypo- or isointense on T2WI, with a fine line of hypointense signal corresponding to the placental-myometrial junction, and a regular pattern of hypointense fine lines corresponding to normal septa. Placental signal intensity is homogeneous during early pregnancy and becomes more heterogeneous with maturation. Subplacental vascularity and the umbilical cord insertion site in the placenta appear as flow voids [2]. T1WI and DWI are useful to help distinguish hyperintense or hypointense hematomas, depending on the age of the blood products [101].

The second most common posttraumatic injury in pregnant women, after solid organ injury, is placental abruption. With the development of low-dose radiation protocols, CT has become a helpful tool to assess maternal injury in the context of trauma when further evaluation is needed (Fig. 21.19). On CT, the

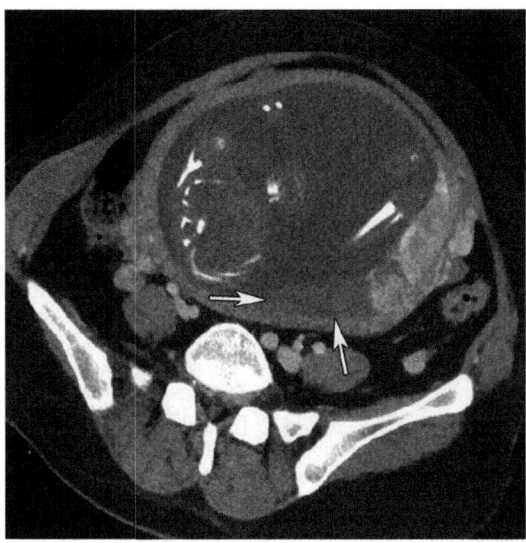

Fig. 21.19 Placental abruption in a 30-year-old woman with profuse vaginal bleeding after a motor vehicle collision at 28 weeks gestation. Axial contrast-enhanced CT image shows a heterogeneously enhancing placenta with devascularized areas (arrows), which represent areas of infarction. Another small nongeographic area of low attenuation forms an acute angle with the myometrium. More than 50% of the placenta shows enhancement; therefore, this is grade 2a on the Trauma Abruptio Placenta Scale (TAPS). From reference [99], with permission

placenta shows homogeneous density during the first and early second trimester, increasing its heterogeneity as pregnancy progresses. From the second trimester onward, placental cotyledons appear as low attenuation foci surrounded by contrast-enhancing placenta. Suspicious findings of placental damage on CT are: the detection of a thick area of reduced contrast enhancement, due to the presence of areas of infarction, and hyperdense amniotic fluid, secondary to placental bleeding into the amniotic cavity. Saphier and Kopelman have developed a 5-grade descriptive classification of placental posttraumatic injuries on CT, the Traumatic Abruptio Placental Scale (TAPS) (Table 21.9) [30].

21.3.3.3 Red Degeneration of Uterine Myomas and Uterine Torsion

Both entities have already been described in their corresponding sections.

Table 21.9 Traumatic abruptio placenta scale (adapted from Ref. [30], with permission)

Grade		CT findings
0		Placenta with normal 100% homogeneous enhancement
1		Geographic hypodense areas involving <50% of placenta surface, due to vascular lakes and cotyledons or age related non-clinically significant infarcts (normal variants)
2	2 a	Non-geographics contiguous hypodense areas that form acute angles with myometrium involving <50% of placental surface
	2 b	Contiguous and/or full-thickness hypodense areas that form acute angles with myometrium involving 50–75% of placental surface
3		Large, contiguous and/or full-thickness hypodense areas involving 50–75% of placental surface

21.3.3.4 Ectopic Pregnancy

An ectopic pregnancy occurs when a fertilized ovum implants outside the uterine endometrium. Nearly 95–98% of cases take place in the ampullary, infundibular, or isthmic segments of the fallopian tube, but other uncommon uterine implantation sites are also possible, including the cervix (in less than 1% of cases), the interstitial segment of the fallopian tube (2–4% of cases), a cesarean or other uterine surgery scar (less than 1% of cases), or even in the uterine myometrium (in less than 1% of cases) [2, 102–104].

Risk factors for ectopic pregnancy include venereal disease, adenomyosis, assisted reproductive techniques, use of IUD, prior cesarean delivery or other uterine surgery, and Asherman's syndrome [2, 102].

The most common symptoms of ectopic pregnancy are vaginal hemorrhage and abdominal pain, always with a positive pregnancy test result. These symptoms are not specific; hence, diagnostic imaging techniques, especially US, play an important role in its diagnosis. Ectopic pregnancy is ruled out if an intrauterine gestational sac is appreciated, given that in most cases of ectopic pregnancy (except for ectopic pregnancies), images show an empty endometrial cavity. US also helps differentiate these rare sites of ectopic non-tubal pregnancy [102]. MRI is helpful when US findings are not conclusive [2].

Interstitial Ectopic Pregnancy

It is the pregnancy in which the implantation takes place in the intramyometrial segment of the fallopian tube.

Its clinical presentation may be severe, in the form of profuse life-threatening hemorrhage, due to the proximity of the gestational sac to the intramyometrial arcuate vasculature. It is important to distinguish between an interstitial ectopic pregnancy and a normal eccentric intrauterine pregnancy. The following three US findings may aid in this task [102, 104]:

– *The interstitial line sign*: the interstitial segment of the fallopian tube is viewed in the transversal plane, at the level of the fundus, as a fine echogenic line that extends from the superolateral aspect of the endometrium through the myometrium. In an interstitial ectopic pregnancy, the gestational sac is located in this echogenic line, whereas in a normal angular intrauterine pregnancy, it is located medially to it.
– *The myometrial mantle sign*: in an interstitial ectopic pregnancy, the gestational sac is completely surrounded by a thin layer (<5 mm) of myometrium, whereas in a normal intrauterine pregnancy, it is placed in the endometrium, encircled by the endometrialmyometrial junction.
– *The bulging sign*: in sagittal and transverse US planes, the eccentric location of the gestational sac in the interstitial segment of the tube causes an abnormal bulging in the uterine contour.

Cervical Ectopic Pregnancy

This type of pregnancy occurs when the ovum implants in the cervical canal.

Its main differential diagnosis is miscarriage. Misdiagnosis between these two entities can be dangerous, as the cervix lacks a muscular wall, which is essential for hemostasis, and a deep curettage in this area may lead to severe hemorrhage [102].

US findings, such as the presence of an embryo with a heartbeat in the cervical canal, peritrophoblastic flow in a Doppler study, or growth of the gestational sac with embryo development in a follow-up US, in addition to β-hCG levels, are indicators of a cervical ectopic pregnancy [102, 104].

Scar Ectopic Pregnancy

In this case, implantation of the ovum takes place in a surgery scar, usually a cesarean scar, located in the anterior lower segment of the uterus. The gestational sac may grow toward the endometrium, progressing as a normal pregnancy, or toward the abdomen, with an associated risk of severe complications. These complications are: uterine rupture, mass effect over the adjacent bladder, placental bladder invasion, and massive hemorrhage. Early diagnosis is crucial, as the deep implantations of the chorionic villi in the scar tissue or adjacent bladder make curettage especially dangerous, with a high risk of uterine rupture, severe hemorrhage, or bladder injury [102].

On US, the gestational sac is located in the lower anterior wall of the uterus, showing hyperechoic margins and a peritrophoblastic flow. A thinning myometrium located in front of the gestational sac or even a possible defect in the uterine wall can also be observed. The sagittal plane is helpful for the assessment of the relation between the gestational sac and the cesarean scar and its proximity to the bladder. MRI may aid in assessing bladder invasion [96, 102, 104].

Myometrial Ectopic Pregnancy

In this type of pregnancy, the ovum implants within the myometrium clearly separated from the endometrium and the interstitial segment of the fallopian tube. In US, the gestational sac is completely surrounded by the myometrium, as in the case of interstitial ectopic pregnancies [102].

21.3.3.5 Uterine Rupture

Uterine rupture is a very rare catastrophic event causing severe abdominal pain. Its risk factors include prior uterine surgery, congenital uterine anatomic abnormalities, or interstitial ectopic pregnancy. Most cases take place during labor but also can occur before delivery. If imaging is performed, US, CT, or MRI may show herniation of the contents of the gestational sac (Fig. 21.20) [2].

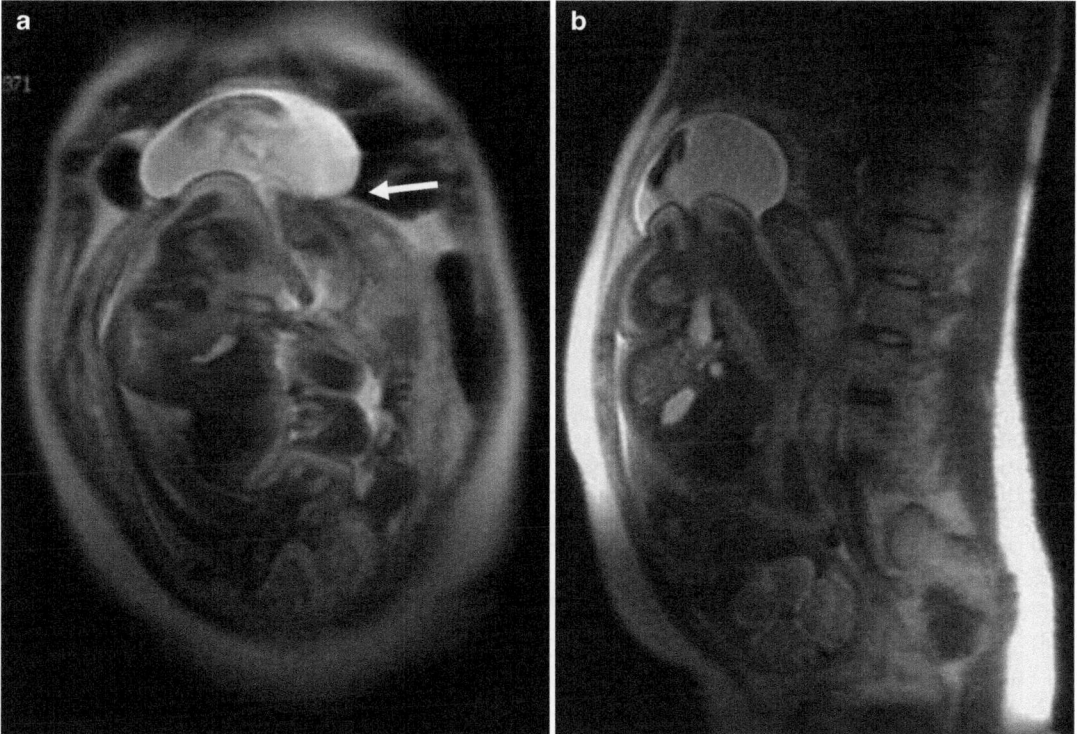

Fig. 21.20 33 year-old pregnant woman with two previous uterine curettages. She presented with abnormal uterine contractions in the 37th week. (**a**) Coronal MR image shows a uterine rupture with extrusion of the gestational sac (*arrow*). (**b**) Sagittal MR image: fetal buttocks plug uterine rupture hole. (Old case from 2005)

Acknowledgment We would like to thank Dr. Marta Rodriguez-Alvarez (radiologist), Dr. Roberto Gonzalez-Boubeta, Emilio Couceiro-Naveira, and Orlando Valenzuela-Besada (gynecologists), all of them from our hospital, for all the help given in the compilation of some images for this chapter. Thank you.

References

1. Knoepp US, Mazza MB, Chong ST, Wasnik AP. MR imaging of pelvic emergencies in women. Magn Reson Imaging Clin N Am. 2017;25(3):503–19.
2. Woodfield CA, Lazarus E, Chen KC, Mayo-Smith WW. Abdominal pain in pregnancy: diagnoses and imaging unique to pregnancy-review. AJR Am J Roentgenol. 2010;194(Suppl 6):14–30.
3. Sala E, Wakely S, Senior E, Lomas D. MRI of malignant neoplasms of the uterine corpus and cervix. AJR Am J Roentgenol. 2007;188(6):1577–87.
4. Behr SC, Courtier JL, Qayyum A. Imaging of Müllerian duct anomalies. Radiographics. 2012;32(6):233–50.
5. Bazot M, Bharwani N, Huchon C, Kinkel K, Cunha TM, Guerra A, et al. European society of urogenital radiology (ESUR) guidelines: MR imaging of pelvic endometriosis. Eur Radiol. 2017;27(7):2765–75.
6. Nougaret S, Lakhman Y, Vargas HA, Colombo PE, Fujii S, Reinhold C, et al. From staging to prognostication: achievements and challenges of MR imaging in the assessment of endometrial cancer. Magn Reson Imaging Clin N Am. 2017;25:611–33.
7. Patel-Lippmann K, Robbins J, Barroilhet L, Anderson B, Sadowski EA, Boyum J. MR imaging of cervical cancer. Magn Reson Imaging Clin N Am. 2017;25(3):635–49.
8. McEvoy SH, Nougaret S, Abu-Rustum NR, Vargas HA, Sadowski EA, Menias CO, et al. Fertility-sparing for young patients with gynecologic cancer: how MRI can guide patient selection prior to conservative management. Abdom Radiol. 2017;42:2488–512.
9. Addley H, Moyle P, Freeman S. Diffusion-weighted imaging in gynaecological malignancy. Clin Radiol. 2017;72(11):981–90.
10. Padhani AR, Liu G, Koh DM, Chenevert TL, Thoeny HC, Takahara T, et al. Diffusion-weighted magnetic resonance imaging as a cancer biomarker: consensus and recommendations. Neoplasia. 2009;11: 102–25.
11. Nougaret S, Tirumani SH, Addley H, Pandey H, Sala E, Reinhold C. Pearls and pitfalls in MRI of gynecologic malignancy with diffusion-weighted technique. AJR Am J Roentgenol. 2013;200(2):261–76.
12. Andreano A, Rechichi G, Rebora P, Sironi S, Valsecchi MG, Galimberti S. MR diffusion imaging for preoperative staging of myometrial invasion in patients with endometrial cancer: a systematic review and meta-analysis. Eur Radiol. 2014;24:1327–38.
13. Nakamura K, Imafuku N, Nishida T, Niwa I, Joja I, Hongo A, et al. Measurement of the minimum apparent diffusion coefficient (ADCmin) of the primary tumor and CA125 are predictive of disease recurrence for patients with endometrial cancer. Gynecol Oncol. 2012;124:335–9.
14. Sala E, Rockall AG, Freeman SJ, Mitchell DG, Reinhold C. The added role of MR imaging in treatment stratification of patients with gynecologic malignancies: what the radiologist needs to know. Radiology. 2013;266(3):717–40.
15. Santos P, Cunha TM. Uterine sarcomas: clinical presentation and MRI features. Diagn Interv Radiol. 2015;21(1):4–9.
16. Thomassin-Naggara I, Dechoux S, Bonneau C, Morel A, Rouzier R, Carette MF, et al. How to differentiate benign from malignant myometrial tumours using MR imaging. Eur Radiol. 2013;23:2306–14.
17. Sala E, Rockall A, Rangarajan D, Kubik-Huch RA. The role of dynamic contrast-enhanced and diffusion weighted magnetic resonance imaging in the female pelvis. Eur J Radiol. 2010;76(3):367–85.
18. Wakefield JC, Downey K, Kyriazi S, de Souza NM. New MR techniques in gynecologic cancer. AJR Am J Roentgenol. 2013;200(2):249–60.
19. Park SB, Moon MH, Sung CK, Oh S, Lee YH. Dynamic contrast-enhanced MR imaging of endometrial cancer: optimizing the imaging delay for tumour-myometrium contrast. Eur Radiol. 2014;24(11):2795–9.
20. Fujii S, Kido A, Baba T, Fujimoto K, Daido S, Matsumura N, et al. Subendometrial enhancement and peritumoral enhancement for assessing endometrial cancer on dynamic contrast enhanced MR imaging. Eur J Radiol. 2015;84(4):581–9.
21. Bennett GL, Slywotzky CM, Giovanniello G. Gynecologic causes of acute pelvic pain: spectrum of CT findings. Radiographics. 2002;22(4):785–801.
22. Masselli G, Derchi L, McHugo J, Rockall A, Vock P, Weston M, et al. Acute abdominal and pelvic pain in pregnancy: ESUR recommendations. Eur Radiol. 2013;23(12):3485–500.
23. The American College of Radiology (ACR): Practice guideline for imaging pregnant or potentially pregnant adolescents and women with ionizing radiation. 2013. https://www.acr.org/-/media/ACR/Files/Practice-Parameters/pregnant-pts.pdf. Accessed 12 Dec 2017.
24. The European Society of Urogenital Radiology (ESUR): 9.0 Contrast media guidelines. 2017. https://www.esur.org/esur-guidelines/. Accessed 20 Nov 2017.
25. The American College of Radiology (ACR): Manual on Contrast Media v10.3, Version 10.3. 2017. https://www.acr.org/-/media/ACR/Files/Clinical-Resources/Contrast_Media.pdf. Accessed 20 Nov 2017.
26. Baheti AD, Nicola R, Bennett GL, Bordia R, Moshiri M, Katz DS, et al. Magnetic resonance imaging of abdominal and pelvic pain in the preg-

nant patient. Magn Reson Imaging Clin N Am. 2016;24(2):403–17.

27. Pedrosa I, Zeikus EA, Levine D, Rofsky NM. MR imaging of acute right lower quadrant pain in pregnant and nonpregnant patients. Radiographics. 2007;27:721–43. discussion 743–53.

28. Spalluto LB, Woodfield CA, DeBenedectis CM, Lazarus E. MR imaging evaluation of abdominal pain during pregnancy: appendicitis and other nonobstetric causes. Radiographics. 2012;32(2):317–34.

29. Leyendecker JR, Gorengaut V, Brown JJ. Imaging of maternal diseases of the abdomen and pelvis during pregnancy and the immediate postpartum period. Radiographics. 2004;24(5):1301–16.

30. Saphier NB, Kopelman TR. Traumatic abruptio placenta scale (TAPS): a proposed grading system of computed tomography evaluation of placental abruption in the trauma patient. Emerg Radiol. 2014;21(1):17–22.

31. Bernardi M, Lazzeri L, Perelli F, Reis FM, Petraglia F. Dysmenorrhea and related disorders. F1000Res. 2017;6:1645.

32. Burnett M, Lemyre M. Primary dysmenorrhea consensus guideline. J Obstet Gynaecol Can. 2017;39(7):585–95.

33. Olpin JD, Moeni A, Willmore RJ, Hellbrun ME. MR imaging of Müllerian fusion anomalies. Magn Reson Imaging Clin N Am. 2017;25(3):563–75.

34. Buttram VC Jr, Gibbons WE. Müllerian anomalies: a proposed classification. (An analysis of 144 cases). Fertil Steril. 1979;32(1):40–6.

35. The American Fertility Society. The American Fertility Society classifications of adnexal adhesions, distal tubal occlusion, tubal occlusion secondary to tubal ligation, tubal pregnancies, Müllerian anomalies and intrauterine adhesions. Fertil Steril. 1988;49:944–55.

36. Oppelt P, Renner SP, Brucker S, Strissel PL, Strick R, Oppelt PG, et al. The VCUAM (Vagina Cervix Uterus Adnex-associated Malformation) classification: a new classification for genital malformations. Fertil Steril. 2005;84(5):1493–7.

37. Grimbizis GF, Gordts S, Di Spiezio Sardo A, Brucker S, De Angelis C, Gergolet M, et al. The ESHRE/ESGE consensus on the classification of female genital tract congenital anomalies. Hum Reprod. 2013;28(8):2032–44.

38. Grimbizis GF, Di Spiezio Sardo A, Saravelos SH, Gordts S, Exacoustos C, Van Schoubroeck D, et al. The Thessaloniki ESHRE/ESGE consensus on diagnosis of female genital anomalies. Gynecol Surg. 2016;13:1–16.

39. Hall-Craggs MA, Williams CE, Pattison SH, Kirkham AP, Creighton SM. Mayer-Rokitansky-Kuster-Hauser syndrome: diagnosis with MR imaging. Radiology. 2013;269(3):787–92.

40. Van der Byl G, di Giacomo V, Miele V. Herlyn Werner Wunderlich syndrome (HWWS): an unusual presentation of acute abdominal pain. J Ultrasound. 2014;17(2):171–4.

41. Letts M, Haasbeek J. Hematocolpos as a cause of back pain in premenarchal adolescents. Pediatr Orthop. 1990;10:731–2.

42. Agostinho L, Cruz R, Osório F, Alves J, Setúbal A, Guerra A. MRI for adenomyosis: a pictorial review. Insights Imaging. 2017;8(6):549–56.

43. Rainhold C, Tafazoli F, Mehio A, Wang L, Atri M, Siegelman ES, et al. Uterine adenomyosis: endovaginal US and MR imaging features with histopathologic correlation. Radiographics. 1999;19: 147–60.

44. Kassam Z, Petkovska I, Wang CL, Trinh AM, Kamaya A. Benign gynecologic conditions of the uterus. Magn Reson Imaging Clin N Am. 2017;25(3):577–600.

45. Sielgeman ES, Oliver ER. MR imaging of endometriosis: ten imaging pearls. Radiographics. 2012;32(6):1675–91.

46. Bazot M, Cortez A, Darai E, Rouger J, Chopler J, Antoine JM, et al. Ultrasonography compared with magnetic resonance imaging for the diagnosis of adenomyosis: correlation with histopathology. Hum Reprod. 2001;16(11):2427–33.

47. Dueholm M, Lundorf E, Hansen ES, Sorensen S, Ledertough S, Olensen F. Magnetic resonance imaging and transvaginal ultrasonography for the diagnosis of adenomyosis. Fertil Steril. 2001;76(3): 588–94.

48. Murase E, Siegelman ES, Outwater EK, Perez-Jaffe LA, Tureck RW. Uterine leiomyomas: histopathologic features, MR imaging findings, differential diagnosis, and treatment. Radiographics. 1999;19(5):1179–97.

49. Gupta S, Jose J, Manyonda I. Clinical presentation of fibroids. Best Pract Res Clin Obstet Gynaecol. 2008;22(4):615–26.

50. Deshmukh SP, Gonsalves CF, Guglielmo FF, Mitchell DG. Role of MR imaging of uterine leiomyomas before and after embolization. Radiographics. 2012;32(6):251–81.

51. Revzin MV, Mathur M, Dave HB, Macer ML, Spektor M. Pelvic inflammatory disease: multimodality imaging approach with clinical-pathologic correlation. Radiographics. 2016;36(5):1579–96.

52. Soper DE. Pelvic inflammatory disease. Obstet Gynecol. 2010;116(2 Pt 1):419–28.

53. Centers for Disease Control and Prevention: Pelvic inflammatory disease (PID): CDC fact sheet—detailed version. 2014. http://www.cdc.gov/std/pid/stdfact-pid-detailed.htm. Accessed 25 Nov 2017.

54. Wildenberg JC, Yam BL, Langer JE, Jones LP. US of the nongravid cervix with multimodality imaging correlation: normal appearance, pathologic conditions, and diagnostic pitfalls. Radiographics. 2016;36:596–617.

55. Okamoto Y, Tanaka YO, Nishida M, Tsumoda H, Yoshikawa H, Itai Y. MR imaging of the uterine cervix: imaging-pathologic correlation. Radiographics. 2003;23(2):525–45.

56. Choi PW. Colouterine fistula caused by diverticulitis of the sigmoid colon. J Korean Soc Coloproctol. 2012;28(6):321–4.

57. Rezvani M, Shaaban AM. Fallopian tube disease in the nonpregnant patient. Radiographics. 2011;31(2):527–48.

58. Silberzweig JE, Powell DK, Matsumoto AH, Spies JB. Management of uterine fibroids: a focus on uterine-sparing interventional techniques. Radiology. 2016;280(3):675–92.

59. Roche O, Chavan N, Aquilina J, Rockall A. Radiological appearances of gynaecological emergencies. Insights Imaging. 2012;3(3):265–75.

60. Munro MG, Critchley HO, Fraser IS. FIGO Menstrual Disorders Working Group. The FIGO classification of causes of abnormal uterine bleeding in the reproductive years. Fertil Steril. 2011;95(7):2204–8.

61. Iraha Y, Okada M, Iraha R, Azama K, Yamashiro T, Tsubakimoto M, et al. CT and MR imaging of gynecologic emergencies. Radiographics. 2017;37(5):1569–86.

62. Casillas J, Joseph RC, Guerra JJJ. CT appearance of uterine leiomyomas. Radiographics. 1990;10(6):999–1007.

63. Cancer center treatment of America: Uterine cancer symptoms. https://www.cancercenter.com/uterine-cancer/symptoms/. Accessed 20 Nov 2017.

64. Cancer.net: Uterine Cancer: Symptoms and Signs. https://www.cancer.net/cancer-types/uterine-cancer/symptoms-and-signs. Accessed 20 Nov 2017.

65. World Health Organization Classification of Tumours. In: Tavassoli FA, Devilee P, editors. Pathology and genetics of tumours of the breast and female genital organs. Lyon: IARC Press; 2003.

66. Meissnitzer M, Forstner R. MRI of endometrium cancer - how we do it. Cancer Imaging. 2016;16:11.

67. Kinkel K, Forstner R, Danza FM, Oleaga L, Cunha TM, Bergman A, et al. Staging of endometrial cancer with MRI: guidelines of the European Society of Urogenital Imaging. Eur Radiol. 2009;19(7):1565–74.

68. Pecorelli S. Revised FIGO staging for carcinoma of the vulva, cervix, and endometrium. Int J Gynaecol Obstet. 2009;105(2):103–4.

69. Union for International Cancer Control (UICC). TNM classification of malignant tumours. 8th ed. Oxford, UK, Hoboken, NJ: John Wiley & sons, Inc; 2017.

70. Freeman SJ, Aly AM, Kataoka MY, Addley HC, Reinhold C, Sala E. The revised FIGO staging system for uterine malignancies: implications for MR imaging. Radiographics. 2012;32(6):1805–27.

71. Nougaret S, Reinhold C, Alsharif SS, Addley H, Arceneau J, Molinari N, et al. Endometrial cancer: combined MR volumetry and diffusion-weighted imaging for assessment of myometrial and lymphovascular invasion and tumor grade. Radiology. 2015;276(3):797–808.

72. Colombo N, Preti E, Landoni F, Carinelli S, Colombo A, Marini C, et al. Endometrial cancer: ESMO clinical practice guidelines for diagnosis, treatment and follow-up. Ann Oncol. 2013;24(Suppl 6):33–8.

73. Bhatla N, Aoki D, Sharma DN, Sankaranarayanan R. Cancer of the cervix uteri. FIGO Cancer report 2018. Int J Gynecol Obstet (2018);143(Suppl. 2): 22–36.

74. Patel-Lippmann K, Robbins JB, Barroilhet L, Anderson B, Sadowski EA, Boyum J. MR imaging of cervical cancer. Magn Reson Imaging Clin N Am. 2017;25(3):635–49.

75. Noël P, Dubé M, Plante M, St-Laurent G. Early cervical carcinoma and fertility-sparing treatment options: MR imaging as a tool in patient selection and a follow-up modality. Radiographics. 2014;34(4):1099–119.

76. Dappa E, Elger T, Hasenburg A, Düber C, Battista MJ, Hötker AM. The value of advanced MRI techniques in the assessment of cervical cancer: a review. Insights Imaging. 2017;8(5):471–81.

77. Wu TI, Yen TC, Lai CH. Clinical presentation and diagnosis of uterine sarcoma, including imaging. Best Pract Res Clin Obstet Gynaecol. 2011;25(6):681–9.

78. Prat J. FIGO staging for uterine sarcomas. Int J Gynaecol Obstet. 2009;104:177–8. (Prat J. Erratum in: Int J Gynaecol Obstet. 2009;106:277).

79. Lakhman Y, Veeraraghavan H, Chaim J, et al. Differentiation of uterine leiomyosarcoma from atypical leiomyoma: diagnostic accuracy of qualitative MR imaging features and feasibility of texture analysis. Eur Radiol. 2017;27(7):2903–15.

80. Frey NV, Svoboda J, Andreadis C, Tsai DE, Schuster SJ, Elstrom R, et al. Primary lymphomas of the cervix and uterus: the University of Pennsylvania's experience and a review of the literature. Leuk Lymphoma. 2006;47(9):1894–901.

81. Alves Vieira MA, Cunha TM. Primary lymphomas of the female genital tract: imaging findings. Diagn Interv Radiol. 2014;20:110–5.

82. Mazur MT, Hsuch S, Gersell DJ. Metastases to the female genital tract: analysis of 325 cases. Cancer. 1984;53(9):1978–84.

83. Limoine NR, Hall PA. Epithelial tumors metastatic to the uterine cervix. A study of 33 cases and review of the literature. Cancer. 1986;57(10):2002–5.

84. Jeong YY, Kang HK, Park JG, Choi HS. CT features of uterine torsion. Eur Radiol. 2003;13(Suppl 6):249–50.

85. Karavani G, Picard R, Elami-Suzin M, Mankuta D. Complete uterine torsion diagnosed during an elective caesarean section following failed external cephalic version: a case report. J Obstet Gynaecol. 2017;37:673–4.

86. Salani R, Theiler RN, Lindsay M. Uterine torsion and fetal bradycardia associated with external cephalic version. Obstet Gynecol. 2006;108(3 Pt 2):820–2.

87. Ulu I, Günes MS, Kiran G, Gülsen MS. A rare cause of placental abruption: uterine torsion. J Clin Diagn Res. 2016;10(1):6–7.

88. Kremer JA, van Dongen PW. Torsion of the pregnant uterus with a change in placental localization on ultrasound; a case report. Eur J Obstet Gynecol Reprod Biol. 1989;31(3):273–5.

89. Peri N, Graham D, Levine D. Imaging of intrauterine contraceptive devices. J Ultrasound Med. 2007;26:1389–401.

90. Nowitzki KM, Hoimes ML, Chen B, Zheng LZ, Kim YH. Ultrasonography of intrauterine devices. Ultrasonography. 2015;34(3):183–94.

91. Potter AW, Chandrasekhar CA. US and CT evaluation of acute pelvic pain of gynecologic origin in nonpregnant pre-menopausal patients. Radiographics. 2008;28:1645–59.

92. Petta CA, Faundes D, Pimentel E, Diaz J, Bahamondes L. The use of vaginal ultrasound to identify copper T IUDs at high risk of expulsion. Contraception. 1996;54(5):287–9.

93. Morales-Rosello J. Spontaneous upward movement of lowly placed T-shaped IUDs. Contraception. 2005;72(6):430–1.

94. Goswami D, Ravi AK, Sharma A. Missing IUCD strings: role of Imaging in locating the misplaced device. J Clin Diagn Res. 2017;11(4):1–2.

95. Kaislasuo J, Suhonen S, Gissler M, Lähteenmäki P, heikinheimo O. Uterine perforation caused by intrauterine devices: clinical course and treatment. Hum Reprod. 2013;28(6):1546–51.

96. Plunk M, Lee JH, Kani K, Dighe M. Imaging of postpartum complications: a multimodality review. AJR Am J Roentgenol. 2013;200:143–54.

97. Doubilet PM, Benson CB, Bourne T, Blaivas M, The Society of Radiologists in Ultrasound Multispecialty Panel on Early First Trimester Diagnosis of Miscarriage and Exclusion of a Viable Intrauterine Pregnancy, et al. Diagnostic criteria for nonviable pregnancy early in the first trimester. N Engl J Med. 2013;369(15):1443–51.

98. Rodgers SK, Chang C, DeBardeleben JT, Horrow MM. Normal and abnormal US findings in early first-trimester pregnancy: review of the society of radiologists in ultrasound 2012 consensus panel recommendations. Radiographics. 2015;35(7):2135–48.

99. Fadl S, Moshiri M, Fligner CL, Katz DS, Dighe M. Placental imaging: normal appearance with review of pathologic findings. Radiographics. 2017;37(3):979–98.

100. Elsayes KM, Trout AT, Friedkin AM, Liu PS, Bude RO, Platt JF, et al. Imaging of the placenta: a multimodality pictorial review. Radiographics. 2009;29(5):1371–91.

101. Masselli G, Brunelli R, Di Tola M, Anceschi M, Gualdi G. MR Imaging in the evaluation of placental abruption: correlation with sonographic findings. Radiology. 2011;259(1):222–30.

102. Chukus A, Tirada N, Restrepo R, Reddy NI. Uncommon implantation sites of ectopic pregnancy: thinking beyond the complex adnexal mass. Radiographics. 2015;35(3):946–59.

103. Zucchini S, Marra E. Diagnosis of emergencies/urgencies in gynecology and during the first trimester of pregnancy. J Ultrasound. 2014;17(1):41–6.

104. Lee R, Dupuis C, Chen B, Smith A, Kim YH. Diagnosing ectopic pregnancy in the emergency setting. Ultrasonography. 2018;37(1):78–87.

Imaging of Ovarian Disease-Related Pain

22

Kirsi Härmä and Philippe Vollmar

Abbreviations

ADC	Apparent diffusion coefficient
CRP	C-reactive protein
CT	Computed tomography
DCE	Dynamic contrast enhanced
DMN	Default mode network
DWI	Diffusion-weighted imaging
DW-WB/MRI	Diffusion-weighted whole-body MRI
EP	Ectopic pregnancy
ESUR	European Society of Urogenital Radiology
EUG	Extrauterine gravidity
FHC	Fitz-Hugh-Curtis syndrome
FIGO	The International Federation of Gynecology and Obstetrics
FOV	Field of view
FSHR	Follicle Stimulating Hormone Receptor
hCG	Human chorionic gonadotropin
ITT	Isolated tubal torsion
IUD	Intrauterine device
Ki-67	Cell proliferation-associated Ki-67 antigen
MRI	Magnetic resonance imaging
NCS	Nutcracker syndrome
OC	Ovarian cancer
OHSS	Ovarian hyperstimulation syndrome
OP	Ovarian pregnancy
OT	Ovarian torsion
PD	Primary dysmenorrhea
PET/CT	Positron-emission tomography
PID	Pelvic inflammatory disease
SLE	Systemic lupus erythematosus
SRY Gene	Sex-determining region Y
T1W/T2W	T1 weighted, T2 weighted
TDF	Testis-determining-factor
TOA	Tubo-ovarian abscess
TV-US	Transvaginal ultrasonography
UO	Utero-ovarian
US	Ultrasonography
VEGF	Vascular endothelial growth factor
WHO	World Health Organization

Electronic Supplementary Material The online version of this chapter (https://doi.org/10.1007/978-3-319-99822-0_22) contains supplementary material, which is available to authorized users.

K. Härmä (✉) · P. Vollmar
Department of Diagnostic, Interventional and Pediatric Radiology, Inselspital, Bern University Hospital, University of Bern, Bern, Switzerland
e-mail: kirsihannele.haermae@insel.ch; Philippe.Vollmar@insel.ch

22.1 Embryology and Anatomy of Ovaries

Until the sixth week of gestation, embryo's gonads are indifferent, meaning the determination to female or male gonads, which will later develop from the sex cord, has not occurred yet.

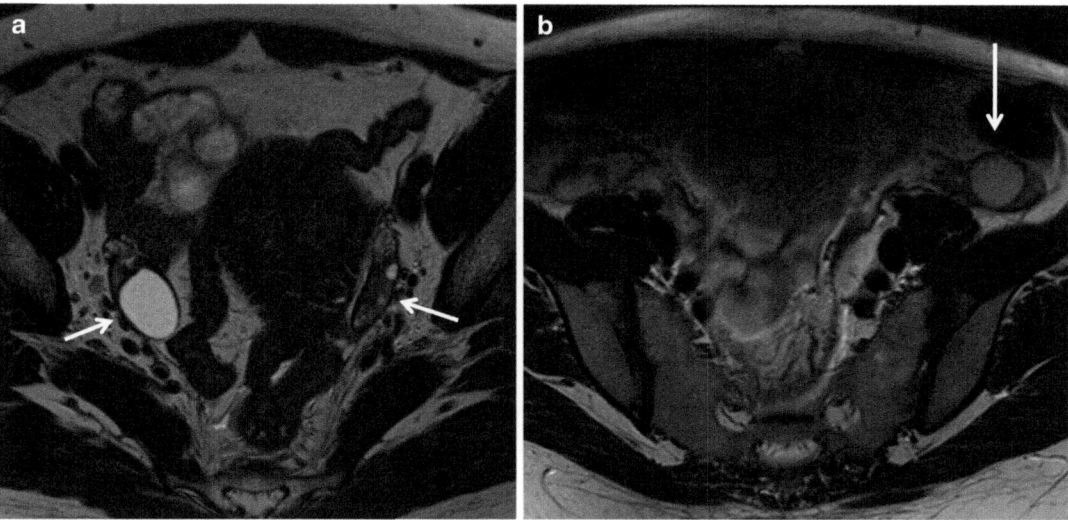

Fig. 22.1 Normal bilateral ovarian location in the pelvis in a 40-year-old patient with a 23 mm follicle cyst in the right ovary (**a**, arrows). Ectopic ovary on the left upper pelvic side wall (arrow) after ovariopexy in a 25-year-old patient with cervical cancer. Ovariopexy was proceeded before radiation (**b**)

The sex-determining region (SRY Gene) of a male embryo on the Y-chromosome leads to the expression of the "testis-determining factor" (TDF) further leading to the development of the testicles. In female embryos, based on the missing Y-chromosome and TDF, indifferent gonads will evolve to ovaries. During development, they move slightly downward to their final position. This migration results from the gubernaculum and the pronounced growth of the upper abdominal region compared to the pelvic area.

The ovaries are glandular, often ovoid, almond-shaped organs, weighing about 10 g each. When stimulated, they contain several follicular cysts. Normally they lie within the pelvis either posterolateral or lateral to the uterus. The broad ligament (ligamentum latum uteri) and the ovarian ligament (ligamentum ovarii proprium) connect the ovaries to the uterus. The first one is a peritoneal duplicature that coats the uterus and the containing ligaments, and the latter one originates from the medial part of the ovary to the lateral part of the uterus. The suspensory ligament of the ovary (ligamentum suspensorium ovarii) rises from the gubernaculum, goes from the lateral part of the ovary to the inner abdominal wall, and contains the ovarian artery and vein, plexus, and lymph vessels.

Because the ovaries are attached to the broad ligament, the easiest way to find them in a pelvic CT scan is to follow the broad ligament from the uterus toward the lateral part. Often they are recognizable as an oval thickening of the broad ligament in the lateral part with sometimes definable cysts. On MRI the ovaries are easiest to find as multicystic structures in T2-weighted images on both sides of the uterus (Fig. 22.1a). On axial images, they are not always depicted on the same level, which makes it important to be sure having them both within the field of view. In transabdominal sonography, a full bladder offers an optimal sonographic window to depict the ovaries behind the bladder on both sides of the uterus. If the bladder is empty, they are often not visible because of intestinal air laying between the ovaries and the abdominal wall. In transvaginal sonography, a bimanual technique can sometimes be helpful to move away the bowel, especially occasionally disturbing the visibility of the ovaries on the left side.

22.2   Ovarian Ectopy

True ectopic ovarian tissue is a very rare condition. In 2003, there were less than 40 reported cases in the literature, beginning in 1959 [1]. Watkins et al. describe several classification systems of ectopic ovaries including the earlier nomenclature of supernumerary and accessory ovaries. The new suggestion includes the term "ectopic ovary" and the subclassifications "postsurgical implant," "post-inflammatory implant," and "true (ectopic) ovarian tissue." A malposition of the ovaries due to an incomplete ovarian descent above the pelvic brim seems to have an association with uterine mullerian duct anomalies [2]. Secondary ovarian reposition may occur both due to postoperative adhesions and moderate to severe endometriosis leading to "kissing ovaries," meaning closely spaced ovaries behind the uterus due to endometrial implants, adhesions, and inflammation.

Intended transposition of ovaries is called "ovariopexy," which can be performed permanently or transient depending on the underlying pathology. In patients with pelvic tumors and planned radiotherapy, a transient ovariopexy with reposition to the lateral abdominal wall, out of the radiation field, can be indicated to preserve ovarian function and fertility [3] (Fig. 22.1b). Transient abdominal ovariopexy is a controversial indication in patients with severe endometriosis [4, 5]. A permanent ovariopexy may be indicated in patients with recurrent ovarial torsion and can be performed unilateral or bilateral, normally to the pelvic side wall.

22.3 Ovarian Disease-Related Pain

A number of different conditions, from ovarian or adnexal benign cysts to tumors, can result in ovarian-related pain. Most likely the ovarian-caused pain is felt in the true pelvis and in the lower abdomen. Visceral pain is diffusely localized and referred to deep somatic tissues, skin, and viscera. It is correlated with the excitation of spinal, thoracolumbar, and sacral visceral afferents, which can be sensitized, e.g., by inflammation [6]. Nociceptor inputs can trigger a prolonged but reversible increase in the excitability and synaptic efficacy of neurons in central nociceptive pathways, the phenomenon called central sensitization [7]. Abdominal wall pain is common in women with pelvic pain and may contribute specifically to the symptom of chronic pelvic pain but not with other symptoms including dysmenorrhea, deep and superficial dyspareunia, or bowel and bladder symptomology [8]. In case of large ovarian tumors or widespread peritoneal metastases, pain or bloating can be experienced in the upper abdomen or even in the shoulder due to irritation of the phrenic nerve (Fig. 22.2). Due to pudendal, obturator, or sacral plexus nerve

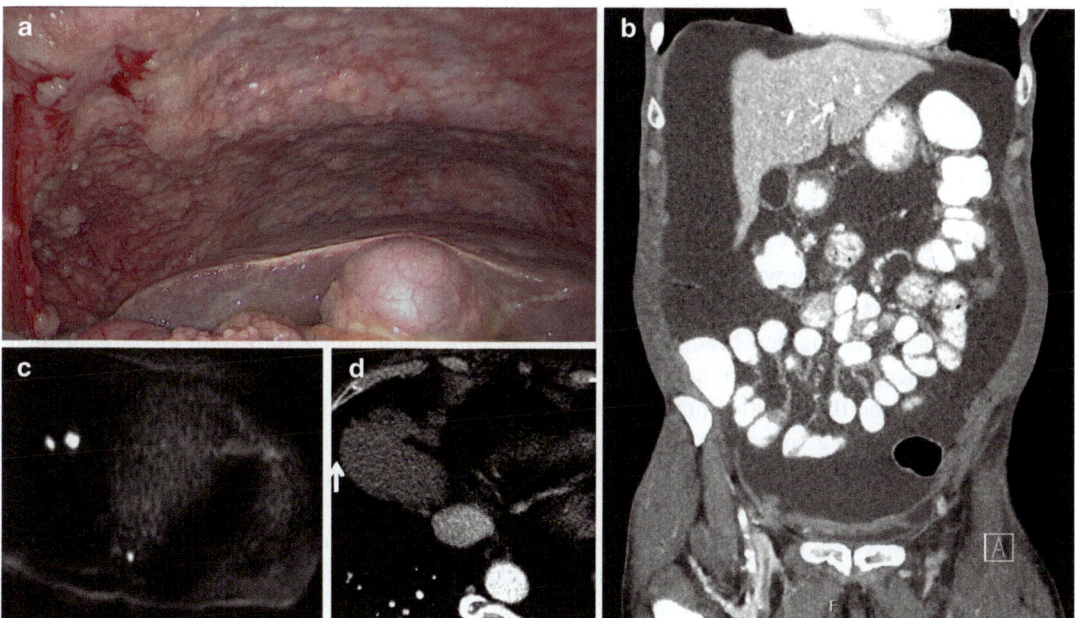

Fig. 22.2 High-grade serous ovarian carcinoma of advanced stage with peritoneal carcinosis and ubiquitous carcinomatosis of the right diaphragma intraoperatively (**a**), thus not clearly depicted on corresponding CT coronal plane (**b**). Another ovarian carcinoma patient with histologically proven diaphragmal metastases clearly seen on diffusion-weighted sequence (**c**, arrow) but missed on CT (**d**) and on T2W imaging (not shown)

irritation of the pelvic lesions, the pain can radiate to lower extremities and vulvar or perineal region. Further, simplified, due to viscero-visceral convergence of different pelvic organ afferent fibers, an inflammation of one organ, for example, of the bowel, may influence the sensitivity of the ovary.

Adnexal pain can be caused either by acute, subacute, or chronic conditions. Acute ovarian pain appears on quickly, over a few minutes or days, and, if not temporary, goes away in a short period of time. For example, women, later diagnosed with ovarian cyst rupture, sometimes describe to be suddenly awaken in the night because of the acute pain. Chronic ovarian pain usually starts more gradually, lasting then for several months. The time point of the menstrual cycle can give us a diagnostic clue when imaging patients with pelvic pain. To mention the "Mittelschmerz," the mid pain that women can experience when ovulating, as the remnants of the follicle called corpus luteum can be depicted in imaging (Fig. 22.3). Severe mid pain is known to be associated with endometriosis.

In this chapter, we describe mostly pathologic conditions, which are or can be related to ovarian-caused pain by means of different imaging modalities, not at last by magnetic resonance imaging (MRI). MRI is well known to be superior to many other imaging modalities in female pelvic imaging, in possessing an excellent soft tissue contrast and spatial and temporal resolution and is further lacking ionizing radiation. Compared to ultrasonography, MRI possesses a larger field of view (FOV). Advances in MR imaging techniques, along with the growing role of the radiologist as part of a multidisciplinary treatment-planning team, have become central in tailoring treatment options and frequently lead to modifications in the therapeutic approach, especially in patients with gynecologic malignancies [9]. In the past decade, the diffusion-weighted imaging (DWI) has technically developed and become less time-consuming and can further be easily incorporated into standard MRI. Accordingly, it is widely used in the daily clinical routine in the imaging of the female pelvis. As the DWI is measuring the random Brownian motion of water molecules voxel by voxel, it is possible to win information about the cellularity of tissues, which helps in differentiation between benign and malignant tumors or infectious conditions, even when imaging without contrast media. In the future, there is potential to broaden the indications of DWI in tumor diagnostics, treatment management decision, treatment monitoring, and prognosis assessment in oncologic patients.

Female patients with suspected pelvic or ovarian pain referred to radiologic department for imaging can challenge us as the interpreters not only in depicting the pathologies. Also overinterpreting the imaging findings can result in harm, misleading clinicians' decision of treatment management. Consequently, it is good to be aware about few clinical conditions associated with pelvic pain as a symptom but typically missing pelvic organ pathological imaging findings. For example, the painful menstruation, dysmenorrhea, is a common gynecological condition that affects between 45 and 95% of menstruating women [10]. It is speculated, whether effectively blocking dysmenorrheic pain ameliorates risk for the development of chronic pain disorders in adolescent girls. Consequently, excluding ovarian or pelvic pathologies such as infections, endometriomas, adenomyosis, cysts, or tumors supports the diagnosis of primary dysmenorrhea (PD). How does PD develop to chronic pelvic pain? It has been suggested that PD had trait changes of the white matter integrities in the cingulum bundle that persisted beyond the time of menstruation in females with known primary dysmenorrhea, so that altered anatomical connections may lead to less-flexible communication within the default mode network (DMN) and/or between the DMN and other pain-related brain networks, which may result in the central susceptibility to develop chronic pain conditions in PD females' later life [11, 12].

To the same category, pelvic pain but missing circumscribed imaging lesion belongs to the "nutcracker syndrome" (NCS): so don't forget to check the ovarian veins. Typical imaging findings of the NCS are presented in

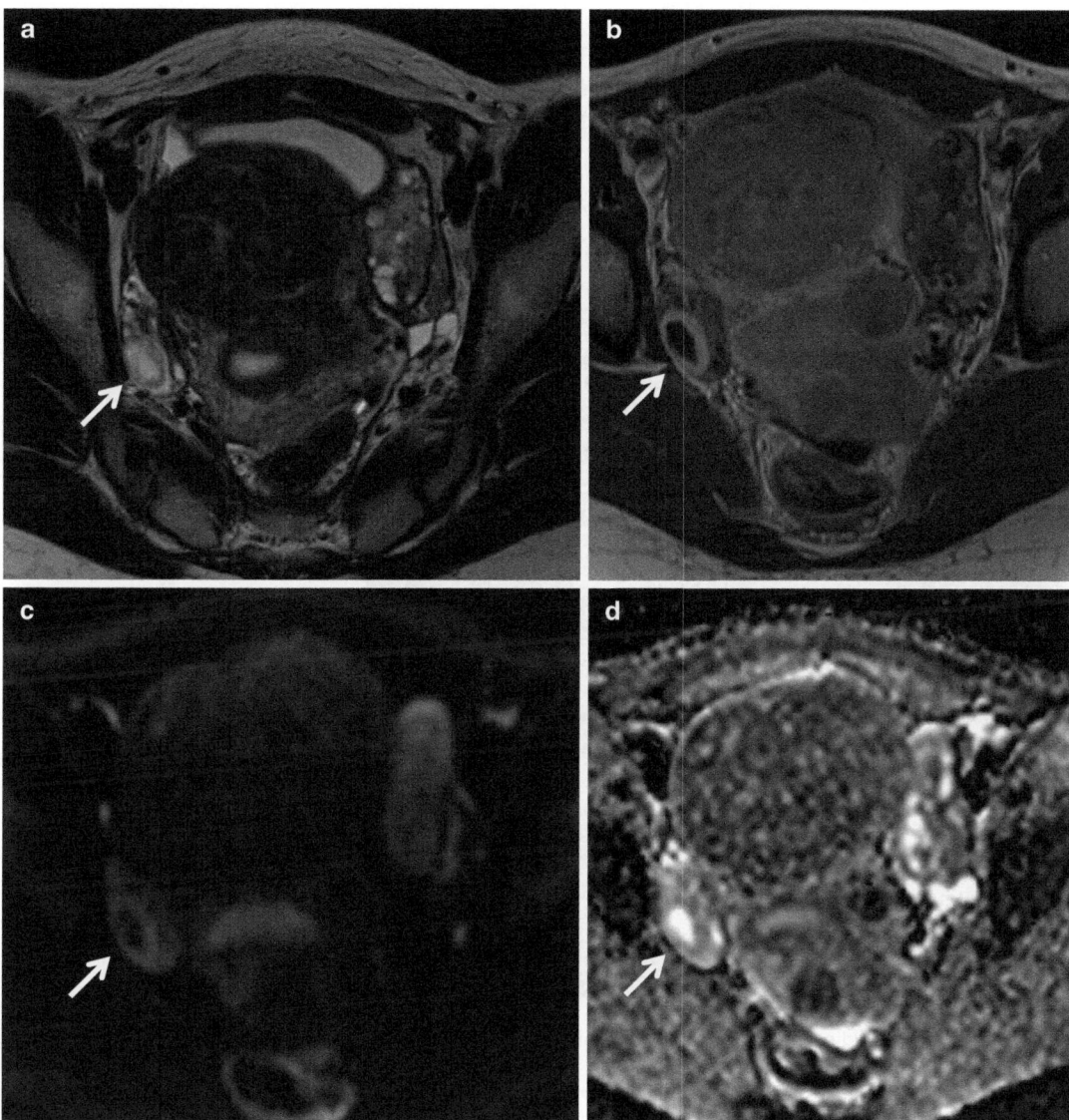

Fig. 22.3 Corpus luteum cyst. The imaging was proceeded because of uterine fibroids. Axial T2-weighted image shows a central hyperintense cystic lesion with thickened wall of the right ovary (**a**, arrow). Axial T1-weighted post-GD administration shows a thick rim enhancement of the right corpus luteum cyst (**b**, arrow). Corpus luteum cyst wall shows an intermediate diffusion restriction on DWI and on ADC map (**c** and **d**)

Fig. 22.4. The findings of NCS can be overseen in different modalities, such as US, CT, or MRI diagnosis being commonly delayed. In symptomatic patients, open laparoscopic and endovascular techniques have been developed to decrease the venous outflow obstruction of the left renal vein [13].

Female patients suspected to have an ovarian disease-related pain are often initially diagnosed by transvaginal ultrasonography (TV-US) by a gynecologist colleague before referred to radiology. The communication between radiologists and gynecologists or other clinicians as referee is underlined. Combining the gynecologic US findings, including valuable morphologic information of the pelvic lesion or information of the blood flow (power Doppler examination), is of importance. Further helpful

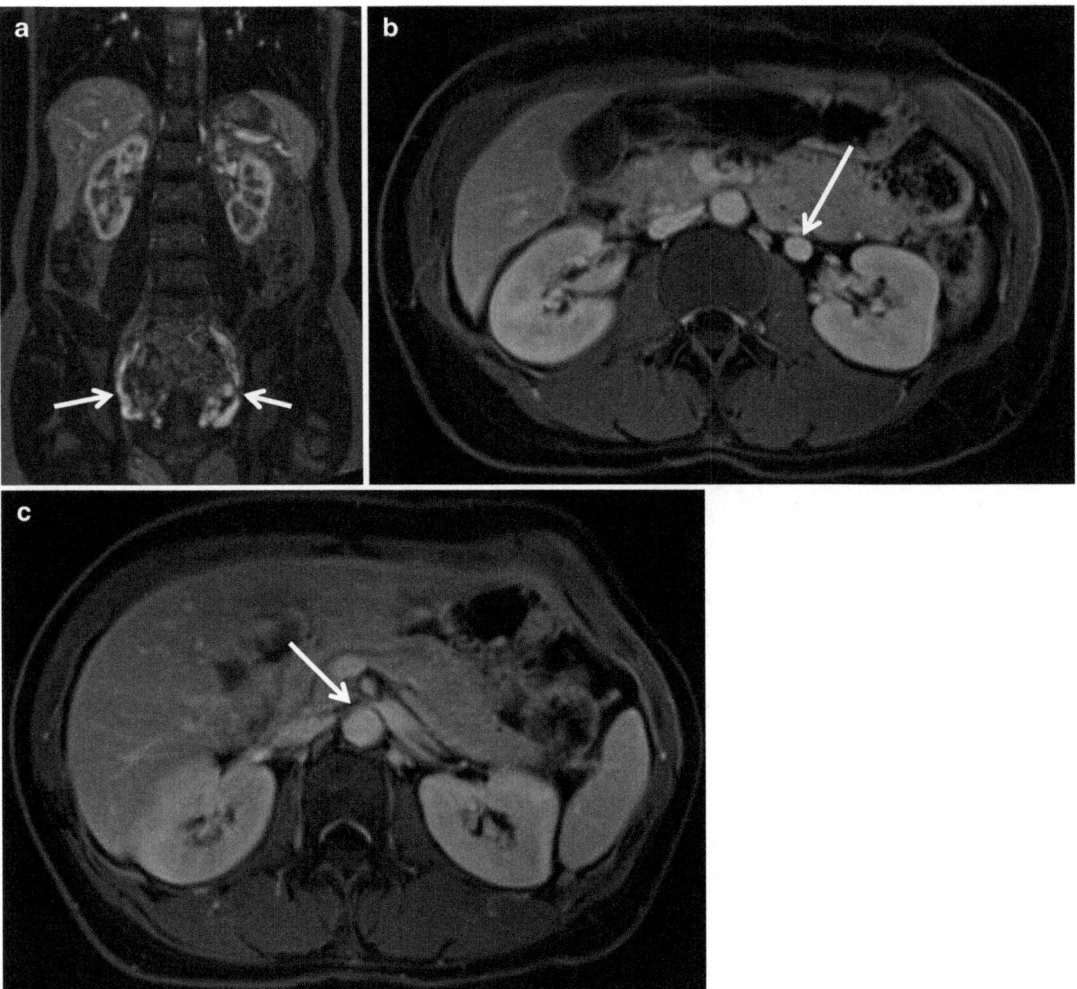

Fig. 22.4 A 35-year-old patient with chronic abdominal and pelvic pain without microhematuria. Parauterine and paracervical varicosis (**a**, arrows). Thickened left ovarian vein 11 mm in diameter (**b**, arrow). Left renal vein is compressed between the aorta and the superior mesenteric artery with a distension of the hilar part of the vein (**c**, arrow). Nutcracker syndrome causative for the pelvic pain was suggested

and supporting the radiological diagnosis are clinical findings, to mention existing peritoneal irritation or a palpable lump or elevation of serum tumor markers. The pelvic inflammatory disease (PID), for example, is in the first line a clinical diagnosis based on anamnesis, bimanual palpation, cervical smear results, and laboratory findings, imaging findings mostly being subtle in the early stadium. Available and accurate imaging modalities in diagnosing ovarian-related pain are further discussed in this chapter under different specific conditions and are also taken from Table 22.1.

22.4 Adnexal Torsion

Adnexal torsion is a rare emergency condition, accounting for 2.7% of female acute pelvic pain [14]. If not accurately diagnosed and rapidly treated, the torsion leads to ovarian ischemia and necrosis, threatening the ovarian function and fertility. The symptoms can vary a lot, and torsion can occur in female patients of all ages, including infants and postmenopausal women. A typical case history, such as acute onset of the pain after sports or coitus with vomiting and nausea, is

Table 22.1 Clinical characteristics and leading imaging features of different modalities in conditions with ovarian-related pain

Condition	Symptoms/pain character	US	MRI	CT	Infant	Adolescent	Pre Menop.	Post Menop.	Labor/tumor marker
Adnexal torsion	Acute Intermittent Pain +++ Vomiting (Ovarian mass)	Enlarged ovarian stroma Twisted pedicle (decreased ovarian perfusion)	Enlarged, T2 hyperintense ovarian stroma Twisted pedicle Thickened tube T1 bright in hemorrhage necrosis	Mass between the uterus and ovary	+	+	+	+	CRP Leu
Pelvic inflammatory disease	Subacute (Chronic) Pain ++ Discharge	Free fluid TOA Thickened tube Early stages	See US features	See US features	(+)	+	++	(+)–+	CRP Leu Cervical smear +
Ectopic pregnancy	Acute Subacute Chronic Pain + to +++	Pseudogestational sac Tubal ring structure (or in other sites) Hemoperitoneum	See US features		–	(+)	+	–	Beta hCG HB
Ovarian cysts	Acute Chronic Pain +	Thin walled	No diffusion restriction	HU > DD serous/ mucinous	+	++	++	+	HB if ruptured
Ovarian carcinoma	Symptoms in early stage lacking or indifferent Pain –,+	Cystic solid Papillary structures Increased perfusion Ascites, PC	Diffusion-restriction (in solid parts without necrosis) Type 3 curves PC	Papillary structures PC, ascites Distant metastases	+	+	++	+++	CA 125 Tati Other TM

US ultrasound, *CT* computed tomography, *MRI* magnetic resonance imaging, *Menop.* menopause, *TM* tumor marker, *DD* differential diagnosis, *PC* peritoneal carcinosis, *HU* Hounsfield unit, *Leu* leucocytes, *TOA* tubo-ovarian abscess, *hCG* human chorionic gonadotropin

often missing. It is not uncommon that symptoms can mimic other disorders such as appendicitis, pyelonephritis, and nephrolithiasis. An elevated blood cell count (>11,000 cells/mL) or C-reactive protein (CRP) can occur. In case of the spontaneous detorsion, symptoms may be intermittent and more seldom chronic. Torsion involves mostly both the ovary and the fallopian tube (tubo-ovarian torsion) though tubal torsion alone is rare. The ovarian vessels are located in the infundibulopelvic ligament, ovarian pedicle, attaching to the pelvic sidewall. Ovaries receive a dual blood supply from the ovarian artery and uterine artery. As adnexal tissue is not being fixed, tumorous growth or enlargement of the ovary can induce the twisting (Fig. 22.5). The other side of the ovary is connected to the uterus by the utero-ovarian (UO) ligament, which connects the ovary to the uterus and support it, and it also supplies blood from the uterine artery to the ovary. An ovarian mass, benign or malignant, can predisponate to the torsion. More than 80% of patients with ovarian torsion had ovarian masses of 5 cm or larger, indicating that the primary risk in ovarian torsion is an ovarian mass [15]. In proven ovarian torsion patients, torsion was suspected preoperatively in 23–66%, and 50% of the patients with suspicious torsion have got different final diagnoses [16]. Normal arterial blood flow on ultrasonography does not rule out ovarian torsion, and not every patient will have a mass on imaging or a palpable mass on examination. The patients also may have symptoms for several hours or days, and thus, ovarian torsion may be present even with a longer

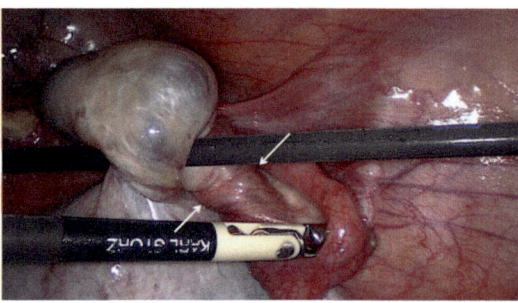

Fig. 22.5 Torsion of the right ovarian pedicle (arrows). Courtesy of Sara Imboden

duration of symptoms. Surgery is the definitive treatment and may still be effective after several hours of symptoms [17].

22.5 Imaging of Torsion

Transvaginal ultrasonography proceeded by gynecologists serves often as the first-line modality in the torsion diagnosis and is rapidly proceeded if conclusive. A trans-rectal or transabdominal US can serve as an alternative imaging modality in virgin females and in children, if MRI is not available or cannot be proceeded. Presence of free pelvic fluid, ovarian edema, or suspicious benign cystic teratoma on US has been described as sign for torsion. On the other hand, ultrasound findings suggestive of hemorrhagic corpus luteum cyst were negatively associated with adnexal torsion [18]. The sensitivities of ultrasonography for adnexal torsion vary from 46 to 74% [19] of course, dependent on the experience of the sonologists. In doubtful cases or as an alternative modality, MR imaging is an accurate technique for the diagnosis of adnexal torsion. The torsion leads to ischemic ovarian stromal edema which can be depicted on MRI as volume growth of the ovary with T2 hyperintense ovarian stroma. Due to ovarian vascular pedicle rotation, a whirlpool sign can be depicted (Fig. 22.6). Tubal structures may be thickened (>10 mm). A hemorrhagic content has clearly been considered dominating in women with proven nonviable ovaries. A vascular pedicle enlargement can also be depicted more cranially of the pelvis [20]. Interval enlargement between two imaging at different points of time and the ovarian stromal T2-weighted signal intensity turning from bright to dark showing bright T1 signal components is consistent with hemorrhagic necrosis.

Although MRI is superior in spatial and temporal resolution and in missing ionizing radiation, the diagnosis of torsion is principally possible on CT, in nonpregnant, adult females. In these cases a torsion may not be suspected in the first line, but diagnosed on the CT proceeded in doubt of another abdominal or pelvic pain etiology but torsion. Imaging features on CT such as a large ovary with a threshold at 80 mm, median

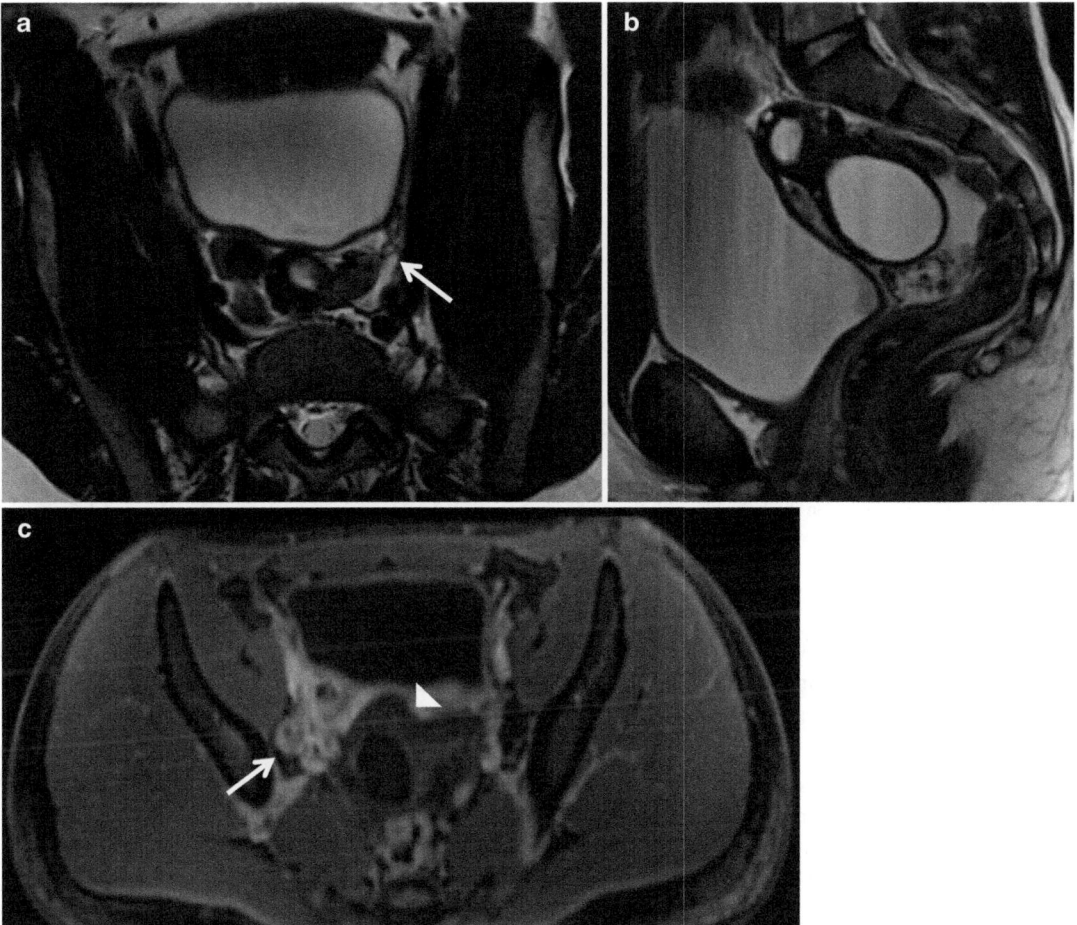

Fig. 22.6 A 14-year-old female patient with left ovarian torsion. Adnexectomy was proceeded, because there was no improvement in ovarian blood supply intraoperatively after detorsion, the ovary remaining darkish blue. Ovarian necrosis was histologically proven. Twisted ovarian pedicle (**a**, arrow). Enlarged, cystic left ovary (**b**). Right ovary on T1 postcontrast sequence (**c**, arrow). Hypoperfusion of the left ovary (**c**, arrow head)

or contralateral displacement of the adnexa, asymmetric wall thickening of the mass, and whirlpool sign are found to be significantly associated with adnexal torsion [21] (Fig. 22.7). Thus, only the finding of an inter-utero-ovarian mass was independently associated with adnexal torsion on CT.

22.6 Torsion in Pregnancy

About 10–22% of ovarian torsion occurred in pregnancy [22]. The incidence is higher at 10–17 weeks of gestation with ovarian masses larger than 4 cm [23]. The accurate diagnosis is crucial; thus, consequently both mother and fetus will undergo the operation and anesthesia. In stimulated pregnancies, where the ovaries are larger, the torsion diagnostic may be challenging. Average normal ovarian length in not stimulated pregnancies is considered 3.2 cm, compared to 5.6–8.8 cm in all following three groups: stimulated and not stimulated pregnancies with torsion and stimulated pregnancies without torsion. However, after inconclusive US, ovarian torsion could not be confidently diagnosed or excluded retrospectively with noncontrast MRI in pregnant patients with stimu-

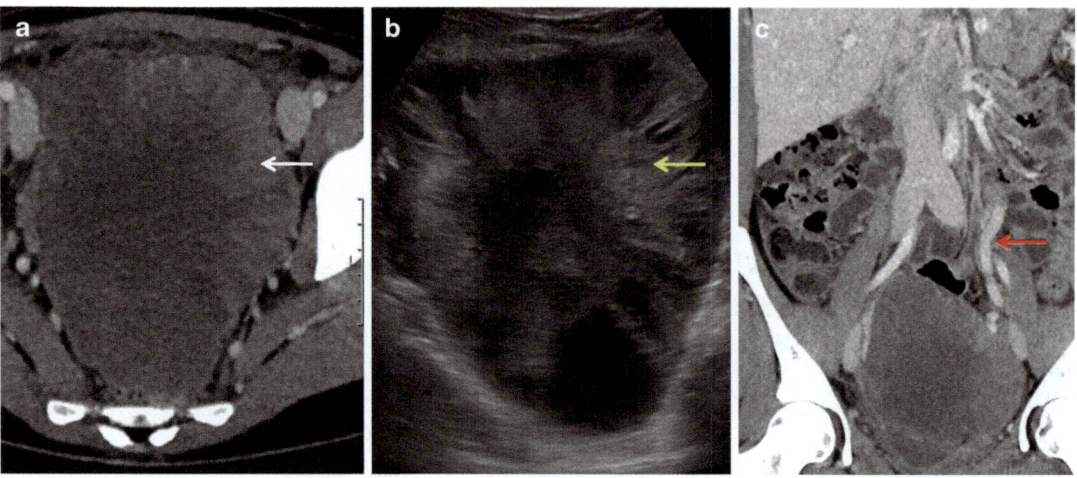

Fig. 22.7 Ovarian torsion on the left side with the severe enlarged ovary. Ovarian stroma central is showing hypodense necrosis on CT (**a**, white arrow) and on ultrasonography (**b**, yellow arrow). Thickened left ovarian vein (**c**, red arrow)

lated ovaries referred for MRI [24]. Ovarian hyperstimulation syndrome (OHSS) is very rare in spontaneous, not stimulated pregnancy; thus, multiple pregnancies, gestational trophoblastic disease, primary hypothyroidism, thyroid-stimulating hormone or gonadotropin-secreting adenomas, and mutations of the FSHR gene may trigger spontaneous OHSS with the risk of torsion [25].

22.7 Torsion in Childhood and in Adolescent

Approximately 3% of all cases of children with acute abdominal pain are diagnosed with torsion requiring immediate surgical intervention [26]. Vomiting, short duration of abdominal pain, and elevated CRP level have been described as a predictive value for the diagnosis of OT in a study with total of 80 patients with acute adnexal pathologies in order to develop a predictive score for the torsion diagnosis. Ovarian torsion patients were younger, median 11 years, compared to the patients with ovarian cysts only, 14 years [27]. Being prior to menarche was a further feature in OT patients but not in patients with cysts only. As

the treatment, a laparoscopy and detorsion should be proceeded without delay, to avoid oophorectomy or salpingectomy if still finding a viable ovary intraoperatively. In rare cases, an ovarian enlargement can occur due to precocious puberty encountering as a causative factor for OT (Fig. 22.8).

In the adolescent, a rare cause of abdominal pain includes isolated tubal torsion (ITT) and high occurrence of paratubal cysts suggesting pathologic predisposition for ITT [28]. Further predisposing intrinsic and extrinsic factors have been reported. The intrinsic factors are congenital anomalies (excessive length or spiral course of the tube); acquired pathology as hydrosalpinx, hematosalpinx, neoplasm, or surgery; and autonomic dysfunction or abnormal peristalsis. The extrinsic factors include changes in the neighboring organs as neoplasms or adhesions, mechanical factors, movement or trauma to pelvic organs, and pelvic congestion. However, ITT can also be found in a normal fallopian tube [29, 30]. Imaging findings in any modality of convoluted adnexal structures and twisted pedicle with paraovarian or fimbrial cyst in the presence of normal ipsilateral ovary are suggestive of isolated fallopian tube torsion.

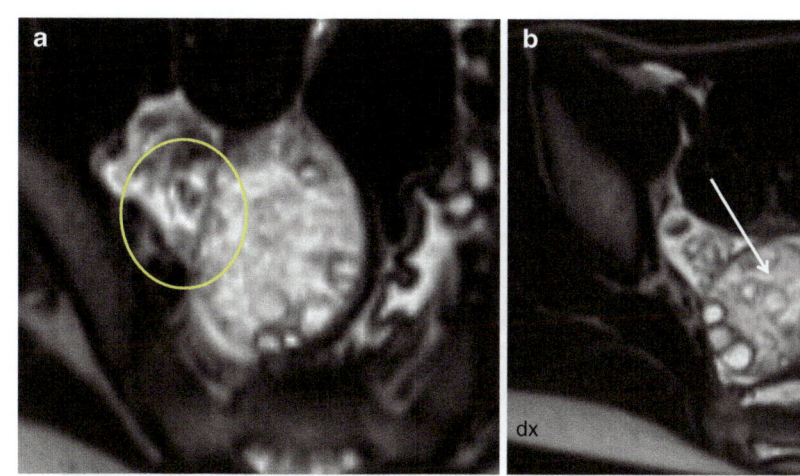

Fig. 22.8 A 7-year-old patient with elevated anti-mullerian hormone and precocious puberty with abdominal pain and defense in lower abdomen bilaterally. Ovarian volume of (right) 39 ml and (left) 7 ml. Twisted pedicle (**a**, circle). T2 hyperintense ovarian stroma right compared to left (**b**, arrows)

22.8 Torsion in Postmenopausal Women

In postmenopausal women, OT is rare, but there are a few examples in the literature, and they may both be a challenge to diagnose and be associated with increased morbidity and malignancy risk. However, ovarian torsion is more likely with a benign tumor than in a malignancy. The incidence of ovarian torsion with ovarian malignancy was <2% in reported case series [31].

22.9 Pelvic Inflammatory Disease

Pelvic inflammatory disease (PID) is defined as an ascending infection of the upper genital tract in women with wide possible spectrum of inflammatory conditions like endometritis, parametritis, salpingitis, oophoritis, tubo-ovarian abscess (TOA) or peritonitis. Infectious agents can be either sexual transmitted or not sexual transmitted pathogens, the severity of PID varying from asymptomatic to life-threatening illness. The onset of symptoms, such as discharge, pelvic, or ovarian pain, occurs more frequently postmenarcheal, which can be used as a diagnostic clue. Further symptoms might exist, such as deep dyspareunia, cervical motion tender-

ness on bimanual vaginal examination, intermenstrual bleeding, postcoital bleeding as a sign of cervicitis, or fever >38 °C. By right hypochondrial pain Fitz-Hugh-Curtis (FHC) syndrome, a perihepatitis linked to inflammatory pelvic disease is to consider, caused mostly by *Neisseria gonorrhoeae* or *Chlamydia trachomatis* infections. Even extensively studied in last decades, the relationship between PID and intrauterine device (IUD) carriers remains controversial. The evidence suggests a very low risk of PID among IUD users; thus, the insertion procedure may increase the risk [32]. A serum complement deficit as a risk factor may predispose to severe forms of PID. Low serum complement level is a frequent manifestation of active systemic lupus erythematous (SLE) [33].

The high prevalence of adverse outcomes following PID or TOA, such as infertility (25.5%), recurrent PID (16%), or chronic pelvic pain (13.8%), should alert clinicians for proper long-term care [34].

22.10 Imaging of PID

Ultrasonography is not recommended to every woman with suspicious PID but practically proceeded always, especially if the female patient is

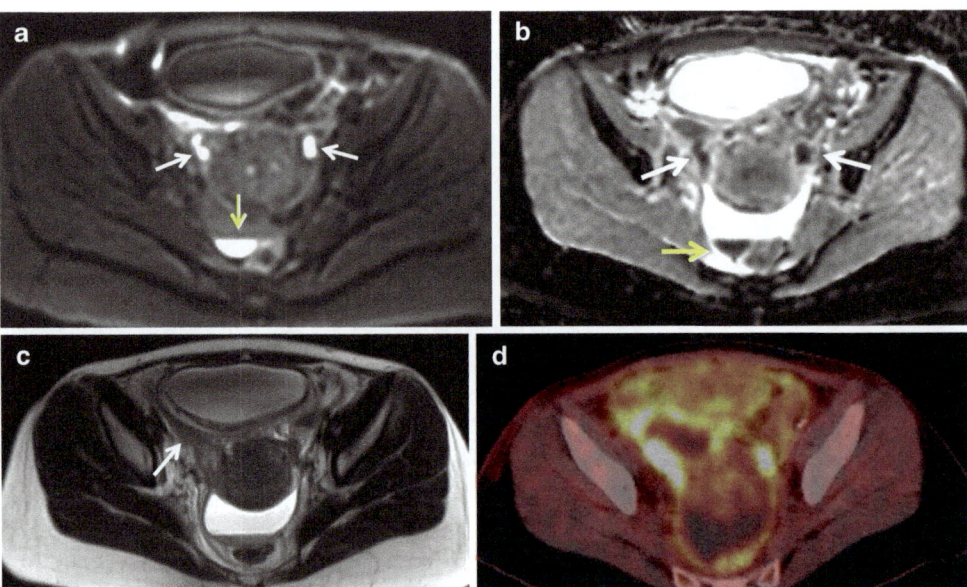

Fig. 22.9 A 31-year-old female patient with the history of cervical cancer and radiation several years ago. MRI was proceeded by subacute pelvic pain to exclude the recurrence. Bilateral tubo-ovarian abscess, clearly diffusion restricted on DWI (**a**, white arrows) and ADC map (**b**, white arrows). Thickened fallopian tube on the right side (**c**). Free fluid in Douglas pouch with diffusion-restricted fluid-fluid level (**a**, **b**, yellow arrows). Correlating findings in PET/CT (**d**). Intraoperative biopsies showed an infection without malignancy

referred to gynecologic ambulatory or emergency with acute or subacute symptoms. Further, the diagnosis of PID does not require an imaging finding, which depends on the severity of the PID.

In ultrasonography, free fluid, thickened fallopian tube, or uni- or bilateral tubo-ovarian abscess (TOA) with increased perilesional blood flow in power Doppler may be depicted. TOA may sometimes mimic a tumor, especially, if obvious infectious symptoms, which can develop gradually, are missing initially. TOA can cause a ureter compression leading to the hydronephrosis. Checking the ureters and renal pelvis is good to remember if diagnosing the PID. An ectopic pregnancy can be ruled out by a pregnancy test.

On MRI, typical features of PID are free fluid and fluid-fluid levels containing pus or debris (Fig. 22.9). An abscess formation is typically central diffusion restricted, hyperintense on DWI, and hypointense on ADC map. The peripheral rim, capsule of the abscess shows contrast enhancement. A pyosalpinx, the fallopian tube filled with pus, or hydrosalpinx can be diagnosed due to a typical "waist sign" (Fig. 22.10). In case

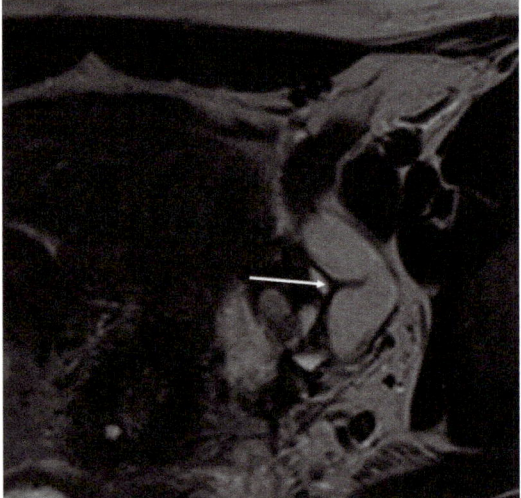

Fig. 22.10 A 30-year-old patient with hydrosalpinx. Notice the so-called waist sign

of advanced diseases, a pyometra, uterine cavum filled with pus, can be seen, also showing diffusion restriction.

Due to frequently vague and indeterminate clinical presentation of PID, CT imaging is not seldom proceeded. Unlike in mild PID, in advanced disease following imaging features, which are partly similar to those depicted in US, may occur: free pelvic fluid; thickened, over 5 mm, uni- or bilateral hyperemic fallopian tube; haziness in the periovarian fatty tissue; untypical enhancement of the myometrium; or sometimes coexisting ovarian abscess or endometrial cavity filled with pus (pyometra). In Fitz-Hugh-Curtis (FHC) syndrome, mentioned above, perihepatic edema or peripheral hepatic capsular hyperemia can be seen [35].

22.11 Ectopic Pregnancy

1.3–2.4% of all pregnancies show an ectopic implantation. An upward incidence can be seen due to utilization of assisted reproductive technology, increasing number of fallopian tube operations, rising maternal age, and more sensitive methods of diagnostic [36]. The symptoms of ectopic pregnancy (EP) not seldom last over few menstrual cycles, characterized through the intermitting lower quadrant abdominal pain, amenorrhea, and vaginal bleeding or spotting and in advanced gestation also through a hypovolemic shock. Because EP can cause severe morbidity and mortality, it is crucial to rule out the pregnancy in fertile aged females with pelvic pain symptomatic. As soon as the pregnancy test is positive and no uterine intracavitary pregnancy is seen in the imaging, ectopic pregnancy has to be excluded or suspected. In uncertain cases, the blood level of beta hCG must definitely be repeated in order to differentiate between very early normal pregnancy, failed pregnancy, and EP. Most common localization of EP is in the ampulla of the fallopian tube (Fig. 22.11). Unusual implantation sites may occur, such as angular, interstitial, cornual, cervical, ovarian, or cesarean scar sites. Ovarian pregnancy (OP) is a rare form of ectopic pregnancy, being found in only 3% of all ectopic pregnancies [37].

Ectopic pregnancy findings are seldom seen on MRI, because the patients with suspected EP are usually referred directly to the gynecologic department and rapidly treated after clinical and US diagnostic. Of course, unintentionally, CT or MRI can be proceeded if other diagnoses than EP are suspected. However, magnetic resonance imaging has gained popularity as an imaging tool for evaluating pregnant patients and as a problem-solving tool in special circumstances, including ectopic pregnancy [38]. MRI can confirm abnormal implantation site and distinguish rupture from non-rupture cases before management. Other benefits include absence of ionizing radiation, superb soft tissue contrast, and sensitivity sufficient for identifying hemorrhage and its stages. A gestational saclike structure within the ovary frequently containing acute hemorrhage with low signal intensity on T2-weighted images and normal fallopian tubes is a suggestive imaging feature of ovarian pregnancy on MRI [39]. To establish a correct diagnosis may still be challenging by several existing ovarian conditions other than OP mimicking it, such as corpus luteal cyst, endometrioma, ovarian tumor, or distal tubal ectopic pregnancy. Of course, if the embryo or clear yolk sac is visible, the diagnosis will be easier to make; otherwise, it will be assured at surgery. Abdominal cavity or retroperitoneal pregnancies occur extremely rare; for the last mentioned, interventions such as cesarean section, induced abortion, or embryo transfer are being hypothesized as causative mechanisms [40]. At advanced gestation age, the risk of the rupture of ectopic pregnancy increases, leading consecutively to intra-abdominal bleeding, diagnosed on emergency CT, showing hemoperitoneum with or without contrast extravasation surrounding the uterus but lacking the identification of the gestational sac due to low soft tissue resolution (Fig. 22.12).

22.12 Ovarian Cysts and Indeterminate Adnexal Masses

Ovarian functional cysts are common adnexal masses of female patients, especially in women in reproductive age. They are often asymptomatic and depicted as imaging for other pelvic or

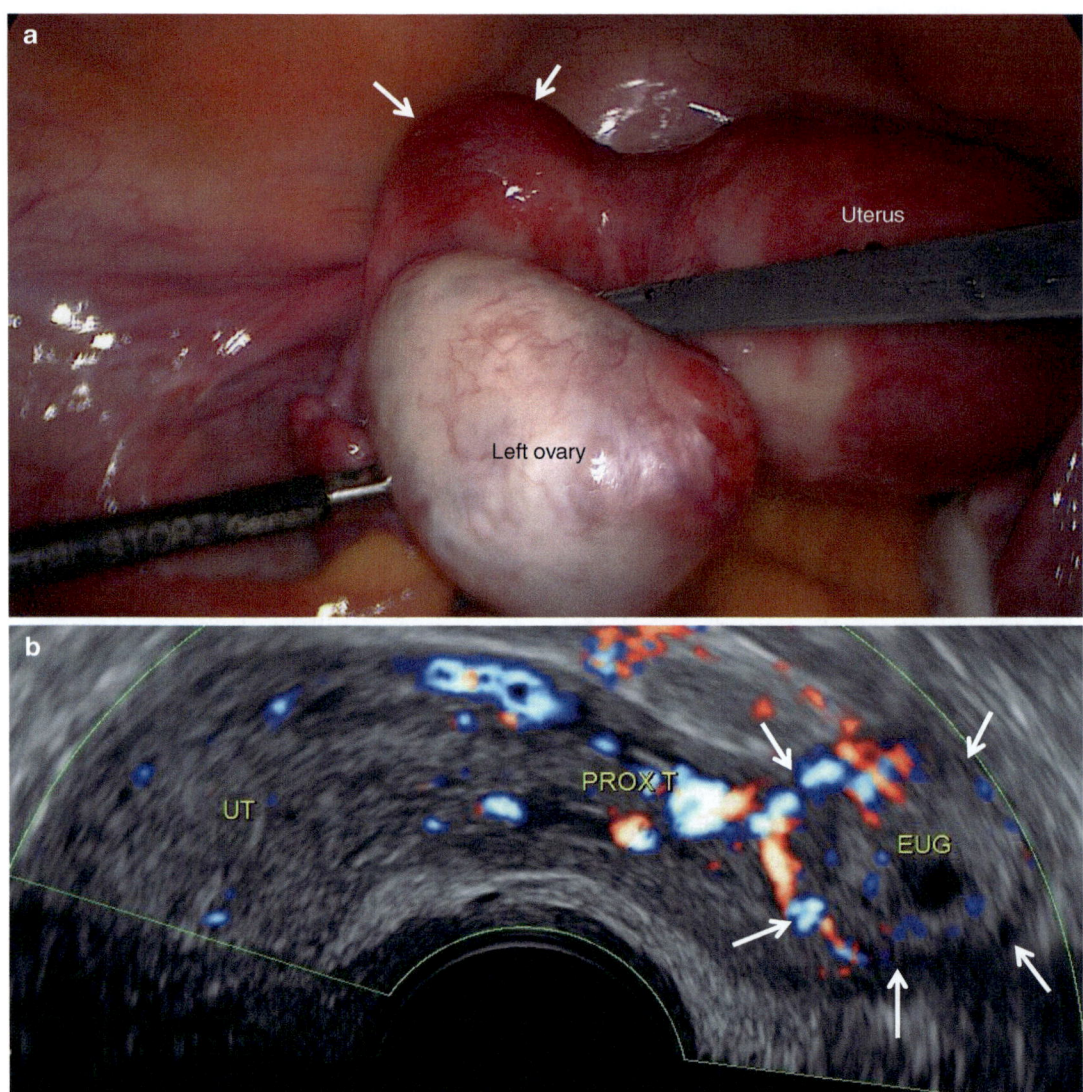

Fig. 22.11 A 22-year-old woman presented with pelvic pain and ectopic pregnancy intraoperatively (**a**, arrows). Ultrasonography shows an ectopic pregnancy = extrauterine gravidity (EUG) in the left fallopian tube with an echogenic ring showing the typical "ring of fire" peripheral vascularity on color Doppler, with internal echoes (**b**, arrows). Courtesy of Sara Imboden

abdominal conditions is proceeded. Gynecologists are not keen to call simple ovarian follicles measuring under 30 mm as cysts. Most common benign, not functional, ovarian cysts are ovarian serous and ovarian mucinous cystadenoma (Fig. 22.13). With the growing size or due to torsion or hemorrhage or even rupture, ovarian cysts can show a pain symptomatic. Typical morphologic imaging features for simple ovarian cysts and benign ovarian cystic lesions are thin, non-irregular internal septa or wall, missing papillary structures, and missing perfusion inside the lesion. Benign cysts are un- or hypo-echogenic in the ultrasonography and T2 bright in the MRI. T1 fat-saturated hyperintense, endometriotic chocolate cysts are handled in their own chapter. The Female Pelvic Imaging Working Group of the European Society of Urogenital Radiology (ESUR) published an update of their recommendations of MRI of the sonographically indeterminate adnexal

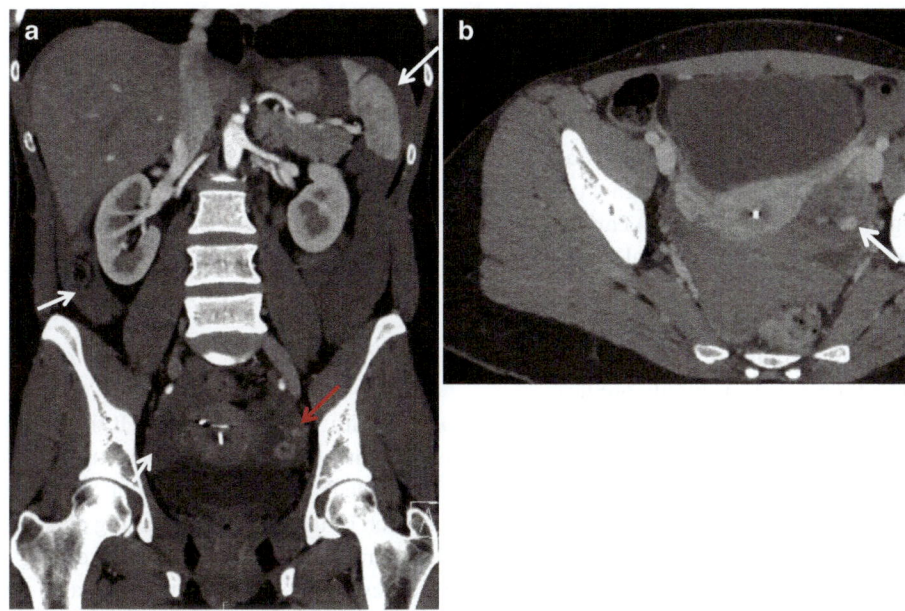

Fig. 22.12 A 31-year-old woman with major peritoneal irritation was referred to emergency CT, on which a massive hematoperitoneum was diagnosed (**a**, arrows). An inhomogeneous mass in the fossa ovarica showed a contrast extravasation, an active bleeding component, in the arterial phase (**a**, red arrow), consequently pooling in the venous phase (**b**, arrow). Intraoperatively, an ectopic pregnancy was proven. Retrospectively, beta hCG was elevated

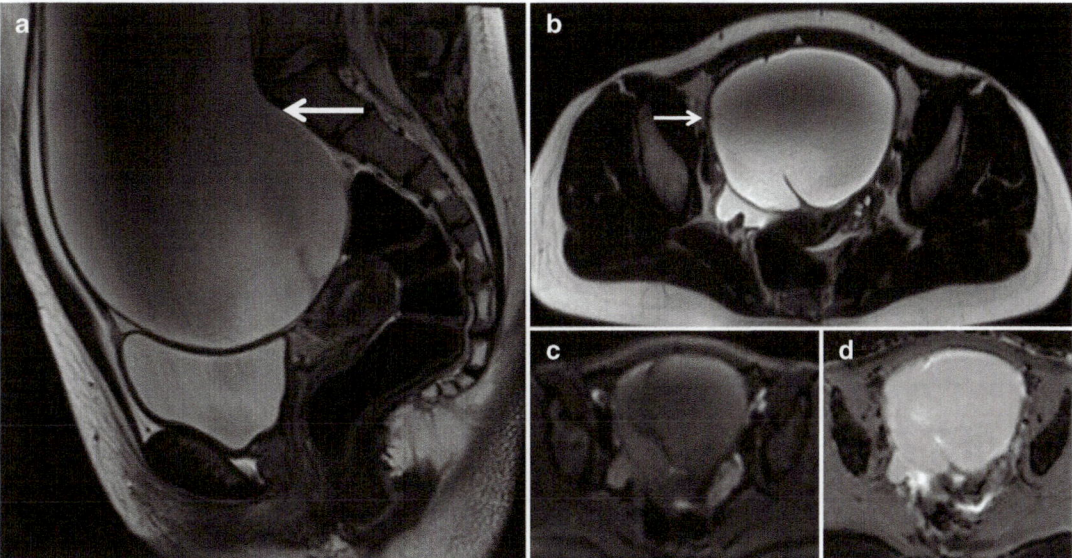

Fig. 22.13 A 16-year-old female patient with histopathologically proven benign mucinous cystadenoma. T2W coronal and axial plane show a large hyperintense cystic tumor (**a, b**, arrows) with small amount of free fluid and a normal contralateral ovary. No diffusion restriction or papillary structures were depicted (**c** and **d**, DWI ($b = 800$) and ADC map), ADC value 3.0×10^{-3} mm^2/s

mass: "An algorithmic approach using sagittal T2 and a set of transaxial T1 and T2WI allows categorization of adnexal masses in three types according to its predominant signal characteristics. T1 'bright' masses due to fat or blood content can be simply and effectively determined using a combination of T1W, T2W and FST1W imaging. When there is concern for a solid component within such a mass, it requires additional assessment as for a complex cystic or cystic-solid mass. For low T2 solid adnexal masses, DWI is now recommended. Such masses with low DWI signal on high b value image (e.g. > b 1000 s/mm^2) can be regarded as benign. Any other solid adnexal mass, displaying intermediate or high DWI signal, requires further assessment by (CE) T1W imaging, ideally with dynamic contrast-enhanced MR (DCE MR), where a type 3 curve is highly predictive of malignancy. For complex cystic or cystic-solid masses, both DWI and CET1W—preferably DCE MRI—is recommended. Characteristic enhancement curves of solid components can discriminate between lesions that are highly likely malignant and highly likely benign" [41]. Neither CT nor MR contrast media is recommended to pregnant patients. Therefore, the diffusion-weighted imaging can be helpful to characterize adnexal lesions in pregnant women (Fig. 22.14).

Also you need to bear in mind that when characterizing ovarian masses, they have to be proven to originate from the ovary or the adnexa. In differentiation of ovarian versus uterine origin, the so-called beak sign may be helpful (Fig. 22.15). Lesions embracing from the uterus, bowel, mesenterium, or presacral space can also mimic lesions of ovarian origin.

22.13 Ovarian Cancer

The World Health Organization (WHO) revised the classification of ovarian, fallopian tube, and primary peritoneal cancer, in parallel with the implementation of the new FIGO staging classification (the International Federation of Gynecology and Obstetrics, Fédération Internationale de Gynécologie et d'Obstétrique), taking account the recent findings on the origin, pathogenesis, and prognosis of different ovarian cancer subtypes. The tubal origin of hereditary and some non-

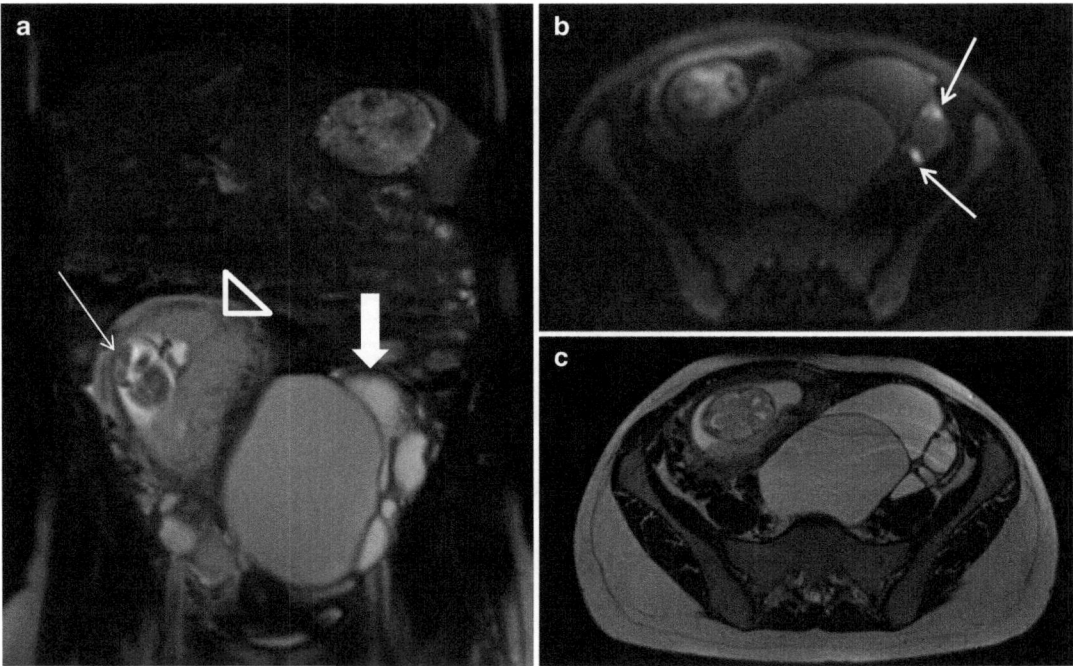

Fig. 22.14 Histopathologically proven multilocular, cystic borderline tumor in a pregnant woman of 16 weeks gestational age. The differential diagnosis on the basis on MR alone would include decidualized endometriosis and luteoma, a "do not touch" lesion. Coronal T2W (**a**, placenta, arrowhead; fetus, arrow; tumor, thick arrow). On axial DWI hyperintense restricted cystic wall structures (**b**, arrows), which can be seen on axial T2W as smooth nodules (**c**)

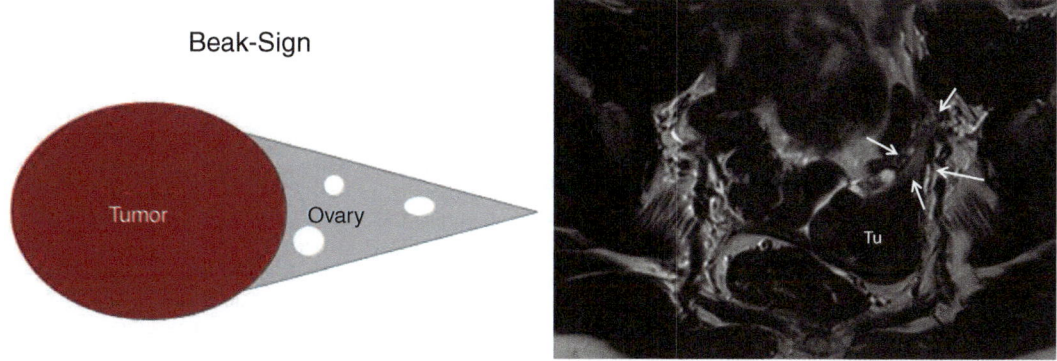

Fig. 22.15 Ovarian dysgerminoma left with "beak sign." Ovary (arrows). Tumor (Tu)

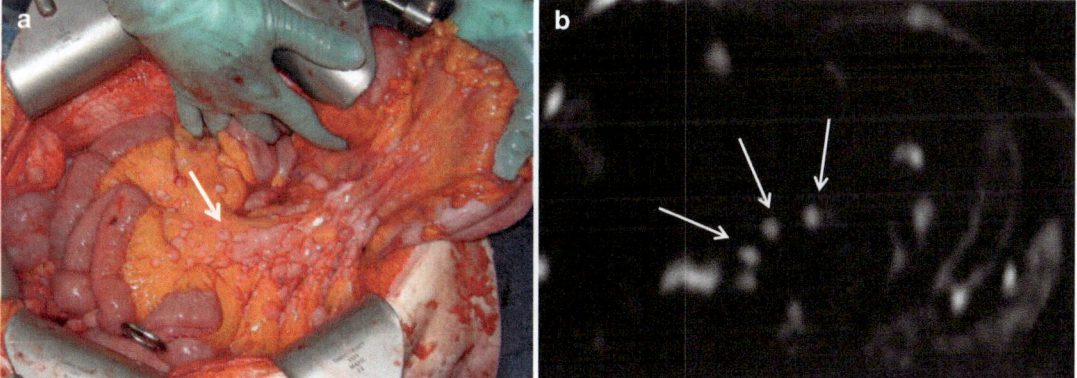

Fig. 22.16 Histopathologically proven mesenterial metastases in a patient with ovarian carcinosarcoma. Intraoperative situs with multiple carcinomatous mesenterial lymph nodes (**a**). Preoperative diffusion-weighted sequence (b = 800) shows prominent hyperintense mesenterial lymph nodes (**b**, arrows)

hereditary high-grade serous cancers is mentioned in contrast to hitherto theory of mesothelial origin of ovarian cancer [42]. A new subgroup are seromucinous tumors.

Unfortunately, the pain is not a common symptom in ovarian cancer patients, and further signs and symptoms are known to be unspecific, not often mimicking symptoms caused by other pathologic conditions such as gall bladder or irritable bowel disease or urinary problems. Consequently about 75% of ovarian cancers are found in advanced stages III or IV (Fig. 22.16). Imaging plays a very important role in the pretherapeutic staging, which guides the clinicians to the treatment strategy in ovarian cancer. Diffusion-weighted whole-body MRI (DW-WB/MRI) was recently shown to be significantly

superior to contrast-enhanced CT imaging in differentiating between benign and malignant ovarian lesions, in staging accuracy, and in assessment of operability [43]. This consequently leads to upstaging of the OC by MRI, possibly changing the choice of treatment, for example, between the neoadjuvant chemotherapy and the primary debulking surgery. The functional imaging technique DWI delivers not only qualitative but quantitative information of the primary tumor characteristics and the metastatic sites, capturing the biological heterogeneity of the ovarian cancer disease group. Moreover, correlating with tissue cellularity, lower ADC values in ovarian cancer primary tumors are shown to be significantly associated with high Ki-67 and low VEGF expression showing poorer 3-year survival in ovarian cancer patients [44]. If proven in larger studies, these new considerations may have potential to broaden the indications of diffusion-weighted imaging in tumor diagnostic, treatment management decision, treatment monitoring, and prognosis assessment in oncologic and also in ovarian cancer patients. Consequently, the future tumor boards may not just show pictures, but the broad expertise of radiology will be a part of the data, analyzed by the specific methods of the data science.

References

1. Watkins BP, Kothari SN. True ectopic ovary: a case and review. Arch Gynecol Obstet. 2004;269(2):145–6.
2. Allen JW, Cardall S, Kittijarukhajorn M, Siegel CL. Incidence of ovarian maldescent in women with mullerian duct anomalies: evaluation by MRI. AJR Am J Roentgenol. 2012;198(4):W381–5.
3. Moawad NS, Santamaria E, Rhoton-Vlasak A, Lightsey JL. Laparoscopic ovarian transposition before pelvic cancer treatment: ovarian function and fertility preservation. J Minim Invasive Gynecol. 2017;24(1):28–35.
4. Poncelet C, Ducarme G, Yazbeck C, Madelenat P, Carbonnel M. Safety of transient abdominal ovariopexy in patients with severe endometriosis. Int J Gynaecol Obstet. 2012;118(2):120–2.
5. Darai E, Touboul C, Ballester M, Poncelet C. Can ovariopexy at the end of surgery for endometriosis be recommended? A case report. J Reprod Med. 2012;57(1–2):81–4.
6. Janig W, Habler HJ. Physiology and pathophysiology of visceral pain. Schmerz. 2002;16(6):429–46.
7. Woolf CJ. Central sensitization: implications for the diagnosis and treatment of pain. Pain. 2011;152(3 Suppl):S2–15.
8. Mui J, Allaire C, Williams C, Yong PJ. Abdominal wall pain in women with chronic pelvic pain. J Obstet Gynaecol Can. 2016;38(2):154–9.
9. Sala E, Rockall AG, Freeman SJ, Mitchell DG, Reinhold C. The added role of MR imaging in treatment stratification of patients with gynecologic malignancies: what the radiologist needs to know. Radiology. 2013;266(3):717–40.
10. Iacovides S, Avidon I, Baker FC. What we know about primary dysmenorrhea today: a critical review. Hum Reprod Update. 2015;21(6):762–78.
11. Liu J, Liu H, Mu J, Xu Q, Chen T, Dun W, et al. Altered white matter microarchitecture in the cingulum bundle in women with primary dysmenorrhea: a tract-based analysis study. Hum Brain Mapping. 2017;38(9):4430–43.
12. Liu P, Liu Y, Wang G, Li R, Wei Y, Fan Y, et al. Changes of functional connectivity of the anterior cingulate cortex in women with primary dysmenorrhea. Brain Imaging Behav. 2017;12(3):710–7.
13. Velasquez CA, Saeyeldin A, Zafar MA, Brownstein AJ, Erben Y. A systematic review on management of nutcracker syndrome. J Vasc Surg Venous Lymphat Disord. 2018;6(2):271–8.
14. Hibbard LT. Adnexal torsion. Am J Obstet Gynecol. 1985;152(4):456–61.
15. Huang C, Hong MK, Ding DC. A review of ovary torsion. Ci Ji Yi Xue Za Zhi. 2017;29(3):143–7.
16. Anders JF, Powell EC. Urgency of evaluation and outcome of acute ovarian torsion in pediatric patients. Arch Pediatr Adolesc Med. 2005;159(6):532–5.
17. Robertson JJ, Long B, Koyfman A. Myths in the evaluation and management of ovarian torsion. J Emerg Med. 2017;52(4):449–56.
18. Melcer Y, Maymon R, Pekar-Zlotin M, Pansky M, Smorgick N. Clinical and sonographic predictors of adnexal torsion in pediatric and adolescent patients. J Pediatr Surg. 2017;53(7):1396–8.
19. Wilkinson C, Sanderson A. Adnexal torsion -- a multimodality imaging review. Clin Radiol. 2012;67(5):476–83.
20. Beranger-Gibert S, Sakly H, Ballester M, Rockall A, Bornes M, Bazot M, et al. Diagnostic value of MR imaging in the diagnosis of adnexal torsion. Radiology. 2016;279(2):461–70.
21. Mandoul C, Verheyden C, Curros-Doyon F, Rathat G, Taourel P, Millet I. Diagnostic performance of CT signs for predicting adnexal torsion in women presenting with an adnexal mass and abdominal pain: a case-control study. Eur J Radiol. 2018;98:75–81.
22. Ding DC, Chen SS. Conservative laparoscopic management of ovarian teratoma torsion in a young woman. J Chin Med Assoc. 2005;68(1):37–9.
23. Yen CF, Lin SL, Murk W, Wang CJ, Lee CL, Soong YK, et al. Risk analysis of torsion and malignancy for adnexal masses during pregnancy. Fertil Steril. 2009;91(5):1895–902.
24. Asch E, Wei J, Mortele KJ, Humm K, Thornton K, Levine D. Magnetic resonance imaging performance for diagnosis of ovarian torsion in pregnant women with stimulated ovaries. Fertil Res Pract. 2017;3:13-017-0040-2. eCollection 2017.
25. Gil Navarro N, Garcia Grau E, Pina Perez S, Ribot Luna L. Ovarian torsion and spontaneous ovarian hyperstimulation syndrome in a twin pregnancy: a case report. Int J Surg Case Rep. 2017;34:66–8.
26. Breech LL, Hillard PJ. Adnexal torsion in pediatric and adolescent girls. Curr Opin Obstet Gynecol. 2005;17(5):483–9.
27. Bolli P, Schadelin S, Holland-Cunz S, Zimmermann P. Ovarian torsion in children: development of a predictive score. Medicine (Baltimore). 2017;96(43):e8299.
28. Webster KW, Scott SM, Huguelet PS. Clinical predictors of isolated tubal torsion: a case series. J Pediatr Adolesc Gynecol. 2017;30(5):578–81.

29. Gross M, Blumstein SL, Chow LC. Isolated fallopian tube torsion: a rare twist on a common theme. AJR Am J Roentgenol. 2005;185(6):1590–2.

30. Krissi H, Shalev J, Bar-Hava I, Langer R, Herman A, Kaplan B. Fallopian tube torsion: laparoscopic evaluation and treatment of a rare gynecological entity. J Am Board Fam Pract. 2001;14(4):274–7.

31. Rotoli JM. Abdominal pain in the post-menopausal female: is ovarian torsion in the differential? J Emerg Med. 2017;52(5):749–52.

32. Hubacher D. Intrauterine devices & infection: review of the literature. Indian J Med Res. 2014;140(1):S53–7.

33. Rueda DA, Aballay L, Orbea L, Carrozza DA, Finocchietto P, Hernandez SB, et al. Fitz-Hugh-Curtis syndrome caused by gonococcal infection in a patient with systemic lupus erythematous: a case report and literature review. Am J Case Rep. 2017;18:1396–400.

34. Chayachinda C, Rekhawasin T. Reproductive outcomes of patients being hospitalised with pelvic inflammatory disease. J Obstet Gynaecol. 2017;37(2):228–32.

35. Spain J, Rheinboldt M. MDCT of pelvic inflammatory disease: a review of the pathophysiology, gamut of imaging findings, and treatment. Emerg Radiol. 2017;24(1):87–93.

36. Taran FA, Kagan KO, Hubner M, Hoopmann M, Wallwiener D, Brucker S. The diagnosis and treatment of ectopic pregnancy. Dtsch Arztebl Int. 2015;112(41):693–703.

37. Lin EP, Bhatt S, Dogra VS. Diagnostic clues to ectopic pregnancy. Radiographics. 2008;28(6):1661–71.

38. Srisajjakul S, Prapaisilp P, Bangchokdee S. Magnetic resonance imaging in tubal and non-tubal ectopic pregnancy. Eur J Radiol. 2017;93:76–89.

39. Tamai K, Koyama T, Togashi K. MR features of ectopic pregnancy. Eur Radiol. 2007;17(12):3236–46.

40. Deng MX, Zou Y. Evaluating a magnetic resonance imaging of the third-trimester abdominal pregnancy: what the radiologist needs to know. Medicine (Baltimore). 2017;96(48):e8986.

41. Forstner R, Thomassin-Naggara I, Cunha TM, Kinkel K, Masselli G, Kubik-Huch R, et al. ESUR recommendations for MR imaging of the sonographically indeterminate adnexal mass: an update. Eur Radiol. 2017;27(6):2248–57.

42. Meinhold-Heerlein I, Fotopoulou C, Harter P, Kurzeder C, Mustea A, Wimberger P, et al. Erratum to: the new WHO classification of ovarian, fallopian tube, and primary peritoneal cancer and its clinical implications. Arch Gynecol Obstet. 2016;293(6):1367.

43. Michielsen K, Dresen R, Vanslembrouck R, De Keyzer F, Amant F, Mussen E, et al. Diagnostic value of whole body diffusion-weighted MRI compared to computed tomography for pre-operative assessment of patients suspected for ovarian cancer. Eur J cancer. 2017;83:88–98.

44. Lindgren A, Anttila M, Rautiainen S, Arponen O, Kivela A, Makinen P, et al. Primary and metastatic ovarian cancer: characterization by 3.0T diffusion-weighted MRI. Eur Radiol. 2017;27(9):4002–12.

Imaging of Endometriosis-Related Pain

23

Lucia Manganaro, Valeria Vinci, Federica Capozza,
Amanda Antonelli, and Serena Satta

23.1 Epidemiology and Pain Pathogenesis

Endometriosis is a benign chronic inflammatory disease and often debilitating disorder, characterized by the presence of endometriotic-like tissue outside the uterine cavity and whose pathogenesis is still unclear. Several theories have been proposed such as retrograde menstruation, embryonic rest, and immunologic pathogenesis [1]; however, none of those would explain the heterogeneity of presentation which characterizes the disease, both in terms of clinical symptoms and type of lesions: peritoneal implants, ovarian cysts, and deep infiltrating endometriosis.

Endometriosis is estimated to affect about 10–15% of women in reproductive age [2]. This percentage rises up to 70% when considering women referring chronic pelvic pain which has a negative impact on the social life constituting a major public health concern [3].

From a clinical point of view, endometriosis is associated with infertility and chronic pelvic pain, the latter comprehensive of several forms, i.e., dysmenorrhea, dyspareunia, noncyclic chronic pelvic pain (NCPP), and, less frequently, dysuria or dyschezia [4, 5].

Several authors have investigated the relationship between endometriosis and pelvic pain, and different theories have been hypothesized, but still causes and mechanisms of pain in patients with endometriosis remain unclear. Interestingly, severity of disease does not correlate with pain; in fact patients with extensive disease may not refer severe pain; on the contrary, small foci of endometriosis can cause debilitating symptoms. Further studies reported no significant correlation between the rASRM stage of endometriosis and pain, while the adnexal adhesions and the presence of deeply infiltrating endometriosis (DIE) significantly correlate with pain symptoms [6–8]. However usually advanced endometriosis is more frequently related to dysmenorrhea and deep dyspareunia in comparison to early disease. In this regard, few studies have investigated a correlation between the location of endometriotic implants and type of pain (i.e., dyspareunia for the involvement of uterosacral ligaments, dyschezia for the rectum and vagina, noncyclic pelvic pain for the intestinal endometriosis, and dysmenorrhea for the pelvic adhesions in Douglas pouch).

Investigating the genesis of pain, many factors have been studied that can explain its pathogenesis such as nociceptive, inflammatory, angiogenetic, and neurovascular factors, oxidative stress,

Electronic Supplementary Material The online version of this chapter (https://doi.org/10.1007/978-3-319-99822-0_23) contains supplementary material, which is available to authorized users.

L. Manganaro (✉) · V. Vinci · F. Capozza
A. Antonelli · S. Satta
Department of Radiological Sciences,
Sapienza University of Rome, Rome, Italy
e-mail: lucia.manganaro@uniroma1.it

neuropathic mechanisms, and anatomic distortion [9]. Histological studies show that chronic inflammation promotes neoangiogenesis, neurogenesis, scars, and adhesion formation. In fact, histological analysis of endometriotic lesions, both in rat model [10] and women [11], shows increased expression of neural biomarkers (neurofilament and NGF). In agreement with this, Wang et al. [12] reported a higher density of nerves fibers within the lesions, thus demonstrating that endometriotic lesions can develop their own nerve supply, with a two-way interaction with the central nervous system [13]. Another mechanism that can be directly involved was proposed by Anaf et al., who showed a direct compression and infiltration of the subperitoneal nerves [14, 15]: a long-term compression may be implied in the genesis of chronic pelvic pain. On the contrary, Stratton et al. [16] suggested the involvement of central nervous system in endometriotic-related pain.

23.2 Imaging Modality

Unfortunately, the diagnosis of endometriosis is still delayed of 6–7 years; most women present with a negative result on clinical examination referring cyclic or acyclic pelvic pain as the only manifestation. In these cases, other causes of pain must be ruled out (mainly gastrointestinal or urologic disorders).

The definitive diagnosis of endometriosis is still represented by histologic confirmation on diagnostic laparoscopy.

However, nowadays, for a presumptive diagnosis, two different noninvasive modalities are routinely used: Transvaginal Ultrasound and Magnetic Resonance Imaging.

Ultrasound examination using transvaginal approach (TVUS) represents the first modality of choice to investigate a patient with clinical suspicion of endometriosis; few meta-analyses show a good overall diagnostic performance although it is reported that TVUS is highly operator dependent.

Magnetic Resonance Imaging (MRI) represents a second-level examination, and in the recent period, its role has been demonstrated. There isn't consensus in literature about the application of MRI and its indication, but surely deep infiltrating endometriosis (DIE) represents the most important indication [17]. Some authors recommend MRI before a surgical treatment to have a complete mapping of endometriosis lesions.

Other more invasive diagnostic modalities such as barium enema, pelvic endoscopy (bladder or rectal), and computed tomography urography are now limited to selected cases.

23.2.1 Ultrasound

TVUS is widely available, cost-effective, and therefore broadly used as first imaging approach for all pelvic pathologies.

Concerning the usefulness of TVUS in the diagnosis of endometriosis, its best results regard the diagnosis of ovarian endometriomas, usually appearing as unilocular cyst with homogeneous low-level echogenicity (ground glass echogenicity) [18]. In cases of endometriomas, TVUS show a sensibility and specificity of approximatively 80 and 95% [19].

However, in a consistent group of women, endometriosis presents an extra-ovarian localization mostly represented by adhesions and deep infiltrating implants.

Adhesions still represent a diagnostic challenge for TVUS; these can be suspected in case of reduced mobility of the pelvic organs or can be directly visualized in case of thin septa within pelvic fluid [20]. When evaluating the Douglas pouch obliteration (POD), this can be suspected in case of an absent sliding sign or in presence of the kissing ovaries sign with both ovaries fixed posteriorly to the uterus and adjacent to each other.

Regarding deep infiltrating endometriosis, US can evaluate the different locations and give several information about size and involvement of different structures. DIE refers to the presence of endometriotic implants which infiltrate >5 mm below the peritoneal surface.

Endometriotic nodules are usually reported as hypoechoic nodules with irregular borders and

Table 23.1 MRI protocol

Sequence	TR (msec)	TE (msec)	FOV (mm)	Matrix	Thickness (mm)	B (s/mm²)
T2 TSE	3000	68	260 × 260	320 × 256	4	
T1 TSE with and without FS	500	Min	320 × 280	192 × 256	4	
DWI	5000	50	240 × 240	128 × 128	4	0, 1000
Non-CE and CE T1 VIBE	150	Min	320 × 280	256 × 256	4	

DWI Diffusion weighted imaging, *FOV* Field of view, *TSE* Turbo spin echo, *TE* Echo time, *TR* Repetition time, *CE* Contrast enhanced, *VIBE* Volumetric interpolated breath-hold examination

shadowing effect. According to Chapron et al. [21], in order to guide the surgeon and provide a surgical mapping, the pelvis can be divided into two main compartments: the anterior one, including the bladder, and the posterior one, including the vagina, uterosacral ligaments, and intestine. In both locations TVUS has shown good diagnostic performance, with highest results in case of bladder involvement (accuracy of 100%) [22].

Regarding the posterior compartments, few studies have reported an overall good diagnostic accuracy of TVUS in the diagnosis of DIE (range 80–95%), especially when evaluating rectosigmoid implants [23]; however, its evaluation is strictly connected to the experience of the sonographer as shown by the great variability in results reported in literature.

When presuming bowel endometriosis, it has been proposed to perform TVUS after proper bowel preparation, which consists of an assumption of oral laxative, low-residue diet, and rectal enema; this is thought to increase the diagnostic performance of TVUS on the detection of bowel implants with results that are eventually better than MRI [24]. However, there is still no consensus about the routinely use of bowel preparation.

23.2.2 Magnetic Resonance Imaging

The role of MRI in the evaluation of endometriosis has been widely demonstrated especially in complex cases as preoperative planning [25, 26].

Its increased application has moved the European Society of Urogenital Radiology to develop a standard MRI protocol for the study of endometriosis [17]. The emerging evidences concerning technique are that there is no preference regarding the use of 1.5T or 3T magnet, but the administration of antiperistaltic agent before the examination is highly recommended. Regarding protocol, T2 nonfat-saturated sequences are essential for anatomical details and for detection of fibrotic component of endometriotic implants; on the other hand, T1 fat-saturated sequences are mandatory to identify the bloody foci which characterize active lesions (Table 23.1).

In order to understand imaging features of endometriosis in MRI, it is necessary to briefly recall its pathological characteristics; the nodules consist of endometrial glands and stroma which undergo cyclical variations in accordance with the fluctuation of hormone levels which causes chronic bleeding surrounded by a fibromuscular inflammatory reaction. The fibromuscular component is responsible for the low signal intensity on T1- and T2-weighted sequences; the glandular component determines hyperintense cystic appearance on T2-weighted sequences; finally, chronic bleeding is responsible for the visible signal alterations on T1-weighted sequences; depending on the time of bleeding, this finding will be more or less marked.

23.3 Adnexal Endometriosis

MRI can depict two different types of adnexal location: the most common endometrioma and the superficial implants along the serosal surface.

Regarding the detection of smaller superficial implants, MRI revealed to be more accurate if compared to US.

In case of a typical US appearing endometrioma, MRI should not be requested; however, it can add other information when a malignant transformation is suspected or in case of inconclusive US. In these cases when solid components, clots, or thick septa are visualized within the cyst, ESUR guidelines suggest the administration of medium contrast agent to evaluate postcontrast enhancement of the papillary projection which would be considered as early sign of transformation [27].

Specific MRI features of endometrioma are hypointense signal on T2-weighted images and hyperintense signal on T1-weighted images with and without fat saturation (Fig. 23.1) (Videos 23.1a, 23.1b). The low signal on T2-weighted images compared to other static fluid (e.g., bladder or simple ovarian cyst) is defined by "shading effect" and is explained by the presence of blood products and protein content; this sign is highly specific for the diagnosis of endometriomas

(Fig. 23.2) (Videos 23.2a, 23.2b, 23.2c). However, blood products might be present in other conditions such as hemorrhagic cysts; in these cases another helpful sign is the "T2 dark spot sign," defined as a marked hypointense focus within the cyst which is characteristic of chronic hemorrhage [28]. Cyclic bleeding is also responsible of the fluid-fluid level variably present in case of endometriomas.

Endometriomas can be multiple or single, of different sized, rarely larger than 5–6 cm [29].

Focusing on the adnexal region, endometriosis can affect also the salpinx presenting with hematosalpinx.

Hematosalpinx is usually seen as an elongated tube with hemorrhagic content (Fig. 23.3) (Videos 23.3a, 23.3b, 23.3c). The presence of hyperintense fluid seen on T1-weighted images in a dilated tube, even if not associated with other

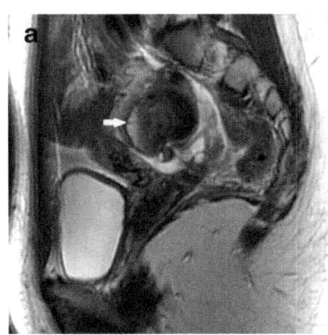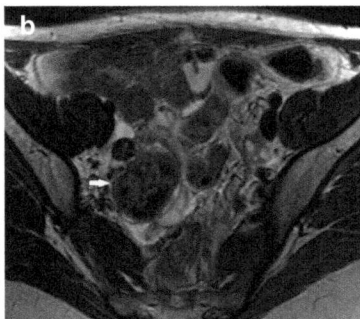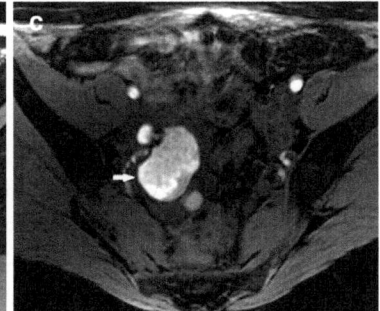

Fig. 23.1 Endometrioma: (**a**) sagittal T2-weighted image, (**b**) axial T2-weighted image, (**c**) fat-suppressed axial T1-weighted image. These images show an endometrioma of the right ovary (arrows), with low signal intensity on T2-weighted images (**a**, **b**) and typical high signal intensity on T1-weighted image (**c**) caused by the presence of blood in subacute stage

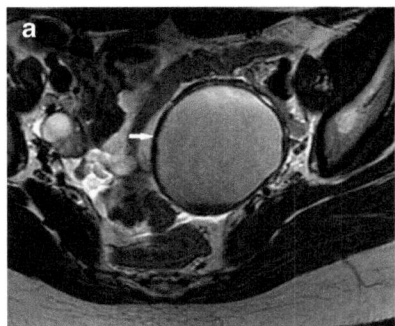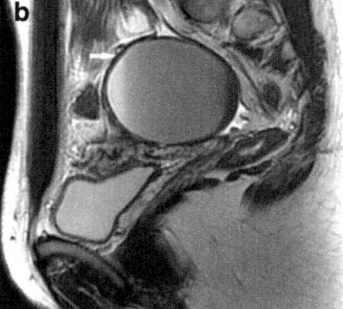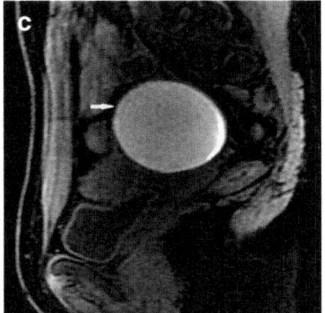

Fig. 23.2 Endometrioma with shading sign: (**a**) axial T2-weighted image, (**b**) sagittal T2-weighted image, (**c**) fat-suppressed sagittal T1-weighted image. The first two images (**a**, **b**) show "shading sign," the fluid-fluid level caused by the presence of blood products in different phases of degradation (arrows)

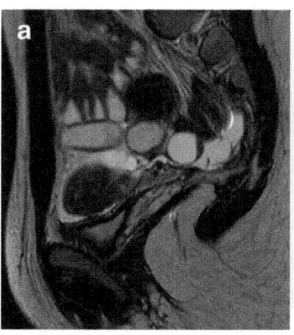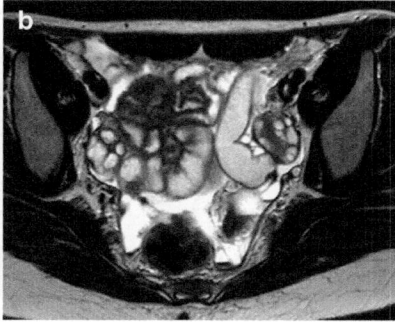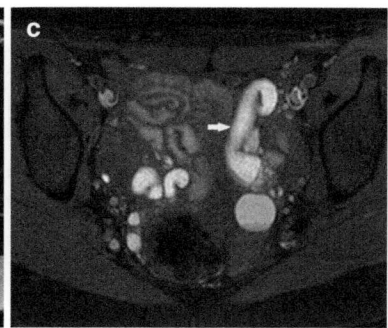

Fig. 23.3 Tubal and ovarian endometriosis: (**a**) sagittal T2-weighted image, (**b**) axial T2-weighted image, (**c**) fat-suppressed axial T1-weighted image. Condition of severe bilateral tubal dilatation. On T1 fat-suppressed image (**c**) the hyperintense signal is suggestive for hematosalpinx (arrow). A large amount of fluid is recognized (**a, b, c**)

implants within the pelvis, is suggestive of tubal endometriosis and may be the only indicator of the disease [30, 31].

23.4 Peritoneal Endometriosis

It has been suggested that pelvic pain in patients with ovarian endometrioma may be linked to other peritoneal foci. It is in fact possible that an elevated inflammatory reaction and increased production of prostaglandin (PG) can give rise to pain [32].

It may be difficult to identify serosal implants as these lesions are not always easy to recognize. Sensitivity and specificity of MRI are thus approx. 47–61% and 87–97%, respectively. If serosal implants are identified, they will be depicted as small laminar foci on the surface of the pelvic organs showing hyperintense signal on T1-weighted fat-saturated images.

23.5 Adhesions

Endometriosis is an inflammatory disease which often generates adhesions. Pelvic adhesions are thus often found in patients with endometriosis, and pain intensity varies according to the site and degree of adhesions. Redwine reported that peritoneal endometriosis and adhesions are more frequently found than ovarian endometriosis [33]. According to the revised American Fertility Society, the presence of adhesions is a significant indication of endometriosis. Adhesions are gen-

erally less frequent in stage I–II endometriosis than in stage III–IV and in women with endometriomas and peritoneal location. A correlation between adhesions and visual analog scale (VAS) scores has been reported in several studies.

MRI diagnosis of adhesions is a challenge. The most important limitation of MRI as compared to TVUS is the impossibility to perform a real-time dynamic test. MRI T1-weighted and T2-weighted images may show adhesions as spiculated low signal intensity filaments of varying thickness. These may also appear in connection with angulated bowel loops, alteration in loop diameter, fat plane obliteration between adjacent organs, retroflexed uterus, and elevated posterior fornix.

23.6 Deep Endometriosis

Deep infiltrating endometriosis (DIE) is defined as a ≥5 mm deep infiltration of muscular endometriosis implants over the peritoneal surface; 4–37% of patients with endometriosis are affected [35, 36]. The most severe forms of deep endometriosis are located in the intestinal and urinary tracts [37, 38]. In DIE, T2-weighted images show a marked hypointense signal representing the presence of fibrous tissue. The posterior compartment, i.e., the torus uterinus and the uterosacral ligaments, is involved in 70% of patients, followed by the vagina in 14.5%, bowel in 10%, and bladder in 6.5% (Fig. 23.4) (Videos 23.4a, 23.4b, 23.4c).

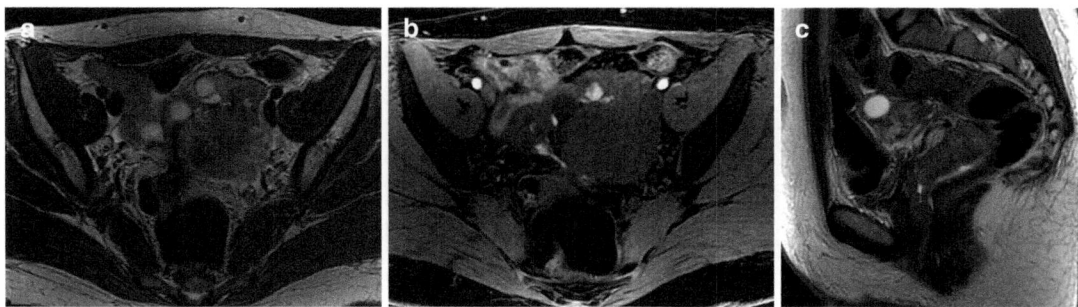

Fig. 23.4 Deep infiltrating endometriosis affecting posterior compartment with rectal wall infiltration, ovarian endometriosis and adenomyosis, T2-weighted image on axial (**a**) and sagittal plane (**c**) and fat-suppressed axial T1-weighted image (**b**). A fibrotic plaque in the rectouterine pouch with extended rectal wall infiltration is depicted in (**c**), with a plaque of adenomyosis infiltrating the serosa causing severe adhesions between the rectosigmoid colon, ovaries, and uterus (**a**). Note also hemorrhagic foci and bilateral ovarian endometriomas (**b**)

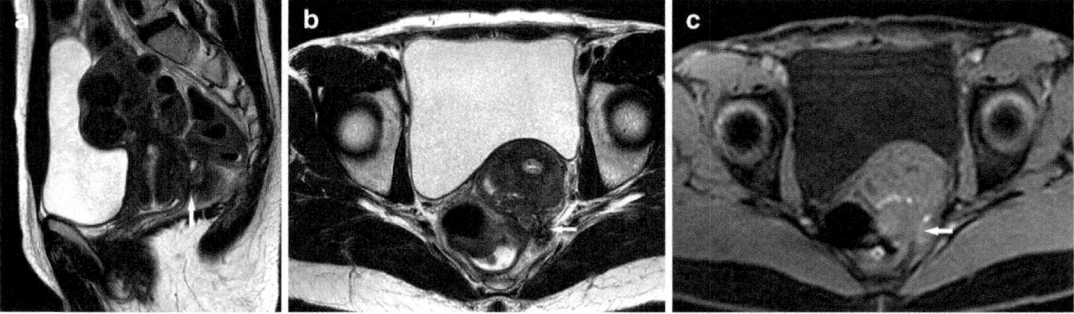

Fig. 23.5 Endometriosis of the posterior compartment with rectal wall infiltration: (**a**) sagittal T2-weighted image, (**b**) axial T2-weighted image, (**c**) fat-suppressed axial T1-weighted image. These images show an endometriotic nodule in the posterior vaginal fornix (**a**, **b**, arrows) involving torus and the uterine sacral ligaments, with typical hemorrhagic foci on T1-weighted image (**c**, arrow); **a**, **b** show infiltration and thickening of the anterior rectal wall in both sagittal and axial planes; (**c**) on axial planes is clearly evident the extent to parametrium and pelvic wall

23.6.1 Posterior Compartment

23.6.1.1 Torus Region and Uterosacral Ligaments

MRI imaging can show various signs of endometriosis in this region:

- Macroscopic endometriosis implants with fibrous plaque.
- Involvement of the rectouterine ligaments is likely if nodular lesions or increased asymmetrical thickness is found associated with tethered and/or abnormal arciform appearance.
- If there are signs of tipped uterus, posterior cul-de-sac obliteration, tethered appearance of the rectum directed toward the uterus, filaments between uterus and bowels, fibrotic plaque covering the serosal surface of the uterus, and/or elevated posterior fornix [34] (Fig. 23.5) (Videos 23.5a, 23.5b).
- MRI signal intensity of the lesions should be evaluated as intensity varies according to the histological characteristics of the ectopic tissue [37].

Three main patterns of signal intensity have been described in literature: (I) hypointense signal on both T1- and T2-weighted sequences with hyperintense foci on T2-weighted sequences which may indicate fibrosis with glandular spots, (II) hypointense signal on T1- and T2-weighted images with hyperintense foci on T1-weighted images which is caused by hemorrhagic foci within the fibrotic tissue, and (III) hypointense signal in both T1- and T2-weighted images in the presence of abundant fibrosis. This last finding may be missed on MRI or be misdiagnosed.

Kataoka et al. reported 1.5T MRI sensitivity 68.4%, specificity 76.0%, diagnostic accuracy 71.9%, positive predictive value (PPV) 76.6%, and negative predictive value (NPV) 68.5% in the diagnosis of posterior cul-de-sac obliteration [34]. Manganaro et al. subsequently reported 3T MRI mean sensitivity 93%, specificity 75%, PPV 93%, and NPV 75%.

23.6.1.2   Vaginal Endometriosis

Diagnosis of vaginal endometriosis is made at physical examination in 80% of cases. MRI appearance of vaginal endometriomas is similar to that of lesions of the *torus* uterinus: hyperintense on T2-weighted images and varying signal intensity on T1-weighted images. If the vagina is involved, MRI will reveal obliteration of the pouch of Douglas in most patients.

23.6.1.3   Bowel Endometriosis

Endometriosis affects the bowel in 3–37% of patients. In 90% of these patients, the rectum and/or sigmoid colon are involved and in descending order the appendix, the cecum, and the distal ileum [21].

Endometriosis lesions infiltrate the bowel walls from the external surface extending toward the muscular layer which becomes hypertrophic and fibrotic.

A rectal nodule with obliteration of the cul-de-sac can cause painful bowel peristalsis, rectal pain during intercourse or while sitting, and rectal pain with passing gas. Furthermore colorectal endometriosis may cause constipation, diarrhea, tenesmus, dyschezia, and sometimes rectal bleeding. Some patients may develop intestinal obstruction or perforation due to endometriosis [39]. Lesions located in the bowels are generally fibromuscular with foci appearing hyperintense on T2-weighted images (Fig. 23.6) (Video 23.6). In some cases, hyperintense foci on T1-weighted images can be recognized. In these patients, contrast enhanced MRI could provide a better differentiation between the lesion and the normal bowel [40].

MRI images showing asymmetrical thickening of the lower sigmoid wall and thickening of the colorectal wall with anterior triangular attraction of the rectum toward the torus uteri are indications of rectal involvement [41] (Fig. 23.7) (Videos 23.7a, 23.7b, 23.7c).

MRI sensitivity 84% and specificity 99% were obtained in a study of 60 patients with bowel invasion [42]. Similar values have been reported in studies using TVUS in patients with rectal lesions. However, lesions above the rectosigmoid junction can only rarely be visualized using TVUS. Endometriosis involving the small bowel is generally located in the distal 10 cm of the ileum. This location is quite rare though, occurring in only 10–15% of patients with intestinal endometriosis, whereas the appendix is involved in up to 18% of cases.

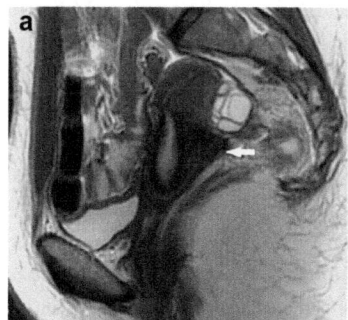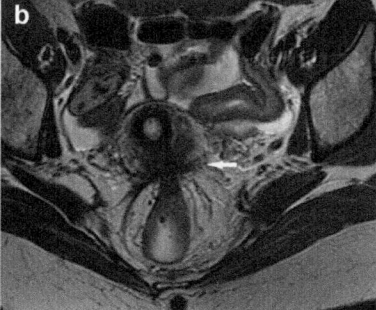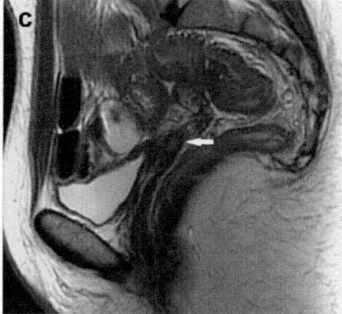

Fig. 23.6 Endometriosis of posterior compartment: (**a, c**) sagittal T2-weighted images, (**b**) axial T2-weighted image. An extended fibrotic plaque in the recto-uterine pouch (**a**, arrow) with torus and uterosacral ligaments involvement and severe adhesions between cervix and rectum/sigmoid colon (**b**, arrow). Wall thickening sign of bowel lesion is showed (**c**, arrow)

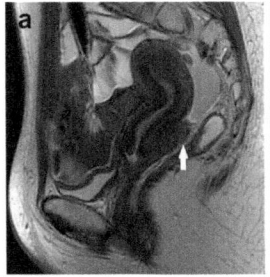 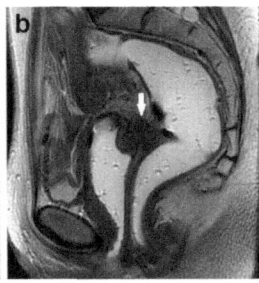 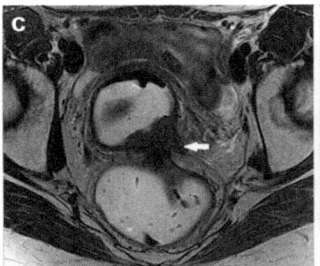 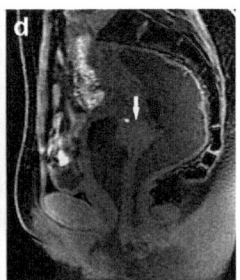

Fig. 23.7 Endometriosis of posterior compartment with rectal wall infiltration: (**a**, **b**) sagittal T2-weighted image, (**c**) axial T2-weighted image, (**d**) fat-suppressed sagittal T1-weighted image, without (**a**) and with (**b**–**d**) gel vaginal and rectal filling. Gel filling can facilitate detection of deep endometriosis in posterior compartment: an extended plaque of fibrous tissue and a nodule in rectovaginal pouch that infiltrates anteriorly the posterior vaginal fornix, vaginal wall, and posteriorly the rectal wall (arrows)

MRI should always be carried out in the study of endometriosis due to the multifocal spread of this disease.

Piketty et al. found that the patients affected by intestinal endometriosis had an increased risk to develop multifocal intestinal locations in up to 55% of patients. Histology furthermore proved association with proximal "right" bowel lesions (cecal or ileal) in 28% of patients with lesions in the rectum and/or sigmoid colon [43].

Some recent studies have been published advocating the use of contrast-enhanced MR colonography (MRC) for diagnosing endometriosis affecting the colon and rectum [44].

Patients undergoing MRC were orally administered 1500 ml of polyethylene glycol (PEG) before the examination, and 1000–2000 ml water solution was subsequently instilled into the colon using a rectal balloon catheter. Pre- and post-gadolinium contrast 3D T1-weighted images with fat saturation for bowel wall study were acquired. The authors reported the following values: sensitivity 95%, specificity 97%, PPV 91%, NPV 99%, and diagnostic accuracy 97% [44].

23.6.2 Anterior Compartment

In up to 50–75% of patients, endometriosis affecting the urinary tract is associated with lesions in other pelvic sites, and involvement of the ureter and/or bladder is usually a sign of advanced stages of the disease, as compared to patients who have not developed urinary tract invasion [29, 37].

Endometriosis affects the bladder in 6% of endometriosis patients [37]. Bladder endometriosis can be divided into two categories: extrinsic and intrinsic lesions.

Extrinsic lesions are the most frequent and confined to serosal surface; they are asymptomatic. However, they may invade the muscular layer and transform into intrinsic lesions [38].

Intrinsic lesions present symptoms in up to 75% of patients and are in many cases related to iatrogenic endometrial injuries. About 43–50% of patients with intrinsic lesions report a medical history of pelvic surgery [37]. MRI reveals focal bladder wall thickening with areas of protrusion into the bladder lumen.

In some patients, a large plaque of fibrous tissue may invade and completely obliterate the vesicouterine space (Fig. 23.8) (Video 23.8). In these cases, the fibrous tissue may be attached to an adenomyotic nodule situated on the anterior wall of the uterus. T2-weighted images acquired on the sagittal plane reveal hypointense tissue, uneven contours of the bladder, and occasional tiny hyperintense spots within the tissue representing cystic dilation of the endometrial glands. T1-weighted images may reveal hyperintense foci, a finding which is highly specific in endometriosis. Bazot et al. carried out a study of 195 patients with suspected endometriosis and obtained MRI sensitivity 88%, specificity 99% (177/179), and diagnostic accuracy 98% in the

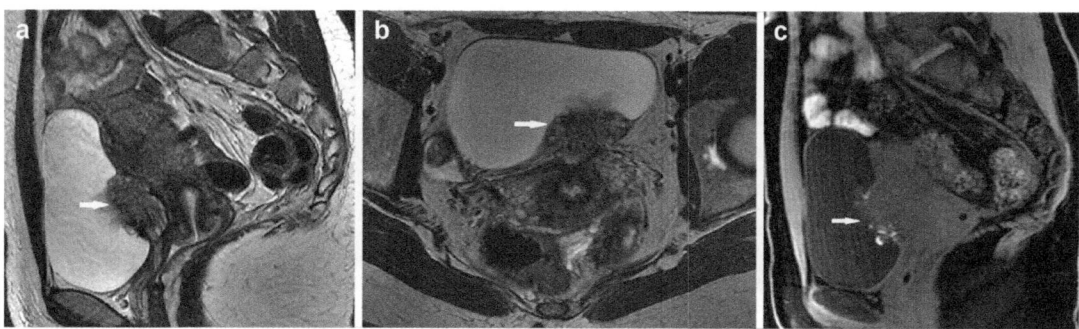

Fig. 23.8 Deep infiltrating endometriosis of anterior compartment: (**a**) sagittal T2-weighted image, (**b**) axial T2-weighted image, (**c**) fat-suppressed sagittal T1-weighted image. T2-weighted images (**a, b**) show a huge nodule in the vesicouterine pouch, between the uterus and posterior bladder wall, with infiltration (arrows); within the nodule there are the typical hemorrhagic foci, hyperintense on T1-weighted images (**c**, arrow)

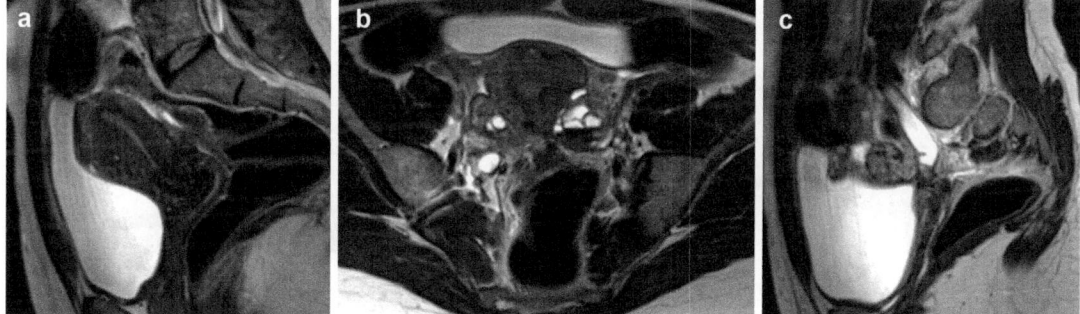

Fig. 23.9 Deep endometriosis affecting posterior and lateral compartments with ureteronephrosis: T2-weighted image on sagittal (**a–c**) and axial plane (**b**). (**a**) Shows a fibro-endometriosis plaque between the torus uterinus and the rectum with signs of infiltration; the plaque extends in the parametric region on the right, causing ureteral stenosis and consequent hydroureteronephrosis; left ovarian endometriosis is also present (**b, c**)

diagnosis of bladder endometriosis. Encasement of the distal ureter is an important problem as this condition requires *ureteral reimplantation surgery* [42] (Fig. 23.9) (Videos 23.9a, 23.9b, 23.9c).

Ureteral endometriosis is usually extrinsic, and encasement of the ureters is generally caused by endometriosis embedded in the ovary, in the broad ligament, or in the parametrium (Fig. 23.10) (Videos 23.10a, 23.10b).

In some patients, the fibrotic scar can lead to ureteral stricture, as direct extension into the ureter may result in luminal narrowing and dilation [37]. If the adipose tissue between the nodule and the ureter is not preserved on T2-weighted images, ureter invasion should be considered.

Hydronephrosis is visible on T2-weighted images, and MR urography using 2D T2-weighted sequences or delayed contrast-enhanced 3D sequences with higher spatial resolution can improve diagnostic accuracy showing the level and severity of the stricture and renal impairment [45].

The round ligaments are less frequently involved, but this region should be routinely evaluated particularly in patients with bladder endometriosis. Substantial thickening of the round ligament (>6 mm) is a significant sign of endometriosis implants. In case of unilateral invasion, the uterus is drawn toward the affected side. T2-weighted sequences usually reveal a hypointense signal, and in rare cases small hyperintense foci are visible on T1-weighted images [29]. In patients with bilateral invasion and bladder endometriosis, the round ligaments appear V-shaped, and they are stiff and thick.

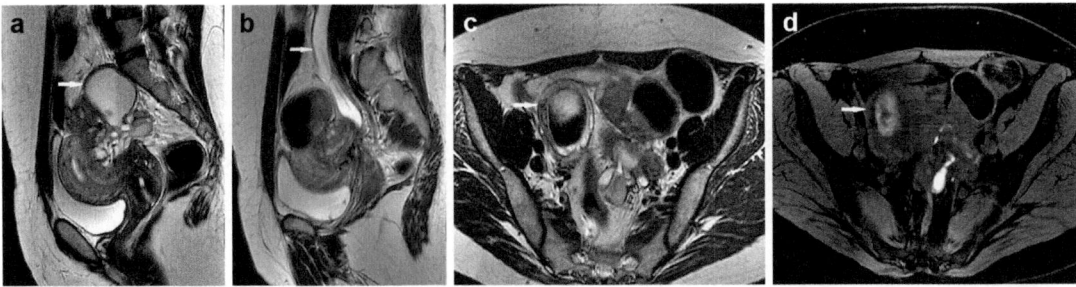

Fig. 23.10 Multifocal deep endometriosis: (**a**, **b**) sagittal T2-weighted images, (**c**) axial T2-weighted image, (**d**) fat-suppressed axial T1-weighted image. Diffuse pelvic endometriosis with bilateral endometriomas, hematosalpinx (**a**, **c**, **d**, white arrows), and left ureter involvement with ureteronephrosis (**b**, yellow arrow)

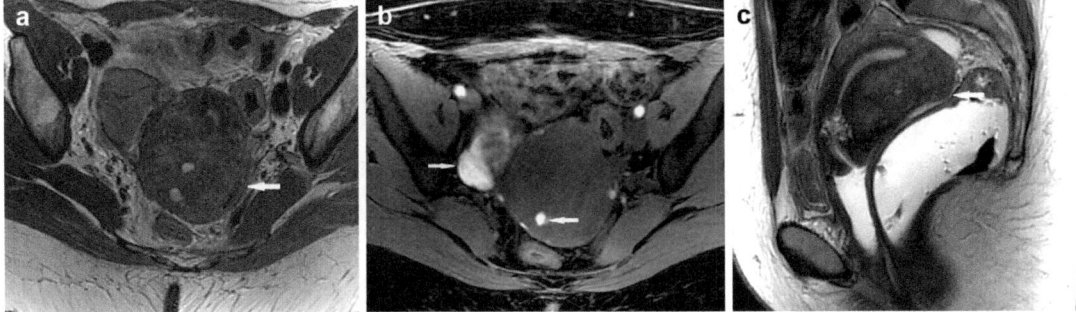

Fig. 23.11 Adenomyosis, tubo-ovarian, and peritoneal endometriosis: (**a**) axial T2-weighted image, (**b**) fat-suppressed axial T1-weighted image, (**c**) sagittal T2-weighted image after gel filling. These images show a thickened junctional zone and asymmetric posterior uterine wall (**a**, arrow), with cystic areas, some of which hyperintense on T1-weighted image (**b**, arrow), specific sign of adenomyosis. Hemorrhagic tubo-ovarian complex on the right side is visualized (**b**, yellow arrow); presence of peritoneal endometriosis on uterine serosa (**b**); a fibrotic plaque in rectouterine pouch with retroflexed uterus (**c**, arrow)

23.7 Adenomyosis

Adenomyosis can be diagnosed using MRI, which is a noninvasive method with elevated specificity (67–99%) and diagnostic accuracy (85–95%) in this pathology.

MRI shows increased junctional zone thickness and a poorly delimited low signal intensity area on T2-weighted acquisitions. Additionally, T2-weighted images may show small high signal intensity areas representing glandular cysts. On T1-weighted images, in some cases, small high signal intensity foci are recognized due to the presence of methemoglobin. These are specific signs of adenomyosis (Figs. 23.11 and 23.12) (Videos 23.11a, 23.11b, 23.11c and 23.12a, 23.12b, 23.12c).

MRI images of endometrial invasion and junctional zone alterations are subjective criteria often used for diagnosing adenomyosis instead of objective criteria which should be preferred. So far three objective MRI criteria for diagnosing adenomyosis have been established: *junctional zone* thickening of *8–12 mm*, junctional zone *ratio, max thickness/*total myometrium >40%, and the difference between max/min thickness of the junctional zone (JZmax-JZmin ¼ JZ dif) >5 mm.

The first two parameters are controversial because the thickness of the junctional zone changes according to the hormonal status and menstrual cycle. The third parameter relies on measurements made in the same hormonal phase and should therefore be independent of hormonal status.

Also other parameters are useful for detecting adenomyosis, such as *asymmetric myometrial*

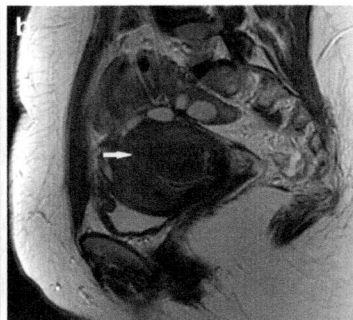
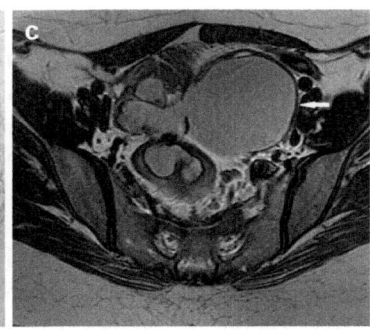

Fig. 23.12 Adenomyosis, hematosalpinx, ovarian and peritoneal endometriosis: (**a**) fat-suppressed sagittal T1-weighted image, (**b**) sagittal T2-weighted image, (**c**) axial T2-weighted image. Adenomyosis signs are thickening of junctional zone, with low signal intensity on T2-weighted images (**b**, arrow) and hyperintense foci on T1-weighted images (**a**, white arrow); a large left ovarian endometrioma near to a dilated fallopian tube is shown (**c**, arrow); presence of hematosalpinx and peritoneal endometriosis of uterine serosal surface (**a**, yellow arrow)

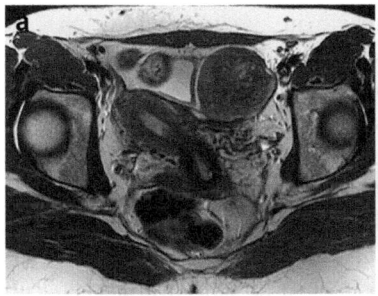
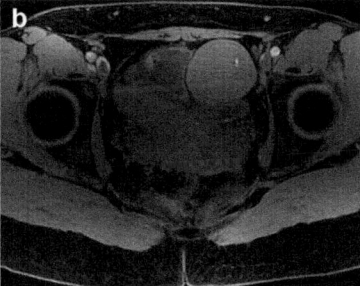
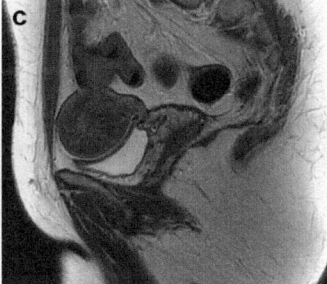

Fig. 23.13 Adenomyoma on (**a**) axial T2-weighted image, (**b**) fat-suppressed axial T1-weighted image, and (**c**) sagittal T2-weighted image. These images show a round-shaped lesion, with regular margins, near the left uterine wall, hypointense with some high-signal spots (**a–c**) and with hemorrhagic foci (**b**)

walls, focal adenomyoma, and macrocystic areas within the myometrium due to cystic adenomyosis (Fig. 23.13) (Videos 23.13a, 23.13b).

23.8 New Perspective in the Study of Pelvic Pain

23.8.1 Neural Involvement in Endometriosis: Pelvic Tractography and Neurography

Since the pathogenesis of pain is still debated, researchers have been going through new paths to try to get as much information as possible that can allow effective explanation and treatment of this invalidating symptom.

Endometriosis is an infrequent cause of peripheral neuropathy.

The involvement of the peripheral system has been theorized in many ways, endometriosis acts with three different mechanisms: producing cytokines and neurogenic factors, directly infiltrating nerves tissue or through chronic bleeding; in fact, lesions were found around the sciatic and under the nerve sheath; as a possible explanation to this, a perineural spread theory was introduced.

Although no final explanation has been proven, we know that sciatica-like pain has a high incidence (50%) in women affected by endometriosis [46] and that endometriosis was the most common cause of sacral radiculopathy of non-spinal origin [47].

Generally, two main causes of "leg pain" have been described: referred pain and neuropathic pain. Large ovarian cysts may be responsible for referred pain in the medial anterior part of the thigh, while neuropathic pain is related to the involvement of the nervous structures. Pain in anterior and medial part of thigh and weakness with adduction has been described in the cases of endometriosis of the obturator nerve. Pain in anterior and lateral part of thigh is related to the invasion of the femoral and femoral cutaneous nerve. Pain at the buttock, extending along the posterior-lateral thigh and calf, is referred in the case of endometriosis of the sciatic nerve or sciatic plexus.

MR Imaging is able to detect the involvement of nervous fibers with hyperintensity on T2, T1 FS and DWI, with a significant and inhomogeneous enhancement after i.v. contrast administration. The presence of adhesions and altered muscle trophism and asymmetry are depicted as indirect signs (Fig. 23.14) (Videos 23.14a, 23.14b).

In this contest, new ways of studying endometriosis were investigated: one that indirectly evaluates the abnormalities of the sacral plexus (tractography) and the other one that directly visualizes the any possible alteration along the neural path (neurography).

Tractography allows us to study the three-dimensional architecture of nerve fibers; in fact it is able to reconstruct nerve fibers starting from diffusion-weighted images. It is routinely used in the study of central nervous system, but its role in the peripheral system has been widely investigated in particular to study major nerves of arms and legs (median, ulnar, radial, sciatic…) [48, 49].

The fundamental principle on which the reconstruction is based is that within the axons,

the movement of the water molecules is not random but hindered by the cell walls; therefore the movement will be facilitated in a direction parallel to the axonal fiber, and a damage in the wall or direction of the nerves pathways is expressed by an altered reconstruction.

Tractography allows an anatomical evaluation both of nervous fibers and also of its microstructural integrity through the analysis of the FA value, whose decrease could indicate acute fiber damage, Wallerian degeneration, involvement of the fiber by extrinsic masses, etc.

Moved by the knowledge that there is an interaction between central nervous system-peripheral nervous system and endometriotic implants, few authors investigated the application of tractography in women affected by endometriosis who referred severe chronic pelvic pain. Interesting results showed that endometriosis-related pain correlated with an altered 3D reconstruction of the sacral plexus [50], as well as pathological DTI is significantly associated with the severity of dysmenorrhea, pain duration and in particular with specific type of endometriosis such as tubo-ovarian and cul-de-sac adhesions, and DIE (Fig. 23.15) [51].

For what concern neurography, already in 1995 Cottier et al. [52] reported a case of endometriotic implant along the sciatic nerve visualized on MRI. Since then other studies have been proposed to show that neurography can help to demonstrate rare location of endometriosis along the nerves pathways especially in women referring with catamenial radiculopathy [53, 54]. These sequences offer an excellent anatomical detail and therefore can be used to visualize small

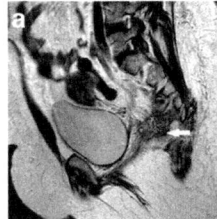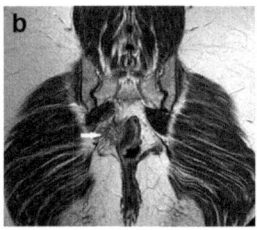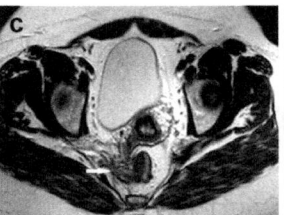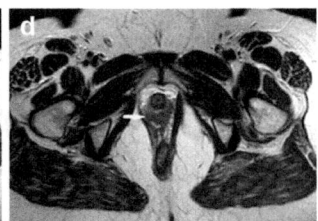

Fig. 23.14 Endometriosis of posterior compartment with muscular and nervous structures infiltration on (**a**) sagittal T2-weighted image, (**b**) coronal T2-weighted image, and (**c, d**) axial T2-weighted images. These images show a fibrotic endometriotic nodule between right vaginal fornix and the rectum, with involvement of the rectal wall, mesorectum, right puborectalis muscle, and ipsilateral sacral nerval roots (arrows)

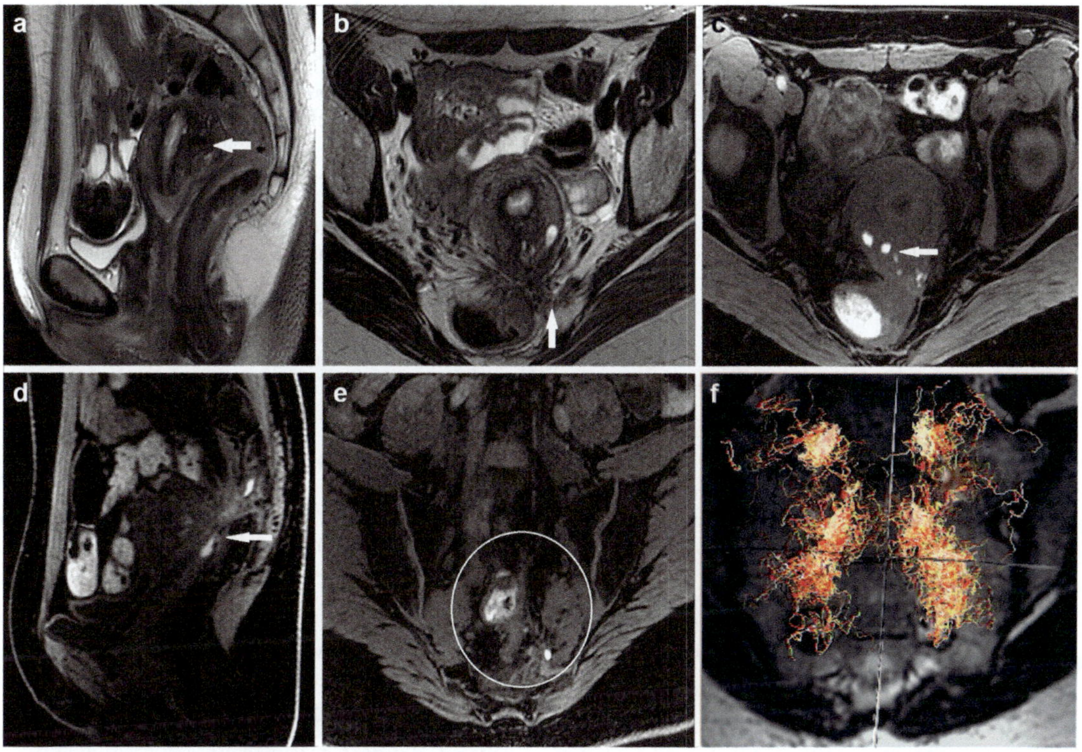

Fig. 23.15 Deep endometriosis of posterior compartment with nerve infiltration: (**a**) sagittal T2-weighted image, (**b**) axial T2-weighted image, (**c–e**) fat-suppressed axial T1-weighted image, (**d**) fat-suppressed sagittal T1-weighted image, (**f**) DTI imaging. These images show an extended fibrotic plaque between cervix, uterosacral ligaments, and bowel (**a–d**, arrows), with high-signal areas on T1-weighted images (**c**, arrow). Infiltration of adipose tissue with active endometriosis in presacral space is shown (**e**, circle) at the third sacral left root level as neural involvement. 3D DTI reconstruction shows irregular and sprouting sacral roots (**f**)

foci along the nerve root or directly evaluate the entrapment of the neural plexus from an endometriotic implants, as well as directly visualize the neuropathic injury.

References

1. Kobayashi H, Higashiura Y, Shigetomi H, Kajihara H. Pathogenesis of endometriosis: the role of initial infection and subsequent sterile inflammation (Review). Mol Med Rep. 2014;9(1):9–15.
2. Giudice LC, Kao LC. Endometriosis. Lancet. 2004;364(9447):1789–99.
3. Nnoaham KE, Hummelshoj L, Webster P, d'Hooghe T, de Cicco Nardone F, de Cicco Nardone C, et al. Impact of endometriosis on quality of life and work productivity: a multicenter study across ten countries. Fertil Steril. 2011;96(2):366–73.
4. Ballard KD, Seaman HE, de Vries CS, Wright JT. Can symptomatology help in the diagnosis of endometriosis? Findings from a national case-control study - Part 1. BJOG. 2008;115(11):1382:91.
5. Apostolopoulos NV, Alexandraki KI, Gorry A, Coker A. Association between chronic pelvic pain symptoms and the presence of endometriosis. Arch Gynecol Obstet. 2016;293(2):439–45.
6. Koninckx PR, Meuleman C, Demeyere S, Lesaffre E, Cornillie FJ. Suggestive evidence that pelvic endometriosis is a progressive disease, whereas deeply infiltrating endometriosis is associated with pelvic pain. Fertil Steril. 1991;55(4):759–65.
7. Porpora MG, Koninckx PR, Piazze J, Natili M, Colagrande S, Cosmi EV. Correlation between endometriosis and pelvic pain. J Am Assoc Gynecol Laparosc. 1999;6(4):429–34.
8. Fauconnier A, Chapron C. Endometriosis and pelvic pain: epidemiological evidence of the relationship and implications. Hum Reprod Update. 2005;11(6):595–606.
9. Kobayashi H, Yamada Y, Morioka S, Niiro E, Shigemitsu A, Ito F. Mechanism of pain generation for endometriosis-associated pelvic pain. Archiv Gynecol Obstet. 2014;289(1):13–21.

10. Berkley KJ, Dmitrieva N, Curtis KS, Papka ER. Innervation of ectopic endometrium in a rat model of endometriosis. Proc Natl Acad Sci USA. 2004;101(30):11094–8.

11. Berkley KJ, Rapkin AJ, Papka RE. The pains of endometriosis. Science. 2005;308(5728):1587–9.

12. Wang G, Tokushige N, Markham R, Fraser IS, et al. Rich innervation of deep infiltrating endometriosis. Hum Reprod. 2009;24(4):827–34.

13. McKinnon BD, Bertschi D, Bersinger NA, Mueller MD. Inflammation and nerve fiber interaction in endometriotic pain. Trends Endocrinol Metab. 2015;26(1):1–10.

14. Anaf V, Simon P, El Nakadi I, Fayt I, Buxant F, Simonart T, et al. Relationship between endometriotic foci and nerves in rectovaginal endometriotic nodules. Hum Reprod (Oxford, England). 2000;15(8):1744–50.

15. Anaf V, Simon P, El Nakadi I, Fayt I, Buxant F, Noel JC. Hyperalgesia, nerve infiltration and nerve growth factor expression in deep adenomyotic nodules, peritoneal and ovarian endometriosis. Hum Reprod. 2002;17(7):1895–900.

16. Stratton P, Berkley KJ. Chronic pelvic pain and endometriosis: translational evidence of the relationship and implications. Hum Reprod Update. 2011;17(3):327–46.

17. Bazot M, Bharwani N, Huchon C, Kinkel K, Cunha TM, Guerra A, et al. European society of urogenital radiology (ESUR) guidelines: MR imaging of pelvic endometriosis. Eur Radiol. 2017;27(7):2765–75.

18. Van Holsbeke C, Van Calster B, Guerriero S, Savelli L, Paladini D, Lissoni AA, et al. Endometriomas: Their ultrasound characteristics. Ultrasound Obstet Gynecol. 2010;35:735–40.

19. Moore J, Copley S, Morris J, Lindsell D, Golding S, Kennedy S. A systematic review of the accuracy of ultrasound in the diagnosis of endometriosis. Ultrasound Obstet Gynecol. 2002;20(6):630–4.

20. Exacoustos C, Manganaro L, Zupi E. Imaging for the evaluation of endometriosis and adenomyosis. Best Pract Res Clin Obstet Gynaecol. 2014;28(5):655–81.

21. Chapron C, et al. Anatomical distribution of deeply infiltrating endometriosis: Surgical implications and proposition for a classification. Hum Reprod. 2003;18(1):157–61.

22. Fedele L, Bianchi S, Raffaelli R, Portuese A. Pre-operative assessment of bladder endometriosis. Hum Reprod. 1997;12(11):2519–22.

23. Hudelist G, English J, Thomas AE, Tinelli A, Singer CF, Keckstein J. Diagnostic accuracy of transvaginal ultrasound for non-invasive diagnosis of bowel endometriosis: Systematic review and meta-analysis. Ultrasound Obstet Gynecol. 2011;37(3):257–63.

24. Chamié LP, Pereira Alves Mendes R, Zanatta A, Serafini PS. Transvaginal US after bowel preparation for deeply infiltrating endometriosis: protocol, imaging appearances, and laparoscopic correlation. Radiographics. 2010;30:1235–49.

25. Chamié LP, Blasbalg R, Goncalves MO, Carvalho FM, Abrao MS, de Oliveira IS. Accuracy of magnetic resonance imaging for diagnosis and preoperative assessment of deeply infiltrating endometriosis. Int J Gynaecol Obstet. 2009;196(3):198–201.

26. Hottat N, Larrousse C, Anaf V, Neol JC, Absil J, Metens T. Endometriosis: contribution of 3.0-T Pelvic MR imaging in preoperative assessment—initial results. Radiology. 2009;253(1):126–34.

27. McDermott S, Oei TN, Iyer RV, Lee SI. MR imaging of malignancies arising in endometriomas and extraovarian endometriosis. Radiographics. 2012;32:845–63.

28. Corwin MT, Gerscovich EO, Lamba R, Wilson M, McGahan JP. Differentiation of ovarian endometriomas from hemorrhagic cysts at MR imaging: utility of the T2 Dark spot sign. Radiology. 2014;271(1):126–32.

29. Siegelman ES, Oliver ER. MR imaging of endometriosis: ten imaging pearls. Radiographics. 2012;32:1675–91.

30. Kim MY, Rha SE, Oh SN, Jung SE, Lee Y, Kim YS, et al. MR imaging findings of hydrosalpinx: a comprehensive review. Radiographics. 2009;29: 495–507.

31. Kaproth-Joslin K, Dogra V. Imaging of female infertility: a pictorial guide to the hysterosalpingography, ultrasonography, and magnetic resonance imaging findings of the congenital and acquired causes of female infertility. Radiol Clin North Am. 2013;51(6):967–81.

32. Khan KN, Kitajima M, Fujishita A, Hiraki K, Matsumoto A, Nakashima M, et al. Pelvic pain in women with ovarian endometrioma is mostly associated with coexisting peritoneal lesions. Hum Reprod. 2013;28(1):109–18.

33. Redwine DB. Ovarian endometriosis: A marker for more extensive pelvic and intestinal disease. Fertil Steril. 1999;72(2):310–5.

34. Kataoka ML, Togashi K, Yamaoka T, Koyama T, Ueda H, Kobayashi H, et al. Posterior Cul-de-Sac obliteration associated with endometriosis: MR imaging evaluation. Radiology. 2005;234(3): 815–23.

35. Scardapane A, Lorusso F, Scioscia M, Ferrante A, Stabile Ianora AA, Angelelli G. Standard high-resolution pelvic MRI vs. low-resolution pelvic MRI in the evaluation of deep infiltrating endometriosis. Eur Radiol. 2014;24(10):2590–6.

36. Lo Monte G, Wenger JM, Petignat P, Marci R. Role of imaging in endometriosis. Cleve Clin J Med. 2014;81(6):361–6.

37. Krüger K, Gilly L, Kreuter-Niedobitek G, Mpinou L, Ebert AD. Bladder endometriosis: characterization by magnetic resonance imaging and the value of documenting ureteral involvement. Eur J Obstet Gynecol Reprod Biol. 2014;176(1):39–43.

38. Medeiros LR, Rosa MI, Silva BR, Reis ME, Simon CS, Dondossola ER, et al. Accuracy of magnetic resonance in deeply infiltrating endometriosis: a systematic review and meta-analysis. Arch Gynecol Obstet. 2015;291(3):611–21.

39. Wolthuis A, Meuleman C, Tomassetti C, D'Hooghe T, Overstraeten Adb M. Bowel endometriosis: Colorectal surgeon's perspective in a multidisciplinary surgical team. World J Gastroenterol. 2014;20(42):15616–23.

40. Rousset P, Peyron N, Charlot M, Chateau F, Glfier F, Raudrant D, et al. Bowel endometriosis: preoperative diagnostic accuracy of 3.0-T MR enterography-initial results. Radiology. 2014;273(1):117–24.

41. Loubeyre P, Copercini M, Frossard JL, Wenger JM, Petignat P. Pictorial review: rectosigmoid endometriosis on MRI with gel opacification after rectosigmoid colon cleansing. Clin Imaging. 2012;36(4):295–300.

42. Bazot M, Darai E, Hourani R, Thomassin I, Cortez A, Uzam S, et al. Deep Pelvic Endometriosis: MR imaging for diagnosis and prediction of extension of disease. Radiology. 2004;232(2):379–89.

43. Piketty M, Chopin N, Dousset B, Millischer-Bellaische AE, Roseau G, Leconte M, et al. Preoperative work-up for patients with deeply infiltrating endometriosis: Transvaginal ultrasonography must definitely be the first-line imaging examination. Hum Reprod. 2009;24(3):602–7.

44. Scardapane A, Bettocchi S, Lorusso F, Stabile Ianora AA, Vimercati A, Ceci O, et al. Diagnosis of colorectal endometriosis: contribution of contrast enhanced MR-colonography. Eur Radiol. 2011;21(7): 1553–63.

45. Lakhi N, Dun EC, Nezhat CH. Hematoureter due to endometriosis. Fertil Steril. 2014;101(6):37.

46. Missmer SA, Bove GM. A pilot study of the prevalence of leg pain among women with endometriosis. J Bodyw Mov Ther. 2011;15(3):304–8.

47. Possover M, Schneider T, Henle KP. Laparoscopic therapy for endometriosis and vascular entrapment of sacral plexus. Fertil Steril. 2011;95(2):756–8.

48. Hiltunen J, Suortti T, Arvela S, Seppa M, Joensuu R, Hari R. Diffusion tensor imaging and tractography of distal peripheral nerves at 3 T. Clin Neurophysiol. 2005;116(10):2315–23.

49. Khalil C, Hancart C, Le Thuc V, Chantelot C, Chechin D, Cotton A. Diffusion tensor imaging and tractography of the median nerve in carpal tunnel syndrome: preliminary results. Eur Radiol. 2008;18(10):2283–91.

50. Manganaro L, Porpora MG, Vinci V, Bernardo S, Lodise P, Sollazzo P, et al. Diffusion tensor imaging and tractography to evaluate sacral nerve root abnormalities in endometriosis-related pain: A pilot study. Eur Radiol. 2014;24(1):95–101.

51. Manganaro L, Vittori G, Vinci V, Fierro F, Tomei A, Lodise P, et al. Beyond laparoscopy: 3-T magnetic resonance imaging in the evaluation of posterior cul-de-sac obliteration. Magn Reson Imaging. 2012;30(10):1432–8.

52. Cottier JP, Descamps P, Sonier CB, Rosset P. Sciatic endometriosis: MR evaluation. AJNR Am J Neuroradiol. 1995;16(7):1399–401.

53. Pham M, Sommer C, Wessing C, Monoranu CM, Perez SG, Bendszus M. Magnetic resonance neurography for the diagnosis of extrapelvic sciatic endometriosis. Fertil Steril. 2010;94(1):351.e11–4.

54. Cimsit C, Yoldemir T, Akpinar IN. Sciatic neuroendometriosis: magnetic resonance imaging defined perineural spread of endometriosis. J Obstet Gynaecol Res. 2016;42(7):890–4.

Imaging of Acute Scrotum

24

Michele Bertolotto, Irene Campo, and Lorenzo E. Derchi

24.1 Introduction

Acute scrotal pain can be determined by many different causes [1]. A number of differential diagnoses must be considered, either scrotal and non-scrotal, some of which requiring emergent management. A correct diagnosis is mandatory and must be obtained in emergency, as treatment options (observation, surgery, antibiotics, etc.) could differ dramatically depending on the disease process.

Testicular torsion, epididymo-orchitis, and torsion of the testicular appendages are the most common causes of acute scrotal pain, but a variety of less common clinical situations can be encountered. Differentiation is a significant diagnostic problem in clinical practice. A firm diagnosis is often difficult based on clinical history and physical examinations only, and imaging is usually requested for this purpose. However, imaging findings are not always easy to understand. They

have to be interpreted in close correlation with clinical information and with knowledge of the possible pathological situations underlying the clinical presentation of the specific patient.

In this chapter, the commonest causes of acute scrotal pain are discussed and illustrated with emphasis to correlation between clinical and imaging findings.

24.2 Testicular Torsion

Torsion of the spermatic cord is a surgical emergency leading to testicular loss, if not timely treated. Torsion results in cessation or marked reduction of blood flow to the testicle causing ischemia and parenchymal necrosis. Intravaginal torsion, caused by a congenital malformation of the processus vaginalis, accounts for 90% of cases. It is related to the bell-clapper deformity, an anatomical variation in which the tunica vaginalis completely encircles the epididymis, distal spermatic cord, and the testis rather than attaching to the posterolateral aspect of the testis. This situation is relatively common, accounting for up to 12% of males in autopsy series [2]. Bell-clapper deformity is often bilateral and leaves the testis free to rotate within the tunica vaginalis [1].

Extravaginal torsion is less common; it occurs in the newborn when the intrascrotal contents are not fixed and are free to move in and out of the scrotal sac.

Electronic Supplementary Material The online version of this chapter (https://doi.org/10.1007/978-3-319-99822-0_24) contains supplementary material, which is available to authorized users.

M. Bertolotto (✉) · I. Campo
Department of Radiology, University of Trieste, Trieste, Italy
e-mail: bertolot@units.it

L. E. Derchi
Department of Health Sciences (DISSAL),
University of Genoa, Genova, Italy
e-mail: derchi@unige.it

24.2.1 Clinical Presentation

Patients with testicular torsion usually present with a sudden acute testicular pain, nausea and vomiting, and ipsilateral lower abdomen pain. Sometimes the onset of symptoms is more gradual and the pain is less severe. In many cases, there is a history of previous episodes of severe, self-limiting scrotal pain and swelling. Careful palpation of the scrotum will assess the asymmetric positioning of the testis within the scrotal sac. The testis may be high-riding in the scrotum in an abnormal transverse position. Cremasteric reflex is absent [3].

24.2.2 Imaging

Grayscale and Doppler modes are the mainstay for the diagnosis of acute testicular torsion [1, 3]. Ultrasonographic features vary with time and with the degree of rotation of the spermatic cord. Early after onset of symptoms, the ischemic testis may appear of normal volume, more often already increased in size due to incoming edema, and with normal echogenicity and echotexture (Fig. 24.1). Within about 4–6 h, the testis becomes swollen and hypoechoic, while a heterogeneous echo pattern is observed much later. A mild hydrocele is

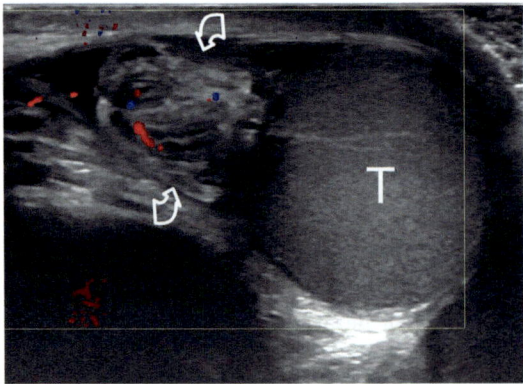

Fig. 24.1 Patient with high-degree testicular torsion investigated early after the onset of symptoms. The testis (T) has normal echogenicity and echotexture, avascular at color Doppler interrogation. The torsion site of the spermatic cord is identified as a lump (curved arrows) above the testis, in which few color signals are identified

generally present. These last changes are secondary to hemorrhage and infarction. After 24–36 h, the testis is markedly hypoechoic, usually with anechoic and patchy hyperechoic areas due to colliquative and hemorrhagic infarction (Fig. 24.2).

It must be underlined that the timing of morphological changes depicted above is only indicative and can vary substantially with the degree of torsion.

In the majority of cases, color Doppler interrogation shows avascular or hypovascular testis, depending on the degree of twisting of the spermatic cord. Blood flow is relatively preserved in the other structures of the scrotal content, though the epididymis could become relatively ischemic. Within a few hours, the paratesticular tissues and the scrotal wall become hyperemic in an attempt to open collaterals.

By using the absence of identifiable intratesticular flow at color Doppler interrogation as the only criterion for detecting torsion, an 86–94% sensitivity, nearly 100% specificity, and 97% accuracy are obtained [4, 5]. This means a false-negative diagnosis in up to 6–14% of patients, most of them with low-degree torsion in which there is only venous occlusion while the arteries are still patent. The clue for diagnosis of low-degree torsion is detection at spectral Doppler analysis of monophasic waveforms, increased resistance index with decreased diastolic flow velocities, or diastolic flow reversal [6–8]. These spectral Doppler changes in the testicular arteries are signs of ischemia caused by swelling and edema occluding the venous flow. Rarely, pulsus tardus et parvus waveforms are recorded, characterized by markedly reduced peak systolic velocities, compared to the contralateral healthy site, slowly accelerating slope, and markedly prolonged acceleration time (Fig. 24.3) [7]. No venous flows are recorded.

In patients with suspicious testicular torsion of any degree, the morphology and vascularization of the spermatic cord must be investigated. The level of twisting of the spermatic cord is displayed at a varying distance above the testis or posterior to the testis by identification of a funicular mass at which the funicular vessels either stop, as occur in high degree torsion, or are characterized by an abrupt change of the normally straight

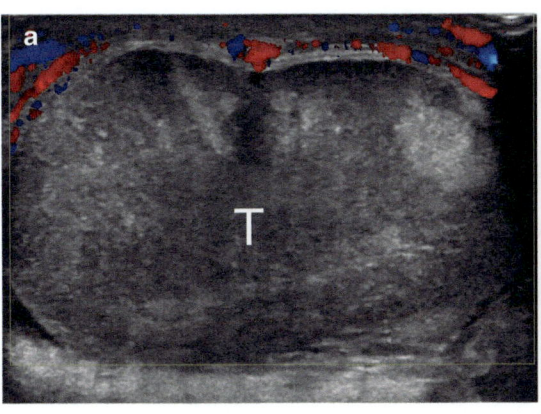
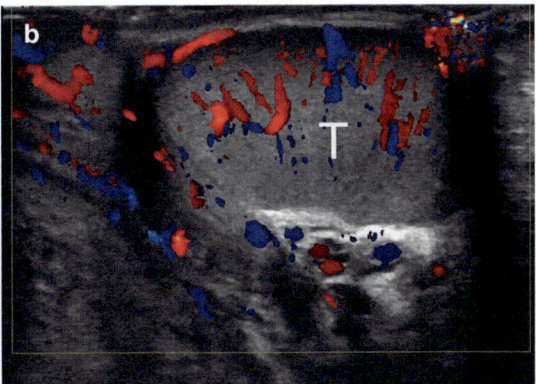

Fig. 24.2 Patient with longstanding high-degree right testicular torsion. (**a**) Right testis. Color Doppler US shows enlarged, inhomogeneously hypoechoic testis (T), with hyperechoic areas consistent with hemorrhagic changes. The testis is completely avascular at color Doppler interrogation. Increased vascularization of the peritesticular tissues is present. (**b**) Left testis (T) with normal appearance

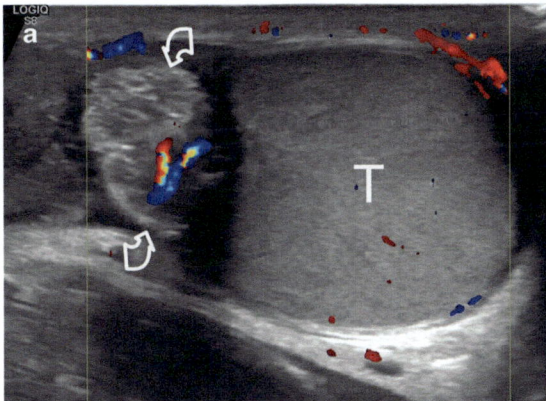
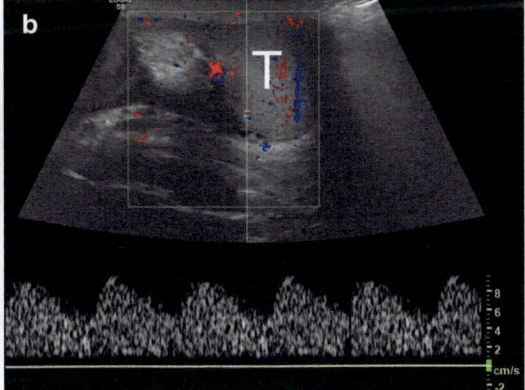

Fig. 24.3 Low-degree testicular torsion. (**a**) The testis (T) has normal echogenicity and echotexture, with few parenchymal vessels displayed at color Doppler interrogation. The torsion site of the spermatic cord is identified as a lump (curved arrows) above the testis, in which spermatic vessels are seen with tortuous course (twirling sign). (**b**) Low-velocity flows with post-stenotic appearance are recorded in the testicular vessels

course. Twirling is demonstrated by the "whirl-pool sign," representing the funicular vessels wrapping around the central axis of the twisted spermatic cord (Fig. 24.3). Moving the probe in cranio-caudal direction along the axis of the spermatic cord eases identification of this sign [9].

24.3 Torsion of Appendages

There are four types of appendages, which are remnants of embryological ducts: the appendix testis (hydatid of Morgagni, remnant of the Müllerian duct), the appendix of epididymis (remnant of Wolffian ducts), the paradydimis (organ of Giraldes, remnant of mesonephric duct), and the vas aberrans of Haller. Appendages become clinically relevant once they undergo torsion.

In appendigeal torsion the onset of the pain can be either insidious, with mild scrotal discomfort, or acute, making differentiation with testicular torsion challenging on clinical basis only. Physical examination may reveal a small (3–5 mm) extratesticular tender nodule at the level of which a bluish change in the skin color appears, due to visualization of the

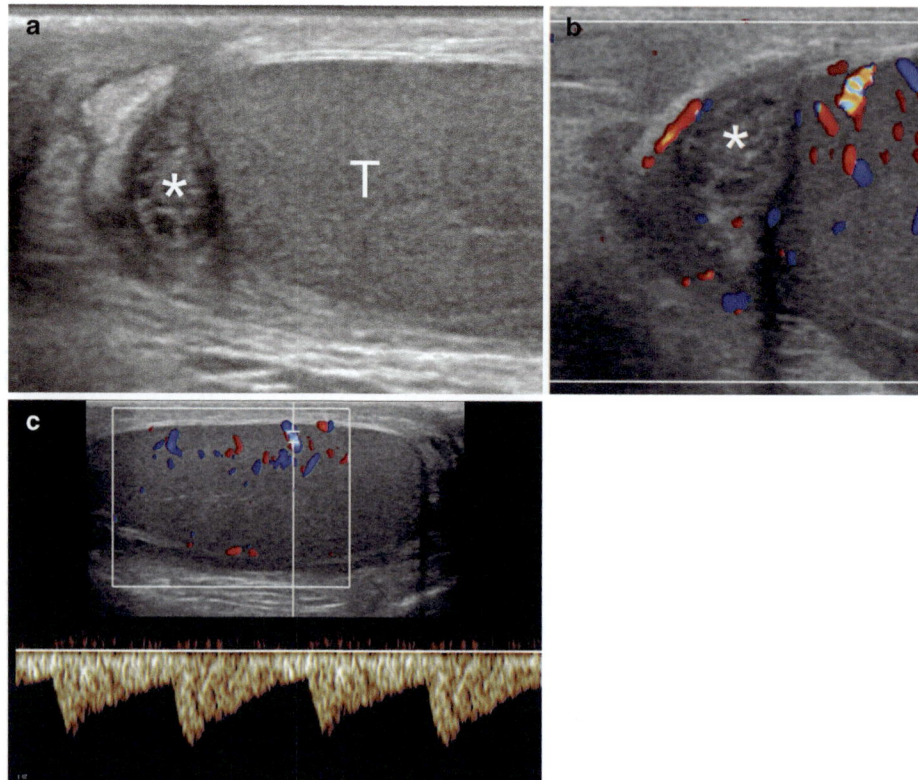

Fig. 24.4 Appendiceal torsion. 11-year-old boy presenting with acute scrotal pain since 7 days. (**a**) Grayscale ultrasonography shows a small mass (asterisk) above the upper pole of the testis. (**b**) The mass (asterisk) is avascular at color Doppler interrogation. Vascularization of the testis (T) is normal. (**c**) Spectral Doppler interrogation of the testicular vessels shows normal arterial flows

infarcted appendage through the skin ("blue dot sign"). The blue dot sign is strongly specific for appendigeal torsion, even though it is detectable in only about 20% of patients.

Twisted appendages are usually 5 mm or larger in size, with variable echogenicity, next to the upper pole of the testis or to the epididymal head [10, 11]. They are avascular at color Doppler interrogation, but perilesional hypervascularization can be present in subacute torsion (Fig. 24.4). Reactive hydrocele and skin thickening are often associated. In chronic appendiceal torsion, shrinking is observed. The appendix can eventually detach or calcify.

24.4 Epididymo-orchitis

Epididymo-orchitis is the most common cause of acute scrotal pain in adults, representing at least 75% of all inflammatory scrotal disease

processes. Complications include abscess, testicular ischemia, and pyocele formation. The infection usually spreads from the urethra, prostate, or bladder. *Chlamydia trachomatis*, *Neisseria gonorrhoeae* and the coliforms, less frequently mycobacteria, brucella, and cryptococcus, are the main pathogens.

24.4.1 Clinical Presentation

Typically, in epididymo-orchitis, scrotal pain and swelling have a gradual onset but occasionally sharp and acute. Fever or other nonspecific signs of inflammation can be associated. Pain may radiate along the spermatic cord and reach the abdomen. Other presenting symptoms include urethral discharge, dysuria, and other irritative lower urinary tract symptoms. Physical examination findings range from painful swelling of the tail of the epididymis to involvement of the entire epididymis, to the testis, which becomes markedly enlarged, hard and tender. The spermatic cord is usually tender and swollen. Also, the wall of the involved hemiscrotum becomes reddish and thicker.

24.4.2 Imaging

Sonography shows diffuse or focally enlarged epididymis, with the epididymal tail most commonly involved. Epididymis usually presents an inhomogeneous echotexture, globally hypoechoic, with hyperechoic areas consistent with edema or hemorrhage. In most of cases, it is markedly hypervascular at color Doppler interrogation compared with the asymptomatic side (Fig. 24.5). When involved the testis is enlarged, usually hypoechoic, hard at elastography, and markedly hypervascular at color Doppler interrogation. Scrotal skin thickening, hyperemia, and a reactive hydrocele are common associated findings.

Focal orchitis can rarely occur, involving only one or few testicular lobules. Color Doppler interrogation shows a hypoechoic, hypervascular area. Differential diagnosis with tumor is performed combining color Doppler appearance, clinics, and presence of signs of inflammation. Diagnosis is confirmed with disappearance of the lesion after appropriate medical treatment.

24.5 Post-inflammatory Testicular Ischemia

In severe inflammation engorgement of the epididymis and testis can produce venous outflow obstruction and, eventually, impairment of the arterial blood supply and tissue ischemia. The disease may progress to segmental or global testicular infarction [8, 12, 13].

While in epididymo-orchitis the testis and epididymis are usually hypervascular, in patients with post-inflammatory ischemia, vascularity of the affected testis is reduced compared with the contralateral one. Intratesticular arteries show high resistance flows or diastolic flow reversal (Fig. 24.6). CEUS improves evaluation of testicular perfusion in these patients differentiating ischemic from viable, hypoperfused testes. It is possible to monitor the efficacy of medical therapy during the follow-up showing progression to global infarction, abscess formation, or, on the contrary, restoration to normal parenchymal vascularization.

24.6 Abscess Formation

Epididymal and intratesticular abscesses can complicate severe epididymo-orchitis [12] and can result from infection of hydroceles or hematoceles or from extension of an intraperitoneal infection into the scrotal sac via a patent process vaginalis. Abscesses present at ultrasonography as heterogeneous, usually hypoechoic, focal lesion with irregular margins, lacking vascularization at color Doppler interrogation and at CEUS (Fig. 24.7). Hypervascularization of the surrounding parenchyma can be observed. Abscess formation may involve the scrotal wall as well, and the inflammatory content can spread into the scrotal sac forming a pyocele. Ultrasonography shows a complex scrotal fluid collection with scrotal skin thickening and hyperemic soft tissues.

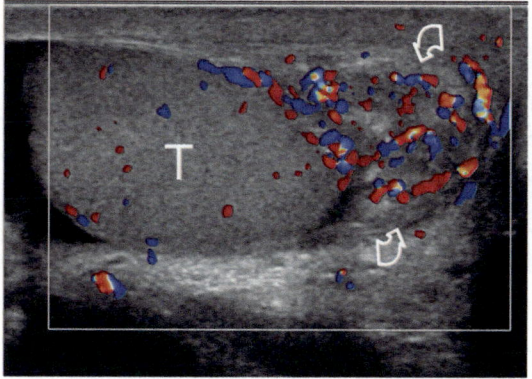

Fig. 24.5 Epididymitis. Color Doppler ultrasonography shows enlarged and heterogeneous, markedly hypervascular epididymal tail (curved arrows). The testis (T) is normal

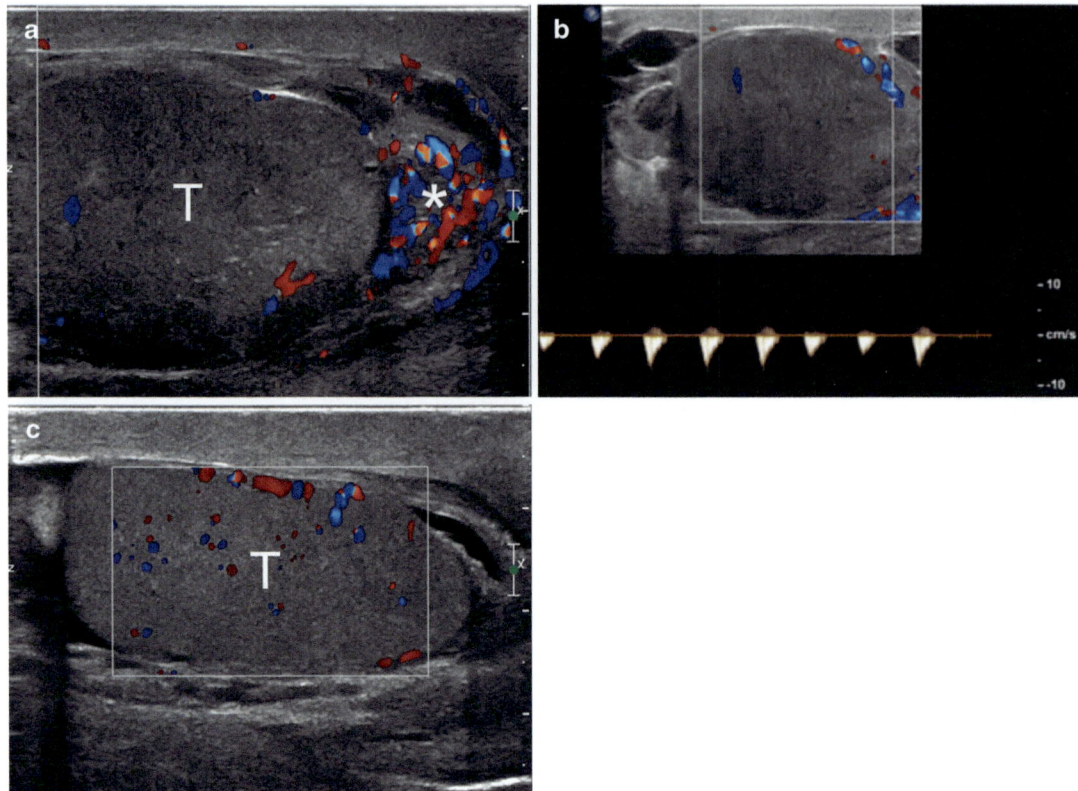

Fig. 24.6 Post-inflammatory testicular ischemia in a patient presenting with severe left epididymo-orchitis. (**a**) Color Doppler ultrasonography shows hypoechoic, hypovascular left testis (T) and hypervascular, enlarged epididymis (asterisk). (**b**) Spectral Doppler analysis shows high resistance testicular flows. (**c**) The contralateral right testis (T) is normal

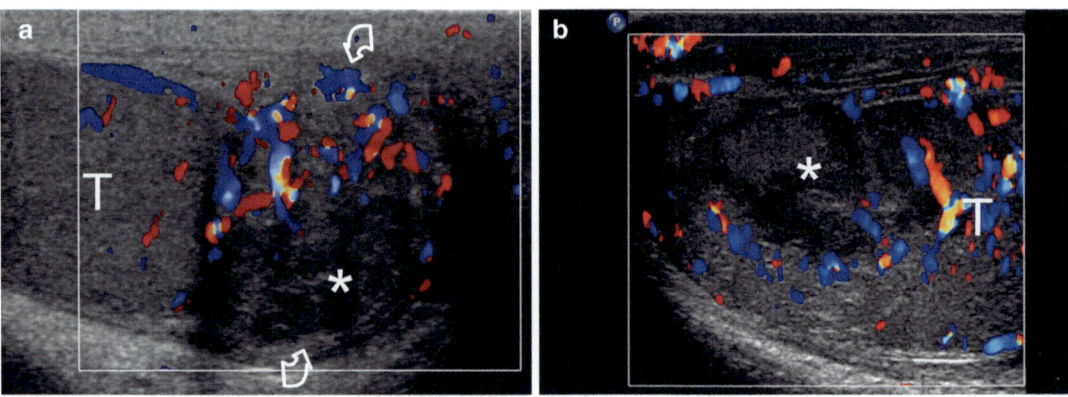

Fig. 24.7 Abscess formation. (**a**) Epididymitis complicated with abscess formation, identified as an inhomogeneous avascular lesion (asterisk) in a globally enlarged, hypervascular epididymal tail (curved arrows). The testis (T) is normal. (**b**) Epididymo-orchitis complicated with testicular abscess formation, identified as a inhomogeneous avascular area (asterisk) within a hypervascular testis (T)

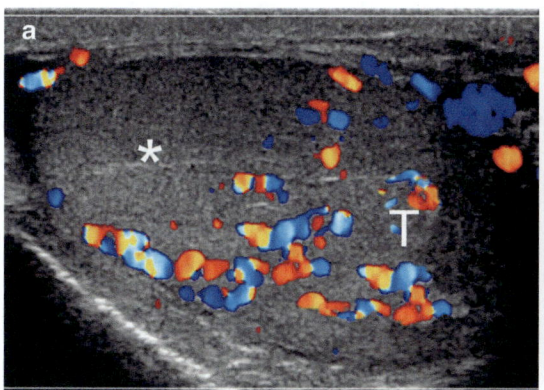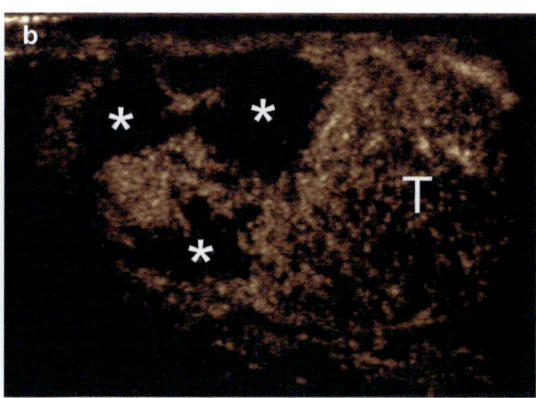

Fig. 24.8 Segmental testicular infarction in a patient presenting with right acute scrotal pain. (**a**) Color Doppler interrogation of the right testis shows avascular upper pole (asterisk). The remaining portions of the testis (T) are normal. (**b**) CEUS confirms presence of ischemic parenchymal lobules (asterisks) in the upper pole of the right testis (T)

24.7 Segmental Testicular Infarction

Segmental testicular infarction presents with acute scrotal pain and may clinically resemble epididymo-orchitis or torsion. A firm diagnosis is important because, if identified, follow-up is advocated. At ultrasonography, segmental testicular infarction presents as a solid intratesticular lesion, hypoechoic or isoechogenic, to the surrounding normal parenchyma, avascular at color Doppler interrogation. The key factor that allows differential diagnosis with tumor is recognition that the lesion is formed by one or more ischemic testicular lobules. When the lesion is wedge-shaped and completely avascular diagnosis is straightforward, but segmental testicular infarction can be round shaped, and may appear not completely avascular at colour Doppler interrogation when viable lobules interleave the ischaemic ones. When intralesional color spots are present, infarction cannot be safely differentiated from hypovascular tumors using conventional Doppler modes. Moreover, perilesional parenchymal flow signals may be prominent in segmental infarction and mimic peripheral vascularization of tumors, especially in small lesions.

Contrast-enhanced MRI has been claimed as the best imaging modality to obtain a firm diagnosis of segmental testicular infarction in equivocal cases [14]. The lesion does not enhance following gado-linium administration. An enhancing perilesional rim can be seen. CEUS provides similar results (Fig. 24.8). It improves characterization of acute testicular segmental infarction showing the morphological features of this lesion which presents as one or more avascular areas occasionally separated by normal vessels or viable areas, consistent with ischemic testicular lobules [15].

24.8 Vasculitides

Testicular vasculitides usually present with acute pain without a history of injury or infection. Symptoms may suggest testicular torsion, leading to non-necessary surgical exploration. They are usually part of a systemic disease, like polyarteritis nodosa (PAN), with damage of medium- and small-size intratesticular arteries resulting in vascular stenoses, thromboses, and micro-aneurysms.

It is important to differentiate between vasculitis and torsion, especially in the context of PAN, because in PAN testicular viability is often preserved and patients usually improve on treatment with cyclophosphamide and corticosteroids. Differential diagnosis, however, is often difficult at imaging in absence of history of PAN, and diagnosis is often made per-operatively by the surgeon or even on histological examination of the orchiectomy specimen.

Both in PAN and in testicular torsion color Doppler ultrasonography can fail to show intratesticular vascularization or can show a marked reduction in arterial blood flow. Echotexture of the involved testis can be heterogeneous, with areas of different echogenicity representing hemorrhage and ischemia. Failure to visualize the twisting of the spermatic cord, however, stands against torsion and helps to consider testicular involvement of PAN, at least in patients with known systemic disease. Churg-Strauss syndrome, a small-vessel necrotizing vasculitis involving the lung, kidneys, and other organs, can also present with acute scrotal pain caused by ischemic changes within the testis. Also, children with Henoch-Schönlein purpura present with acute scrotal pain. Color Doppler ultrasonography shows testes with normal echotexture and vascularity, while epididymides are enlarged, heterogeneous, and hypervascular. Scrotal skin thickening and reactive hydrocele are usually associated. Differential diagnosis with epididymitis may be difficult when scrotal involvement presents before the disease is clinically apparent elsewhere.

24.9 Tension Hydrocele

When the hydrostatic pressure of a hydrocele exceeds the blood pressure in the testicular vessels, parenchymal ischemia develops. Patients present to the emergency department with acute scrotal pain mimicking torsion. This uncommon condition can be observed in men with a long-standing history of hydrocele that undergoes sudden increase in fluid quantity. On physical examination, a large hydrocele is found. Ultrasound confirms the hydrocele and shows the testis, compressed from the fluid, avascular at color Doppler interrogation or with high-resistance flows or diastolic flow reversal [8] (Fig. 24.9). The course of the spermatic cord is normal. Needle aspiration of the hydrocele results in pain improvement, followed by restoration of low-resistance testicular flows.

24.10 Acute Venous Thrombosis

Thrombosis of the pampiniform plexus can present clinically as an acutely painful inguino-scrotal mass mimicking an

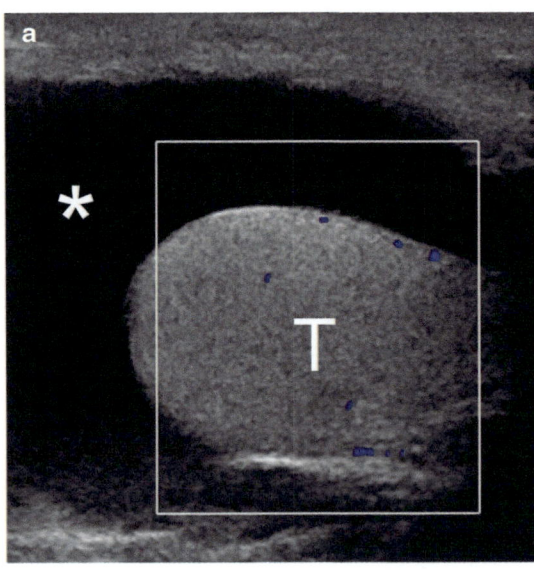
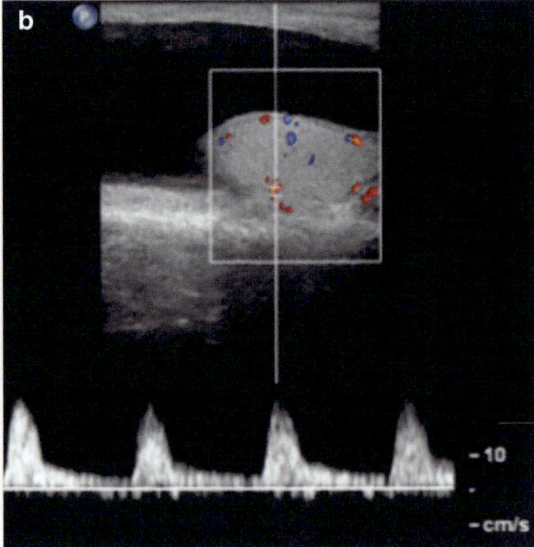

Fig. 24.9 Tension hydrocele. Patient with already known left hydrocele presenting with sudden increase in size of the left hemiscrotum and acute pain. (**a**) Color Doppler ultrasonography shows hydrocele (asterisk) and markedly hypovascular left testis (T). (**b**) Spectral Doppler interrogation of the intratesticular vessels shows high resistance arterial flows

incarcerated hernia. This rare entity can occur spontaneously or secondary to exercise in patients with varicocele or with Henoch-Schonlein purpura.

Ultrasonography and color Doppler interrogation show patent arteries and thrombosed veins, recognized by presence of echogenic, non-compressible material within the lumen [8].

24.11 Spontaneous Intratesticular Hematoma

Testicular hematoma is common in the setting of trauma but rarely can occur spontaneously [16]. Differential diagnosis is important, because this entity is managed conservatively provided that a firm preoperative diagnosis is done. Patients present with acute scrotal pain. Ultrasonography shows an intratesticular mass completely avascular at color Doppler interrogation and at CEUS or at MR imaging (Fig. 24.10). Avascularity and clinical presentation with acute scrotal pain are the clue for the right diagnosis, which is confirmed during the follow-up by change in size and in appearance within few days. Besides demonstrating lack of vascularity, MRI has the advantage to show the characteristic signal intensity of blood and of its changes over time.

24.12 Isolated Torsion of the Epididymis and of a Spermatocele

Isolated torsion of the epididymis and of a spermatocele is a very rare cause of acute scrotal pain, with only few cases described in the literature. In torsion of the epididymis, presence of a long and tortuous epididymis with a long mesorchium or of epididymal-testicular dissociation is the major predisposing factor. Spermatoceles arose from the head of the epididymis and had a distinct pedicle with torsion identified at surgical exploration. This makes differential diagnosis with torsion of a large appendix epididymis difficult, if spermatozoa are not identified within the lesion. At color Doppler ultrasound, the testis is normal. In isolated torsion of the epididymis, the twisted portion is enlarged, with heterogeneous echotexture, lacking vascularization at color Doppler interrogation [17]. On ultrasound, twisted spermatoceles are described as cystic like or heterogeneous lesions, possibly due to hemorrhagic content [18] (Fig. 24.11).

24.13 Testicular Neoplasms

Tumors can occasionally manifest with acute scrotal pain or can be found incidentally in patients examined for a pathology causing acute

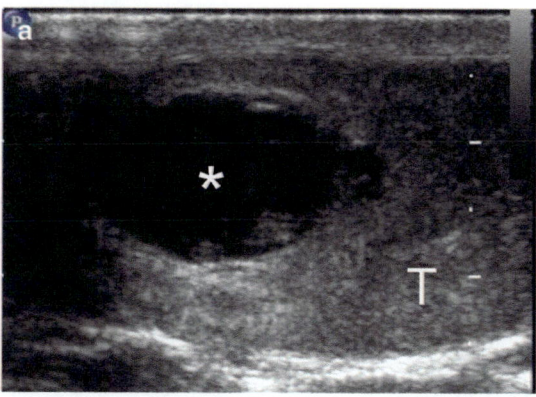
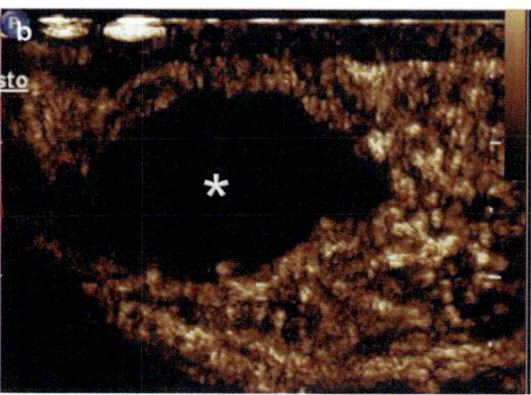
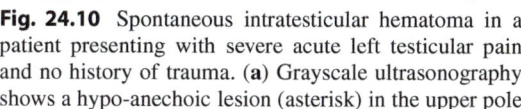

Fig. 24.10 Spontaneous intratesticular hematoma in a patient presenting with severe acute left testicular pain and no history of trauma. (**a**) Grayscale ultrasonography shows a hypo-anechoic lesion (asterisk) in the upper pole of the left testis (T). (**b**) CEUS shows lack of vascularity of the lesion (asterisk). Follow-up investigations showed change in lesion appearance and progressive reduction in size (not shown)

scrotal pain, such as trauma or inflammation [19]. In testicular neoplasms, the pain may be secondary to hemorrhage into the tumor which is spontaneous or secondary to even minor traumas. Tumor markers often help in the differential diagnosis between testicular tumors and nonneoplastic lesions. Virtually all patients with choriocarcinoma have elevated human chorionic gonadotropin (hCG) levels. Serum alpha-fetoprotein (AFP) levels are elevated in approximately half of the patients with nonseminomatous neoplasms. Leydig and Sertoli cell tumors may produce

excessive estrogen or testosterone, resulting in precocious virilization or feminization. The majority of seminomas, however, present with normal serum tumor markers. The ultrasonographic findings of traumatic and inflammatory changes evolve rapidly and may be recognized at short-term follow-up. On the contrary, testicular tumors do not vary or increase in size over time (Fig. 24.12).

24.14 Non-scrotal Causes of Acute Scrotal Pain

A variety of non-scrotal clinical conditions may present with acute scrotal pain, thus entering in differential diagnosis with acute scrotal diseases [8]. The commonest is renal colic which can present, rarely, with severe scrotal pain and very mild (or even absent) flank pain. These patients are referred for a scrotal ultrasonographic examination because clinical attention is given primarily to the testis.

Other extra-scrotal causes for acute scrotal symptoms are infected peritoneal fluid, hemoperitoneum developing in subjects with patent peritoneo-vaginalis duct, retroperitoneal fluid collections following pancreatitis, or adrenal hemorrhage and aortic aneurysm rupture. Having in mind this possibility, in patients with acute scrotal pain and normal scrotal content, extending

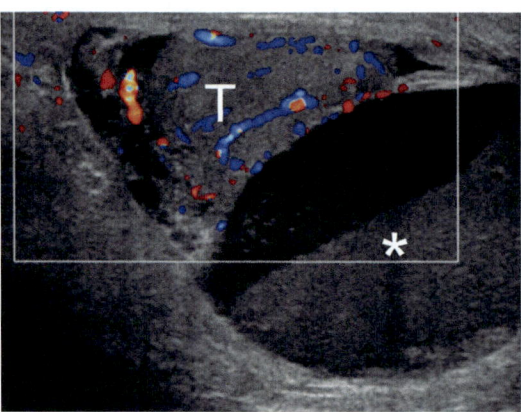

Fig. 24.11 Spermatocele torsion in a patient presenting with sudden right scrotal swelling and acute scrotal pain. The testis (T) has normal appearance and vascularity. A cystic like lesion (asterisk) is found adjacent to testis, with fluid-fluid level. A twisted spermatocele was found at surgery

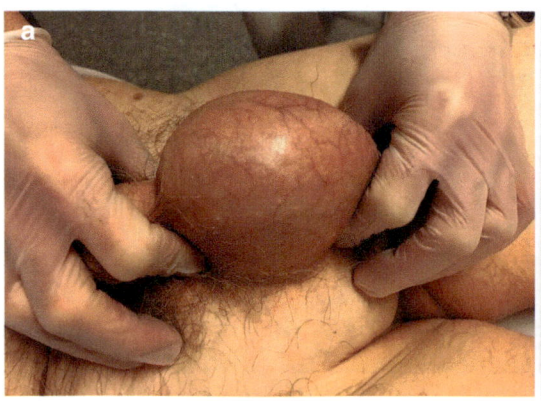

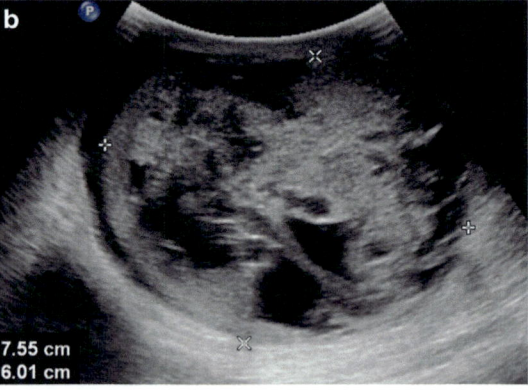

Fig. 24.12 Testicular tumor presenting with acute scrotal pain and swelling. (**a**) Findings at physical examination of painful enlargement of the left hemiscrotum which

developed in a few days. The scrotum was previously normal. (**b**) Ultrasonography reveals presence of a scrotal mass replacing the left testis

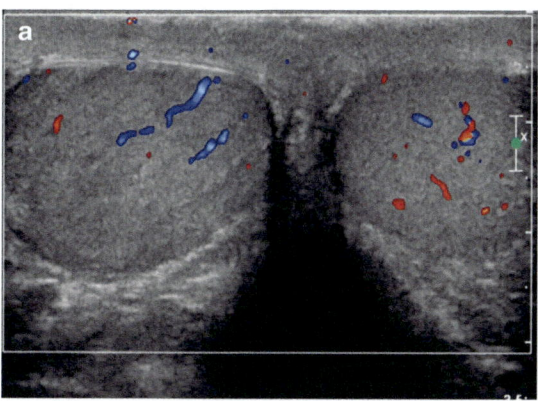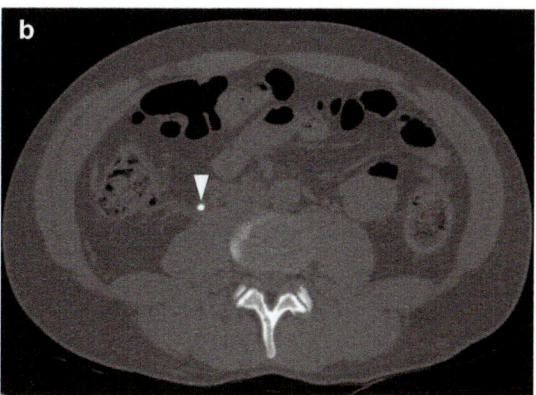

Fig. 24.13 Renal colic in a patient presenting with right acute scrotal pain. (**a**) Color Doppler interrogation of the scrotum, performed to rule out torsion, shows normal testes. (**b**) Unenhanced axial CT shows a stone (arrowhead) in the right ureter

the ultrasound investigation to the abdomen is advised to rule out non-scrotal cause for the symptoms (Fig. 24.13).

24.15 Conclusion

Grayscale and Doppler modes are the imaging modalities of choice for the evaluation of patients presenting with acute scrotal pain. The information provided is vital to discriminate between situations that require immediate surgery, from those that are managed conservatively. It is therefore crucial to perform the study rapidly enough to avoid delay in surgery, when needed. Also, high-end equipment provided with sensitive Doppler modes is essential. The operator must be familiar with clinical presentation of the different scrotal pathologies and trained enough in optimizing Doppler parameters to obtain high-quality imaging.

References

1. Dogra VS, Gottlieb RH, Oka M, Rubens DJ. Sonography of the scrotum. Radiology. 2003;227(1):18–36. https://doi.org/10.1148/radiol.2271001744.
2. Caesar RE, Kaplan GW. Incidence of the bellclapper deformity in an autopsy series. Urology. 1994;44(1):114–6.
3. Lin EP, Bhatt S, Rubens DJ, Dogra VS. Testicular torsion: twists and turns. Semin Ultrasound CT MR. 2007;28(4):317–28.
4. Yagil Y, Naroditsky I, Milhem J, Leiba R, Leiderman M, Badaan S, Gaitini D. Role of Doppler ultrasonography in the triage of acute scrotum in the emergency department. J Ultrasound Med. 2010;29(1):11–21.
5. Burks DD, Markey BJ, Burkhard TK, Balsara ZN, Haluszka MM, Canning DA. Suspected testicular torsion and ischemia: evaluation with color Doppler sonography. Radiology. 1990;175(3):815–21. https://doi.org/10.1148/radiology.175.3.2188301.
6. Dogra VS, Rubens DJ, Gottlieb RH, Bhatt S. Torsion and beyond: new twists in spectral Doppler evaluation of the scrotum. J Ultrasound Med. 2004;23(8):1077–85.
7. Cassar S, Bhatt S, Paltiel HJ, Dogra VS. Role of spectral Doppler sonography in the evaluation of partial testicular torsion. J Ultrasound Med. 2008;27(11):1629–38.
8. Bertolotto M, Cantisani V, Valentino M, Pavlica P, Derchi LE. Pitfalls in Imaging for acute scrotal pathology. Semin Roentgenol. 2016;51(1):60–9. https://doi.org/10.1053/j.ro.2016.02.012.
9. Vijayaraghavan SB. Sonographic differential diagnosis of acute scrotum: real-time whirlpool sign, a key sign of torsion. J Ultrasound Med. 2006;25(5):563–74.
10. Baldisserotto M, de Souza JC, Pertence AP, Dora MD. Color Doppler sonography of normal and torsed testicular appendages in children. AJR Am J Roentgenol. 2005;184(4):1287–92. https://doi.org/10.2214/ajr.184.4.01841287.
11. Yang DM, Lim JW, Kim JE, Kim JH, Cho H. Torsed appendix testis: gray scale and color Doppler sonographic findings compared with normal appendix testis. J Ultrasound Med. 2005;24(1):87–91.
12. Lung PF, Jaffer OS, Sellars ME, Sriprasad S, Kooiman GG, Sidhu PS. Contrast-enhanced ultrasound in

the evaluation of focal testicular complications secondary to epididymitis. AJR Am J Roentgenol. 2012;199(3):W345–54. https://doi.org/10.2214/AJR.11.7997.

13. Yusuf G, Sellars ME, Kooiman GG, Diaz-Cano S, Sidhu PS. Global testicular infarction in the presence of epididymitis: clinical features, appearances on grayscale, color Doppler, and contrast-enhanced sonography, and histologic correlation. J Ultrasound Med. 2013;32(1):175–80.

14. Tsili AC, Bertolotto M, Turgut AT, Dogra V, Freeman S, Rocher L, Belfield J, Studniarek M, Ntorkou A, Derchi LE, Oyen R, Ramchandani P, Secil M, Richenberg J. MRI of the scrotum: recommendations of the ESUR scrotal and penile imaging working group. Eur Radiol. 2018;28(1):31–43. https://doi.org/10.1007/s00330-017-4944-3.

15. Bertolotto M, Derchi LE, Sidhu PS, Serafini G, Valentino M, Grenier N, Cova MA. Acute segmental testicular infarction at contrast-enhanced ultrasound: early features and changes during follow-up. AJR Am J Roentgenol. 2011;196(4):834–41. https://doi.org/10.2214/AJR.10.4821.

16. Gaur S, Bhatt S, Derchi L, Dogra V. Spontaneous intratesticular hemorrhage: two case descriptions and brief review of the literature. J Ultrasound Med. 2011;30(1):101–4.

17. Dibilio D, Serafini G, Gandolfo NG, Derchi LE. Ultrasonographic findings of isolated torsion of the epididymis. J Ultrasound Med. 2006;25(3):417–9. quiz 420–411.

18. Hikosaka A, Iwase Y. Spermatocele presenting as acute scrotum. Urol J. 2008;5(3):206–8.

19. Valentino M, Bertolotto M, Derchi L, Bertaccini A, Pavlica P, Martorana G, Barozzi L. Role of contrast enhanced ultrasound in acute scrotal diseases. Eur Radiol. 2011;21(9):1831–40. https://doi.org/10.1007/s00330-010-2039-5.